Wolfram Bücking

A Dental Treasure Chest

Tips and tricks for daily practice

Wolfram Bücking

A Dental Treasure Chest

Tips and tricks for daily practice

Translated from the German by
Ulrike Heiß and Laura Russell

Quintessence Publishing Co, Ltd

London, Berlin, Chicago, Tokyo, Barcelona,
Beijing, Istanbul, Milan, Moscow, Mumbai, Paris,
Prague, São Paulo, Seoul, Warsaw

Every effort has been made to ensure that the contents of this book are reliable and complete. Nonetheless, readers are strongly advised to consult official product information inserts and other sources deemed to be accurate and reliable. The author and publisher explicitly do not warrant the accuracy of information contained in the book.

British Library Cataloguing in Publication Data
Bucking, Wolfram
A dental treasure chest : tips and tricks for daily practice
1. Dentistry
I. Title
617.6
ISBN-13: 9781850971566
ISBN-10: 1850971560

quintessence books

Translation by *Ulrike Heiß* and *Laura Russell*
Layout and Production: *Andreas Rauschenbach*
Printing: Binding: Bosch-Druck GmbH
Binding: Conzella Verlagsbuchbinderei Urban Meister GmbH & Co. KG

ISBN: 1-85097-156-0
ISBN: 978-1-85097-156-6

Printed in Germany

Table of contents

Dedication

To my dear wife Mia, who has supported me through all of the phases of the treasure chest with lots of love and patience. You are the best wife anyone could have ...

Foreword

In the 30-plus years of my professional career, I have become acquainted with many different kinds of people:

- Loudmouths who never tire of talking about how wonderful they are
- Know-it-alls who always have a theoretical solution to problems, but fail miserably when it comes time to implement their idea
- Tinkerers who manage to make things work in some form or another, but never really know why

It has seldom been my pleasure to encounter someone who truly knows and understands his work down to the last detail and who knows how to put this insight into practice. Wolfram Bücking is one of these exceptional people.

Because of the example of the late Professor Dr André Schroeder, I believe that a restorative dentist has to be a "Renaissance man" in dentistry, in spite of the current trend toward specialization. *Wolfram Bücking* is one of these rare few.

Over the years I have met many dentists who embody the negative clichés of our profession: They do not read the instruction manuals that come with their tools, plow ahead blindly with their work, and improvise with their materials and approaches however it suits them. When I started serving on a board that reviewed formal complaints, I realized once and for all how accurate the negative stereotype could be.

In some ways, *Wolfram Bücking* is a dentist like many others, though you cannot accuse him of not reading his instruction manuals. On the contrary—he reads them all very conscientiously and carefully and expounds on them with the insight and knowledge of a true expert.

This book is his credo. He takes a thoroughly tested problem-oriented approach to devising solutions in all areas of dentistry. These solutions are the result of a profound understanding of the fundamentals combined with imaginative thinking and skillful craftsmanship. This book offers dental colleagues a rich treasure trove of techniques and tips for dealing with many problems not covered in textbooks.

In some regards, this can be seen as an alternative textbook. The current trend in education is "problem-based learning." In general medicine, this has already been practiced for some time. In dentistry, it is only beginning to come into its own,[1] and *Wolfram Bücking* is a pioneer in this trend. The book you hold in your hands is absolutely systematic in its problem-oriented methodology. My congratulations to the author.

Jean-François Roulet, DDS, Dr Med Dent, PhD
Schaan, Liechtenstein

1. Roulet JF. A new concept of dental education. Ann R Australas Coll Dent Surg 2002;16:37–39.

Preface

Many years ago, a class evolved as part of the basic coursework in prosthodontics at the Akademie Praxis und Wissenschaft in Düsseldorf, Germany. The class was called "Prosthetic First Aid—One Practitioner's Suggestions for Emergency Solutions," and it focused on the problematic situations a dentist encounters in everyday life, or rather the major and minor incidents that can make a clinician miserable. These are problems that when you tell someone about the situation later, you are likely to begin by saying, "It was just one of those days where nothing was going right . . ." In delicate situations like these, you do not want to bother with taking pictures, but in many cases I did so anyway. Over time I developed a treasure chest of wide-ranging tips and tricks, and the people who took part in my class became more and more enthusiastic about them. I was invited to hold seminars and presentations about critical situations in a dentist's professional life, and the treasure chest grew larger and larger. Of course, this was also due in part to the tidbits and hints that participants contributed. (After all, you learn the most from the students you teach.)

After I joined the editorial board of Die Quintessenz in Germany, the seminar received its official and final name—"Die dentale Trickkiste" ["A Dental Treasure Chest"]—and it has provided the inspiration for a successful series in the journal since early 2001. Since then, I have received many suggestions and ideas from readers every week, and I am always eager to follow up and integrate these suggestions. There was never a point at which I simply copied something from someone else—there is a bit of Bücking in every chapter. Naturally I included all sorts of input from friends and colleagues, and I wish to thank them warmly for that. It is quite an effort for me to produce a new article for the series each month, especially because I am not what you would call a natural at writing. However, it is always very gratifying to hold the newest Die Quintessenz in my hands and see my work. I receive a great deal of praise for these contributions, and when I feel frustrated or exhausted at the end of a long day in the office, reading these letters makes me feel better right away.

Over time, these first-aid tricks became useful building blocks for all different aspects of dental practice, and this book summarizes and categorizes them for your convenience. This book features 46 treasure chest entries in one compact volume for your reference. An index at the back allows you to look up the topics you need. The next volume will be released after the next 40 entries have been completed. The goal I have set for myself is to write 100 entries altogether; I have already designed a concept for them and will retire when I am finished. This is my plan, although there is one person who does not believe me, and that is my wife. She thinks that as long as I continue to pursue my work as a dentist with such dedication and enthusiasm, I will keep writing and teaching.

I hope that as you read this, you will find a multitude of useful tips and tricks in the dental treasure chest, and I look forward to continuing a lively exchange of ideas with my colleagues. Your comments and input are welcome; I would be pleased to hear about suggestions for improvement, news of your successes or failures, and any new tips and tricks you would care to pass along (w.buecking@t-online.de).

Mr Meenen, my editor, takes my folksy, dialect-tinted style and converts it into standard and eloquent language, for which I am very grateful. I also wish to thank *Mr Rauschenbach*, who is in charge of layout and works with *Mr Kürten*, the graphic designer at Regg Media, to fulfill my wishes patiently and expertly.

Without *Mr Wolters*, the publishing director, who kept everything in his benevolent hands, this book would never have been written—many thanks to him as well.

Many thanks to *Mr H.-W. Haase*, the publisher, whose very unique and paternal manner led me to writing.

Wangen, February
Wolfram Bücking

1

Prosthetic First Aid

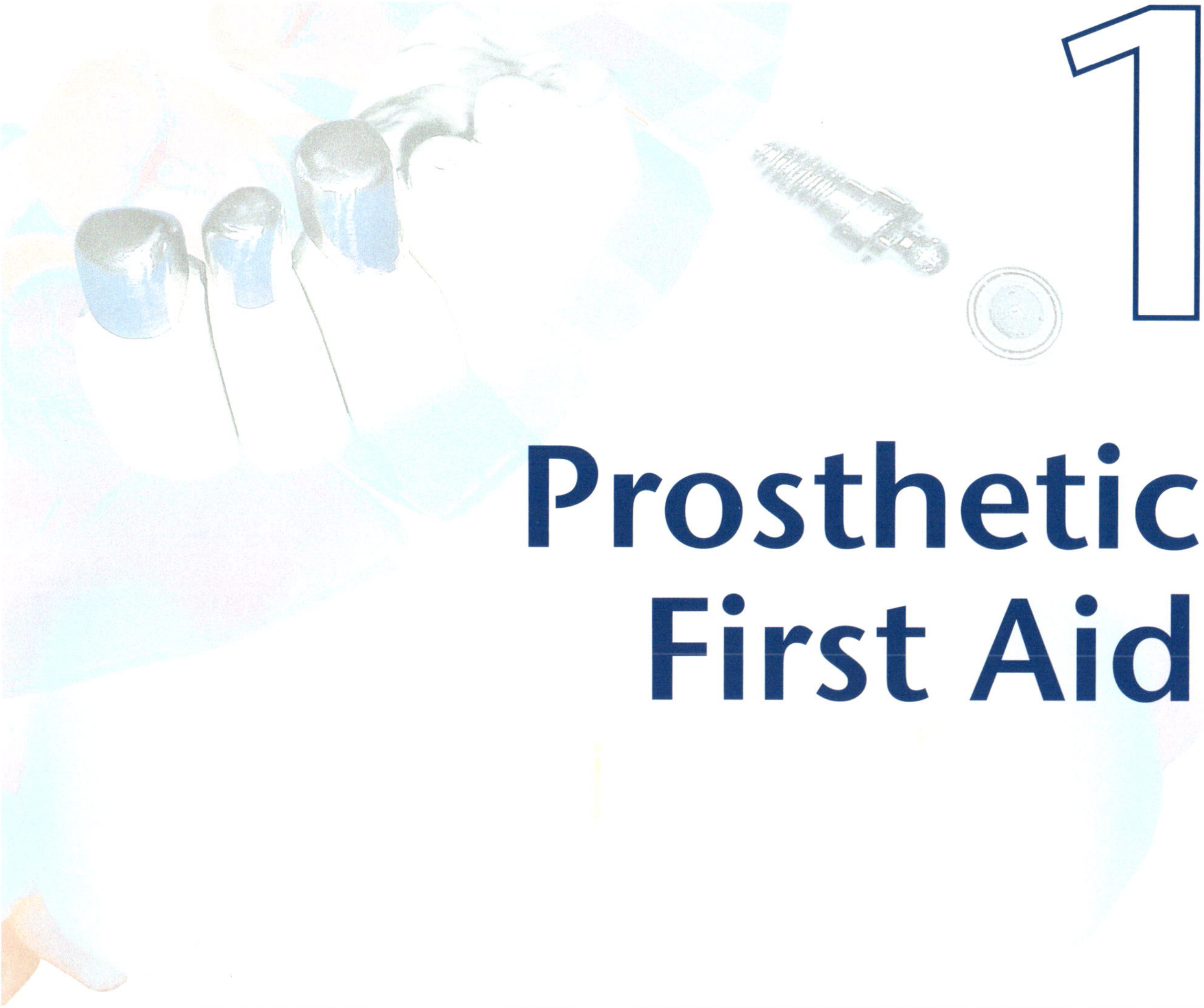

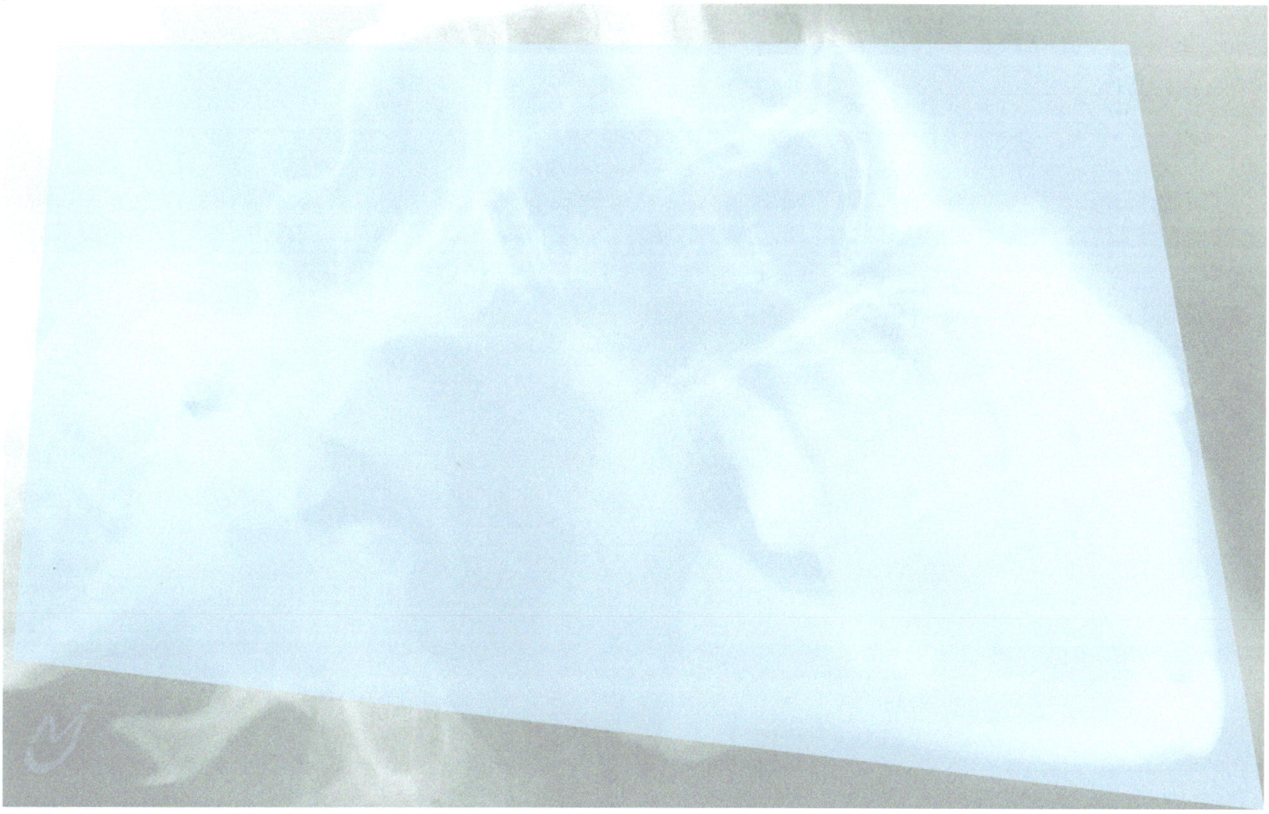

1

Porcelain Fracture

Crown Removal with the Crown Lift System

Removal of a Porcelain-Fused-to-Metal Crown Using Mechanical Tools

Removal of Fixed Partial Dentures

First Aid for Complete Dentures

Fractured Posts

Lost Abutment Teeth

Retention of Telescopic Crowns

Porcelain Fracture

Common problem: Fractured porcelain

Occasionally, the porcelain of a metal-ceramic crown can break or chip off. In such a situation it is important to start by determining why and how the fracture occurred. Possible reasons include:

1. Trauma (eg, accident, impact, or fall).
2. Poor workmanship on the part of the dental laboratory.
3. Malocclusion, usually in association with bruxism.

If the fracture occurred because of trauma, the ceramic can be repaired immediately.

If ceramic breaks off without leaving visible residue of ceramic on the metal and the fracture is a clean break, faulty workmanship is most likely the problem. If poor workmanship is the cause, the metal-ceramic crown usually is promptly replaced by the laboratory.

In the case of malocclusion, the cause should be established and eliminated by selective grinding, reshaping the crown contour, and possibly enhancing the disclusion (developing canine guidance). If there is extensive occlusal interference that cannot be clearly identified in the mouth, a functional analysis should be performed with casts mounted on an articulator.

The following case report describes a proven solution for the problem of porcelain fracture caused by malocclusion.

Proven solution: Direct intraoral repair

In the patient shown in Fig 1-1a, the mesial aspect of the labial porcelain of the maxillary right lateral incisor had broken off. The incisodistal position of the corner of the mandibular right lateral incisor was identified as the cause. In addition, a disturbed mediotrusion was found contralaterally between the maxillary and the mandibular left second molars. Both areas were marked and selectively ground.

After placement of rubber dam with a ligature (Fig 1-1b), an undercut box was milled into the metal for additional retention (Fig 1-1c). The ceramic part of the crown was abraded with a diamond to form a chamfer.

The ceramic was then etched with 9.5% buffered hydrofluoric acid (Porcelain Etch) for 1 minute (Figs 1-1d to 1-1f). While this product causes no damage to the epidermis even after several minutes of contact, it can chemically burn the mucosa (eg, gingiva and eyes). Therefore, the safety precautions used for conventional etching with orthophosphoric acid gel (eg, informed consent, covering the patient's eyes, and use of protective eyewear) should be taken.

Dental ceramics cannot be etched with the orthophosphoric acid included in most repair kits. As an alternative, use of a mini-sandblaster could be considered, but this would only condition the metal.

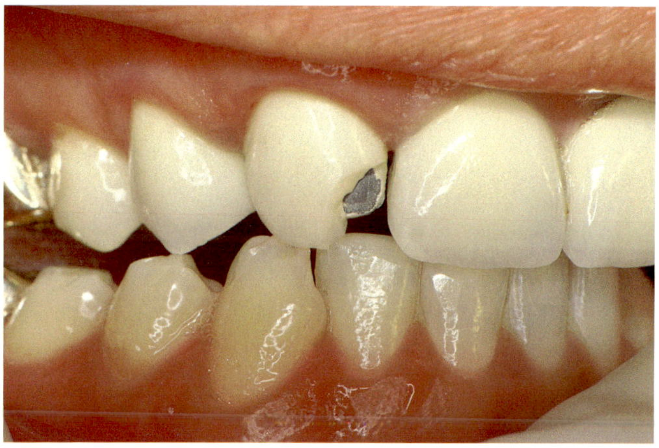

Fig 1-1a The fracture of porcelain on the lateral incisor crown has been caused by malocclusion.

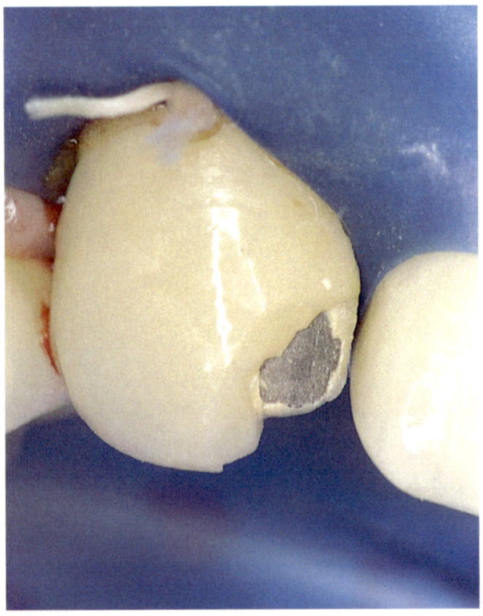

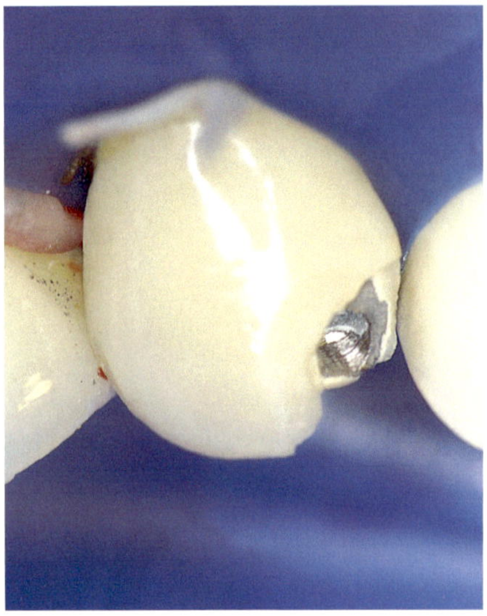

Fig 1-1b *(left)* An entirely dry field is created using rubber dam.

Fig 1-1c *(right)* The retention cavity is prepared.

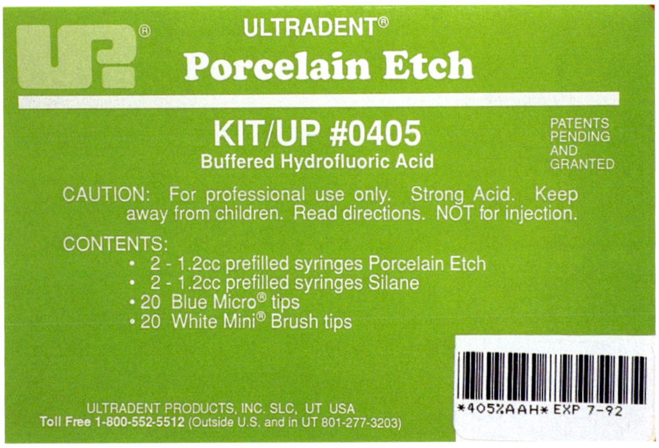

Fig 1-1d Porcelain Etch.

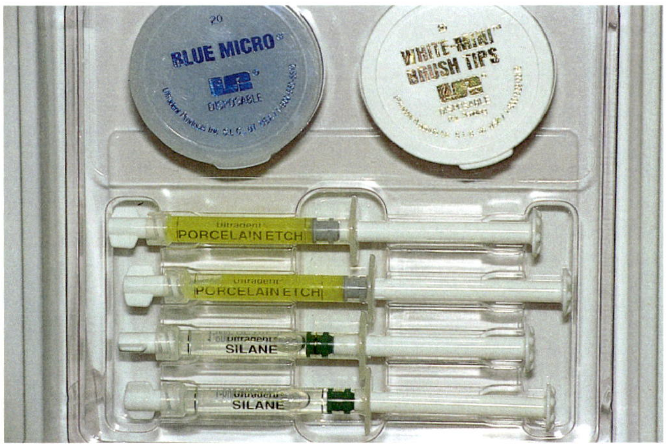

Fig 1-1e Syringes for Porcelain Etch and silane.

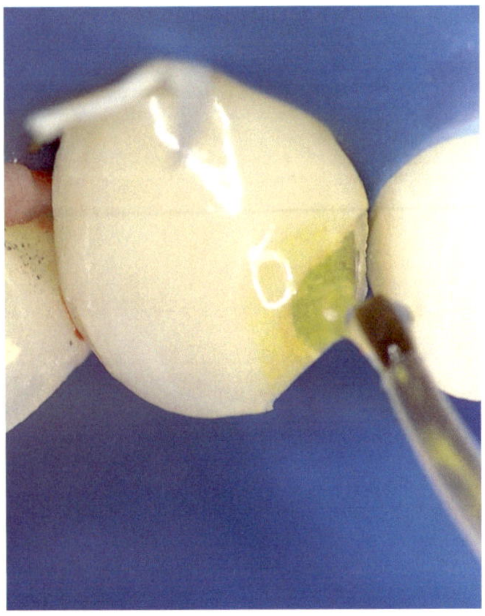

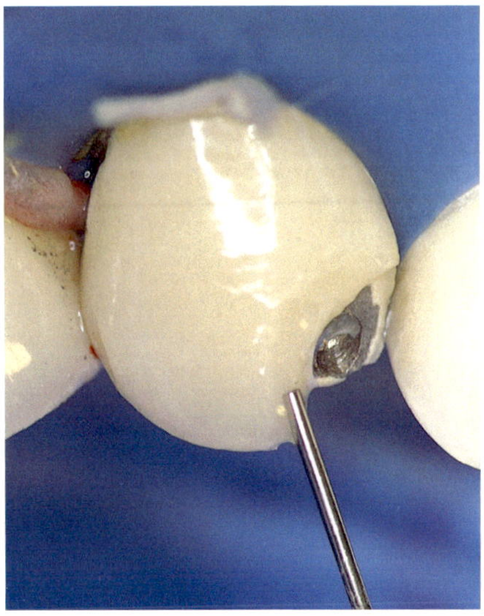

Fig 1-1f *(left)* The ceramic is etched for 1 minute.

Fig 1-1g *(right)* After thorough rinsing with water spray and subsequent drying, the material was silanized for 1 minute, and the metal surface was treated with metal primer.

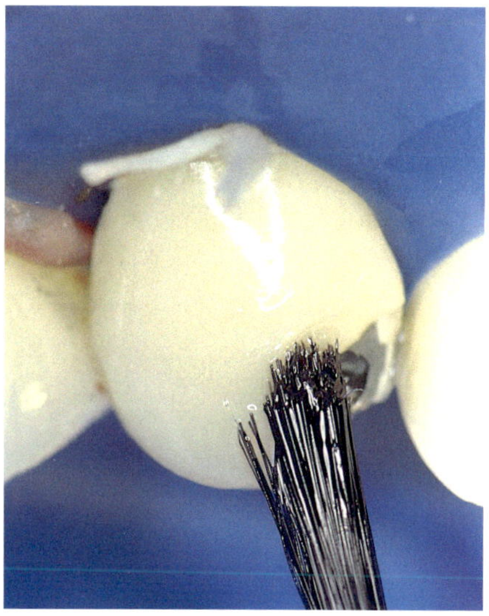

Fig 1-1h Bonding agent is applied.

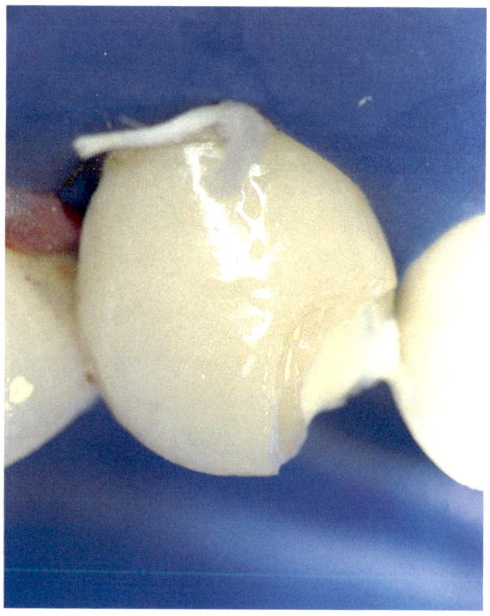

Fig 1-1i Several layers of dentin-colored opaquer are applied to mask the metal.

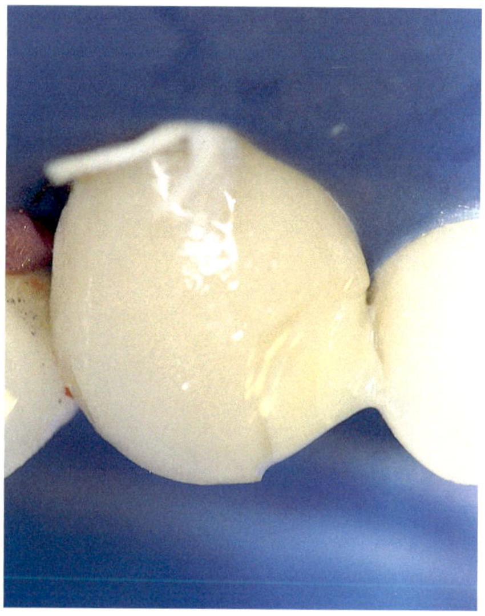

Fig 1-1j Layers of dentin material are applied.

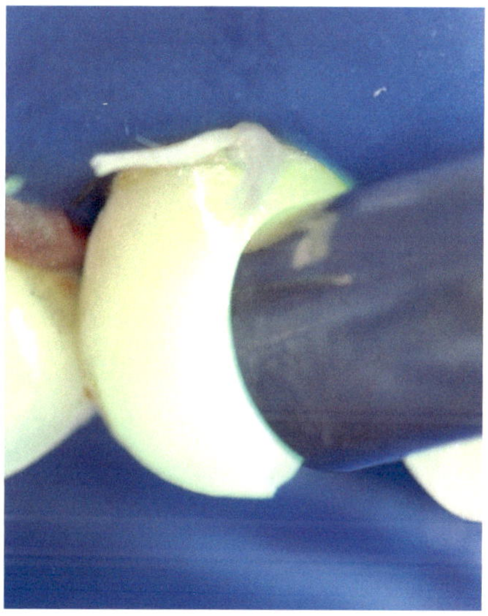

Fig 1-1k The dentin material is polymerized with a curing light.

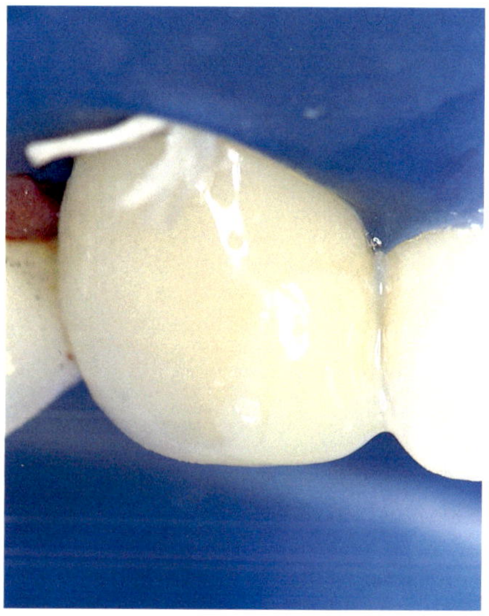

Fig 1-1l Layers of enamel material are applied.

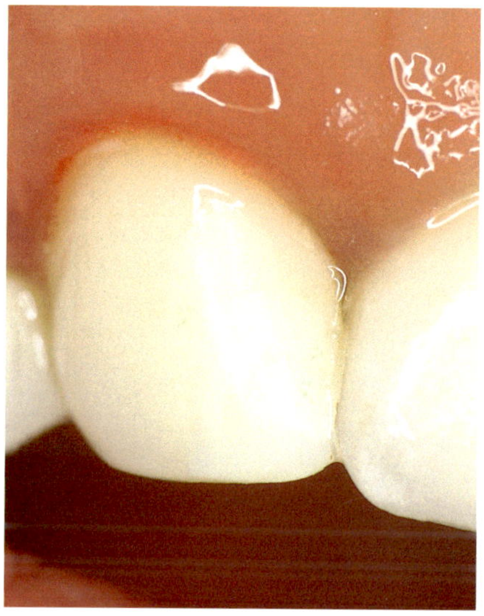

Fig 1-1m Rubber dam is removed to reveal the finished porcelain.

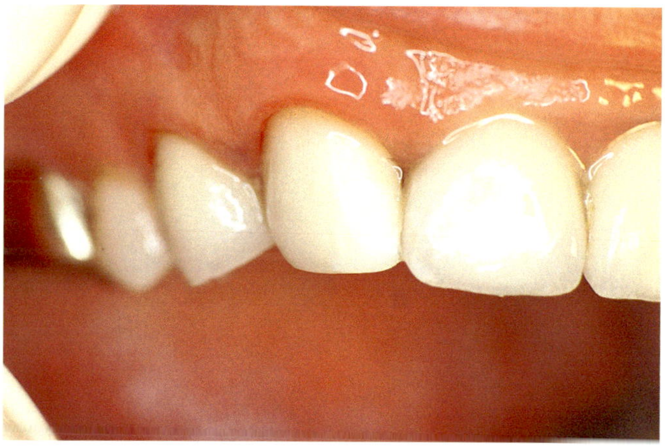

Fig 1-1n The esthetics of the repaired crown is evaluated.

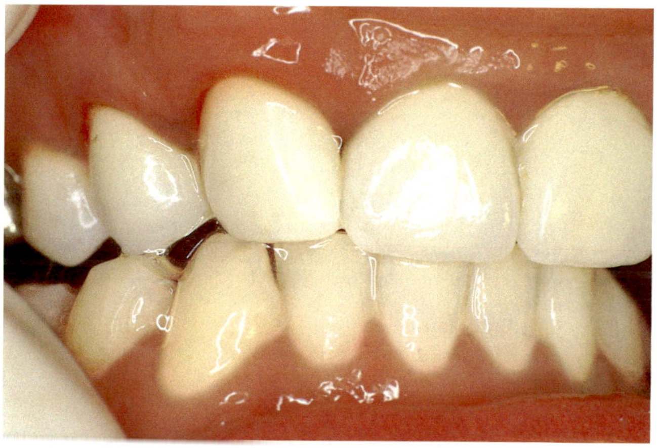

Fig 1-1o Occlusion and articulation are evaluated.

After thorough rinsing with water spray and subsequent drying, the material was silanized for 1 minute (Fig 1-1g), and the metal surface was treated with metal primer. The crown was then ready for reapplication of porcelain with the following technique:

1. The crown was moistened with the bonding agent metal primer (Fig 1-1h).
2. The metal was masked with several layers of dentin-colored opaquer, which received 40 seconds of intermediate polymerization (Fig 1-1i).
3. The dentin shade was applied and polymerized for 40 seconds (Figs 1-1j and 1-1k).
4. The enamel shade was applied and polymerized for 40 seconds (Fig 1-1l).
5. The repaired crown was contoured and finished and rubber dam was removed (Fig 1-1m).
6. Esthetics was evaluated (Fig 1-1n).
7. Occlusion and articulation were evaluated (Fig 1-1o).

Materials

Porcelain Etch and Silane (Ultradent)
Tetric and Tetric Color (Ivoclar Vivadent)
Metal/Zirconia Primer (Ivoclar Vivadent)

Crown Removal with the Crown Lift System

Common problem: Cemented permanent crown requiring removal and recementation

Two years previously, the mandibular right second molar was replaced with a partial gold crown as part of a rehabilitation procedure in a 40-year-old woman (Fig 1-2a). An excellent fit of the crown had been achieved with the help of a magnifying loupe and a stereomicroscope.

The patient paid an emergency visit to the dental office because of throbbing pain in this tooth. The results of the pulp test and sensitivity to percussion indicated the need for endodontic treatment.

In such a case, the occlusal surface of the crown usually is perforated and treatment of the root canal is carried out through the crown. The crown is subsequently sealed with a resin composite restorative material or an occlusal gold inlay.

However, endodontic treatment through a crown (especially in the distal molar region) is extremely difficult or, in many cases, impossible. With this procedure, the fully waxed up occlusal surface would have been destroyed and could have been reconstructed only imperfectly.

Proven solution: Crown removal with the Crown Lift System

This procedure is based on a principle originating in automobile maintenance technology to remove wheel hubs by using a flywheel-puller while applying a carefully regulated force.

Following nerve block anesthesia, the crown was perforated with a fine carbide bur in a high-speed handpiece (FG). The perforation was made in the central fossa as closely as possible along the tooth axis (Figs 1-2b and 1-2c). The central perforation was flared to a predefined diameter with a spiral bur that was part of the Crown Lift System (no longer available; replaced by the Crown Lifter CL, which can be used manually, as shown here, as well as mechanically, as shown in the following section). The bur was used at low speed and with a drop of Vaseline oil (Fig 1-2d). If the resulting cavity is spiral-shaped, the preparation was performed correctly.

Because minor penetration of the remaining natural crown is inevitable, the cavity has to be shaped into a plain surface underneath the artificial crown with the help of an inverted cone bur. Otherwise, the crown would be tightened rather than lifted by the lifting bolt.

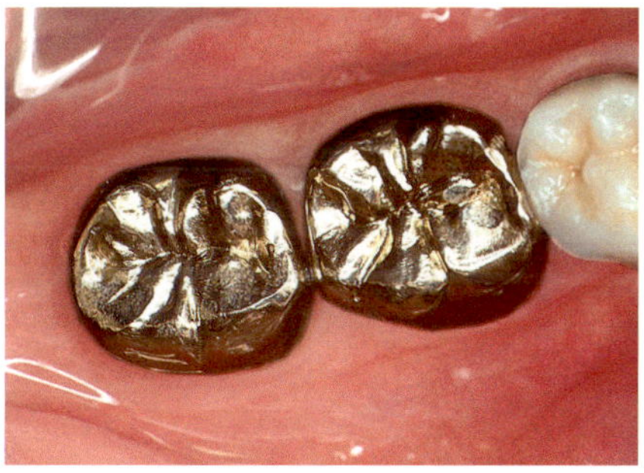

Fig 1-2a Occlusal view of gold crowns on the mandibular right first and second molars.

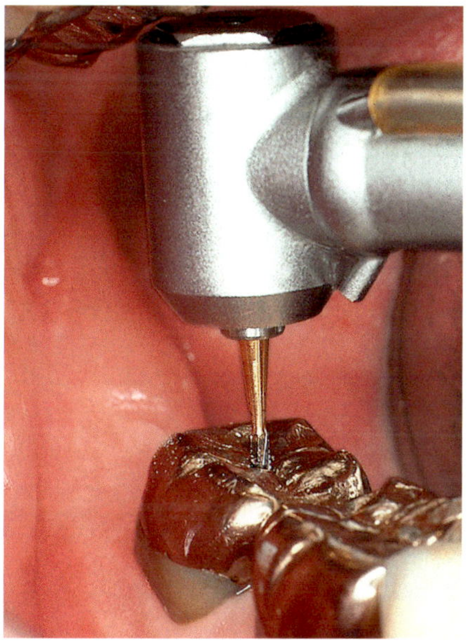

Fig 1-2b Occlusal perforation with the carbide bur.

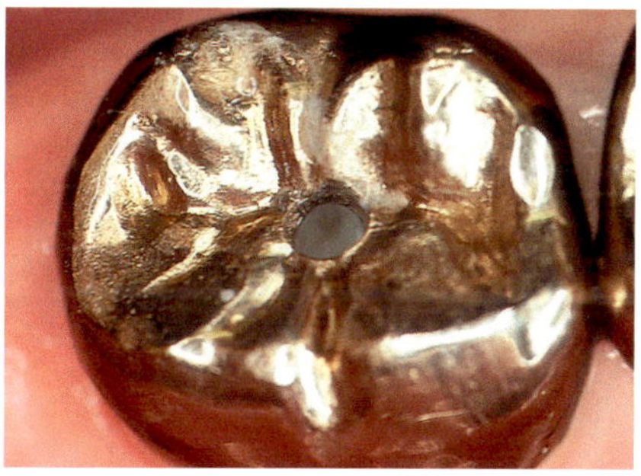

Fig 1-2c Perforated crown.

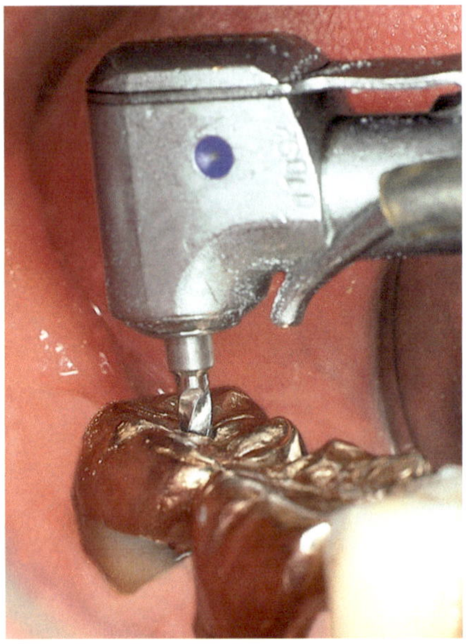

Fig 1-2d Flaring with the Crown Lift System spiral bur.

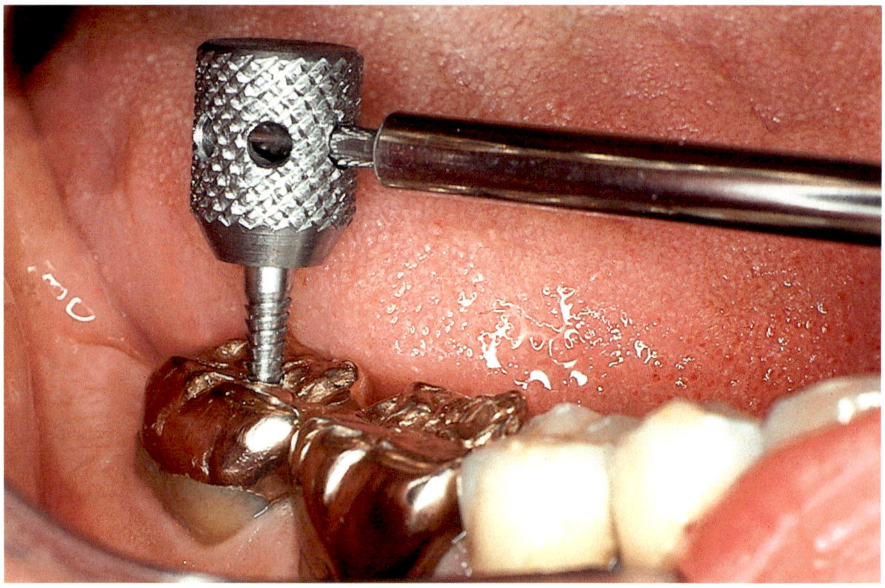

Fig 1-2e Lifting bolt further tightened with the extension lever.

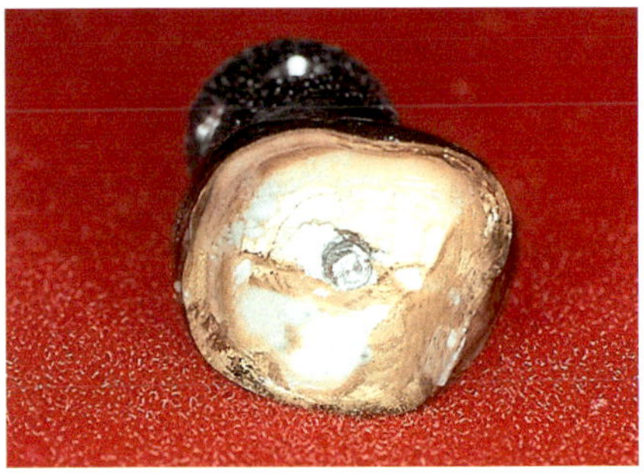

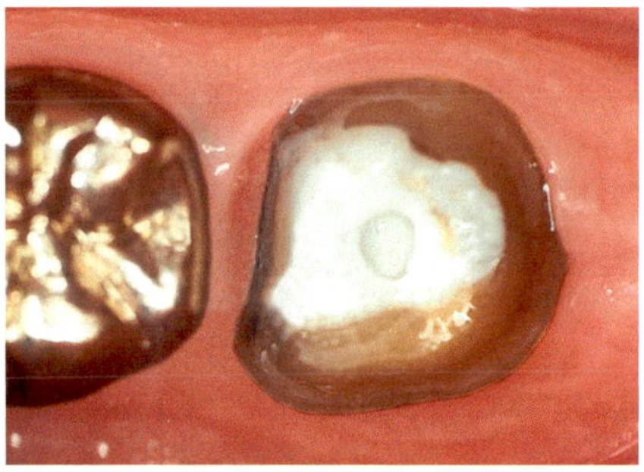

Fig 1-2f *(left)* Interior view of the removed crown.

Fig 1-2g *(right)* Tooth preparation after crown removal.

In this case, a lifting bolt from the Crown Lift System was screwed into the central cavity in the mandibular right second molar. The bolt cut its own thread into the gold of the crown. It was firmly secured. The extension lever from the Crown Lift System was pushed horizontally into the designated holes in the lifting bolt to begin the crown removal (Fig 1-2e). The bolt was tightened with a slow, gentle turning movement while central pressure was applied to the lifting bolt with the other hand to avoid tilting of the crown. The crown margin was carefully monitored through a magnifying loupe. As soon as the margin of the crown was lifted, tightening of the bolt was stopped and the crown and bolt were removed with a tilting movement (Figs 1-2f and 1-2g).

For this patient, the good access to the site meant that endodontic treatment of the tooth could be carried out as usual. The crown was cemented provisionally for subsequent easy removal with the lifting bolt. Three months later, after the endodontic treatment of the mandibular right second molar had been successfully completed, the crown was soldered in the dental laboratory and reintegrated easily, successfully, and permanently, without damaging the crown margins and with minimal impact on occlusal morphology.

Materials

Crown cutter (S. S. White)
Crown Lift System/Crown Lifter CL (Bredent)

Removal of a Porcelain-Fused-to-Metal Crown Using Mechanical Tools

Common problem: Cemented permanent metal-ceramic crown requiring removal and recementation

In a situation where there is not enough contact between, for example, a metal-ceramic crown on the mandibular left first molar and the adjacent teeth, the crown has to be removed, corrected, and reinserted. How can the crown be preserved during this process?

The following case is a mock situation demonstrated on a model, but similar cases are frequently encountered in the dental office, for example, in periodontal patients in the pretreatment stage.

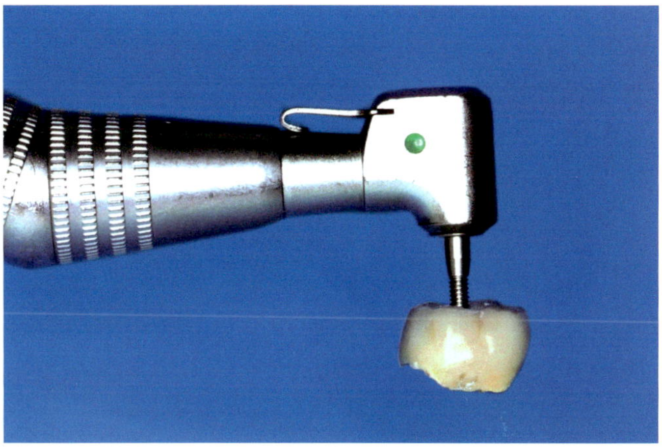

Fig 1-3a Mechanical removal of a metal-ceramic crown.

Proven solution: Crown removal with mechanical tools

The previous section discussed removal and reuse of cast gold crowns. The question arose as to whether metal-ceramic crowns could be removed, repaired, and recemented in the same way.

After many futile attempts, a system was successfully designed following the same principles, and it can very likely solve the aforementioned problem with great precision. Moreover, the instrument has succeeded in mechanically removing metal-ceramic crowns with minimal damage (Figs 1-3a and 1-3b). The method is demonstrated using casts.

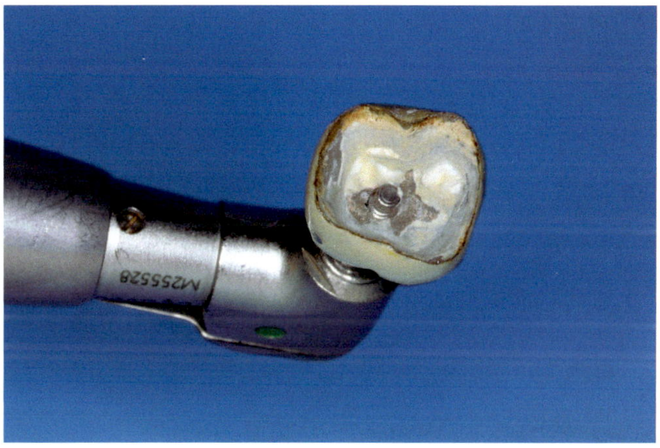

Fig 1-3b Metal-ceramic crown after mechanical removal.

A metal-ceramic crown on the mandibular left first molar had insufficient interproximal contacts and therefore required removal, repair, and recementation (Fig 1-4a). The center of the occlusal surface was marked with a red felt-tip pen (Fig 1-4b). A layer of ceramic material around this central point was to be removed to prevent the resulting strain on the ceramic material from causing fractures of the material while the crown was removed. The area was marked with a green felt-tip pen (Fig 1-4c). The entire marked area of the ceramic was removed with a cylindrical diamond bur (Figs 1-4d to 1-4f).

A special bur, the Multidrill, was used to drill through the metal axially (Figs 1-4g and 1-4h). The Multidrill can be used approximately three times, depending on the hardness of the metal (Fig 1-4i). The central perforation, which should be extended only slightly underneath the metal, is shown in Fig 1-4j. To prevent the lifting bolt from tightening rather than lifting the crown, the cavity is undercut with a small bud bur or an inverted cone bur (Figs 1-4k and 1-4l). This should be done only while the handpiece is moved horizontally (Fig 1-4m), and the undercut should be examined with the magnifying loupe (Fig 1-4n).

The central thread was then cut with a thread cutter moistened with a drop of Vaseline oil (Figs 1-4o to 1-4q).

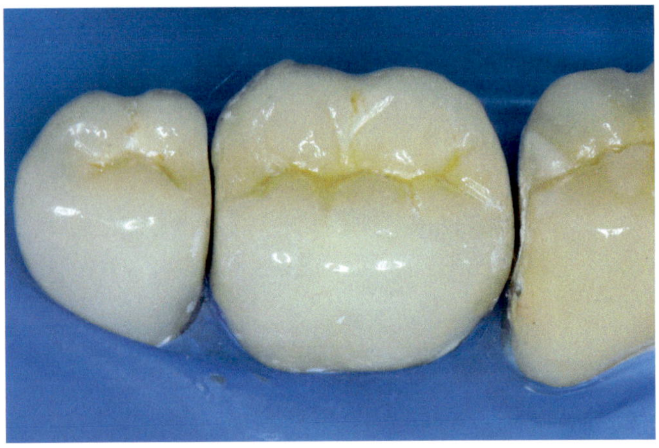

Fig 1-4a The metal-ceramic crown on the mandibular left first molar has to be removed because of insufficient interproximal contacts. It will be corrected in the laboratory and recemented.

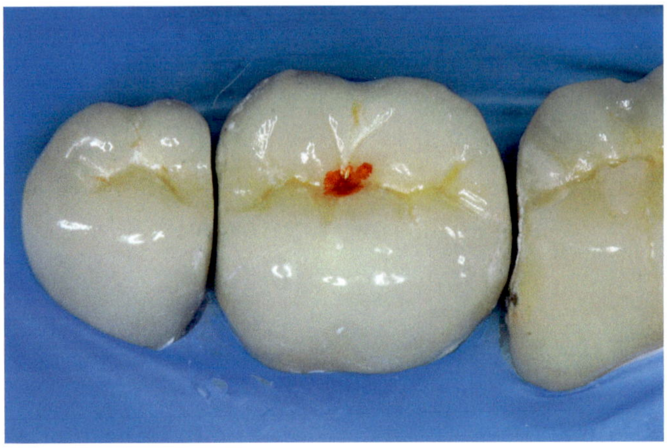

Fig 1-4b The center of the occlusal surface is marked with a red felt-tip pen.

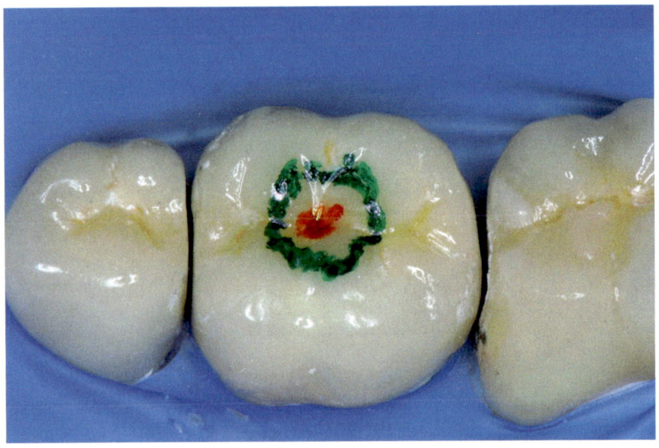

Fig 1-4c A green felt-tip pen is used to mark the area of the ceramic that will be ground off.

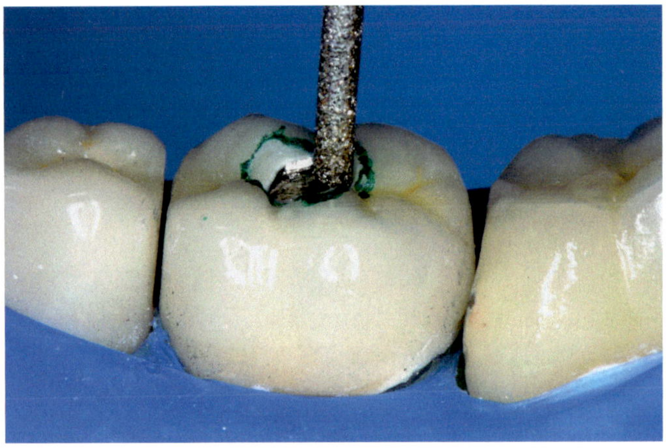

Fig 1-4d The ceramic material around the central point is removed with a cylinder diamond bur.

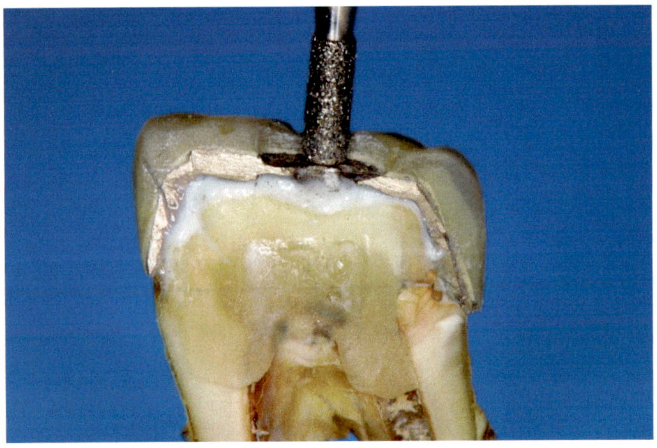

Fig 1-4e Cross section showing depth of penetration.

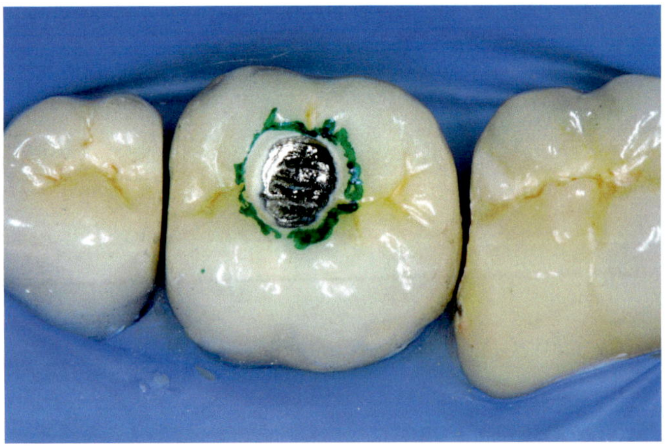

Fig 1-4f The metal is exposed.

It is important to ensure that the cut is not deeper than necessary because the thread should only cut into the metal. To achieve this, the thread cutter was adjusted to a slow speed and torque of 20 Ncm with the help of a torque limiter.

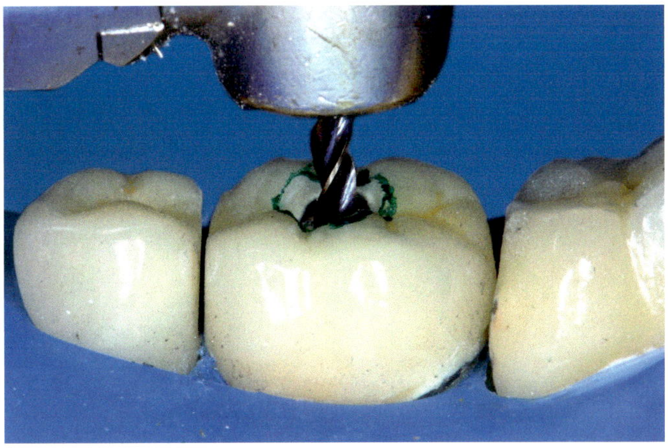

Fig 1-4g The crown is perforated axially with the Multidrill bur.

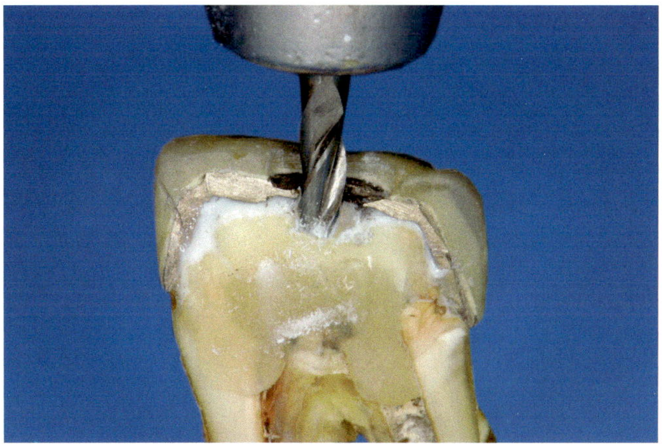

Fig 1-4h Cross section of the perforation.

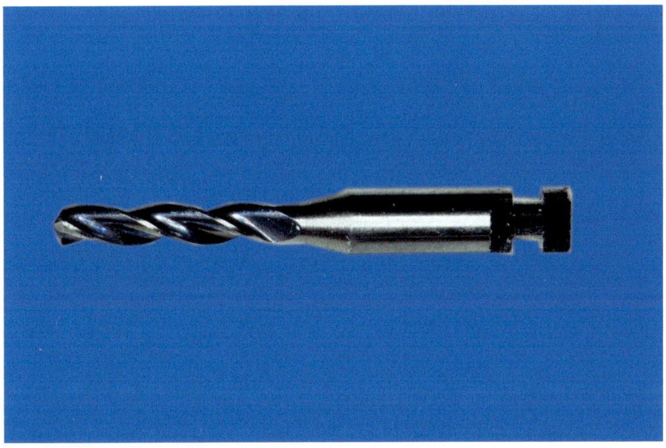

Fig 1-4i The Multidrill is a specially hardened steel spiral bur.

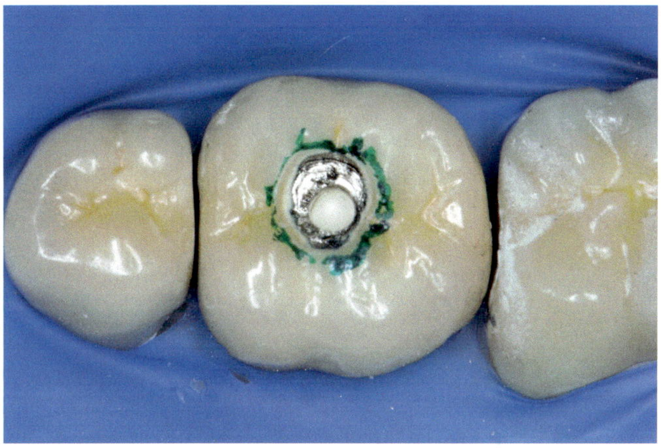

Fig 1-4j The central perforation should extend only slightly beneath the metal.

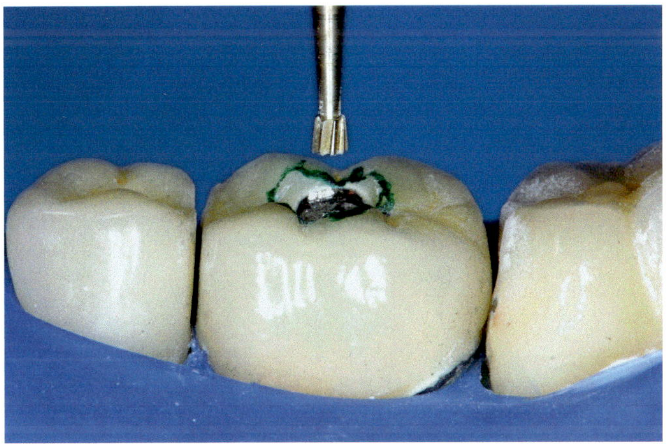

Fig 1-4k The cavity is carefully undercut with an inverted cone or bud bur.

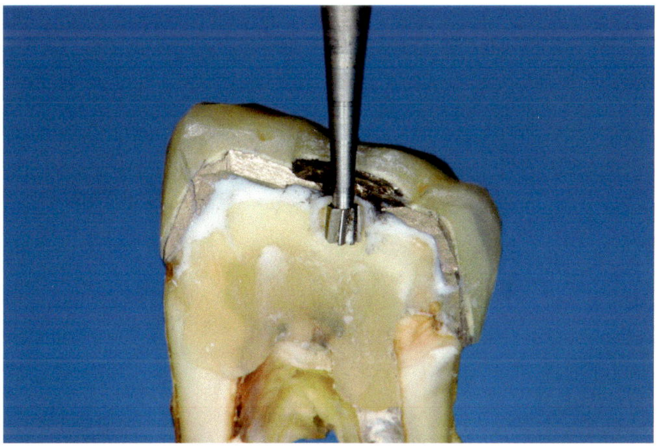

Fig 1-4l Cross section of the undercut.

The thread cutter was replaced with the lifting bolt, which has no thread in the last 2 mm of its tip to prevent it from being screwed into the underlying dentin. The lifting bolt was inserted slowly and steadily (Figs 1-4r to 1-4t), while the cervical crown margin was monitored with the magnifying loupe. It is important to lift the crown

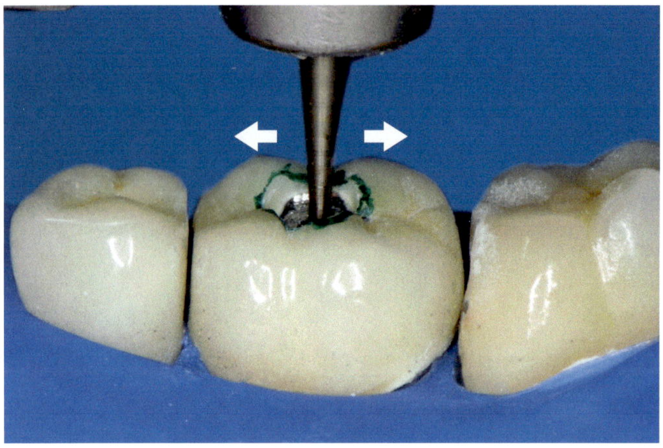

Fig 1-4m The crown is undermined using horizontal movements only.

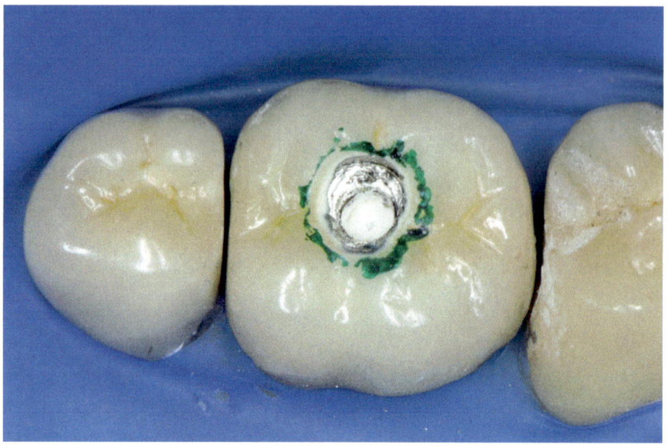

Fig 1-4n Undermined cavity.

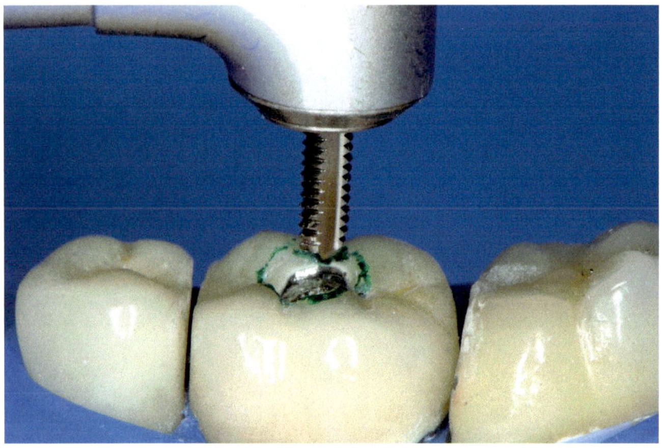

Fig 1-4o A thread cutter at low speed and 20 Ncm torque is used to cut the thread.

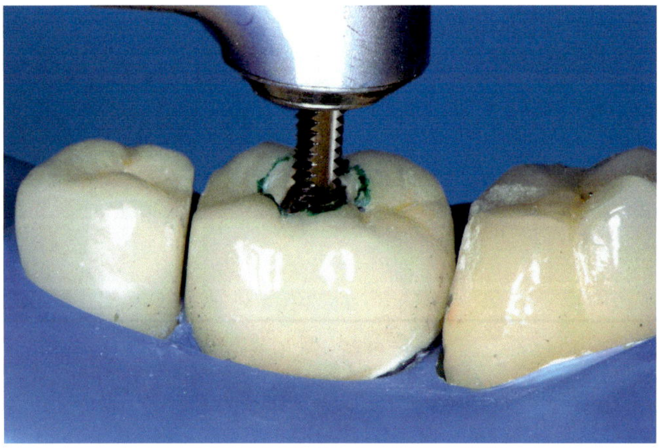

Fig 1-4p The thread cutter is lowered.

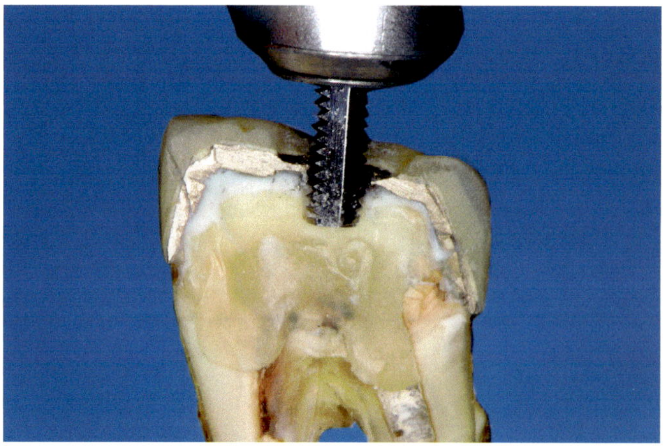

Fig 1-4q Cross section of the thread cutter after penetration. The thread should only cut into the metal.

with a slow and steady movement (Figs 1-4u to 1-4w). The crown, which was attached to the handpiece, was then lifted off (Fig 1-4x). The prepared tooth now had a cavity and an undercut area but was otherwise undamaged (Fig 1-4y). The metal-ceramic crown was then repaired in the laboratory, corrected, and recemented (Fig 1-4z).

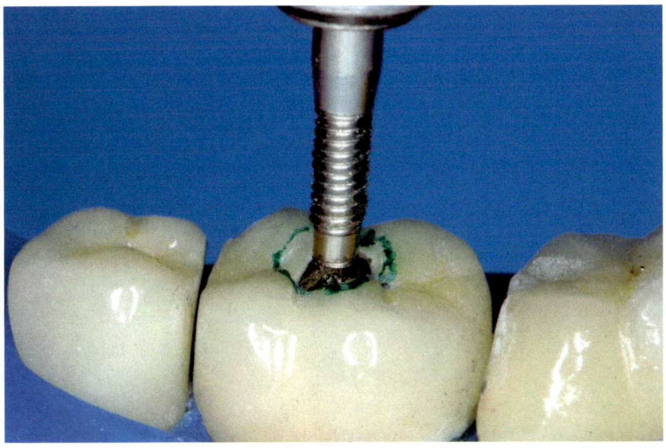

Fig 1-4r The crown is removed with the lifting bolt fastened to the handpiece. The lower section of the lifting bolt has no thread. The cervical crown margin should be monitored with a magnifying loupe.

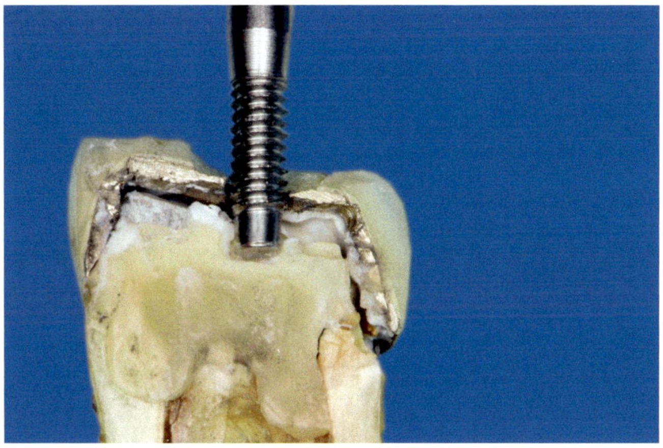

Fig 1-4s Cross section of the lifting bolt in place.

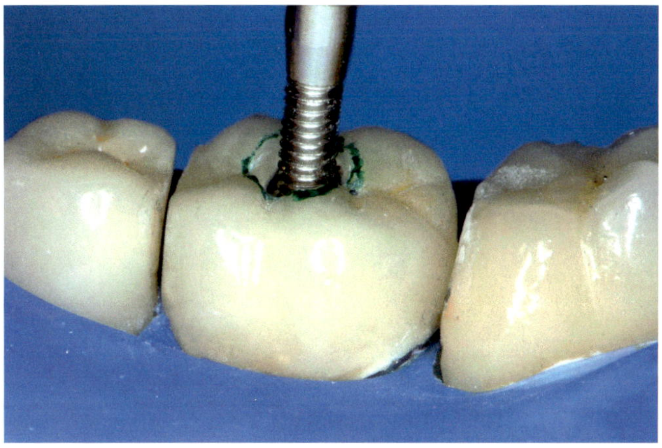

Fig 1-4t The lifting bolt is slowly and steadily screwed into the crown.

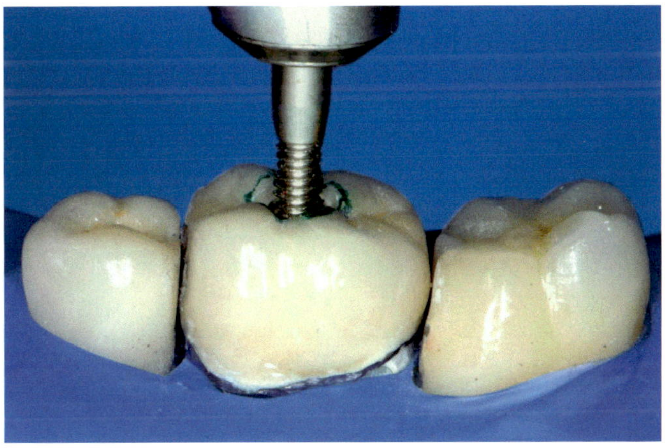

Fig 1-4u The crown is gradually lifted with the lifting bolt.

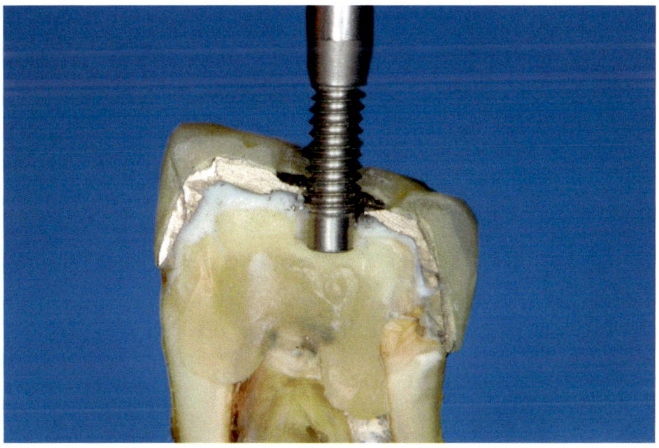

Fig 1-4v Cross section of crown with lifting bolt inserted.

In summary, this system provides prosthodontists with a reliable method for removing crowns (Figs 1-5 and 1-6). However, it is not effective if the occlusal metal surface of the metal-ceramic crown is thinner than 0.5 mm; in the author's experience, thin metal tends to bend, and thus no lifting effect is achieved.

Figure 1-7 lists the indications for the Crown Lifter CI system. The entire procedure can also be carried out man-

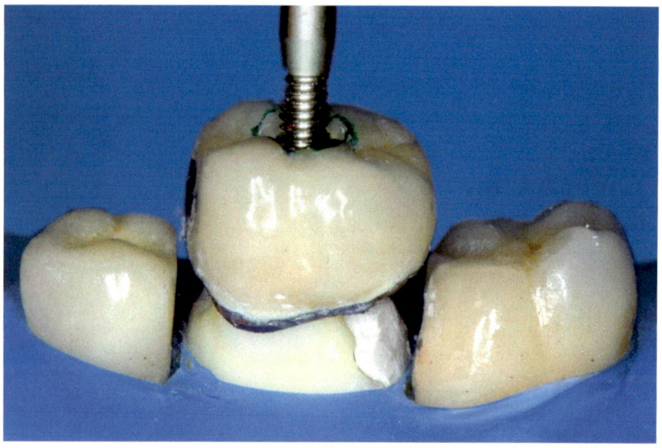

Fig 1-4w The crown is removed from the tooth preparation.

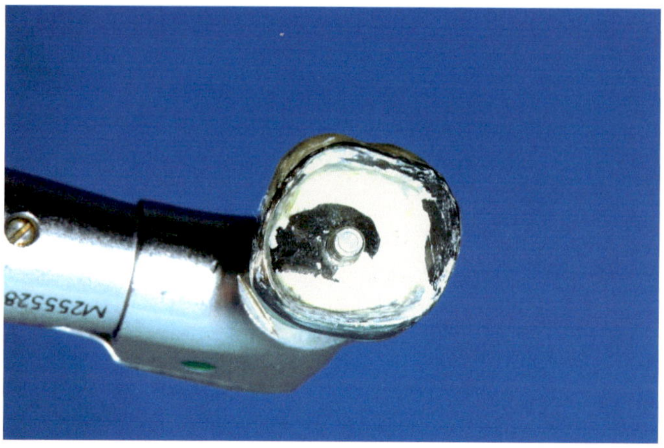

Fig 1-4x Crown attached to the handpiece after removal.

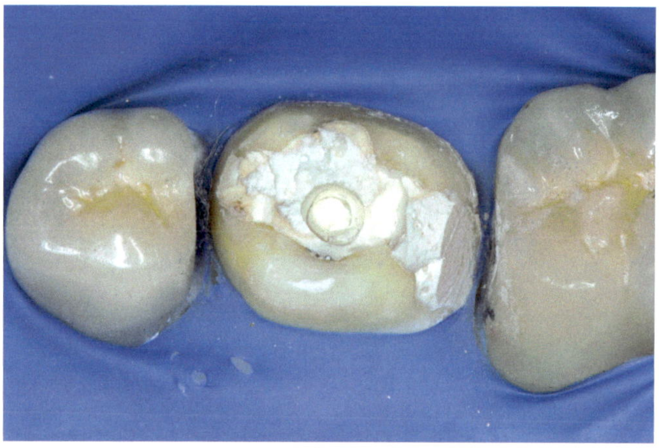

Fig 1-4y Natural tooth after removal of the crown.

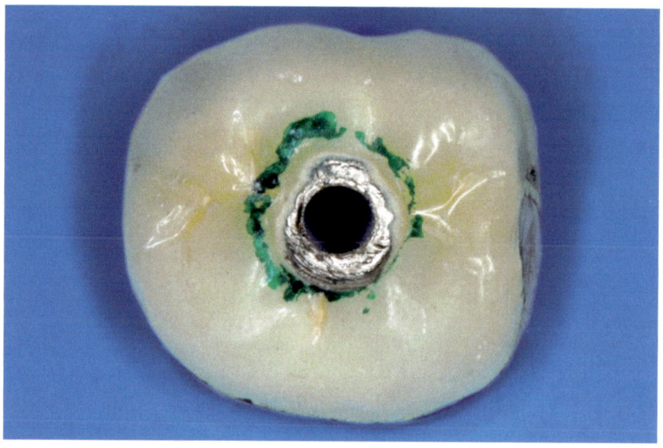

Fig 1-4z The crown can now be corrected, and rebaked and the central perforation can be resealed.

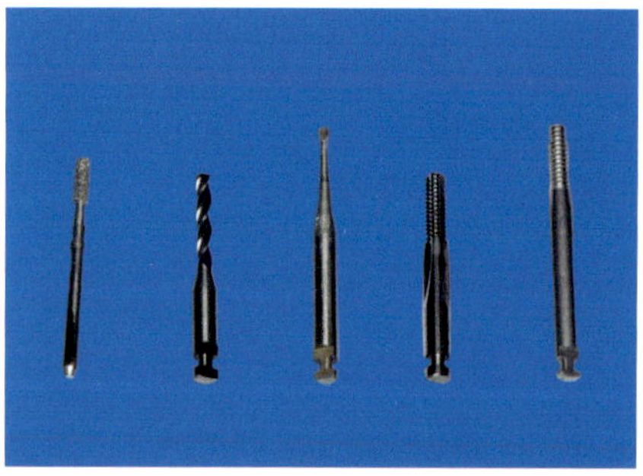

Fig 1-5 Crown Lifter CL instruments used in this procedure *(left to right)*: Cylindrical diamond bur, Multidrill, inverted cone bur, thread cutter, and lifting bolt.

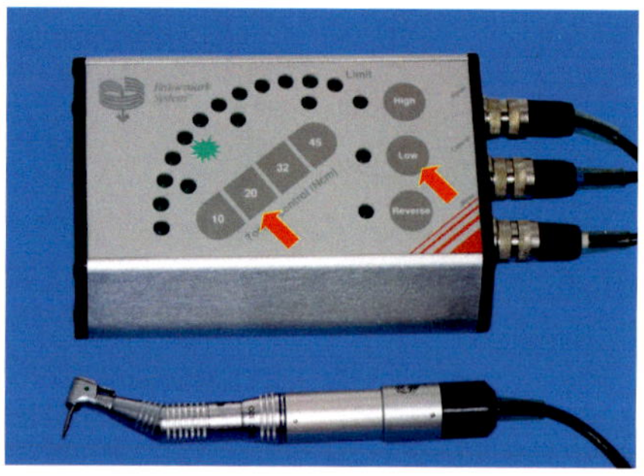

Fig 1-6 Torque limiter with speed and torque adjusted.

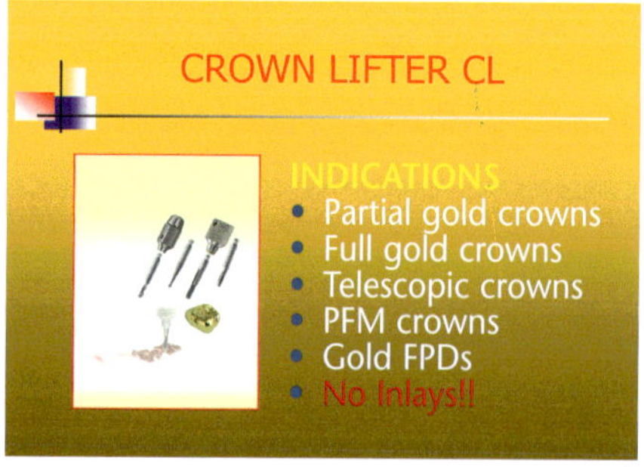

Fig 1-7 Indications for the Crown Lifter CL.

ually with a ratchet and a wrench, but this method is much more time consuming and lacks a mechanically defined force.

Materials

Crown Lifter CL (Bredent)
Multidrill (Bredent)
Torque limiter (eg, Torque Controller, Nobel Biocare)

Removal of Fixed Partial Dentures

Common problem: Fixed or splinted partial dentures requiring removal

In everyday dental practice, a fixed or splinted partial denture occasionally has to be removed and recemented. Possible reasons include:

1. Cementation errors:
   a. The fixed partial denture was tilted during cementing and its fit is not accurate enough. Marginal leakage is visible after the cement has been removed.
   b. The metal-free ceramic shoulder has fractured because of tilting and stress during cementation that went unnoticed until after the cement had hardened.
2. Loss of cementation on individual abutment teeth:
   a. Malocclusion has caused stress.
   b. Partial denture spans are too wide.
   c. Bone torsion has occurred, especially in the mandible.
3. Repair:
   a. Fractured porcelain has to be repaired.
   b. The patient is unhappy with the color or shape of the restoration and wants it to be changed.

Is it possible to remove these cemented or splinted partial dentures without destroying the margins and without fracturing the abutment teeth? What technical options are available?

The dental industry offers an array of removal aids, including the Treymann crown remover and hammer, the Crown Butler (Schuler Dental) with clips and weights, the crown spreader, crown removal claws, the malleable crown and bridge remover, and rubber-coated extraction forceps. However, all of these tools greatly increase the risk of fracture during removal of fixed or splinted partial dentures.

With most denture removal methods, the force that is applied is concentrated on only one point of the partial denture. This often results in uncontrolled chipping of the porcelain finish or deformation of the crown margins, which means that the partial dentures cannot be recemented.

Mechanical considerations prompt the following question: Is it possible to evenly spread the impact (ie, the force that is applied for a very short time) over the whole partial denture and thus minimize the danger of fracture or deformation?

Proven solution: Denture removal through the envelope technique

The following method is intended to remove partial dentures with as little risk as possible to the dentures themselves and to the abutment teeth.

To evenly distribute the impact (the force that is applied) throughout the entire partial denture, the denture to be removed is completely enveloped in slow-curing autopolymerizing acrylic resin, which develops very little heat. An arched hook is polymerized into the center of resistance of the solid partial denture and used as the point where the force can be applied.

The center of resistance is identical to the center of mass of a solid body. A force applied to the center of mass permits the force to act in a linear direction. If a force is applied outside this center of resistance, it could result in uncontrolled rotational movements and thus in the fracture of the abutment teeth. The master cast on which the prosthesis was manufactured can be very helpful in determining the original path of insertion.

Case report

Five years previously, a 50-year-old man had received a metal-ceramic fixed partial denture spanning from the maxillary right canine to the maxillary right first molar. Because of the divergence of the molar abutment tooth, the fixed partial denture was designed with a slide attachment. The anterior part of the fixed partial denture from the maxillary right canine to the maxillary right second premolar slid into the crown of the first molar (Figs 1-8a and 1-8b).

This part of the fixed partial denture became loose at the second premolar but was still firmly cemented to the canine. Knocking off this part of the fixed partial denture with a Treymann crown remover and hammer would

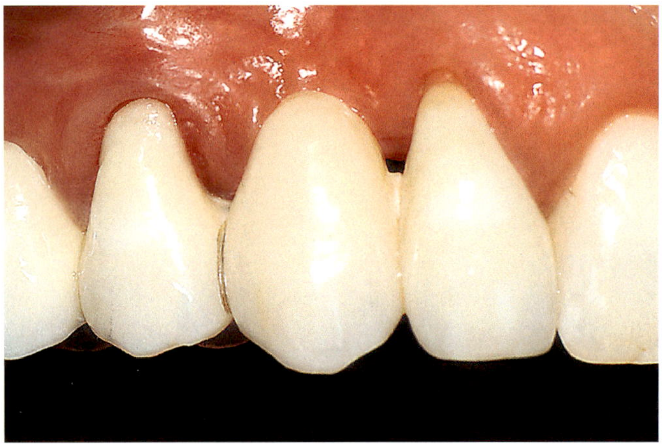

Fig 1-8a Buccal view of loose fixed partial denture.

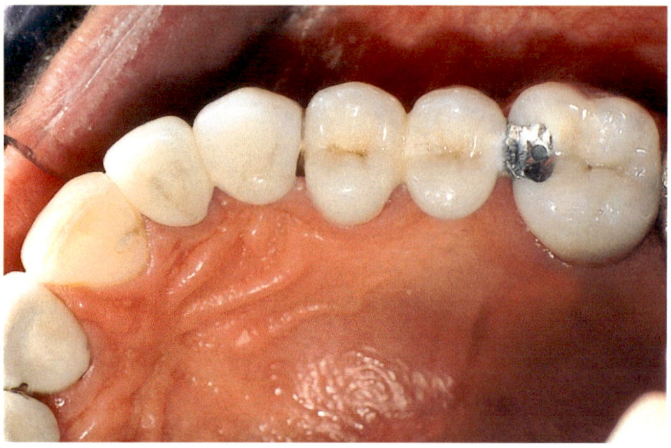

Fig 1-8b Occlusal view of loose fixed partial denture.

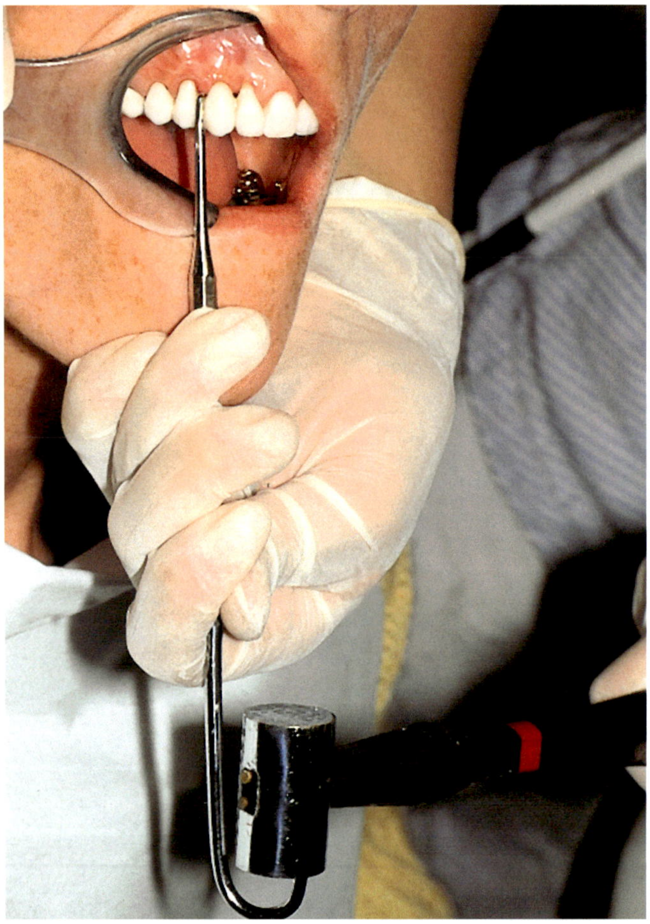

Fig 1-8c Treymann crown remover with lead hammer in position. This technique would most likely result in uncontrolled chipping of the ceramic material.

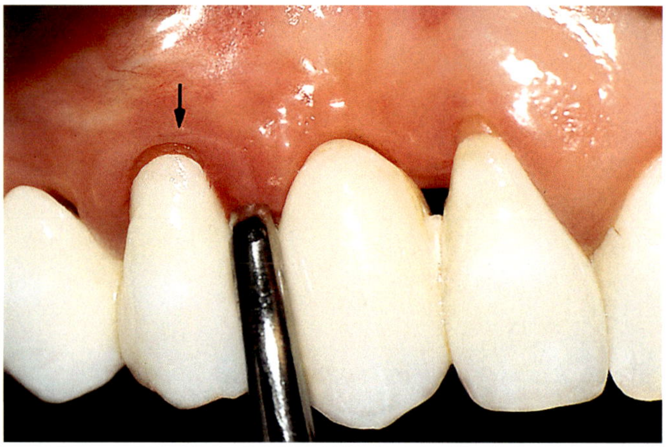

Fig 1-8d Loose crown *(arrow)*.

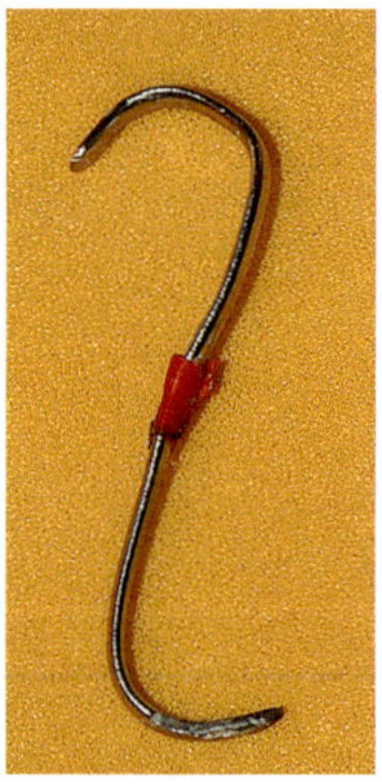

Fig 1-8e S-hook.

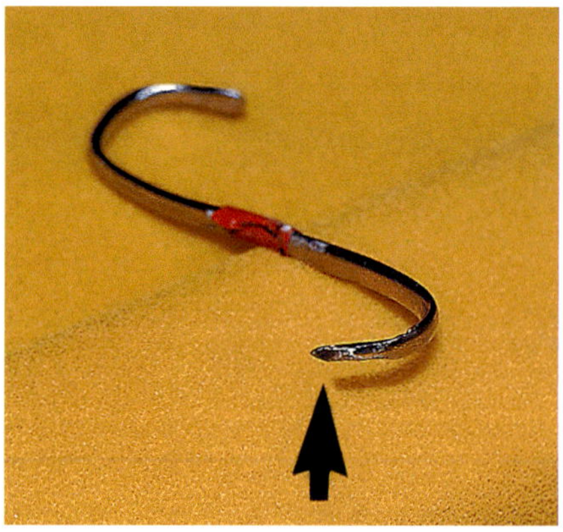

Fig 1-8f S-hook with pointed tip *(arrow)*.

have most likely resulted in uncontrolled chipping of the ceramic material (Figs 1-8c and 1-8d).

The partial denture was removed using a procedure that has proven very useful in the author's own office. A pointed, S-shaped hook made of lingual bar wire for provisional prostheses was inserted into the interproximal space distal to the canine and brought into an upright position (Figs 1-8e to 1-8g). A paste of a slow-curing material for provisional crowns and fixed partial dentures (Dentalon Plus) was mixed, and the entire fixed partial denture was enveloped with the S-hook in place (Figs 1-8h to 1-8j). The material was allowed to cure for 6 min-

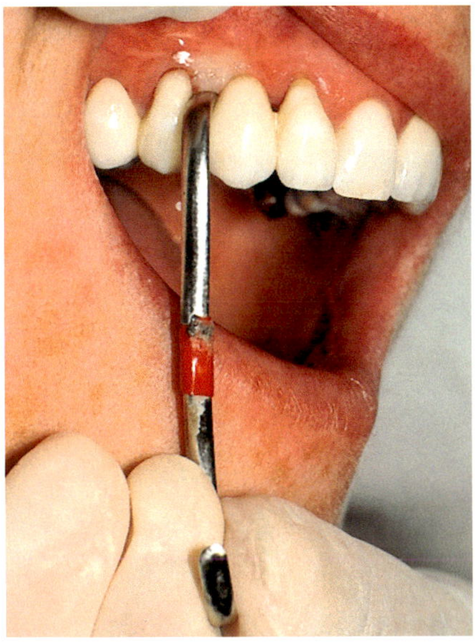

Fig 1-8g S-hook in position.

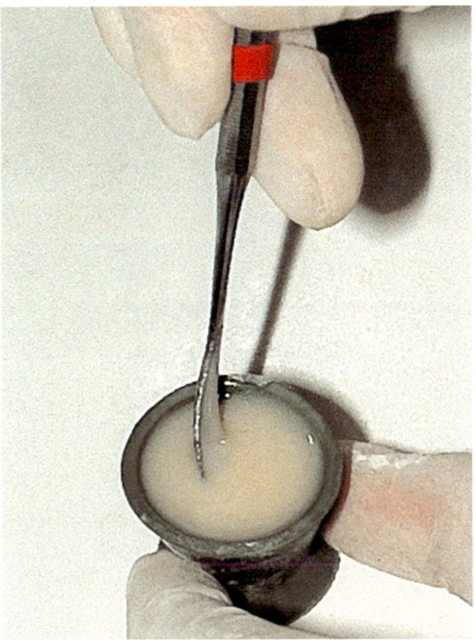

Fig 1-8h The polymer resin is mixed.

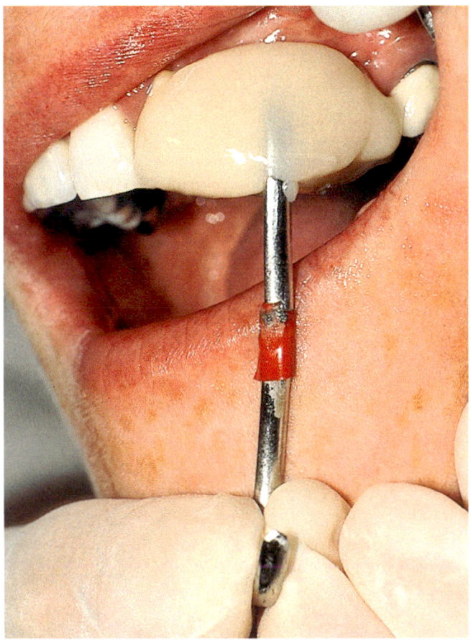

Fig 1-8i Buccal view of the S-hook polymerized into the envelope.

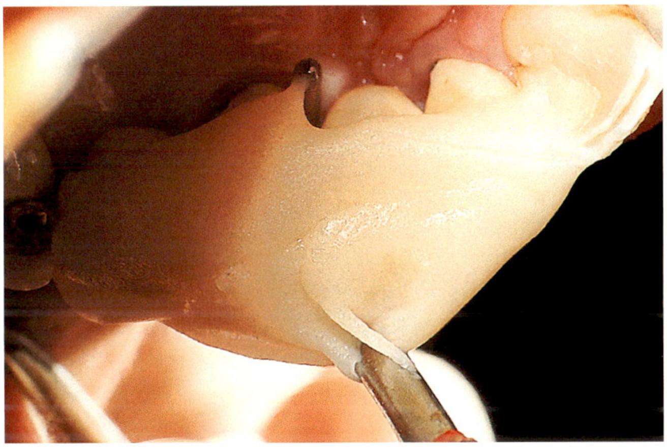

Fig 1-8j Palatal view of the S-hook in place.

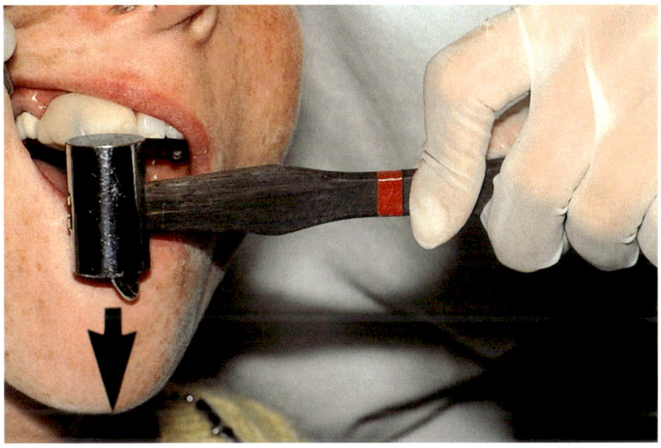

Fig 1-8k The fixed partial denture is knocked off with the lead hammer. *Arrow* indicates direction of hammer force.

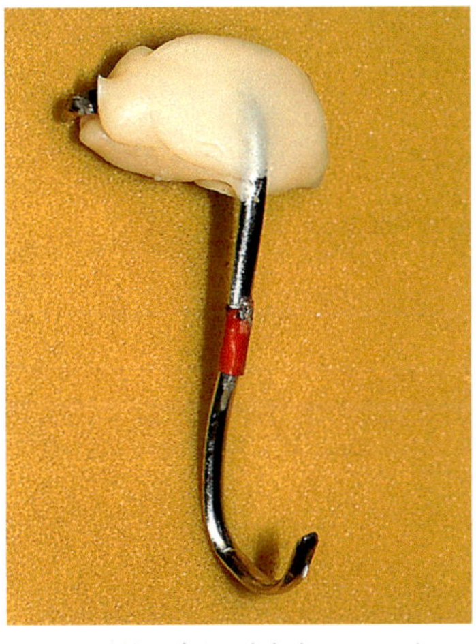

Fig 1-8l Fixed partial denture after removal.

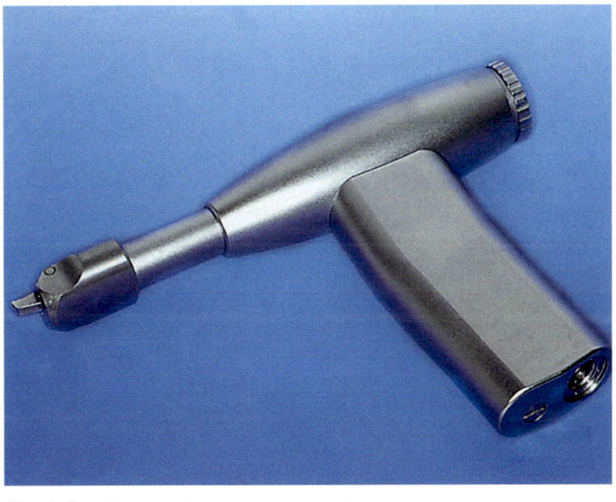

Fig 1-8m Coronaflex pneumatic hammer.

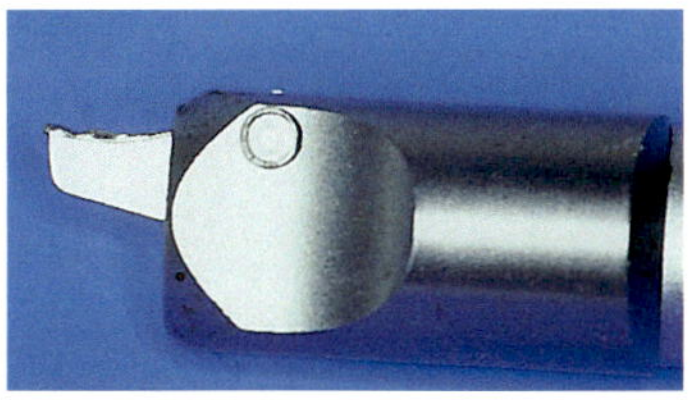

Fig 1-8n Striking pin of the Coronaflex.

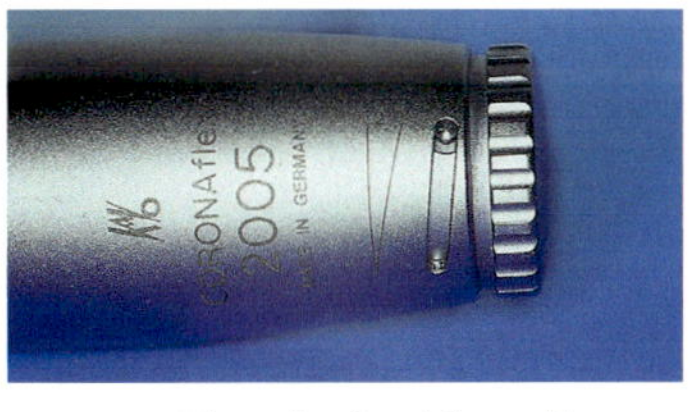

Fig 1-8o Thumbwheel for adjusting the force applied.

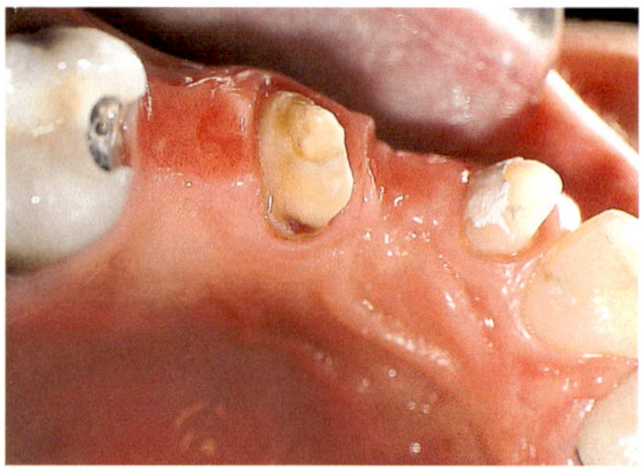

Fig 1-8p Occlusal view of the abutment teeth after removal of the denture.

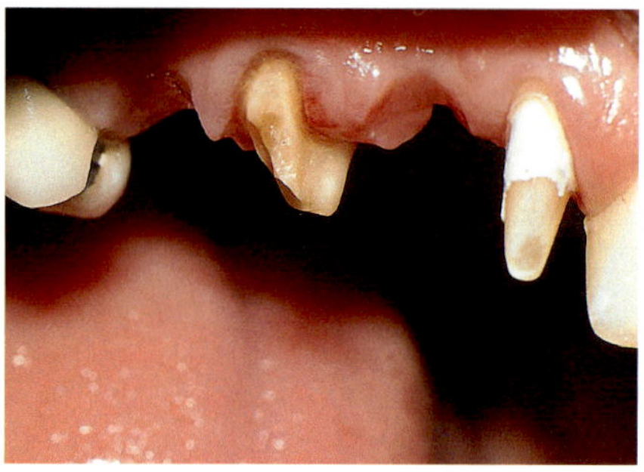

Fig 1-8q Buccal view.

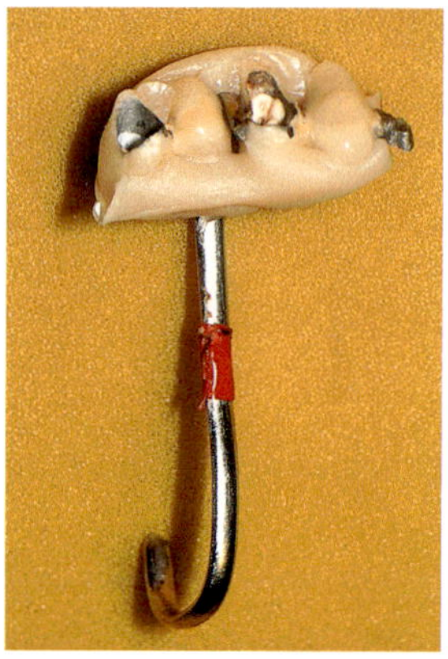

Fig 1-8r S-hook and removed fixed partial denture.

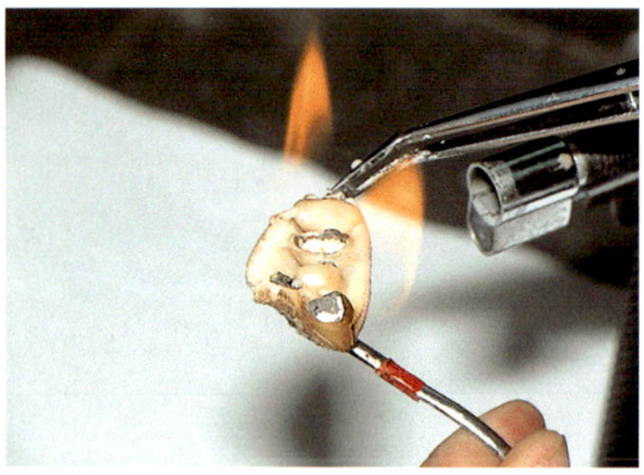

Fig 1-8s The envelope is burned off.

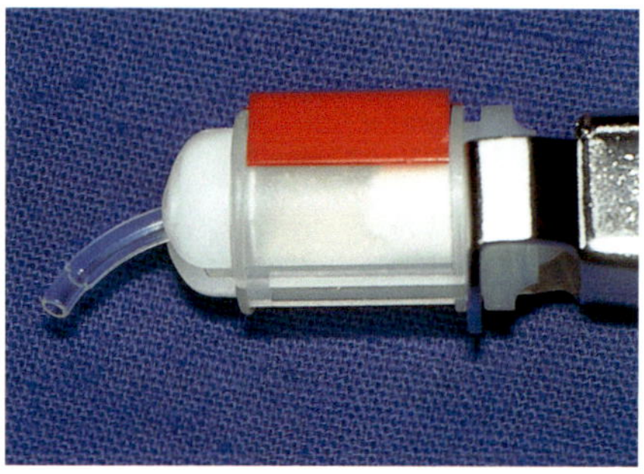

Fig 1-8t The reinserted fixed partial denture will be bonded with glass-ionomer cement.

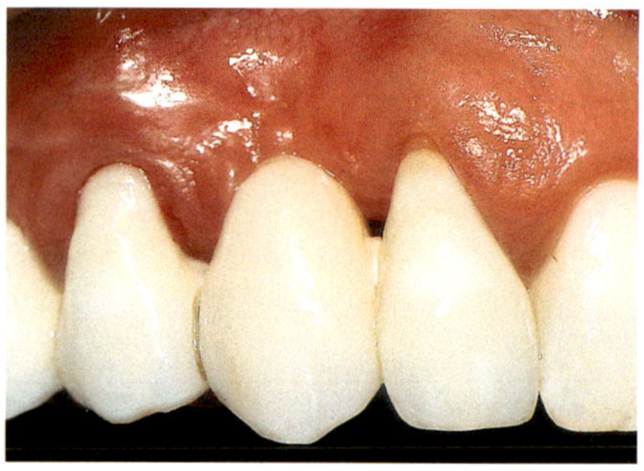

Fig 1-8u Reintegrated fixed partial denture.

utes to reach its final hardness so that the full impact of the blow would be transmitted to the fixed partial denture.

The fixed partial denture was knocked off with a quick but strong blow with a lead hammer (Figs 1-8k and 1-8l). Alternatively, the Coronaflex compressed air system has also proven to be useful in place of the lead hammer. According to the author's own statistics, 87% of fixed partial dentures (some of which were larger units) removed with the Coronaflex system suffered no damage. The device has the advantage of having an impact as fast as a gunshot, making it extremely effective (Figs 1-8m to 1-8o).

The fixed partial denture was removed easily with a few taps (Figs 1-8p to 1-8r). This fixed partial denture originally was cemented with a glass-ionomer cement, but this method may be used for all conventional cementing materials, such as zinc phosphate cement, glass-ionomer cements, carboxylate cement, and hybrid cement materials. Problems could arise with 4-methacryloxyethyl trimellitate anhydride (4-META) cement and with adhesives, but the author has no experience with these cements.

Because it was made of metal-ceramic, the enveloped fixed partial denture could be heated over a flame after removal. The envelope softened and was easily undone (Fig 1-8s). The fixed partial denture was then permanently recemented with glass-ionomer cement mixed in a machine (Figs 1-8t and 1-8u).

Because the loosening of the fixed partial denture presumably was caused by dysfunctional laterotrusion and a too-steep canine guidance, it was important to adjust the canine guidance by careful grinding and to check it thoroughly.

Materials

Lingual bar wire (Dentaurum)
Dentalon Plus provisional crown and bridge resin (Heraeus Kulzer)
Coronaflex crown and bridge remover (KaVo)
Maxi Cem (3M ESPE)

First Aid for Complete Dentures

Common problem: Complete dentures with insufficient retention

A 74-year-old patient was unable to chew or speak while wearing his complete dentures. Denture adhesive creams did not help; both dentures came off with every movement of the mandible. After several attempts to reline the dentures were unsuccessful, the patient gave up. When he smiled in public while wearing his dentures, he pressed them upward and downward with his tongue (Fig 1-9a). Otherwise, he achieved prosthesis "retention" only by clenching his teeth (Fig 1-9b).

The patient planned to celebrate his 75th birthday in 2 weeks' time. His whole family wanted to celebrate the day with him, but he refused because of the poor condition of his prosthesis. The family finally convinced him to see a dentist.

The dental examination revealed flat and edentulous alveolar ridges in the maxilla and mandible and somewhat reduced salivation. The complete dentures were inadequate (Fig 1-9c). These findings raised the following questions:

1. How could we help the patient so he could celebrate his 75th birthday with functioning dentures?
2. What treatment options were available as an interim first-aid measure?
3. With what kind of final prostheses could the patient be treated subsequently?

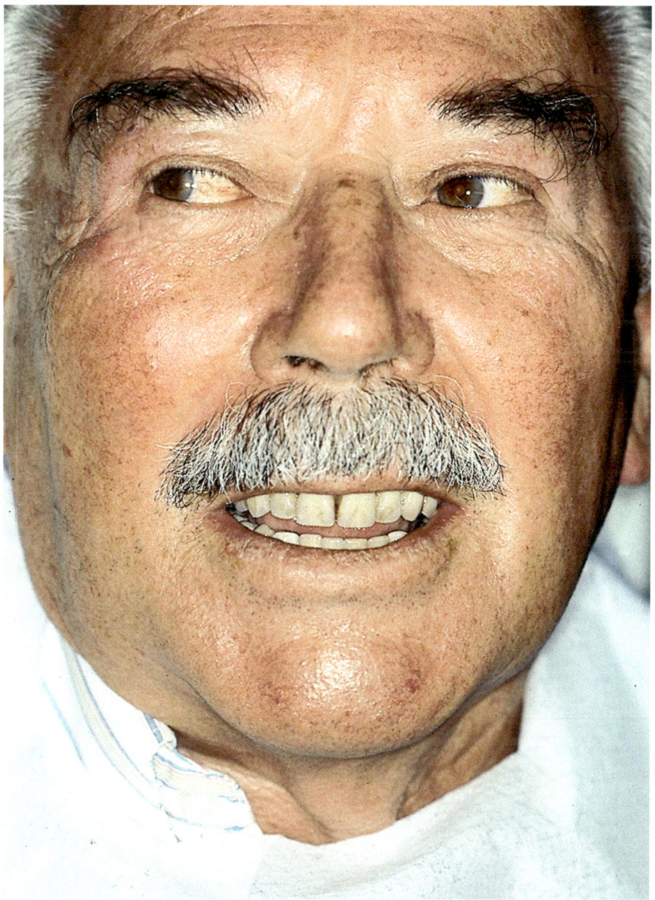

Fig 1-9a The patient is smiling painfully—he has to stabilize his dentures with his tongue.

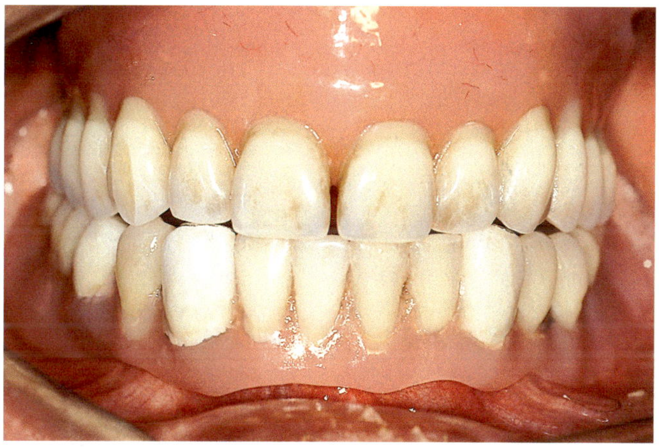

Fig 1-9b The patient has to clench the dentures together to obtain retention.

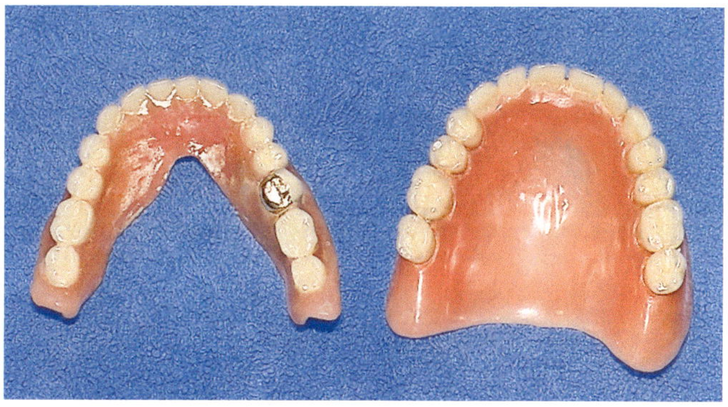

Fig 1-9c Poorly fitting pair of dentures.

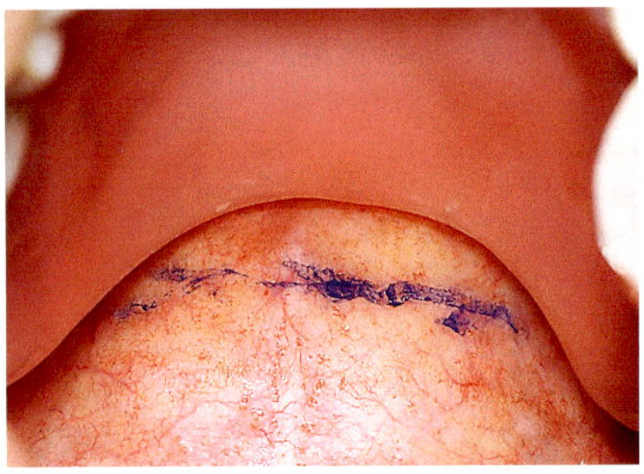

Fig 1-9d The maxillary denture is too short.

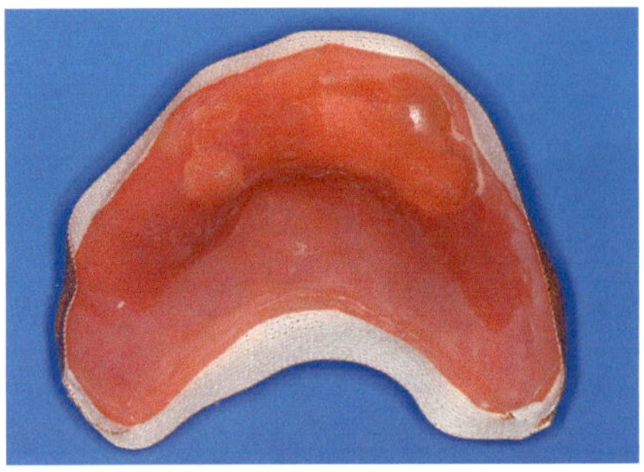

Fig 1-9e Palatal view of the elongated prosthesis masked with tape.

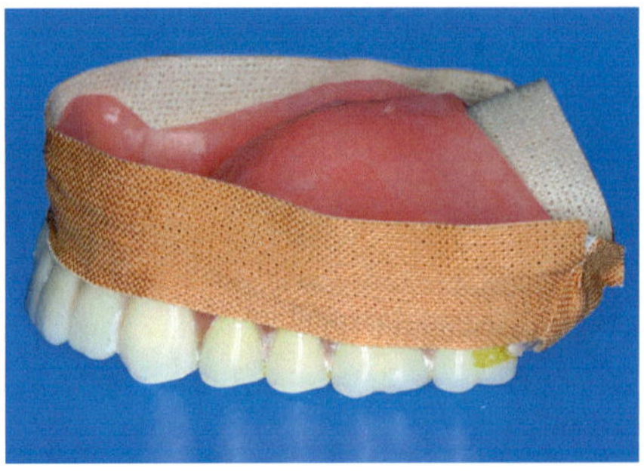

Fig 1-9f Lateral view.

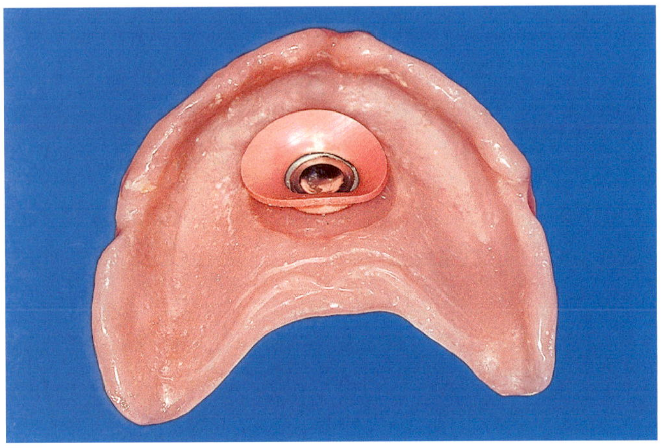

Fig 1-9g Relined maxillary denture with integrated suction cup.

Proven solution: Improved retention through relining and provisional implants

Maxilla

The palatal base of the maxillary denture was too short and had to be elongated (Fig 1-9d). The palatal and vestibular margins of the denture were marked with first-aid tape to prevent methacrylates from running into the patient's throat during relining and, at the same time, to prevent accidental polymerization of the artificial teeth (Figs 1-9e and 1-9f).

The relined complete denture was finalized and polished. A suction cup was then incorporated into the central palatal area. It must be emphasized that this prosthetic first-aid measure was meant only to bridge the few months until final restoration. Suction cups in complete dentures are contraindicated as a permanent solution for denture retention. There have been documented cases of ulceration, perforation of the palate, and tumor formation.[1] However, this has occurred rarely and only after several years' use of a suction cup. Therefore, the patient was required to sign a very detailed informed consent form.

This design provided satisfactory retention of the maxillary denture in the denture-bearing area (Fig 1-9g).

Mandible

Retention of the mandibular denture was improved by relining and by placement of provisional implants. Provisional implants were developed so that even after the insertion of final implants, additional transitional implants could be inserted to help attach provisional fixed dentures. The dental industry offers several systems for this type of application. In this case, the Modular Transitional Implant (MTI) System was used (Figs 1-9h and 1-9i).

After the panoramic radiograph was evaluated, the positions of the provisional implants were marked in the patient's mouth (Fig 1-9j). Blue dots were used to indicate the positions for implant insertion and black dots were used to indicate the mental foramina.

After local anesthesia with articaine (along with a substance which contains hyaluronidase to make the bone more permeable) the implant channel was drilled through the disinfected gingiva using the standardized drill. The drill was carefully moved up and down without much pressure (Figs 1-9k and 1-9l).

Afterward, the provisional implants were placed and the groove was aligned in the upper part of the implant with the help of a template so that it was parallel to the alveolar ridge (Figs 1-9m to 1-9p). The other channels were then drilled (Fig 1-9q), and the provisional implants were mechanically inserted at slow speed (Fig 1-9r).

The implants were aligned parallel to each other with the insertion wrench (Fig 1-9s), and their positions were checked from the labial and occlusal perspectives (Figs 1-

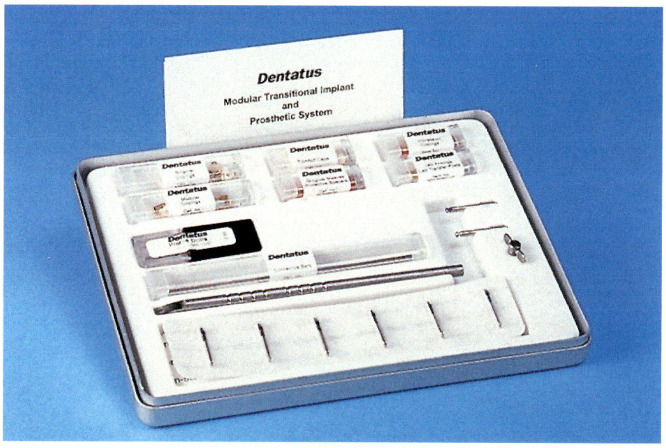

Fig 1-9h MTI System in its tray.

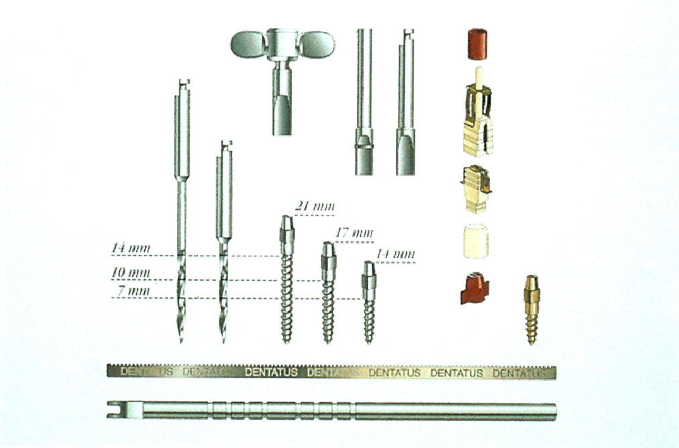

Fig 1-9i Individual components of the MTI System.

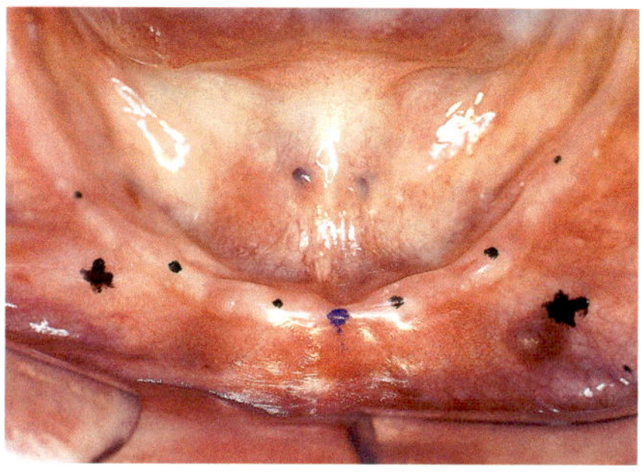

Fig 1-9j Implant positions are marked in blue, and the mental foramina are indicated in black.

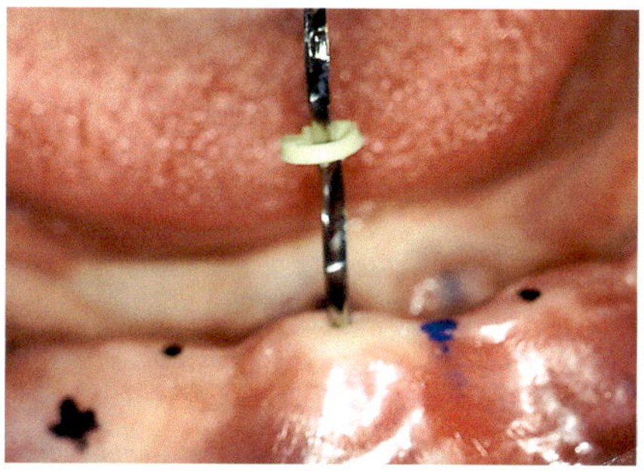

Fig 1-9k First transgingival preparation.

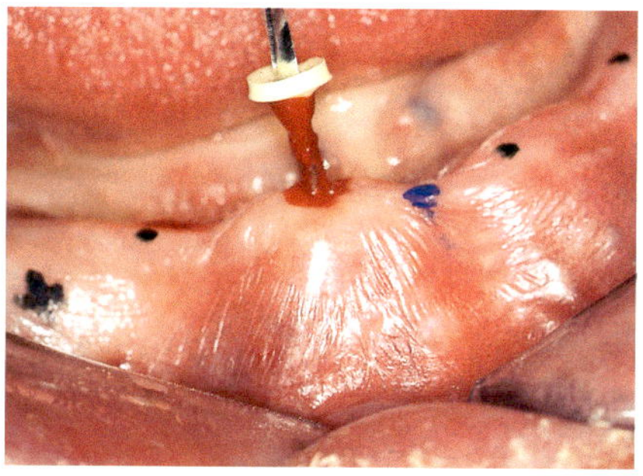

Fig 1-9l The drill is carefully moved up and down in a pumping motion without great pressure.

Fig 1-9m *(left)* The provisional implant is placed with the help of the hand wrench.

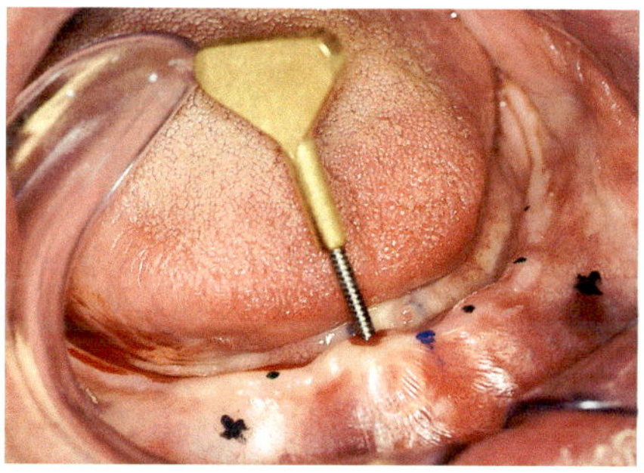

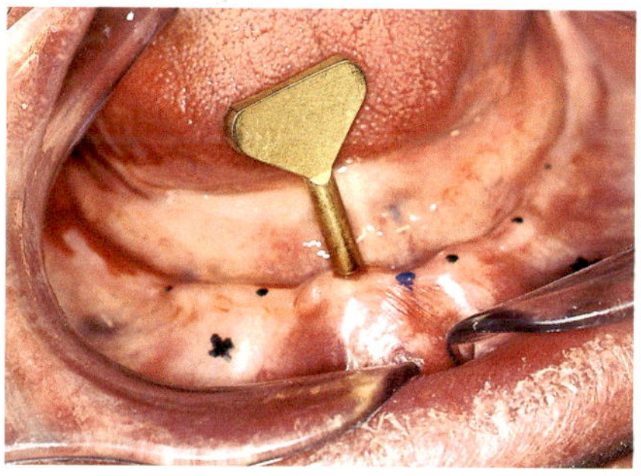

Fig 1-9n *(right)* Provisional implant in place.

Fig 1-9o *(left)* The alignment template is slipped on.

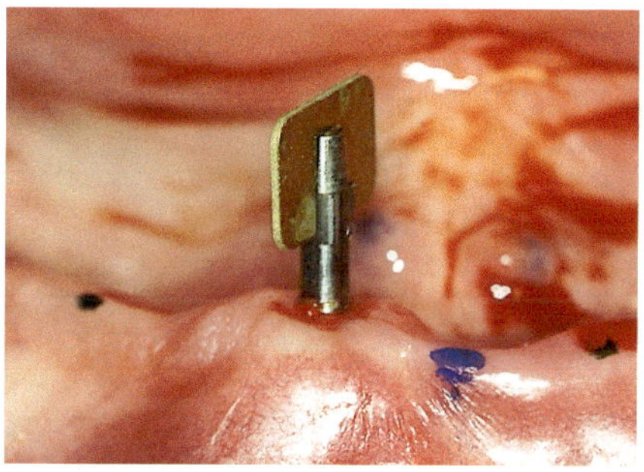

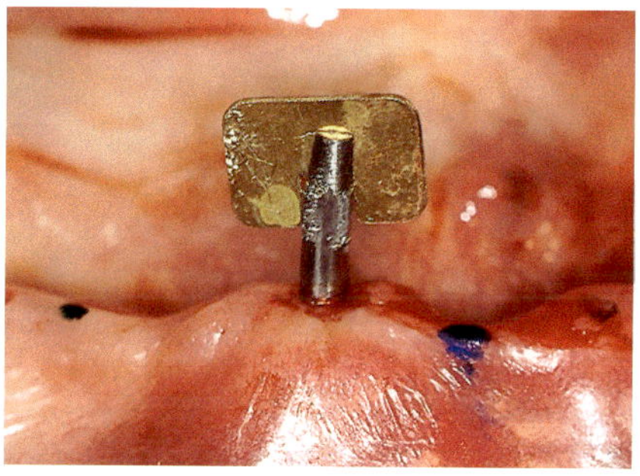

Fig 1-9p *(right)* The implant is aligned so that the groove is parallel to the alveolar ridge.

9t and 1-9u). With the help of templates, the alignment of the implants in a line parallel to the alveolar ridge was confirmed (Fig 1-9v), and a curved bar was fitted into the grooves in the implants (Fig 1-9w). Because the provisional implants did not all reach the same height, the curved bar was ground so that it could be countersunk into the horizontal grooves (Figs 1-9x and 1-9y).

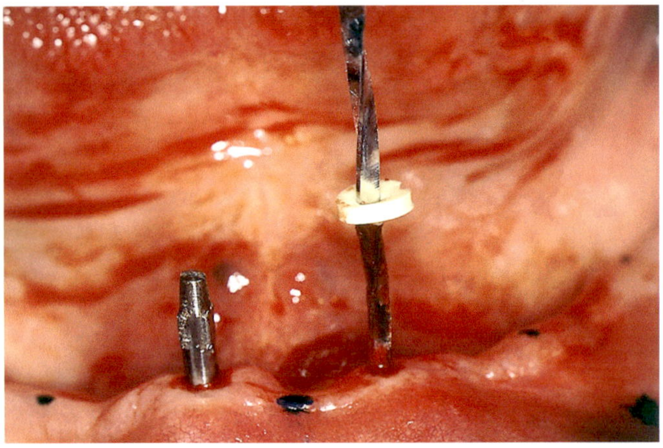

Fig 1-9q Second preparation in the marked position.

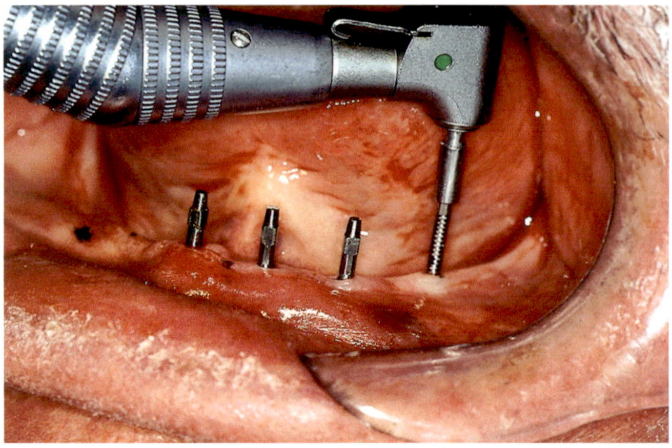

Fig 1-9r Further mechanical insertion of the provisional implants.

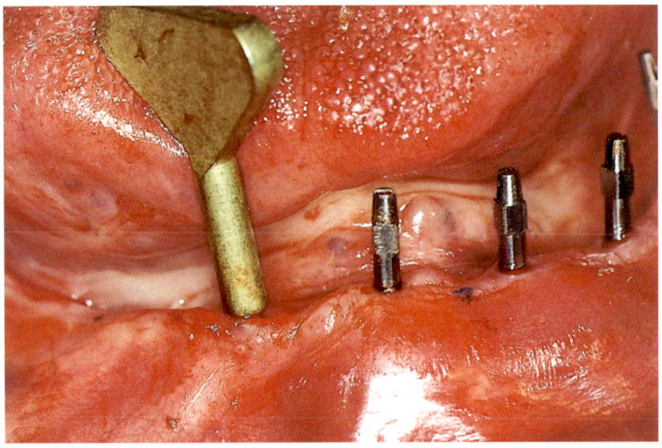

Fig 1-9s The provisional implants are aligned with the help of the hand wrench.

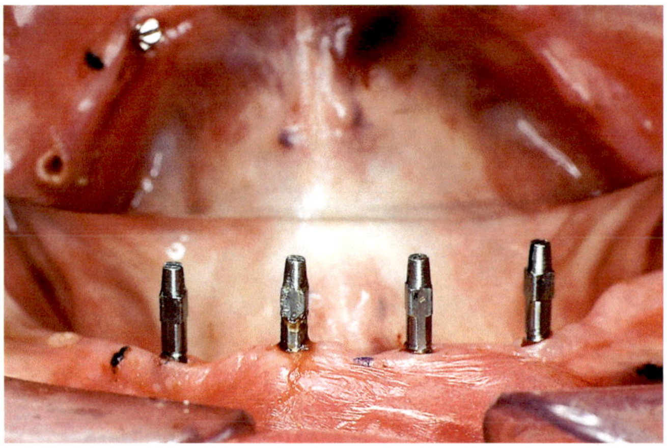

Fig 1-9t The alignment is evaluated from the labial view.

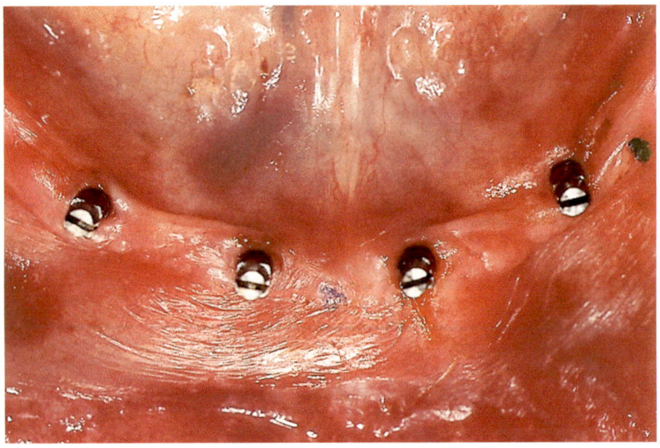

Fig 1-9u The alignment is evaluated from the occlusal view.

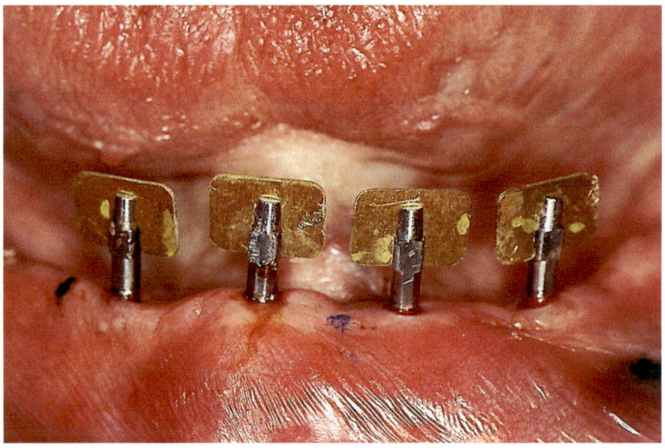

Fig 1-9v All of the provisional implants are reevaluated using the alignment templates.

The white plastic bar alignments were slipped on from above and bonded to the bar with light-curing adhesive (Figs 1-9z to 1-9cc). The existing mandibular denture was selectively ground and adapted (Figs 1-9dd to 1-9ff).

Finally, the mandibular denture was relined with self-curing methacrylate, and the bar was polymerized into the denture. This was accomplished by covering the undercut sections of the implant with red rubber rings

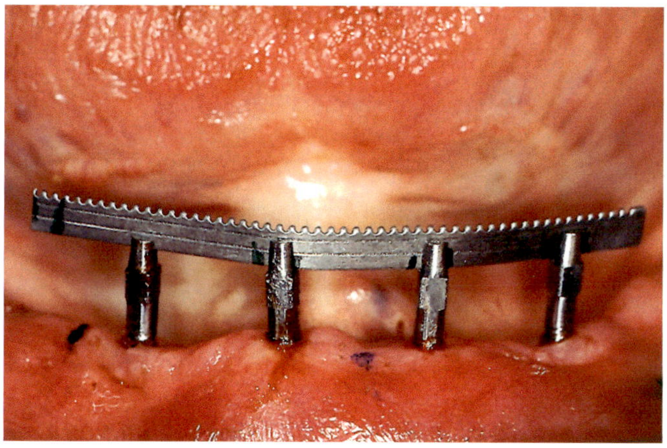

Fig 1-9w First try-in of the preformed bar.

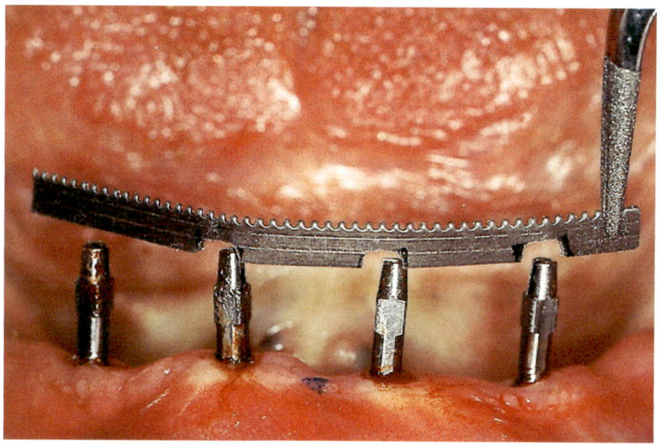

Fig 1-9x Second try-in, with notches ground out of the bar.

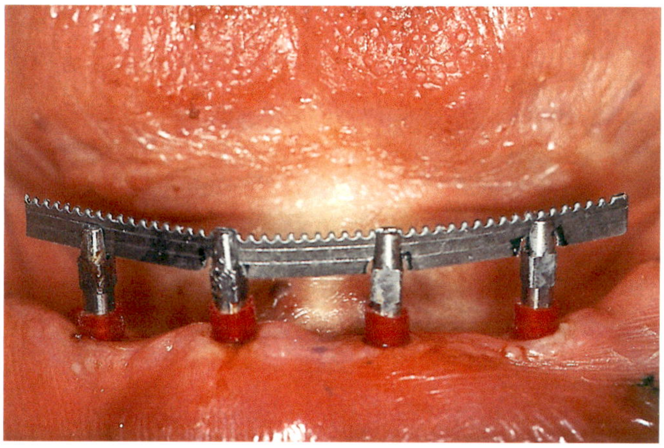

Fig 1-9y The fit of the bar is accurate.

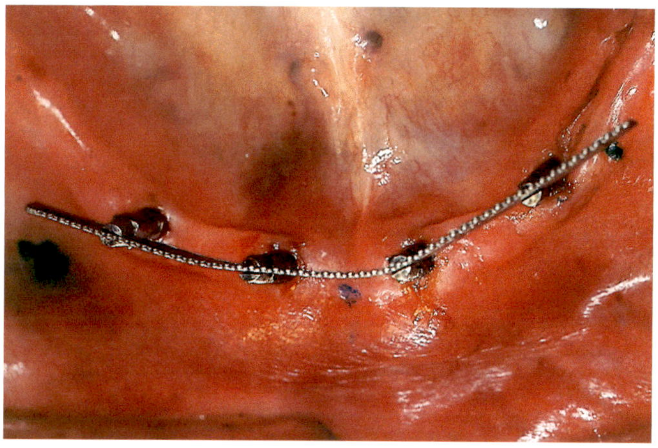

Fig 1-9z The bar is evaluated from the occlusal view.

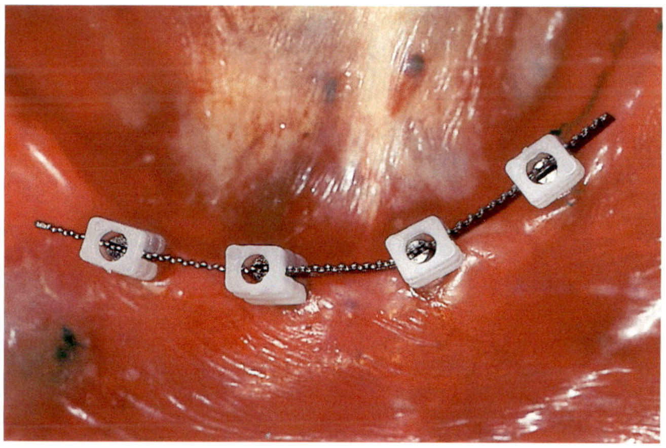

Fig 1-9aa The alignment guides are slid on the bar.

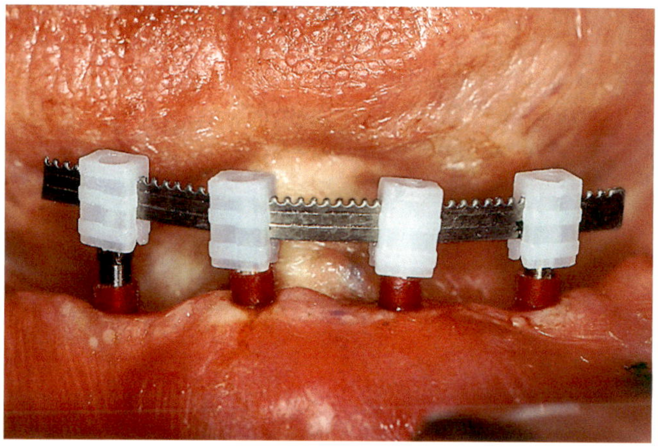

Fig 1-9bb Labial view of the bar alignment guides. The red rubber protectors around the undercuts are visible cervically.

(see Fig 1-9bb). Figures 1-9gg to 1-9ii show the bar guides from below and above after curing, contouring, and polishing. The mandibular denture sat firmly in the patient's mouth (Fig 1-9jj).

These treatment procedures firmly secured the patient's complete dentures, enabling him to eat and speak—and to celebrate his birthday (Fig 1-9kk). The planned final restoration consisted of a maxillary denture

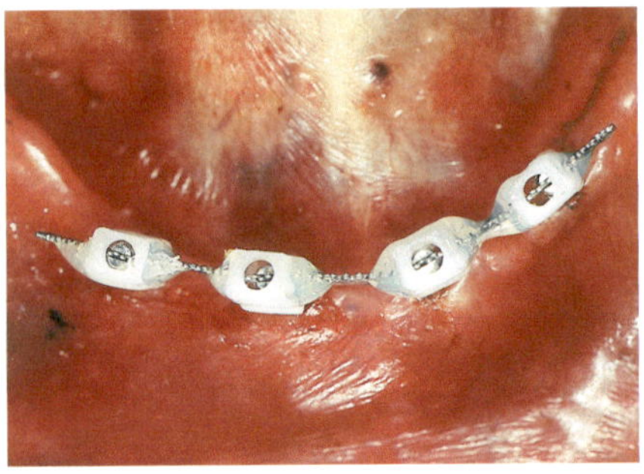
Fig 1-9cc The bar guides are bonded with light-curing adhesive.

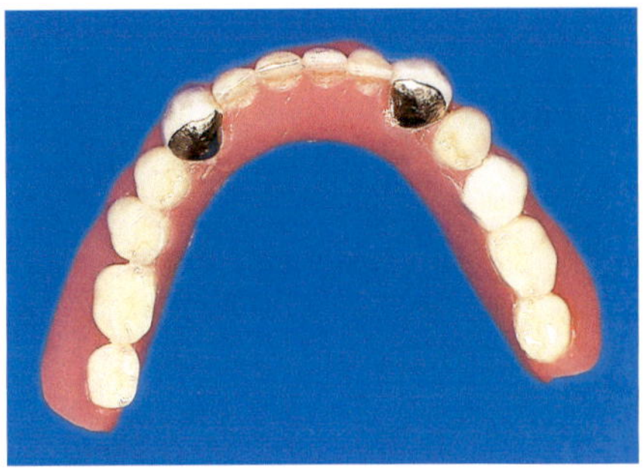
Fig 1-9dd Completed mandibular denture.

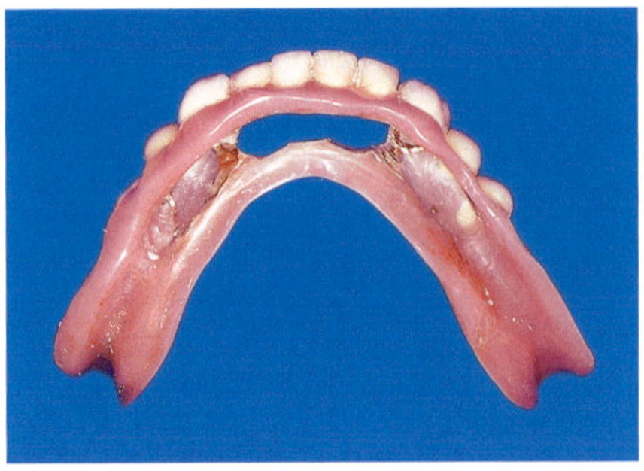
Fig 1-9ee The opening for the bar is ground out.

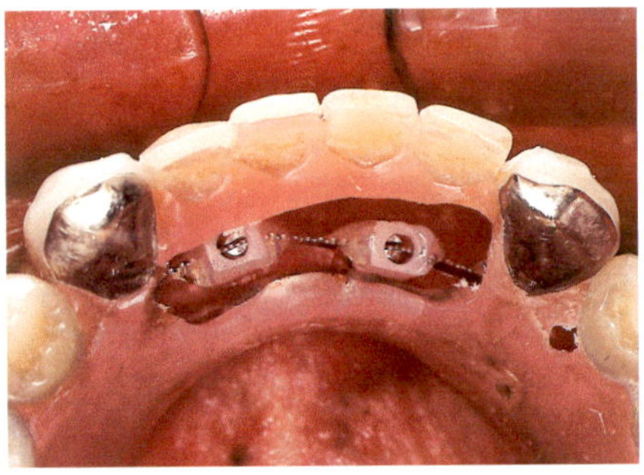
Fig 1-9ff The ground-out prosthesis is tried in the patient's mouth.

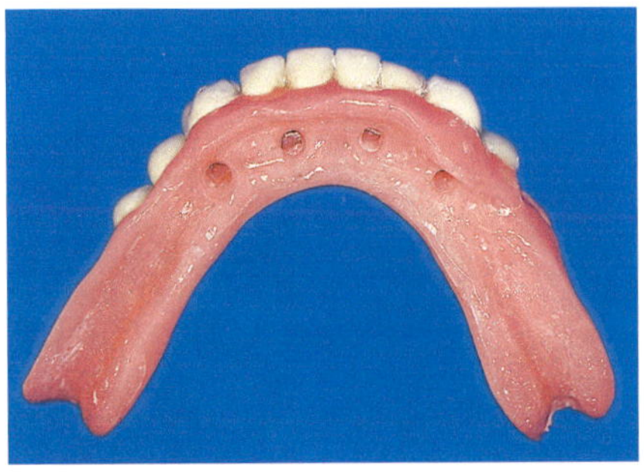
Fig 1-9gg Base of the mandibular denture with the polymerized bar.

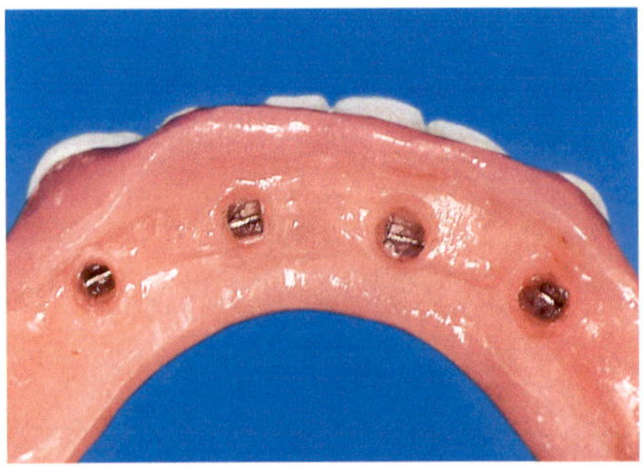
Fig 1-9hh View of the denture base. The bar alignments are clearly visible.

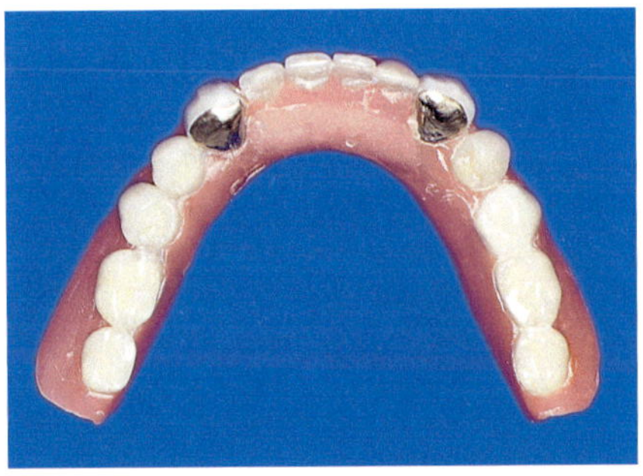
Fig 1-9ii Finalized and polished mandibular denture.

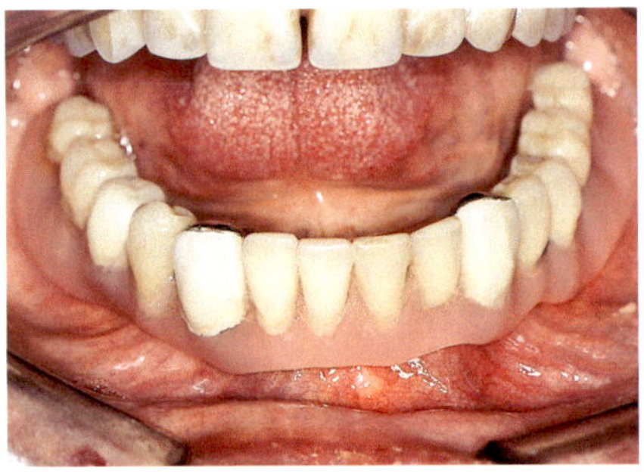
Fig 1-9jj Retention of the prostheses is ensured.

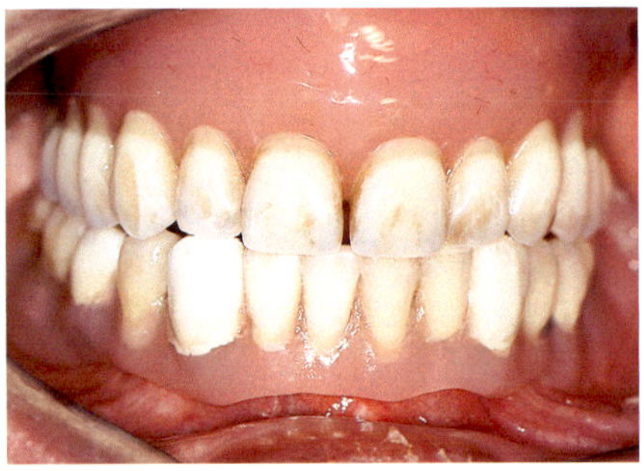
Fig 1-9kk The goal was met: The maxillary and mandibular dentures are kept in place.

(bar retention on four implants) and a mandibular denture (four telescopic attachments on four implants), both manufactured using model casting.

Materials

Leukoplast first-aid tape (BSN Medical)
Impression compound, green or brown (Kerr Dental)
Paladur pink self-curing denture base resin (Heraeus Kulzer)
MTI System (Dentatus)
Heliosit Orthodontic light-curing adhesive (Ivoclar Vivadent)

Fractured Posts

Common problem: Broken root post

In the last couple of years, the dental profession has improved its knowledge a great deal. In the past, many unjustified conclusions were made about core buildups and posts. Among other things, the following mistakes were made:

1. The posts were too long.
2. The posts were too thick.
3. The posts were bonded with conventional instead of adhesive resin cements.
4. The posts for cast cores were cast instead of using prefabricated drawn posts.
5. The root above the gingiva was too short (minimum 2 mm circular).
6. The screws caused stress on the root, guaranteeing fractures.

In the mid-1990s, a study by Velvart et al showed that the post works solely as a retainer for the core but that in no way does it splint the endodontically treated tooth. If the post is too long and too thick, the risk of breakage increases. The fractures may not occur for several years, but at some point they are virtually guaranteed.

In most cases, metal posts that have been bonded with conventional cements can be successfully removed with the trephine system of the Masserann Kit (Fig 1-10). In modern esthetic dentistry, however, posts made of zirconium dioxide are often bonded with adhesive cements. What can be done if such a hard post breaks and its cement cannot be loosened?

Proven solution: Direct restoration using a trephine buildup

A zirconium dioxide post can rarely be removed successfully—in most cases, the root fractures. How can the tooth be saved? How can the fractured crown be provided with a new core and then recemented? Brandau created a titanium trephine post that is manufactured by Brasseler. The following case report demonstrates this last resort for saving a tooth with a zirconium oxide post.

Case report

The crown of the right lateral incisor in a 60-year-old patient had broken at the gingival level due to trauma. The crown had been recemented twice with resin composite, but it held for only a few hours (Figs 1-11a to 1-11f).

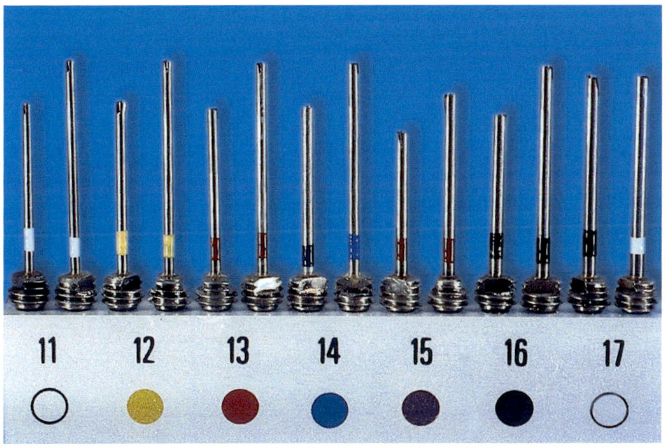

Fig 1-10 Masserann Kit, a set of trephine burs for removing fractured posts and root canal instruments.

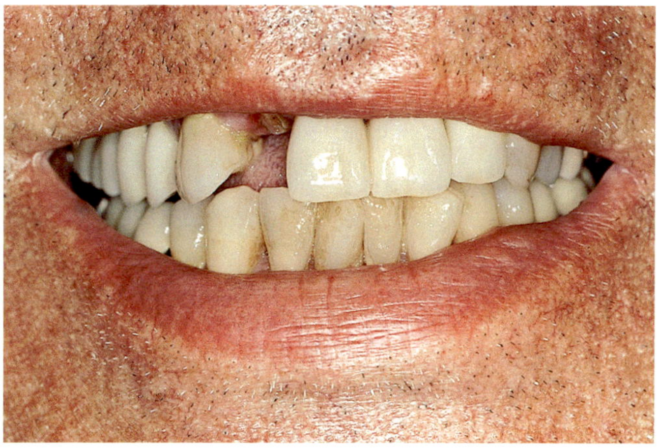

Fig 1-11a The patient's right maxillary lateral incisor is fractured.

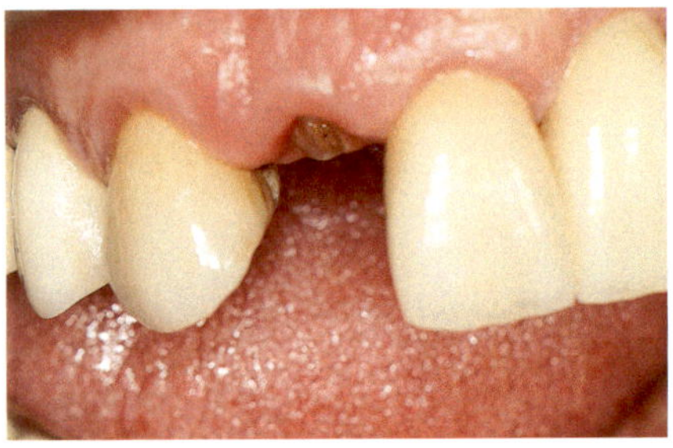

Fig 1-11b The crown has broken off at the gingival level.

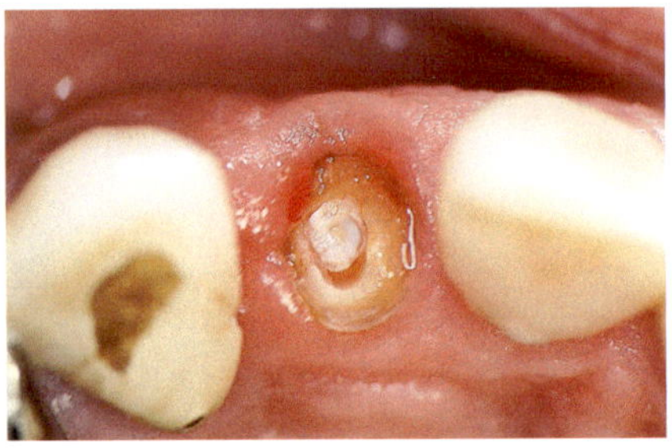

Fig 1-11c The broken zirconium oxide post is visible *(center)*.

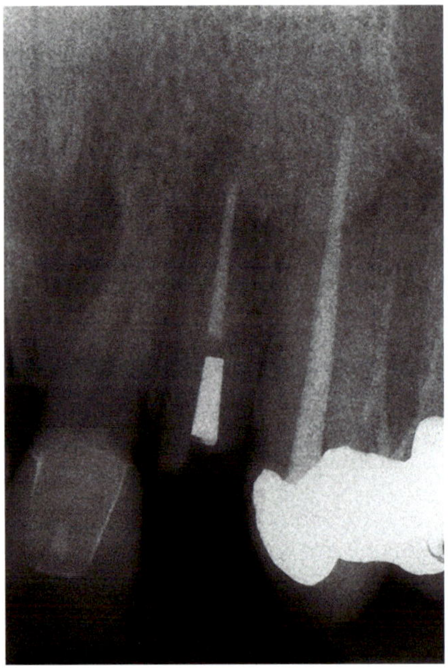

Fig 1-11d Radiograph of the fractured tooth.

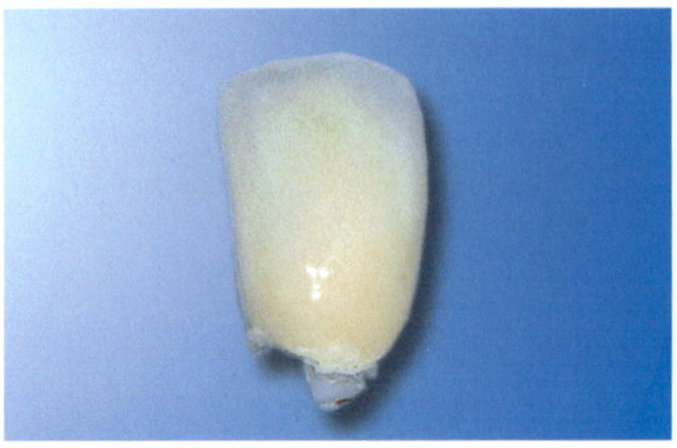

Fig 1-11e Fractured crown.

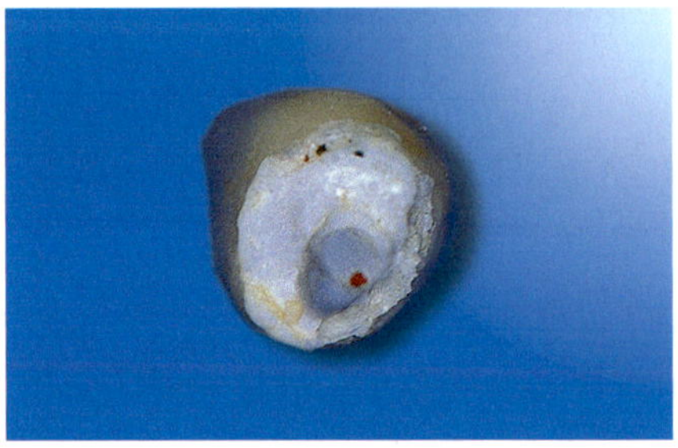

Fig 1-11f Fractured crown with remnants of cement (view of base).

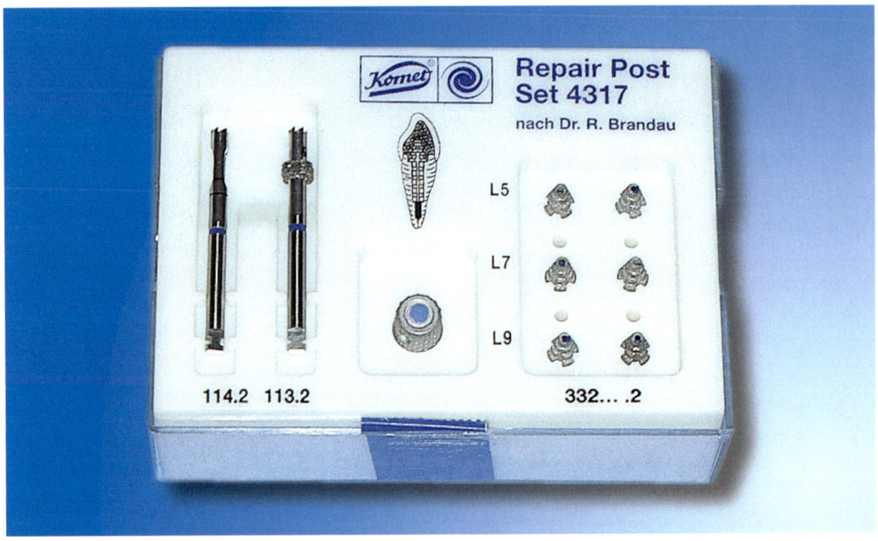

Fig 1-11g Post Repair Kit 4317.

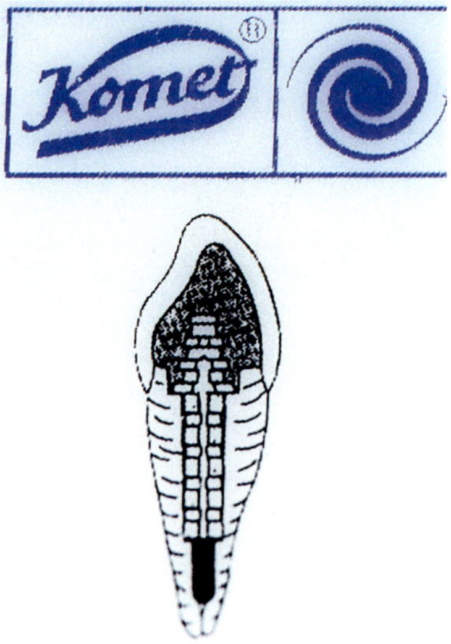

Fig 1-11h Diagram of the trephine buildup.

Underneath the crown there was a direct buildup that could not be removed again; it consisted of a zirconium oxide post bonded with adhesive cement. At one time, the only alternative would have been to extract the tooth and then place either a fixed partial denture or a single-tooth implant. However, with a trephine buildup set (Post Repair Kit 4317), one last attempt could be made to rescue the tooth (Figs 1-11g and 1-11h).

A trephine bur (Figs 1-11i and 1-11j) was used to cut around the fractured zirconium oxide post (Figs 1-11k and 1-11l). The procedure is demonstrated in Figs 1-11m to 1-11q on an extracted tooth. The author recommends always practicing the technique and use of a new system on an extracted tooth before trying it in a patient's mouth.

The trephine post was tried in the patient's mouth (Fig 1-11r). DTK, a special adhesive that can be pre-cured with light (Fig 1-11s) was then used to cement it carefully (Fig 1-11t). The 12-minute curing time should be controlled with a timer. Figures 1-11u and 1-11v show a polished

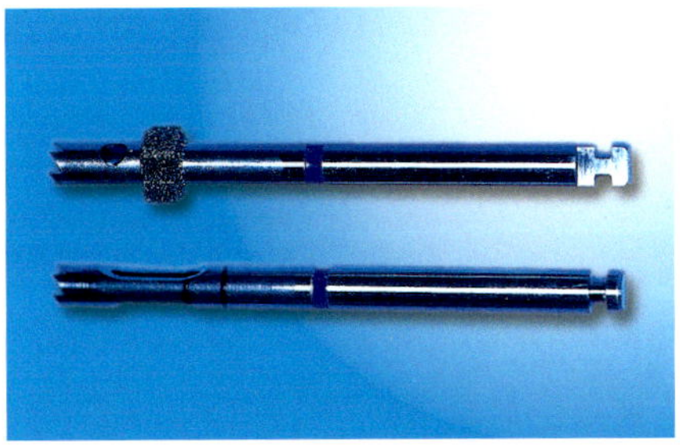

Fig 1-11i Trephine burs included in the repair kit.

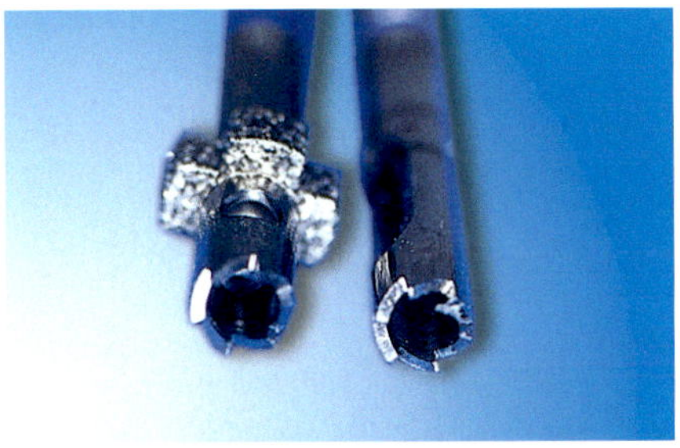

Fig 1-11j Cutting edges of the trephine burs.

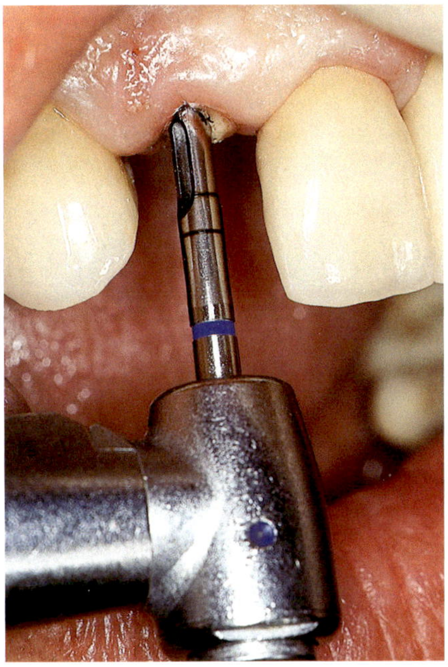

Fig 1-11k A trephine bur is used to cut around the zirconium oxide post in the patient's mouth.

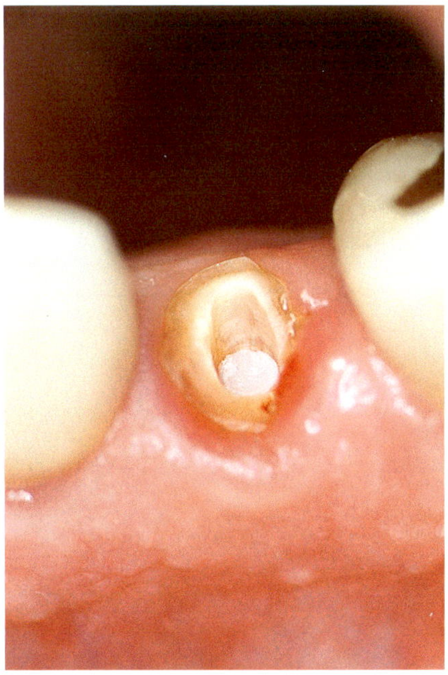

Fig 1-11l Prepared zirconium oxide post.

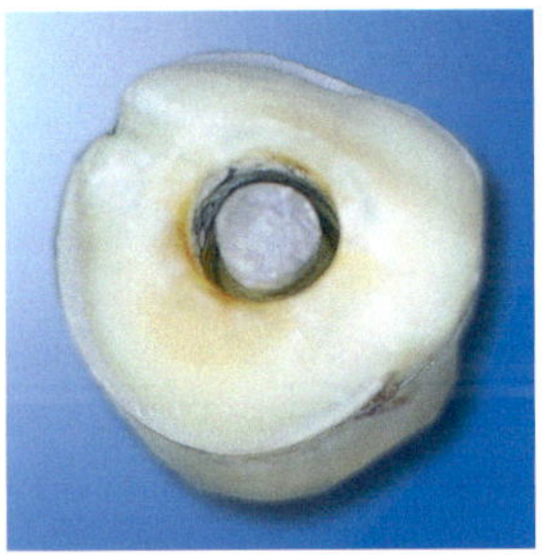

Fig 1-11m Cutting around the post, demonstrated with an extracted tooth.

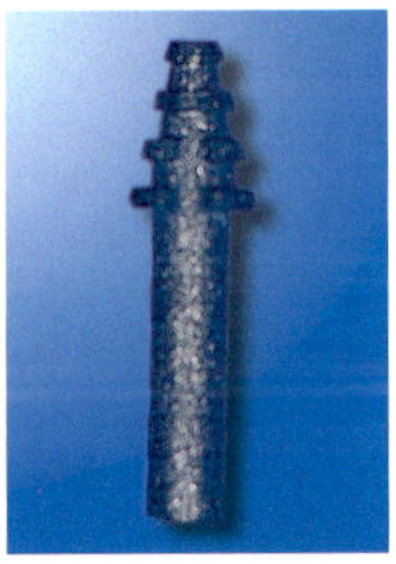

Fig 1-11n Trephine post. The upper part corresponds to the Vlock anchoring system (Brasseler).

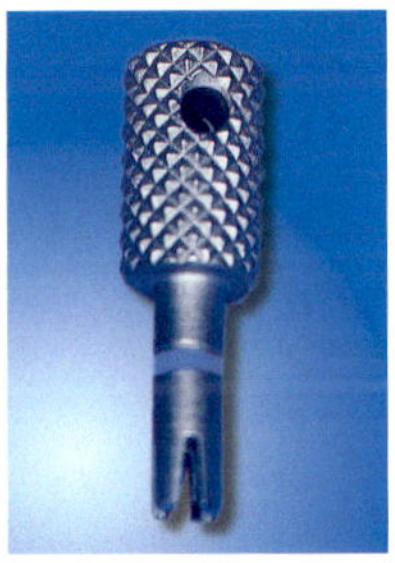

Fig 1-11o Positioner.

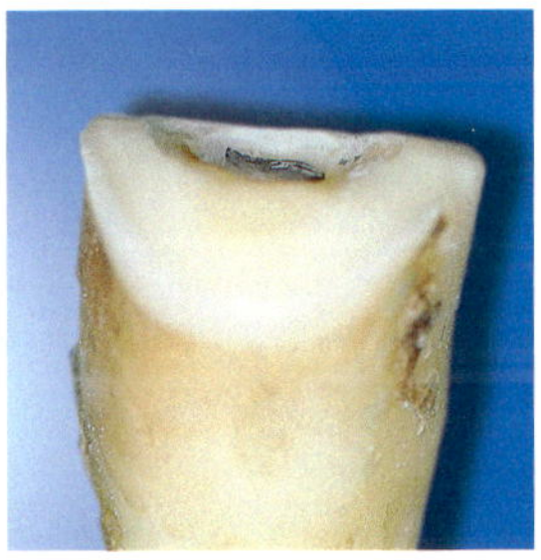

Fig 1-11p The procedure is demonstrated on an extracted tooth.

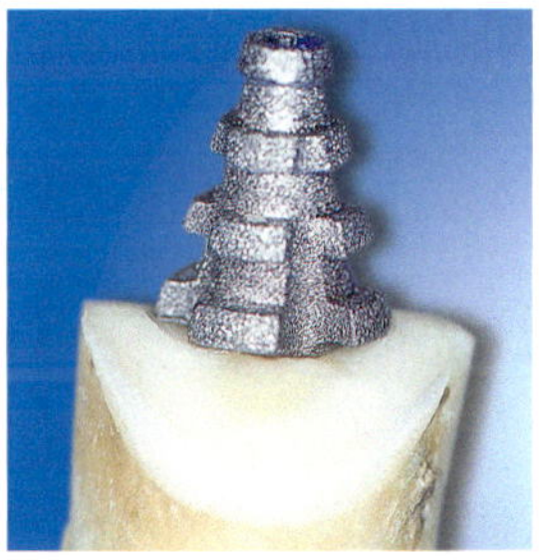

Fig 1-11q The buildup inserted in the extracted tooth.

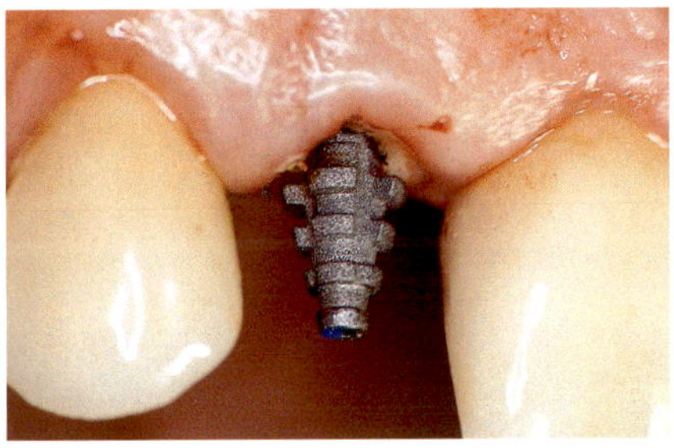

Fig 1-11r The buildup is inserted in the maxillary right lateral incisor to check its length and diameter.

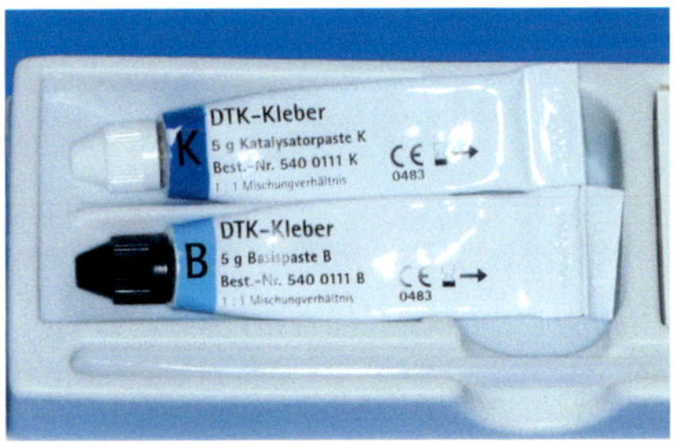

Fig 1-11s DTK adhesive.

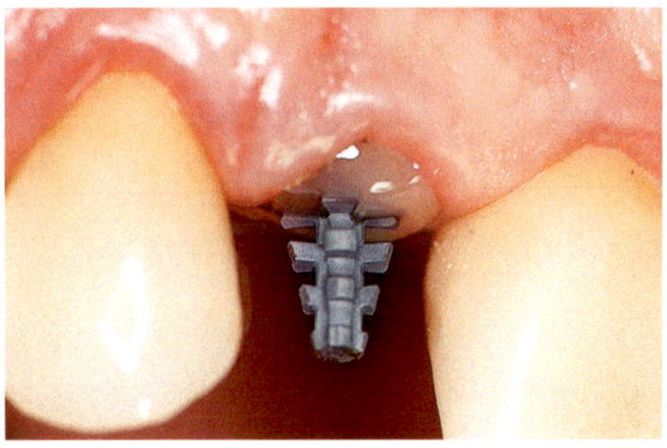

Fig 1-11t Cemented trephine post.

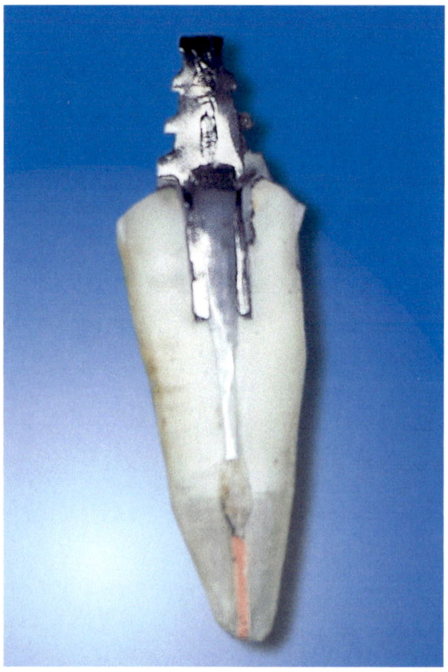

Fig 1-11u Cross section of the tooth with the trephine post in place. The obturated root canal, the zirconium oxide post, and the trephine buildup are clearly visible.

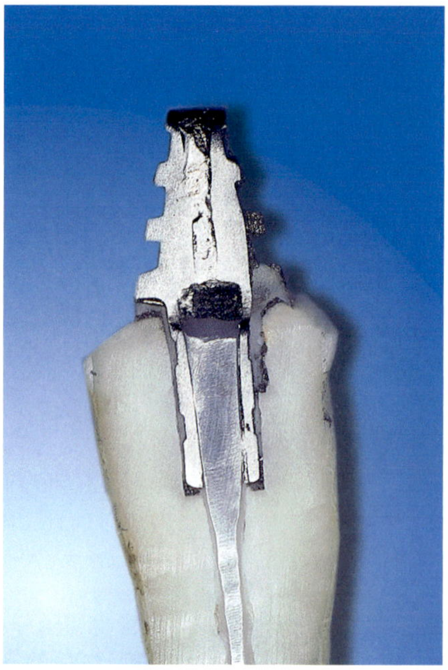

Fig 1-11v Close-up of the cross section. The good fit of the buildup is clearly visible.

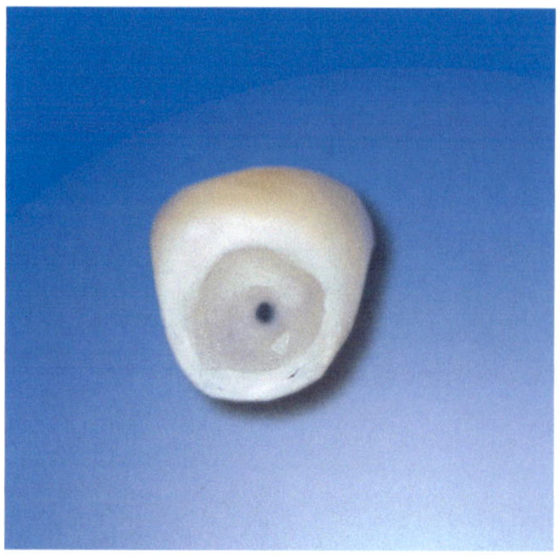

Fig 1-11w Ground-out crown (view of base).

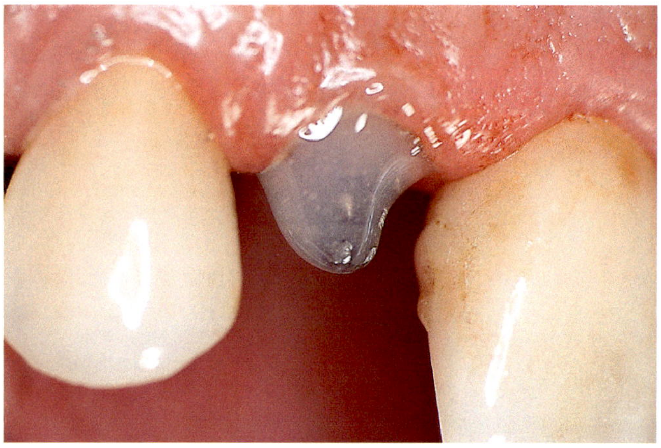

Fig 1-11x Trephine buildup with the resin composite cement applied.

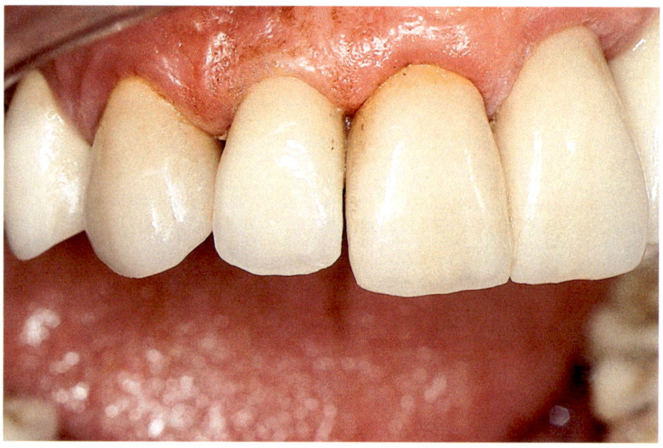

Fig 1-11y Final evaluation.

cross section of the extracted tooth to illustrate the situation in and around the tooth.

The crown was then carefully ground out in the laboratory under a stereomicroscope (Fig 1-11w) and subsequently tried in the patient's mouth. The buildup had to be abraded somewhat. After the DTK adhesive was applied to the cemented buildup, the inside of the crown was brushed and then cemented (Fig 1-11x). If positioning of the crown is difficult, an incisal positioner should be prepared from autopolymerizing acrylic resin (eg, Pattern Resin).

Figure 1-11y shows the repaired crown in situ. The patient was sent home after the occlusion and articulation were carefully checked.

Materials

Post Repair Kit 4317 (Brasseler)
DTK adhesive (Bredent)
Pattern Resin (GC)
Masserann Kit (Micro-Mega)

Lost Abutment Teeth

Common problem: Abutment teeth lost to restoration in a fixed partial denture with several spans

A woman (Fig 1-12a) reported severe pain throughout the area covered by her extensive maxillary fixed partial denture (Figs 1-12b and 1-12c). The examination and the panoramic radiograph (Fig 1-12d) yielded the following findings.

The multispan fixed partial denture had the following abutment teeth: the maxillary right first molar, second premolar, and canine and the maxillary left first premolar and first molar. The denture replaced the right first molar, lateral incisor, and central incisor and the left central incisor, lateral incisor, canine, and second premolar (20-year-old fixed partial denture).

The fixed partial denture exhibited mobility of 0 to 1 degree.

There was purulent discharge around the maxillary left first premolar; root remnants were visible from the palatal view (Figs 1-12e to 1-12g).

A condition consistent with pulpitis was present at the maxillary left second molar (pulp testing: +++).

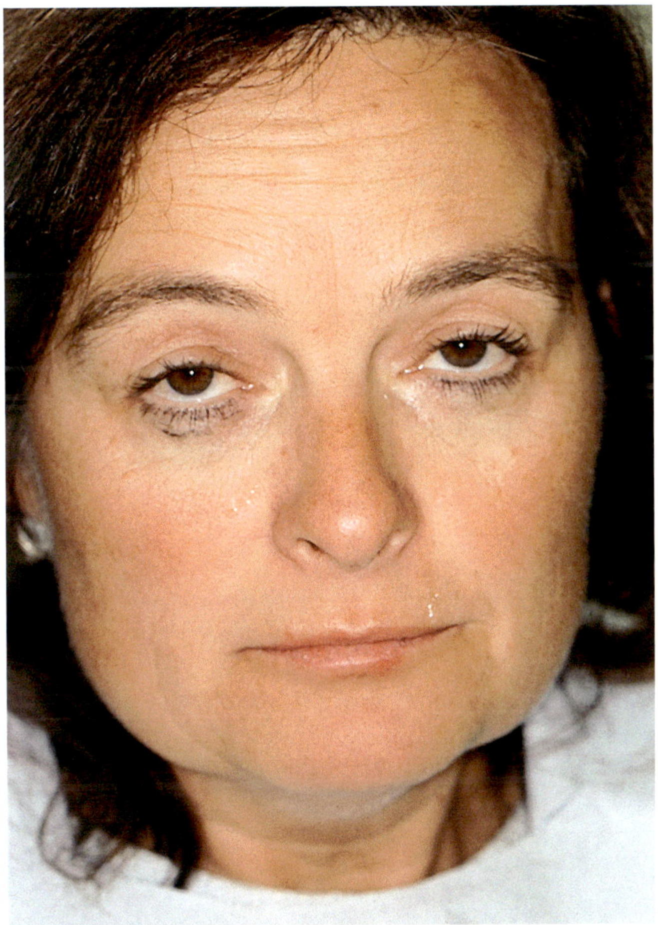

Fig 1-12a Patient with severe pain throughout the area covered by her extensive maxillary fixed partial denture.

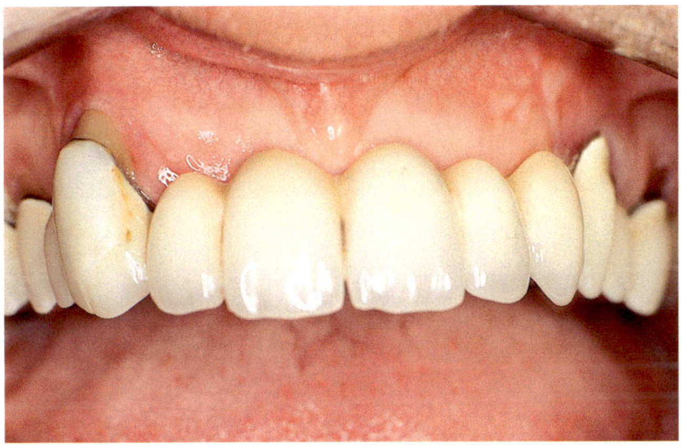

Fig 1-12b View of the fixed partial denture over the problem area.

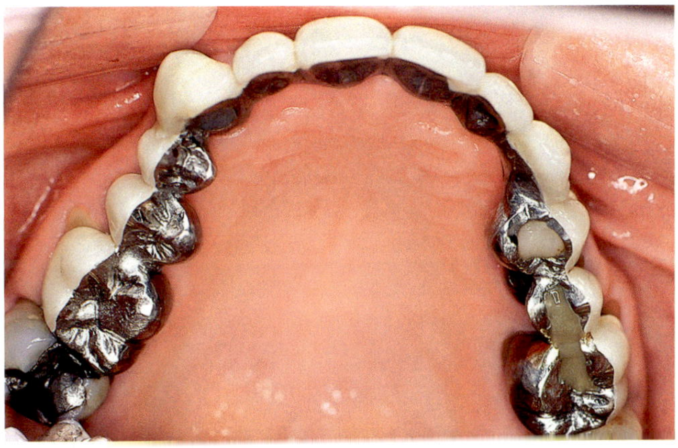

Fig 1-12c Palatal view of the 20-year-old fixed partial denture.

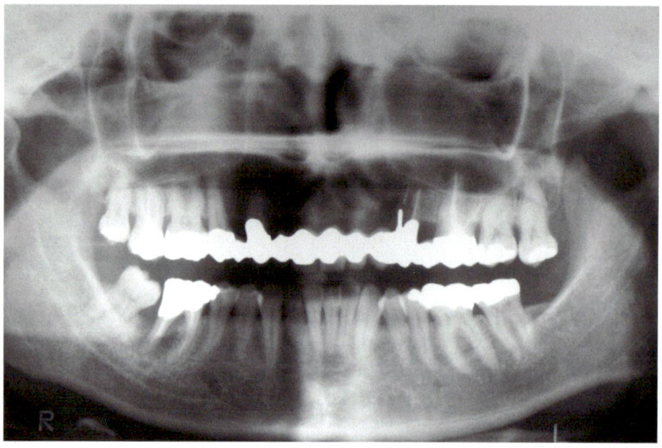

Fig 1-12d Panoramic radiograph showing the initial situation.

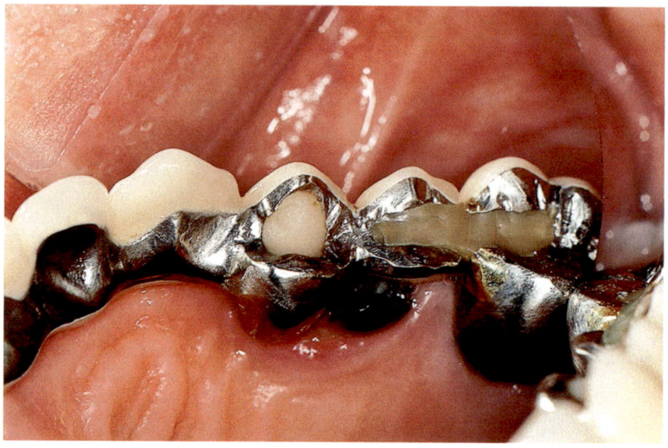

Fig 1-12e The root of the maxillary left first premolar has become visible; it is palatally displaced and carious.

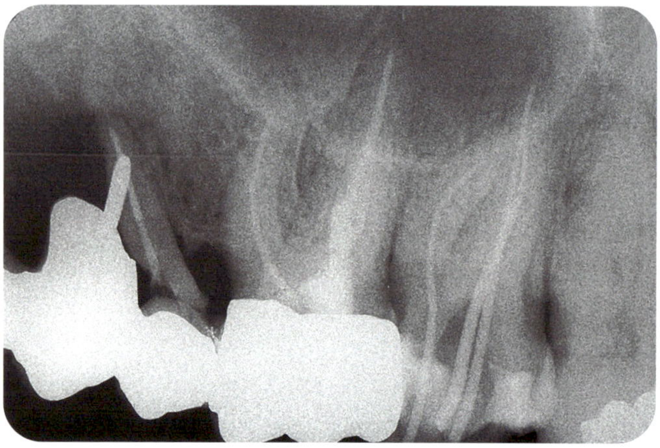

Fig 1-12f Orthoradial radiograph of the maxillary left first premolar.

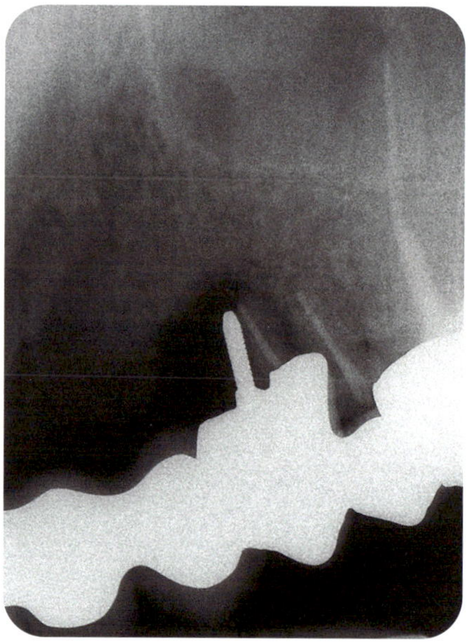

Fig 1-12g Mesial-eccentric radiograph of the maxillary left first premolar.

The patient could not take any time off work, so a quick solution was necessary.

Proven solution: Supporting the fixed partial denture with provisional implants

To support the loosened fixed partial denture, two transitional implants were placed between the positions of the maxillary left central incisor and maxillary left lateral incisor and between the positions of the left lateral incisor and left canine. Two vertical grooves were countersunk into the body of the fixed partial denture as retainers (Fig 1-12h). To prevent metal cuttings from entering the extraction wound, this step must be performed before surgical intervention.

The area around the remnant of the root of the maxillary left first premolar was dissected, and the resulting flap was reflected to expose the residual roots (Fig 1-12i). A luxator was used to cut through the circular fibers with a vertical cutting movement. The root was luxated with a vertical turning movement (Figs 1-12j and 1-12k) and removed with an extraction forceps. The root post was then separated with an extralong diamond bur (Fig 1-12l). The wound was closed with a suture to complete the surgical procedure.

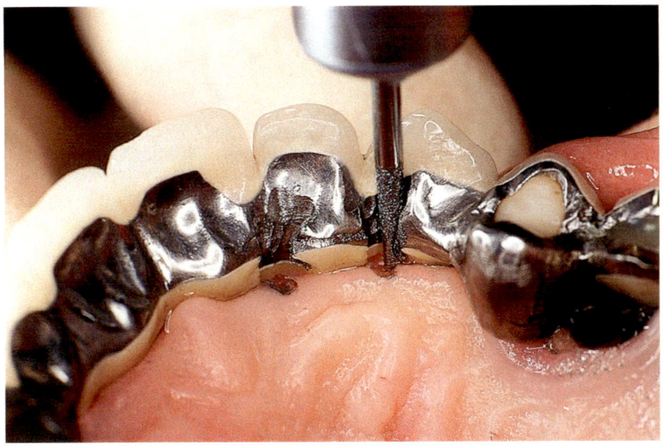

Fig 1-12h Retainer grooves are ground vertically into the fixed partial denture at the palatal side.

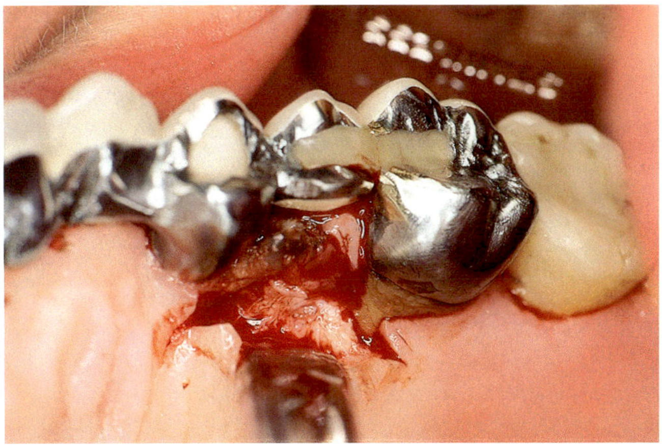

Fig 1-12i Reflected palatal flap.

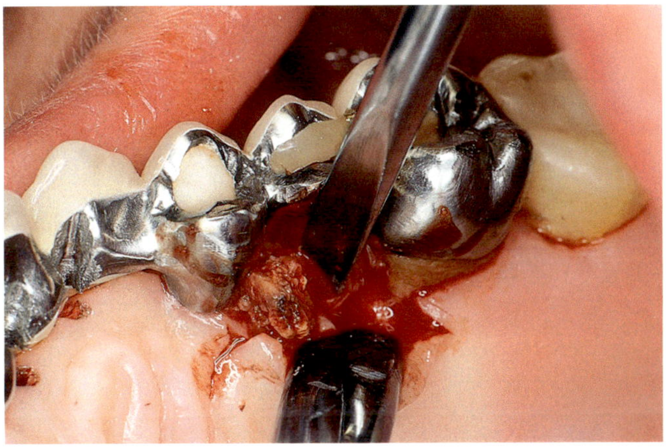

Fig -12j The residual root is luxated.

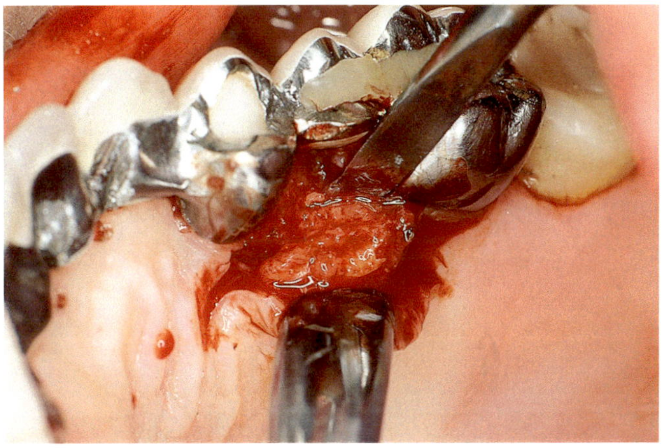

Fig 1-12k The residual root is extracted.

Luxators combine the functions of periotomes and Bein elevators (Fig 1-12m). A sophisticated set of luxators is available for the various tooth shapes and regions of the jaws (Fig 1-12n). They should never be used in a horizontal direction; misuse may result in fractures.

Provisional implants from the MTI System were used to support the fixed partial denture and increase the number of abutments (see Figs 1-9h and 1-9i). The gingiva along the grooves that would serve as retainers for the fixed partial denture was drilled through to a depth of approximately 10 mm (Figs 1-12o and 1-12p). The provisional implants were screwed in with a hand wrench to a depth of approximately 15 mm and the primary stability was checked (Fig 1-12q and 1-12r). The implants were shortened with a bur (Fig 1-12s) and bonded to the fixed partial denture with metal adhesive. The implant restorations were carefully ground to adjust the static and dynamic occlusion, and the fixed partial denture was checked for tilting (Fig 1-12t). Finally, the position of the provisional implants was evaluated on a panoramic radiograph (Fig 1-12u). The patient was then sent home (Fig 1-12v). The second panoramic radiograph was later used to design the final implant-supported fixed partial denture (Fig 1-12w).

Materials

Luxators (Directa Dental)
MTI System (Dentatus)
DTK metal adhesive (Bredent); Nimetic (3M ESPE) can also be used

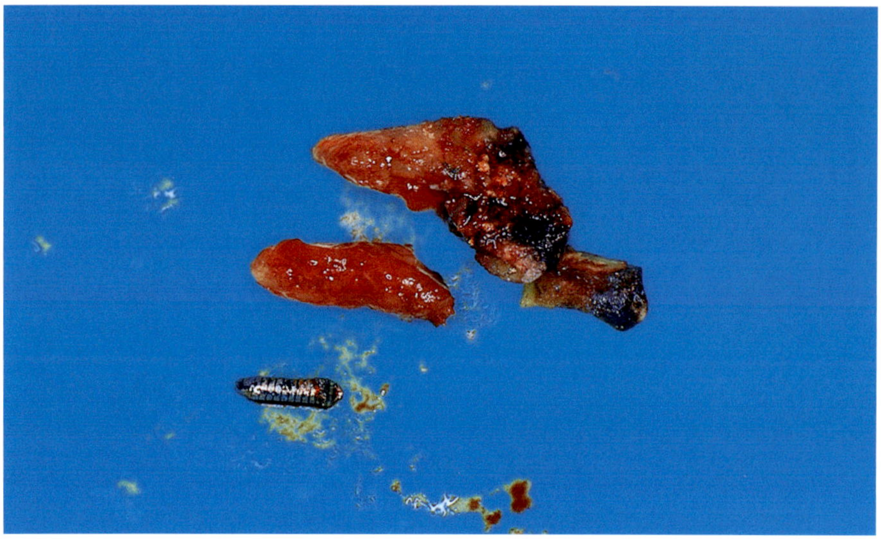

Fig 1-12l Extracted root remnants and severed post of the maxillary left first premolar.

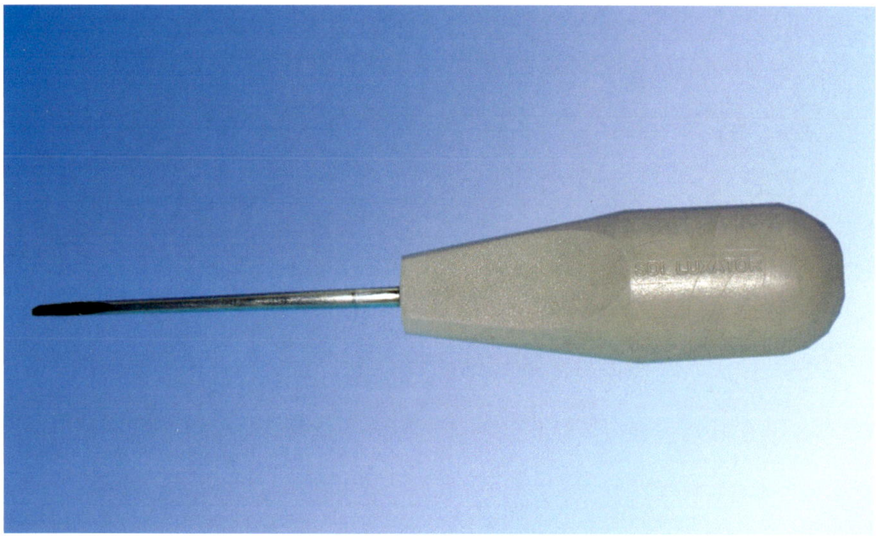

Fig 1-12m Luxator.

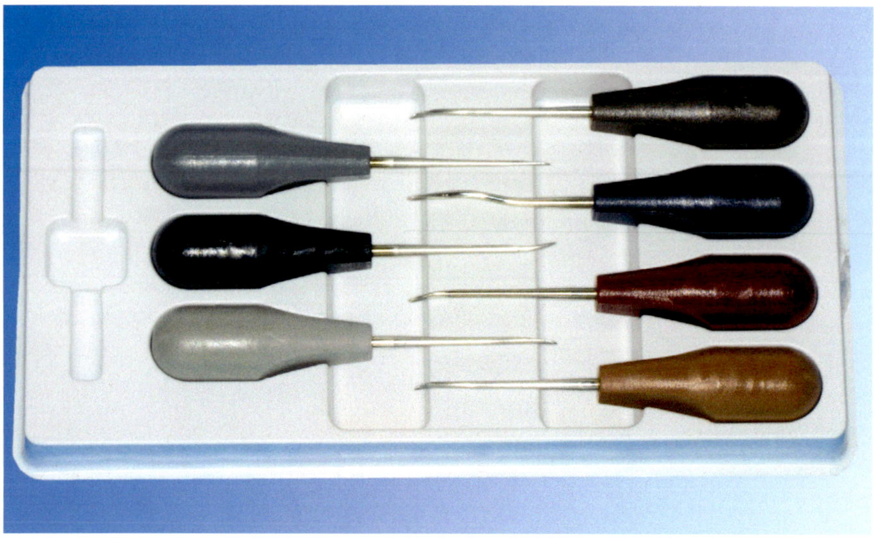

Fig 1-12n A sophisticated set of luxators is available for various tooth shapes and regions of the jaw.

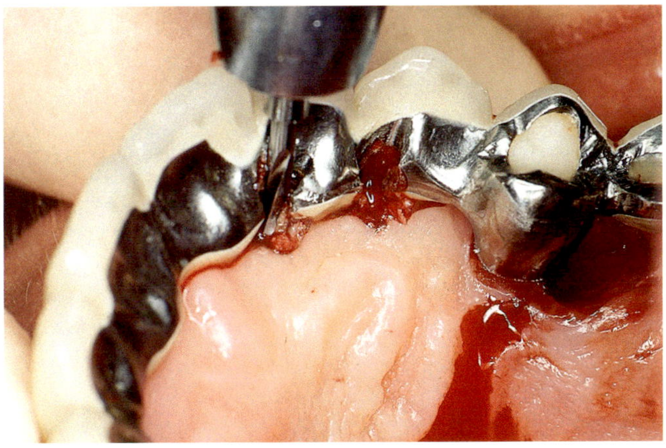

Fig 1-12o The implant is tapped between the maxillary left central and lateral incisors.

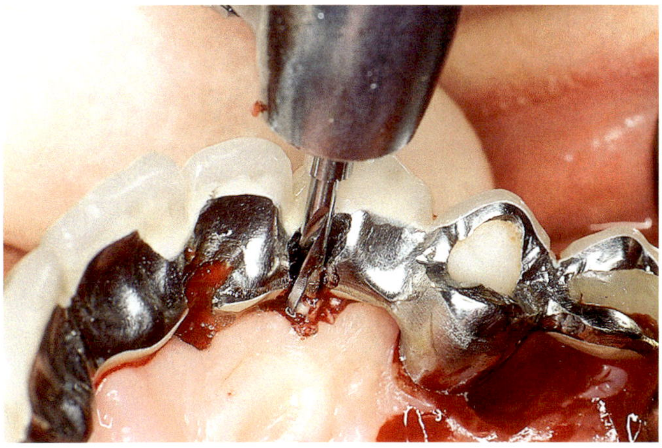

Fig 1-12p The implant is tapped between the maxillary left lateral incisor and canine.

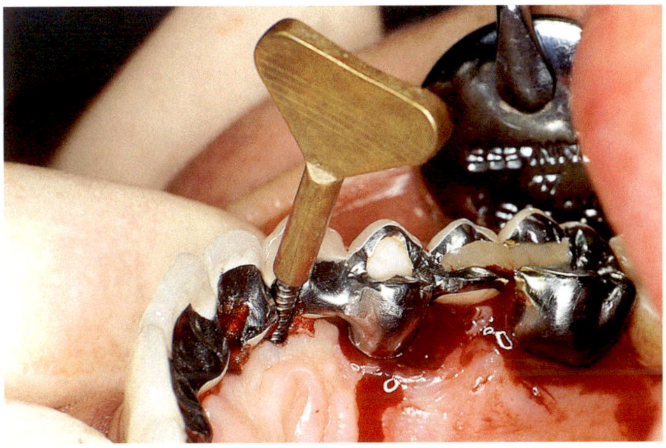

Fig 1-12q The provisional implants are inserted.

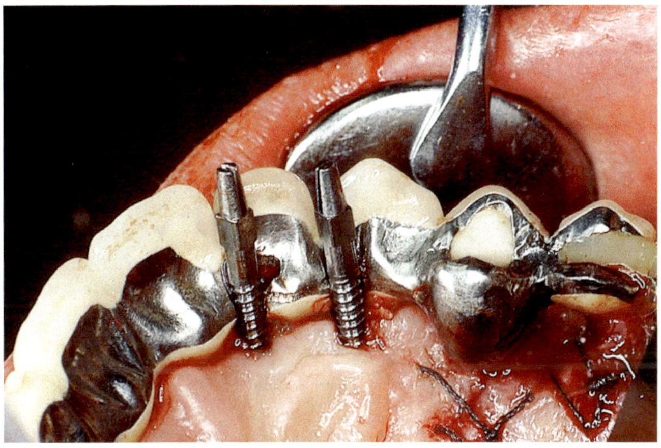

Fig 1-12r Provisional implants in place.

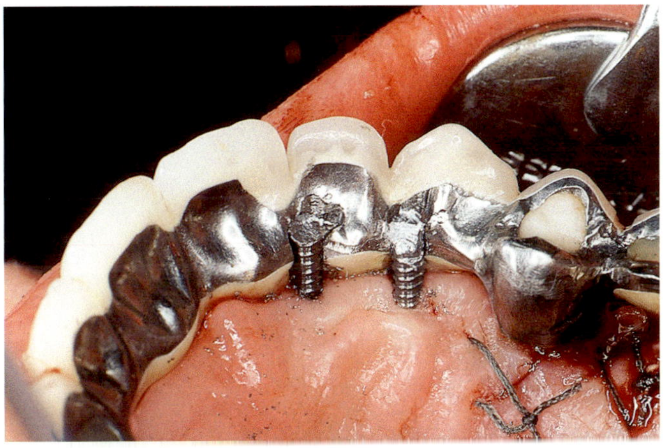

Fig 1-12s The provisional implants are shortened.

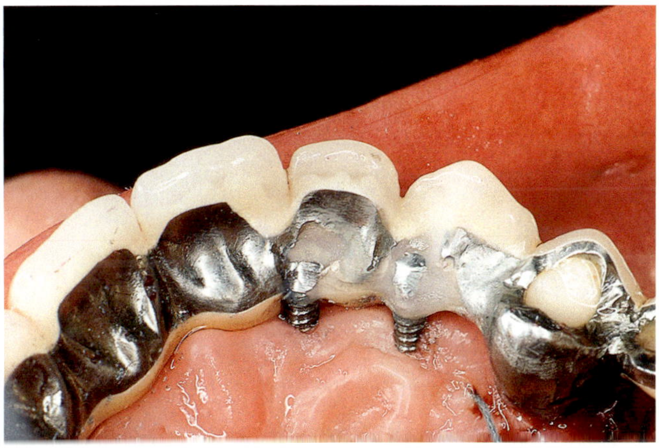

Fig 1-12t The provisional implants are bonded with metal adhesive.

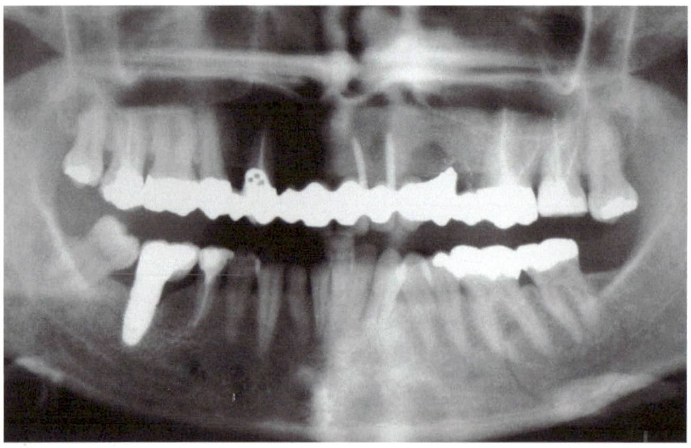

Fig 1-12u The panoramic radiograph is evaluated.

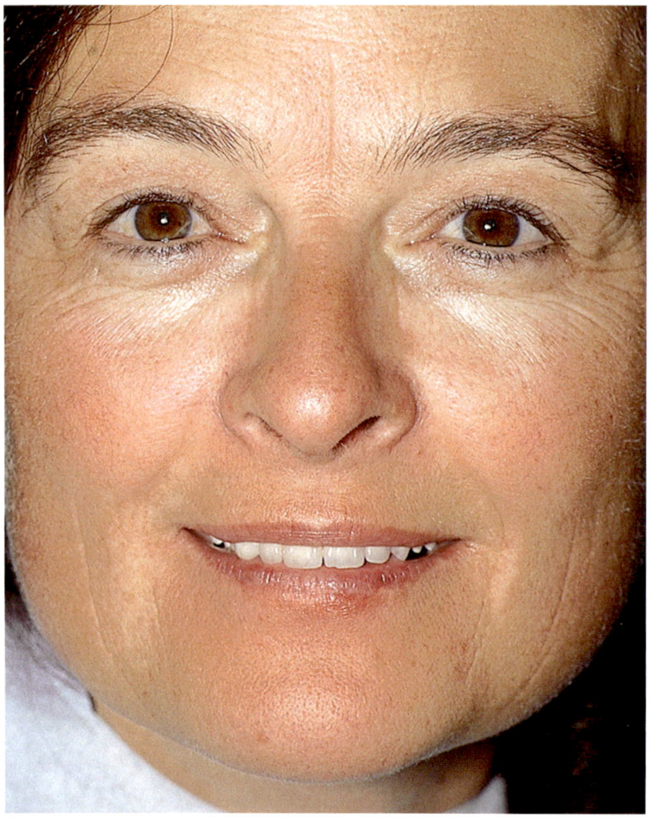

Fig 1-12v Satisfied patient.

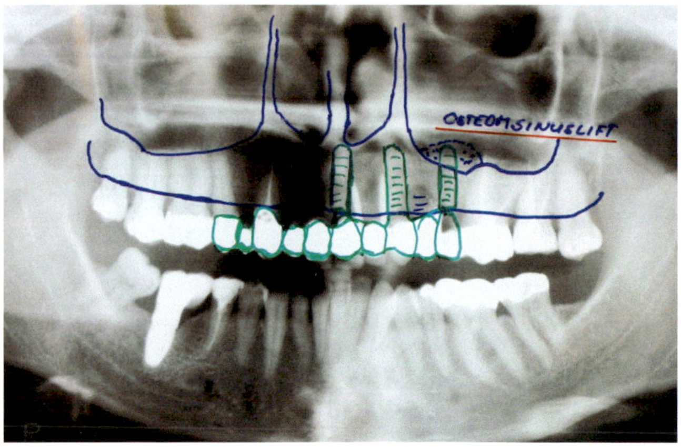

Fig 1-12w The panoramic radiograph is used to design the implant-supported fixed partial denture.

Retention of Telescopic Crowns

Common problem: Inadequate prosthesis retention and loss of friction from telescopic crowns

A man complained about the inadequate retention of his partial denture, which was supported on the residual dentition by telescopic crowns. The patient reported to have seen his dentist about it several times, but the dentist's only advice was to avoid sticky food—apart from that, the patient would "get used to" the partial denture after a while.

What options are available in everyday practice to help patients achieve better retention of their telescopic dentures? Different methods and their possible disadvantages are described below. With the exception of replacing the entire prosthesis, all of these prosthetic first-aid measures can all be performed at chairside.

Proven solutions

Replacement of the prosthesis

If the telescopic denture is new and its retention inadequate, the problem is likely to have been caused by a mistake by the laboratory or the dentist. The entire prosthesis should be replaced, preferably by the same dentist and laboratory.

Simple corrective measures

If the denture was made in your own office and serious errors can be ruled out, the following situation has usually occurred. After the primary copings are cemented, the patient cannot remove the telescopic denture no matter how hard he or she tries. Even the dentist can only remove the denture with the help of a Treymann crown remover or even with light hammer blows. At this point, dentists frequently yield to the temptation of grinding out the secondary copings freehand until the patient can easily remove the telescopic denture. After 2 days or fewer, the same patient will return to the dental office complaining that the denture keeps falling out.

No matter how much the new telescopic denture may be jamming, if the patient wears it for a day without removing it, the abutment teeth will usually adjust to their new position. Ask the patient to return to the dental office the next day to remove and clean the prosthesis. After that, the friction of the telescopic copings nearly always works properly.

If, after a week, one or two telescopic crowns can still only be removed with difficulty, the chloropercha method is recommended. Gutta-percha sticks are dissolved in chloroform to create a milky liquid (Fig 1-13a). This liquid is brushed into the dry secondary coping and dried carefully with a chip blower. The denture is then placed on the primary copings in the patient's mouth while the path of insertion is carefully followed. The denture is, removed

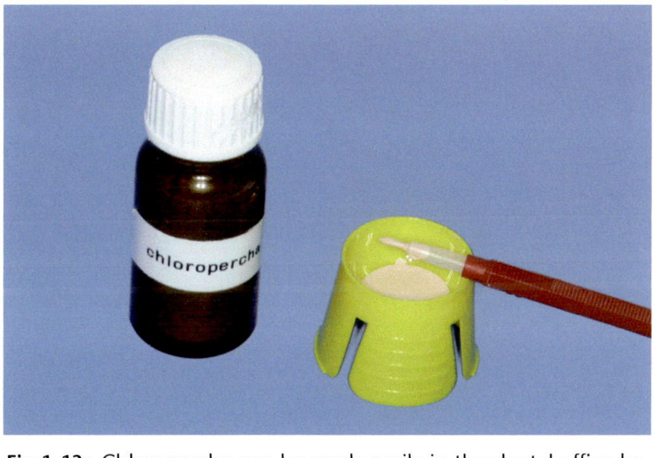

Fig 1 13a Chloropercha can be made easily in the dental office by dissolving gutta-percha sticks in chloroform to create a milky liquid.

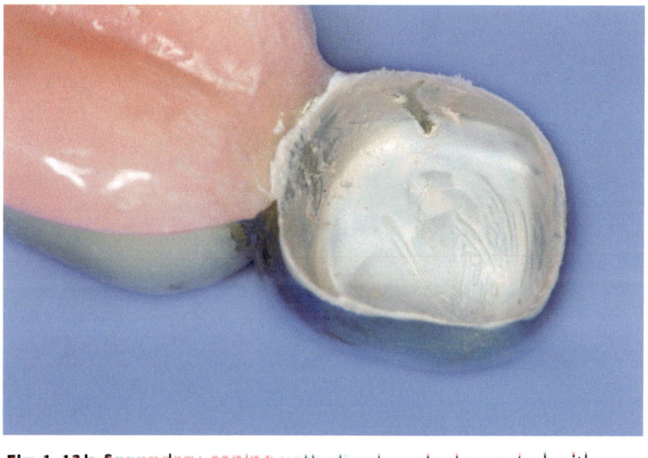

Fig 1-13b Secondary coping with direct contacts, coated with chloropercha.

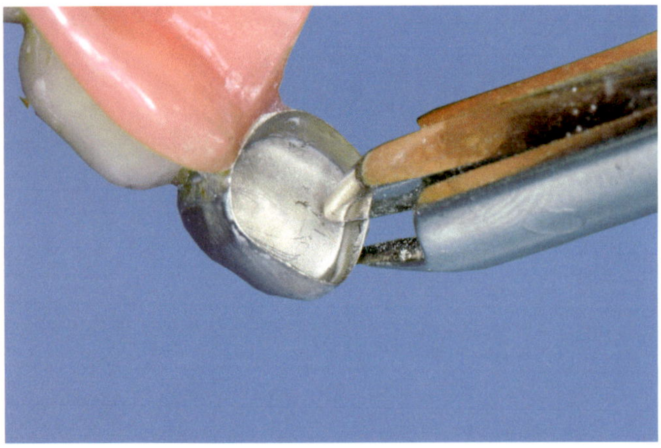

Fig 1-14 The secondary coping is bent with Aderer pliers.

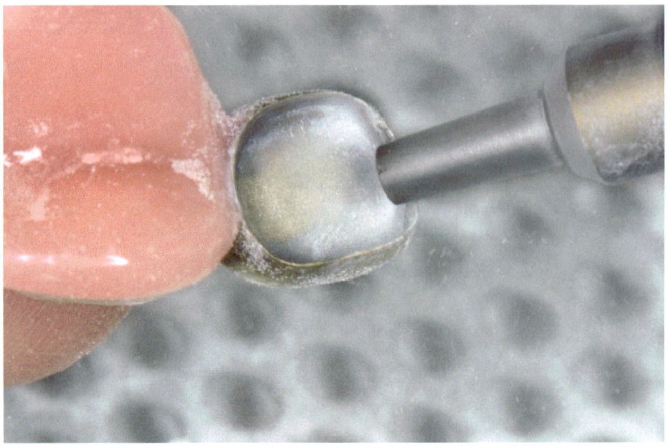

Fig 1-15 The secondary copings are sandblasted.

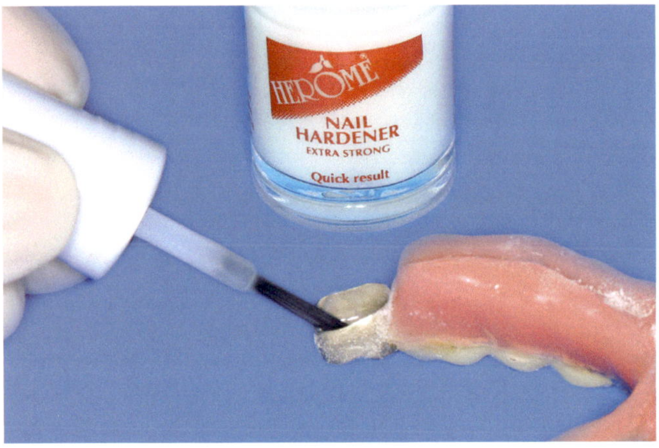

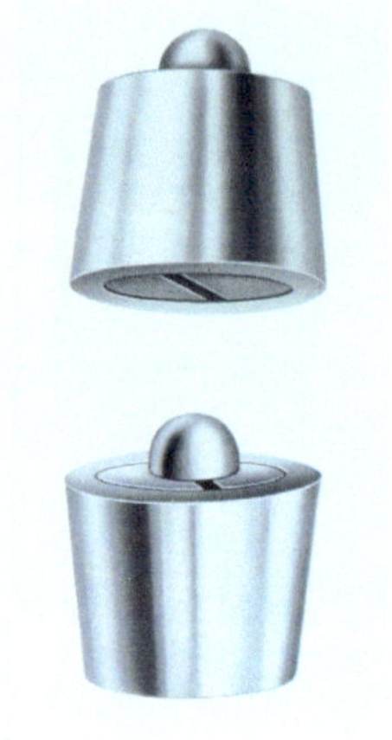

Fig 1-16 *(left)* The secondary copings are brushed with nail polish.

Fig 1-17 *(right)* Spring anchor for integration.

and its insides are examined with the magnifying loupe. Any primary contacts that exist are selectively ground out and polished (Fig 1-13b). After careful cleaning, the telescopic crown should work properly.

Controversial corrective measures

For telescopic dentures that will be in use for some time to come, dentists have resorted to rather adventurous strategies. A few such methods are listed below.

Some practitioners bend the margins of the secondary copings with Aderer pliers to create friction (Fig 1-14). However, the telescopic denture usually cannot be reseated. If the copings are subsequently ground out, denture retention is better for a couple of days, but the patient usually will complain about an unpleasant feeling of tension, and soon after, retention will be lost again.

Some dentists sandblast the secondary telescopic copings to achieve more frictional retention (Fig 1-15). However, this trick also only works for a short time.

Other dentists sandblast the secondary copings, brush them with transparent nail polish, and press them back onto the isolated primary copings. However, because the nail polish flakes off, this method is not very long lasting (Fig 1-16).

Complicated corrective measures

The following methods have been proven successful but are difficult to use:

1. Two points opposite each other are created on the primary copings with a dental laboratory laser. This is very cumbersome, and it takes a long time to achieve a good fit. Very often it does not lead to any improvement at all.
2. A very thin layer of gold is applied by electroplating. This procedure is also difficult to perform, and most of the time, the plated gold layer comes off very soon.

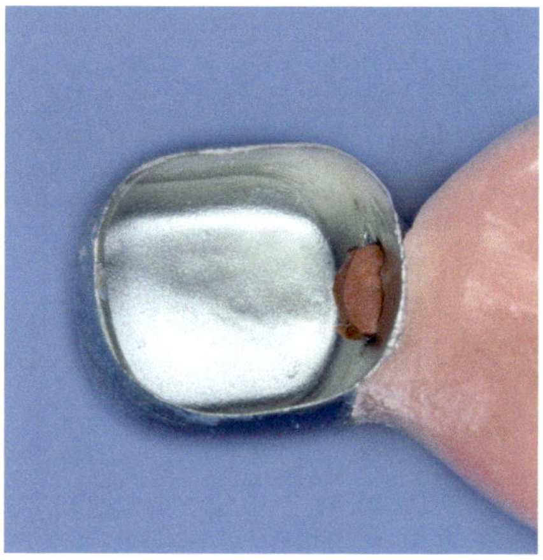
Fig 1-18 Built-in retainer disk.

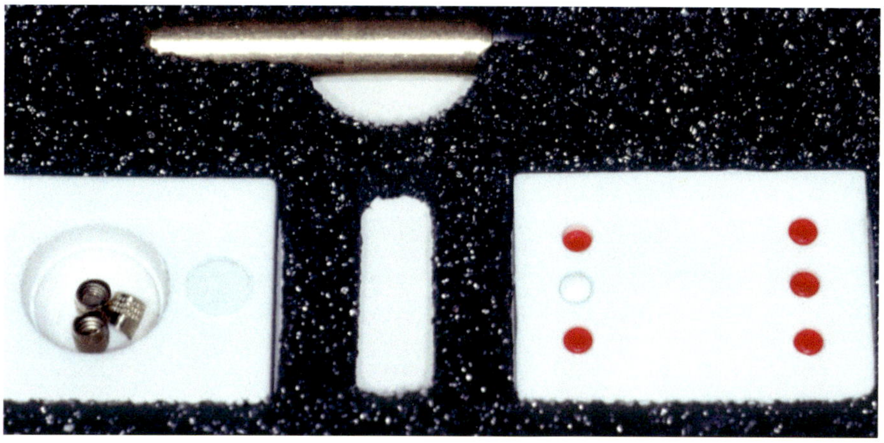
Fig 1-19 Components of the Frisoft System.

Integration of additional retainers

The success of this method depends on the type of retainer used:

1. The integration of an internal spring (as developed at the University of Tübingen, Germany) is an outdated procedure.
2. Resilient snap-fasteners such as the Ipsoclip (Cendres & Metaux) or the similar TK-Snap system (Si-tec) are successful but very difficult to integrate (Fig 1-17).
3. The integration of retainer disks has also been reported to be a very painstaking procedure and is said to have only a short-term effect (Fig 1-18).

Incorporation of attachment screws

Another procedure that usually provides long-term success is to incorporate Frisoft attachment screws (Microtec Dental) into the denture (Fig 1-19). The author has used this method several times with good results. The procedure is demonstrated step by step in the following case report.

Case report

An implant-supported denture was to be inserted in the mandible of a 65-year-old woman. In the meantime she was to continue to wear her existing maxillary telescopic denture (Fig 1-20a). However, its fit was unsatisfactory, and it kept dislodging. Thus it was decided to insert attachment screws into the denture to regain denture retention (Fig 1-20b).

An area of sufficient strength was found in the secondary coping; in this case it was proximal (Fig 1-20c). Then the coping was drilled to the appropriate depth (Figs 1-20d and 1-20e), and the depth was checked with the probe (Fig 1-20f). The fit of the jacket was subsequently checked, and the jacket was bonded into the hole with the special adhesive contained in the Frisoft kit (Figs 1-20g to 1-20l). After 15 minutes of curing, the red plastic friction screw was screwed into the threaded jacket. While the screw has an inner square, it is very hard to use a straight screwdriver to screw it into the threaded jacket, which is already bonded into the hole. Therefore, the author used a probe that was ground to size as a square "head," so that the screw could be placed easily (Fig 1-20m). The plastic friction screw was then inserted as far as required for good retention of the maxillary telescopic denture.

Permanent improvement of friction with the Friction Fit System

The Friction Fit System is a two-component resin (Fig 1-21) that can help to achieve a permanent improvement of friction using telescopes, precision attachments, and bars (Figs 1-22 to 1-24). The manufacturer recommends completely relining the denture directly in the patient's mouth; however, this is a very risky venture and should be carefully considered. The greatest risk is of polymerizing the secondary copings onto the residual teeth when the cured adhesive flows into the undercuts in the anchors of the primary copings. This is an experience to be avoided, because it would mean that the entire denture would have to be disassembled in the patient's mouth. Furthermore, if the secondary copings are completely

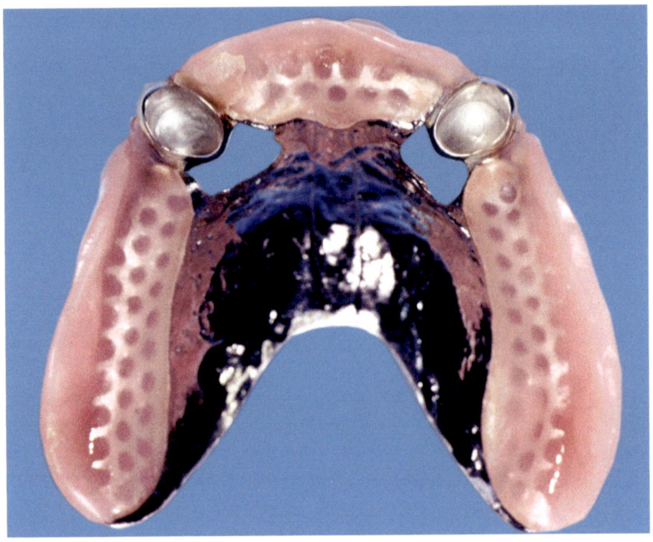

Fig 1-20a Model cast denture with telescopic crowns.

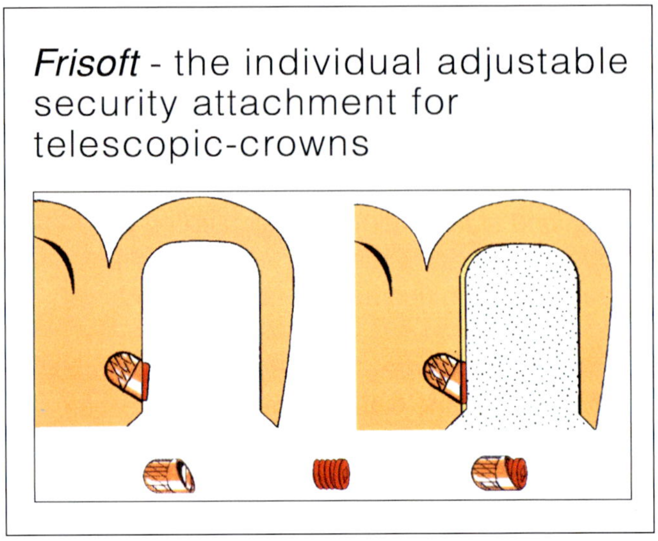

Fig 1-20b Use of the Frisoft System.

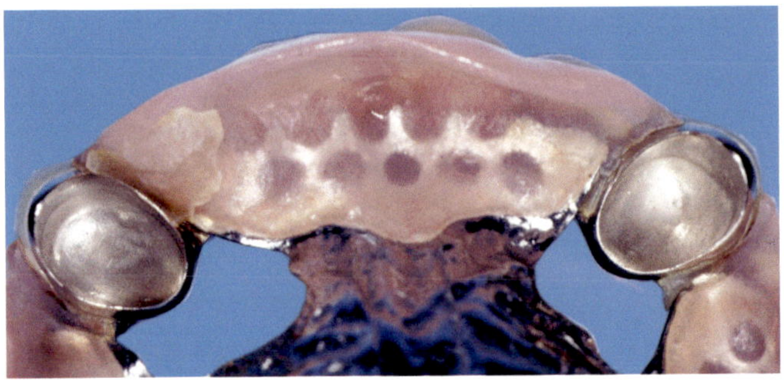

Fig 1-20c The proximal area of the secondary copings has sufficient strength for the insertion of attachment screws.

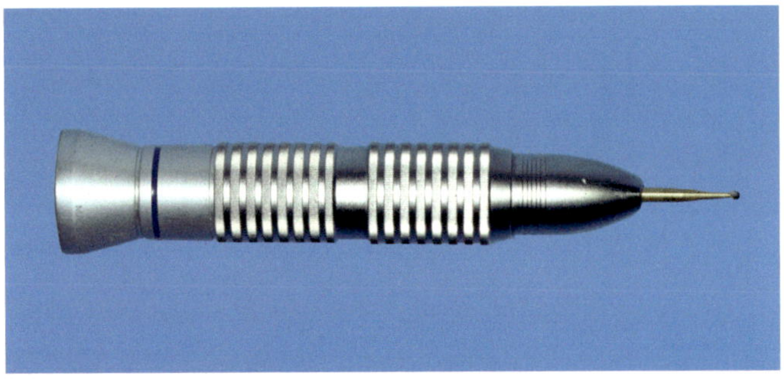

Fig 1-20d Handpiece with bud bur.

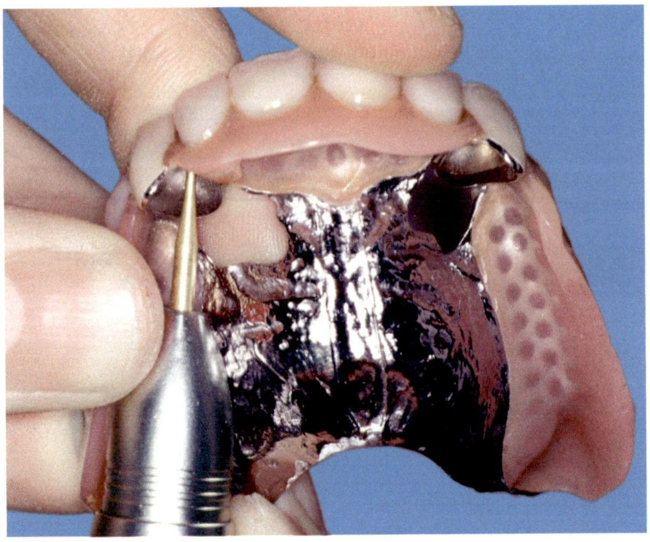

Fig 1-20e A hole is drilled for the threaded jacket.

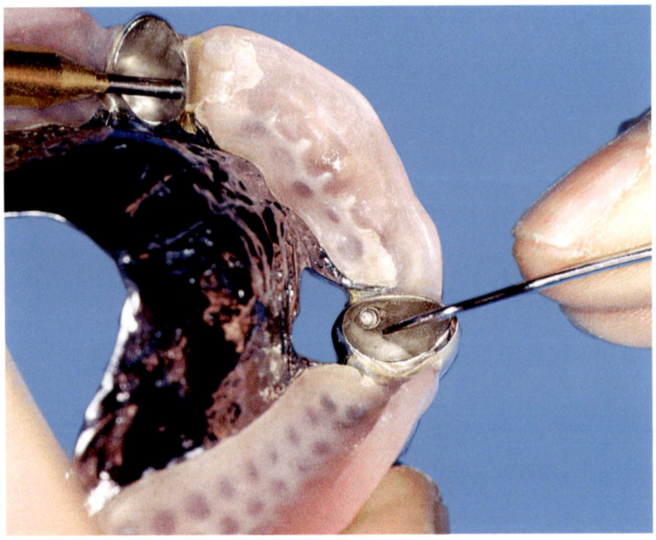

Fig 1-20f The cavity is checked.

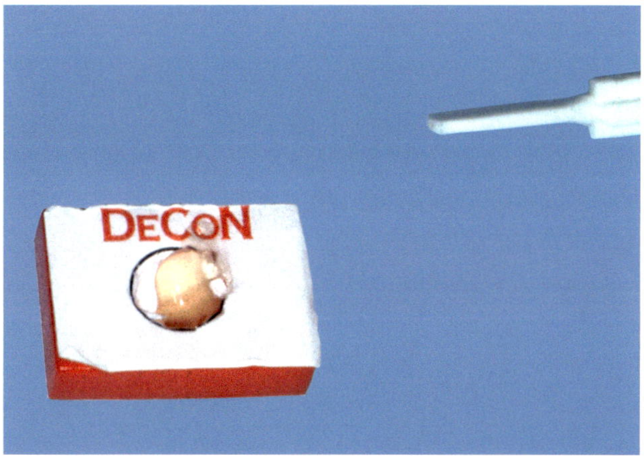

Fig 1-20g *(left)* The adhesive contained in the Frisoft kit is mixed.

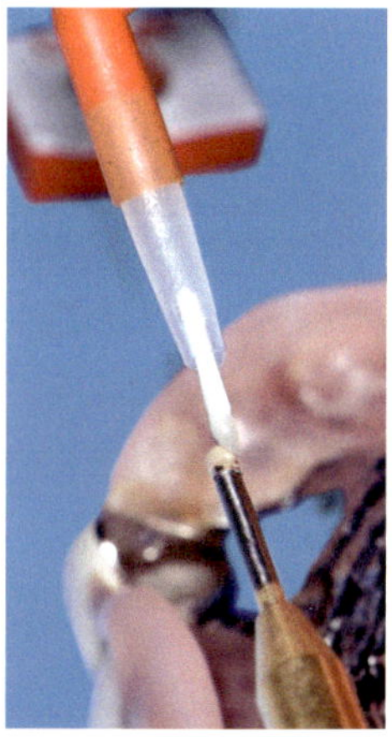

Fig 1-20h *(right)* The adhesive is applied to the threaded jacket.

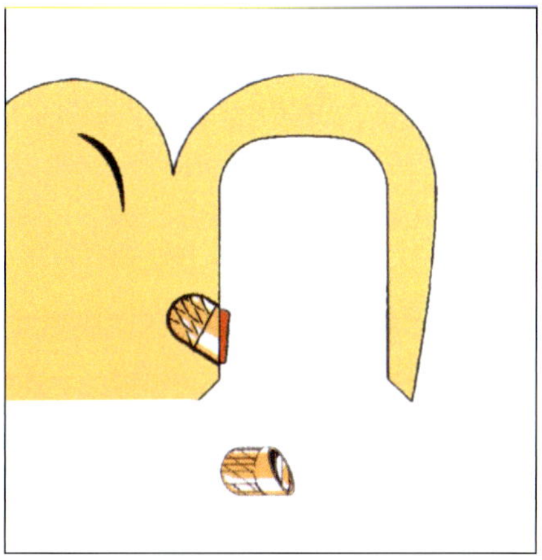

Fig 1-20i Bonding procedure.

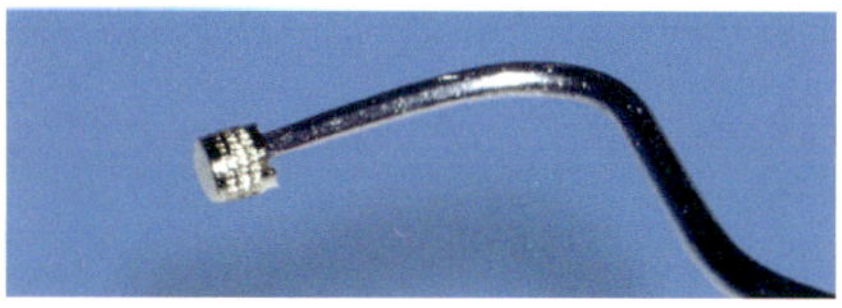

Fig 1-20j Jacket on the probe, ready to be inserted.

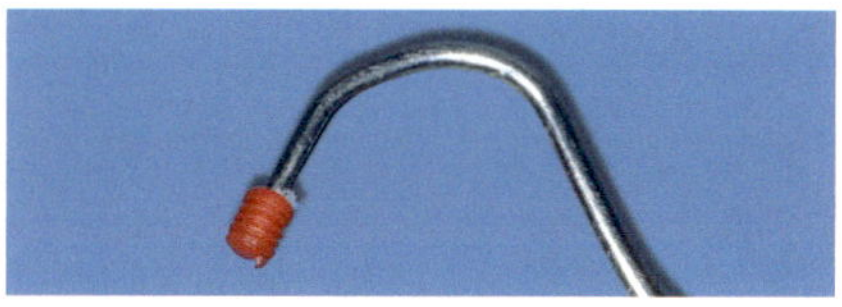

Fig 1-20k Screw before insertion.

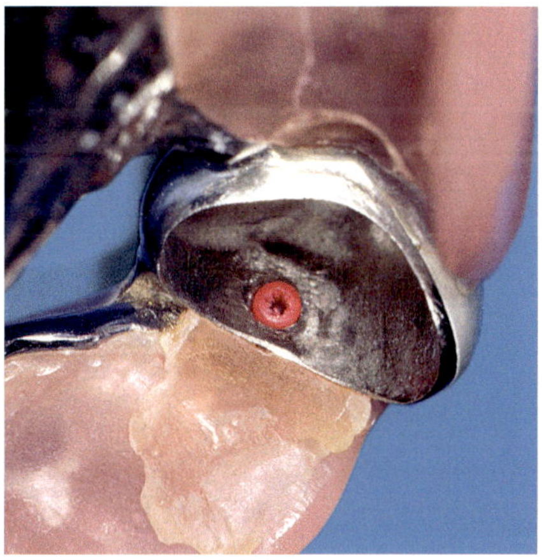

Fig 1-20l *(left)* Screw after insertion.

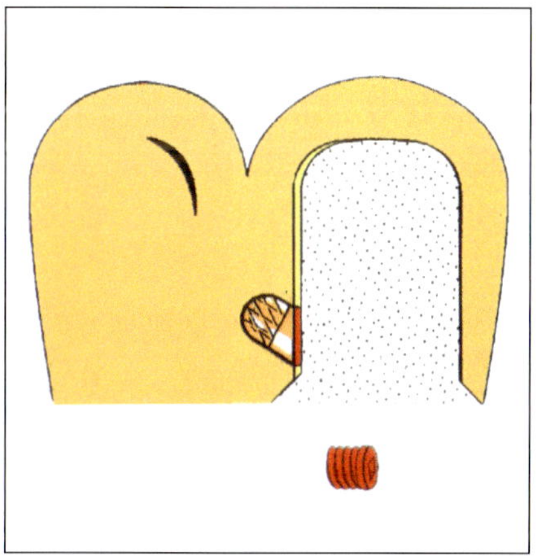

Fig 1-20m *(right)* Screw after insertion.

relined, it will inevitably raise the entire construction. Thus the saddles would also have to be relined, which raises the bite.

To eliminate the danger of polymerizing the denture onto the abutments and to avoid raising the bite, the author recommends countersinking vertical retention grooves into the secondary copings and filling these with the friction resin (Figs 1-25a and 1-25b). This procedure is demonstrated in the following case report.

Case report

A woman wore a denture that was manufactured using model casting technology and had electroformed tele-

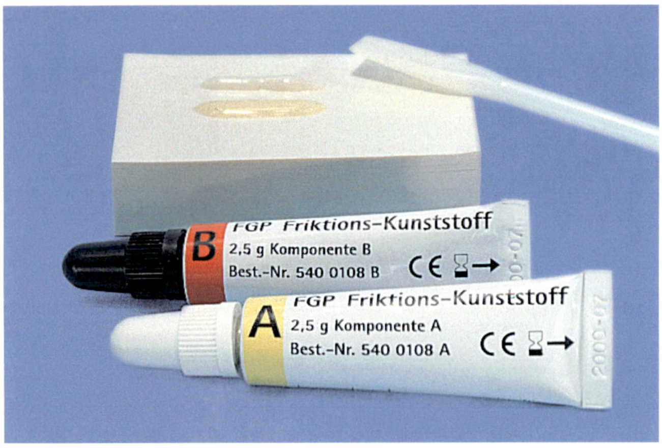

Fig 1-21 Components of the Friction Fit System kit.

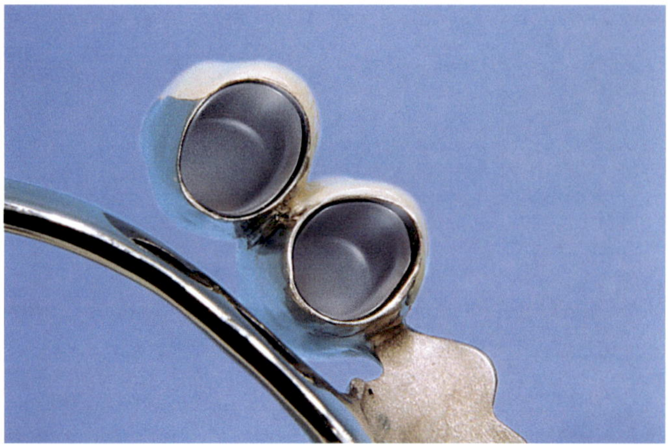

Fig 1-22 The secondary copings are completely relined.

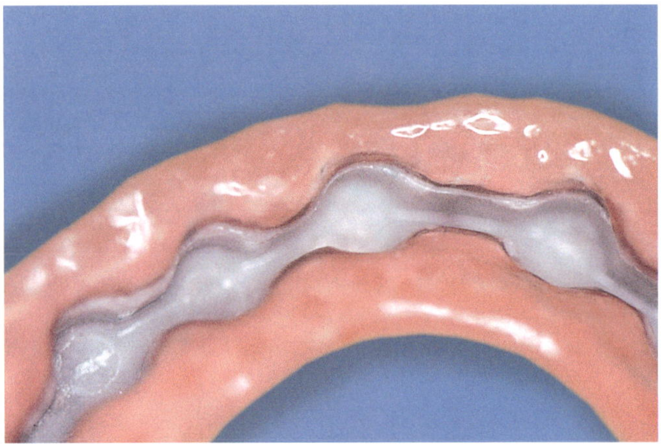

Fig 1-23 The precision attachments are relined.

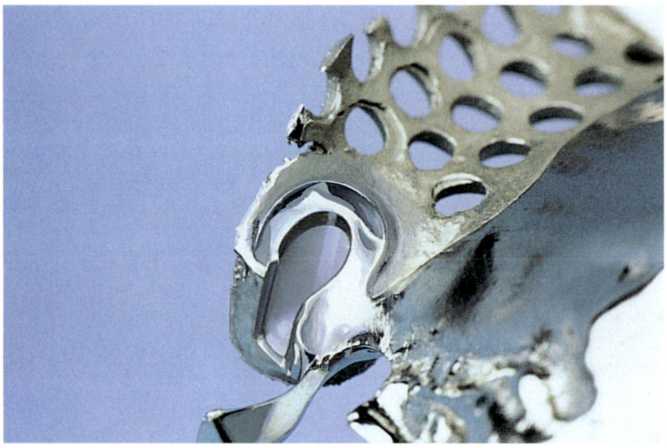

Fig 1-24 A bar attachment is relined.

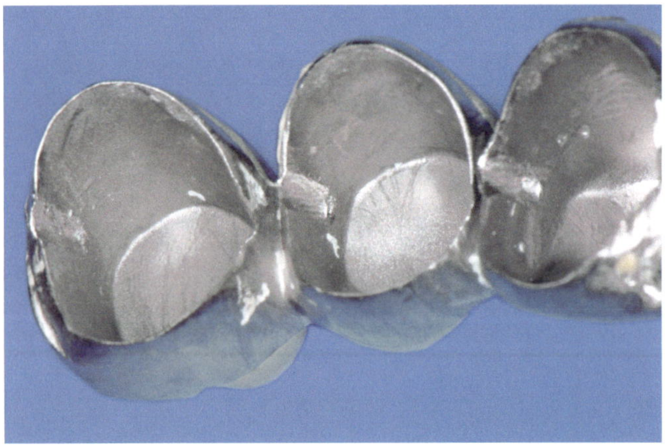

Fig 1-25a Vertical retention grooves are cut into the secondary copings.

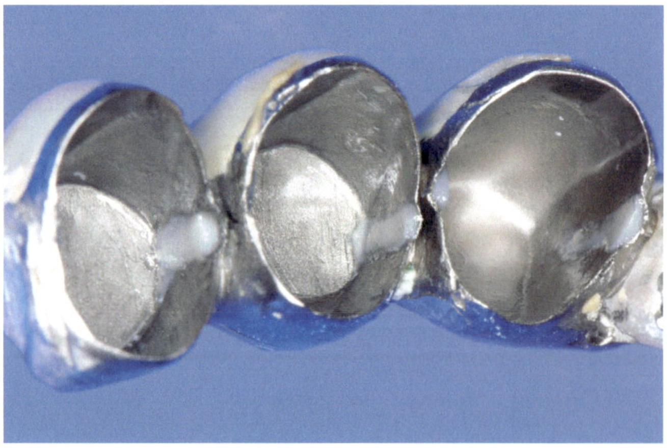

Fig 1-25b The retention grooves are filled with the resin contained in the Friction Fit System.

scopic copings supported by four mandibular implants (Figs 1-26a and 1-26b). After some time, the retention of the telescopic copings had worn off. Traces of abrasion on the inside of the secondary copings were visible with the magnifying loupe (Fig 1-26c). An attempt to completely reline the prosthesis failed, because blocking out the undercuts at the primary copings kept the denture from being exactly repositioned.

Thus the author opted for successive relining with vertical retention grooves without blockout (Fig 1-26d). This

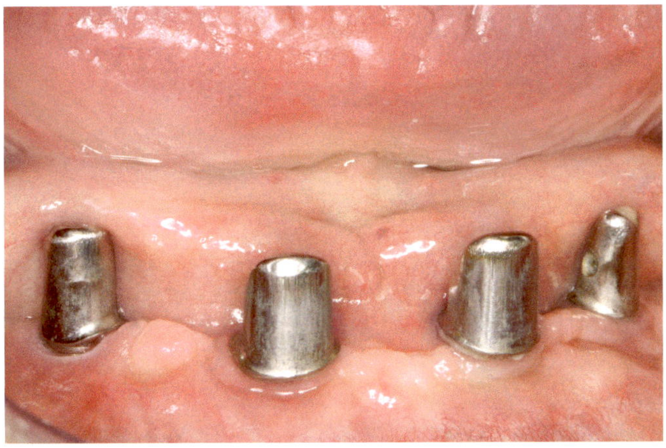

Fig 1-26a Primary copings on implants.

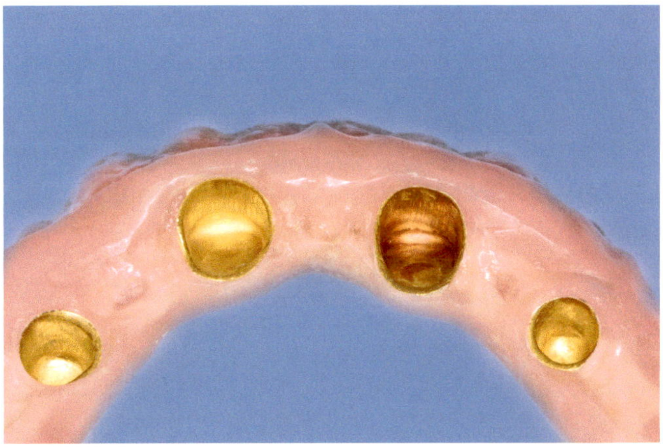

Fig 1-26b The secondary copings are insufficient to retain the denture in the patient's mouth.

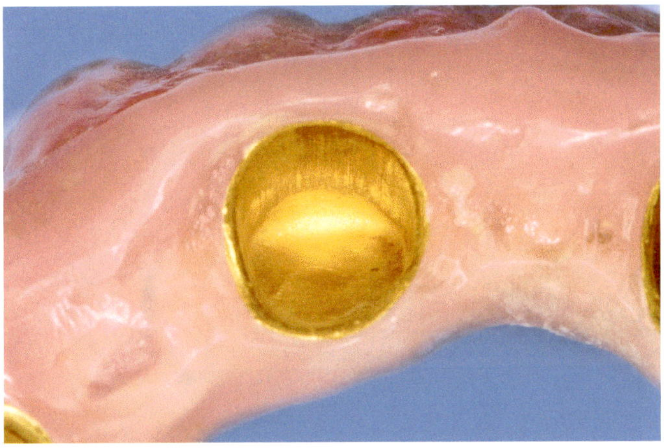

Fig 1-26c Traces of abrasion are visible on the inside of the secondary copings.

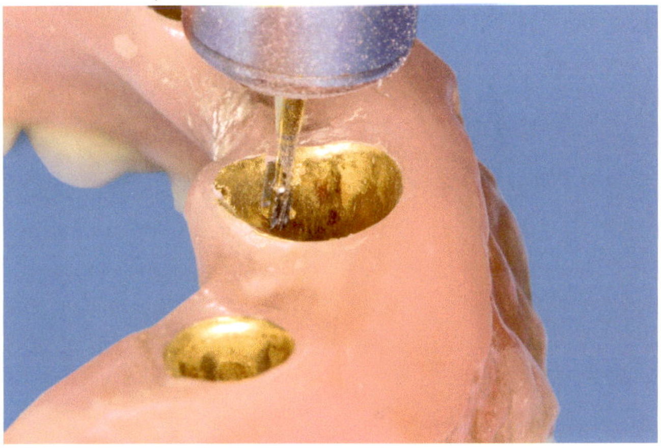

Fig 1-26d Vertical retention grooves are ground into the secondary copings.

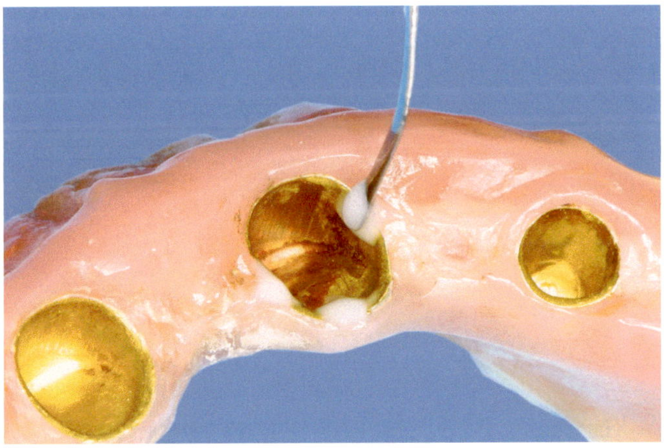

Fig 1-26e The retention grooves are filled with the resin.

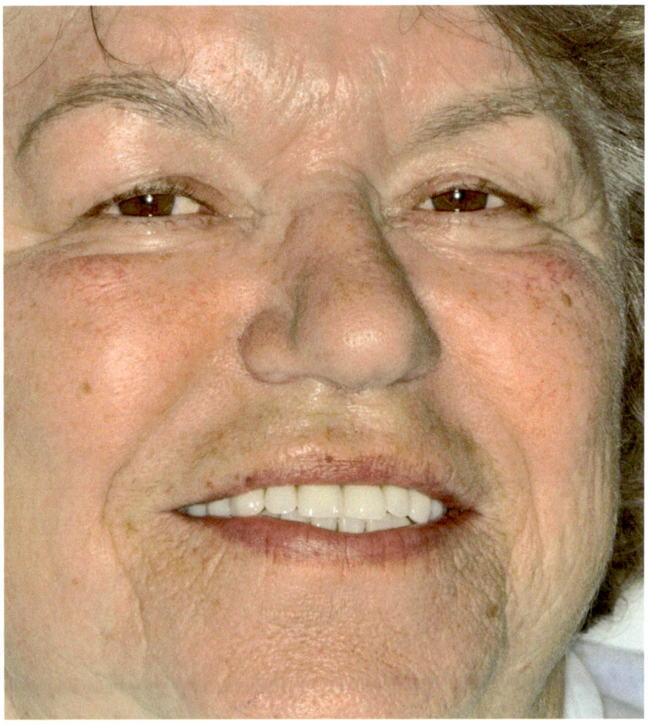

Fig 1-26f The denture has been successfully relined, and the patient is satisfied with the improved retention.

can be done without risk, provided that the procedure is carried out coping by coping, and the denture is lifted briefly after 90 seconds and again after 180 seconds. Sparing use of the adhesive is absolutely imperative (Fig 1-26e). The author also strongly recommends isolating the anchors with Vaseline oil before adaptation.

Successive relining of the denture was easily accomplished, and the patient was very happy with the new retention of her denture (Fig 1-26f).

Materials

Frisoft System (Microtec Dental)
Friction Fit System (Bredent)
Chloropercha can be easily made in the dental office by dissolving gutta-percha sticks in chloroform. Keep the solution in a tightly sealed bottle.
Vaseline oil

2

Restorative Dentistry

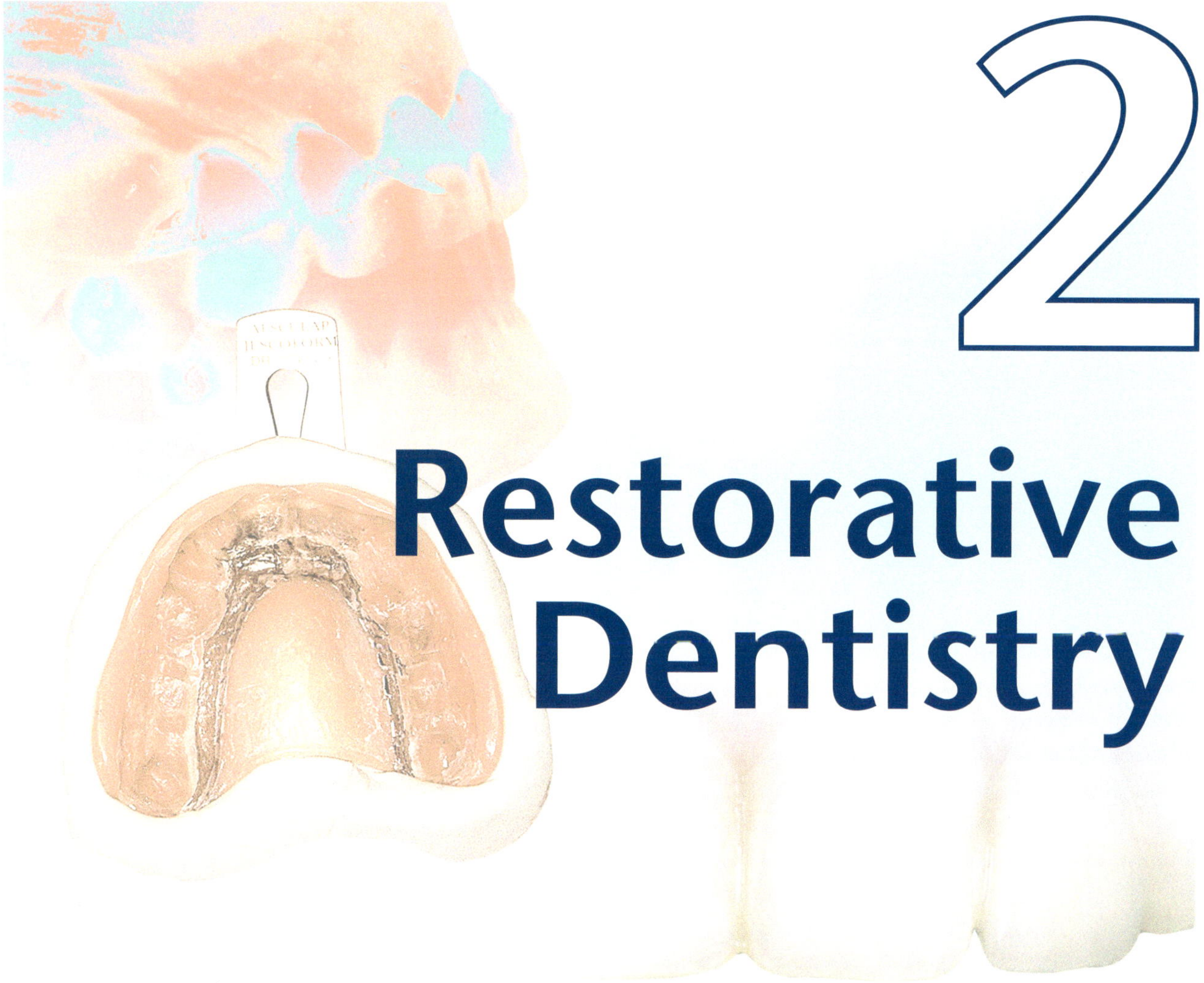

2

Efficient Placement of Rubber Dam for Endodontic Treatment

Efficient Placement of Rubber Dam for Adhesive Bonding Procedures

Class V Restorations

Efficient Adhesive Bonding of Ceramic Inlays

Diastema Closure with a Matrix System and Resin Composite

Efficient Placement of Rubber Dam for Endodontic Treatment

Common problem: Rubber dam is unwieldy and difficult to place

Use of rubber dam is a must in dentistry for endodontic treatment and during direct and indirect bonding.

No one likes to put rubber dam in place, but every dentist loves it once it is in position. Working in a completely moisture-controlled field is much easier for the dentist.

Why is the use of rubber dam not more widespread? At dental school, placement of rubber dam was usually taught and practiced very awkwardly. This has kept many dentists from using rubber dam to the present day.

If a procedure of this kind seems unwieldy, then it is worth thinking about how to make it more efficient. In industrial production, processes are divided into two stages: process planning and the process itself, or preparatory work and the actual execution of the task. One principle of efficient work is to shift as many aspects as possible of the manufacturing process to the process-planning stage, to make the process itself as short as possible. This can be compared with a slight-of-hand magic trick that a magician prepares intensively so that the actual performance is very fast and cannot be seen or reproduced by the spectators. That is another example of 90% preparatory work and 10% execution!

Proven solution: Efficient use of rubber dam in endodontics

To make placement of rubber dam a more efficient procedure, this discussion will also divide this "production" into process planning and the application process itself.

Process planning

The preparatory work, which can be done by the dental assistant before the patient arrives, comprises the following steps:

1. The medium gauge rubber dam should be precut (Fig 2-1).

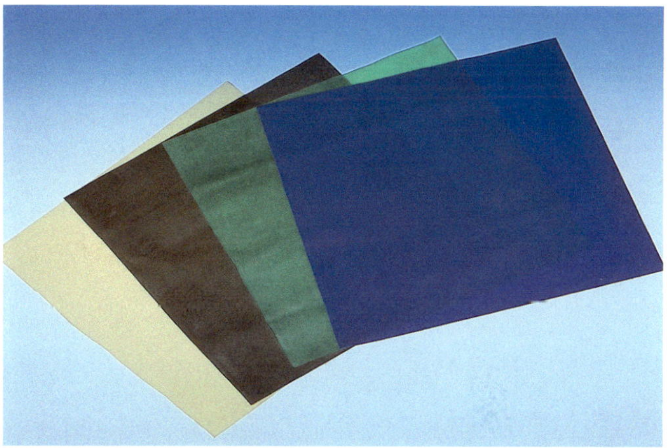

Fig 2-1 Precut rubber dam.

2. Rubber dam should be stamped. The stamp is applied to the matte side. Red stamping ink is more durable than blue (Fig 2-2a).
3. A rubber dam punch is used to punch a hole in rubber dam at the point where the tooth that is to be isolated will be situated (Figs 2-2b and 2-2c).
4. A rubber dam clamp (with wings) is selected and tried on the cast (Fig 2-3a).
5. The rubber dam clamp is adapted to rubber dam carefully to prevent ripping of the dam (Fig 2-3b).
6. Prepared rubber dam is stretched over rubber dam frame (Fig 2-3c).
7. The clamp forceps are placed in the holes in the clamp and locked (Fig 2-3d).

The preparatory work is completed (time required: approximately 3 minutes).

Application process

Rubber dam can be placed in the following manner:

1. The prepared rubber dam set is grasped by the clamp forceps.
2. The clamp is placed on the relevant tooth (Fig 2-4a).
3. The rubber is pushed off the wings of the clamp (Fig 2-4b). Rubber dam may not fit snugly around the tooth because of the pointy edges of the clamp. This

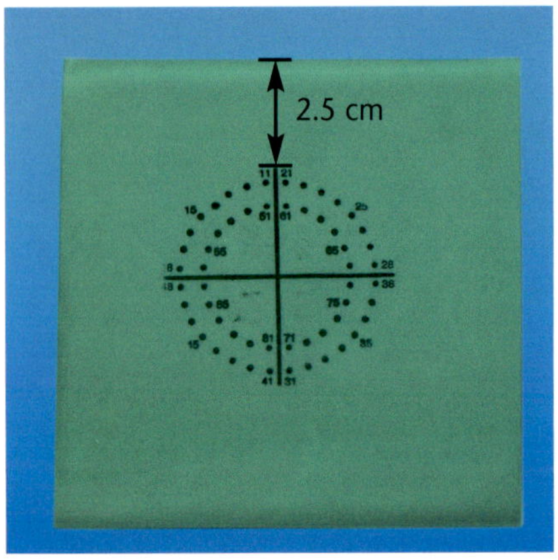

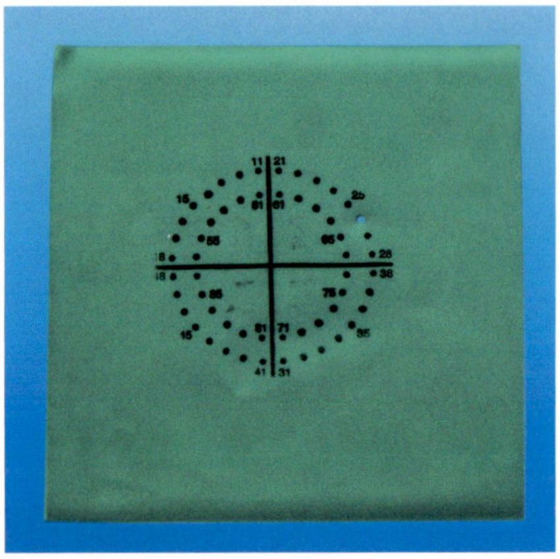

Fig 2-2a *(left)* Stamped rubber dam.

Fig 2-2b *(right)* Punched rubber dam.

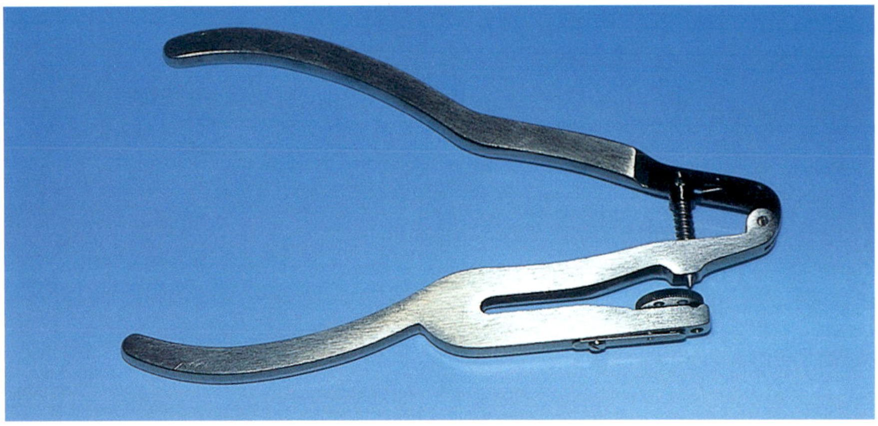

Fig 2-2c Rubber dam punch.

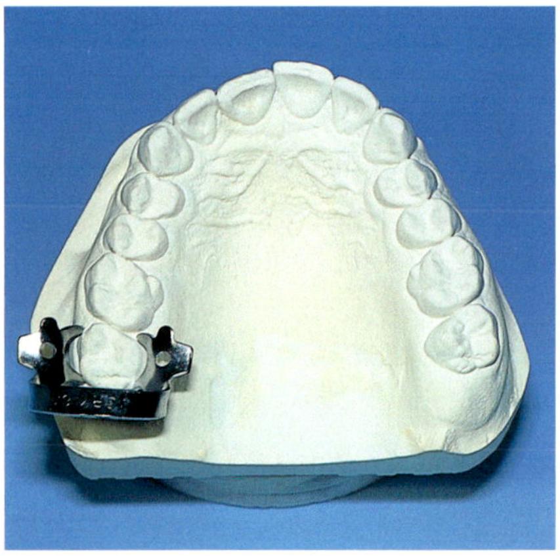

Fig 2-3a The clamps are tried on a cast. Only the tips of the clamps should rest on the tooth.

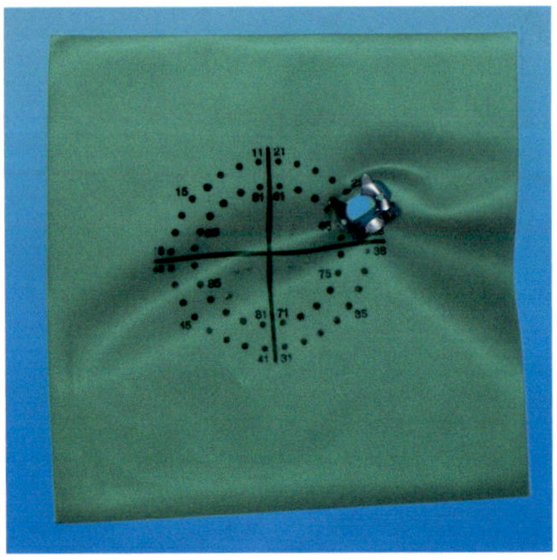

Fig 2-3b The winged clamp is positioned in rubber dam.

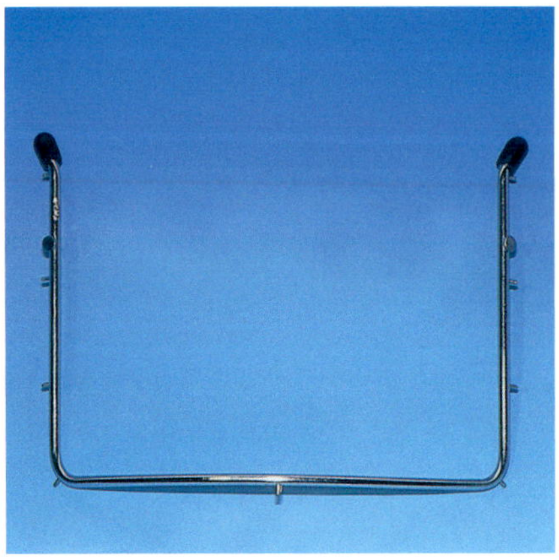

Fig 2-3c Metal rubber dam frame.

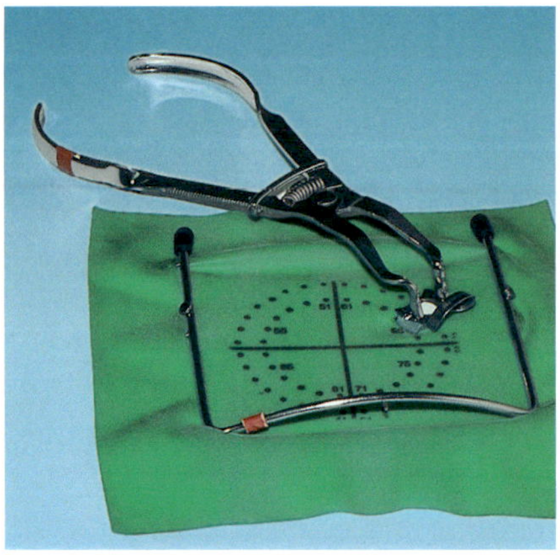

Fig 2-3d The preparatory work is finished. The rubber dam is mounted with the clamp forceps locked in the clamp.

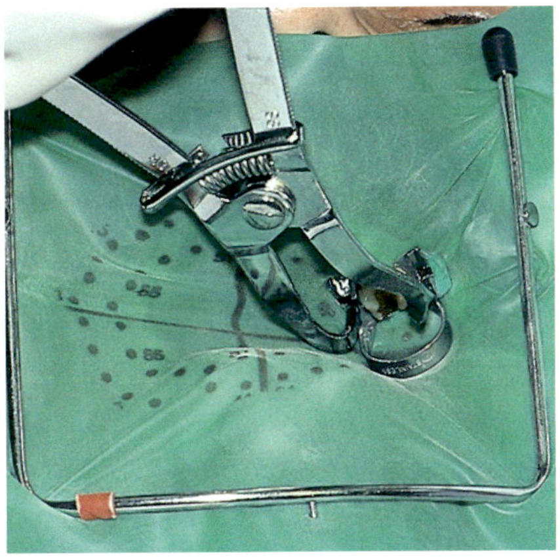

Fig 2-4a The mounted rubber dam set is placed on the tooth that is to be treated endodontically.

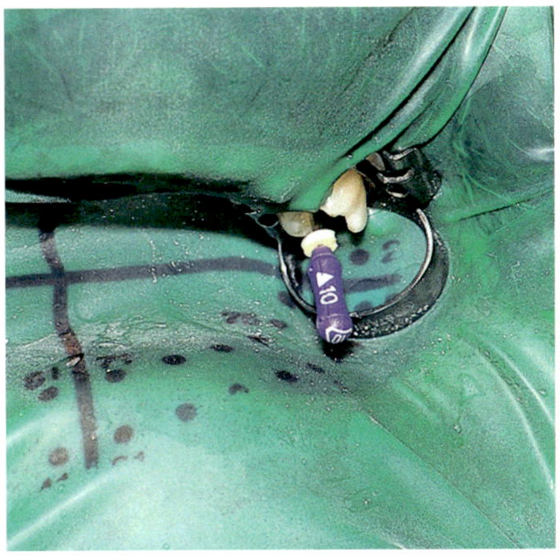

Fig 2-4b Rubber dam is pushed off the wings with a Heidemann spatula.

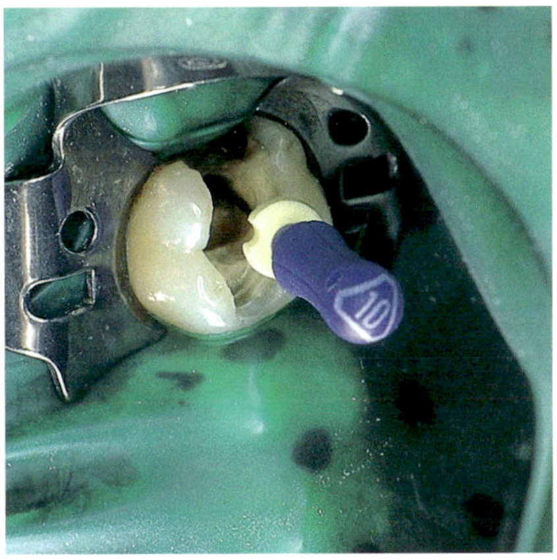

Fig 2-4c The root canal treatment can begin.

can be resolved by lifting the clamp slightly.

4. Rubber dam is adjusted by stretching it over the frame again.

The area is isolated and ready for endodontic treatment (Fig 2-4c; time required: approximately 20 seconds).

Materials

Hygenic rubber dam sheets, precut (Coltène Whaledent)
Rubber dam stamp (Hygenic, Coltène Whaledent)
Ivory rubber dam punch (Heraeus Kulzer)
Ash rubber dam clamps (Dentsply Ash)
Ivory clamp forceps (Heraeus Kulzer)
Frame Type Junior (Coltène Whaledent)

Efficient Placement of Rubber Dam for Adhesive Bonding Procedures

Common problem: Rubber dam is unwieldy and difficult to place

Absolute moisture control is a must for endodontic treatment, repairing ceramic veneers in the patient's mouth, cohesive gold foil restorations, direct bonding with resin composite, and adhesive bonding of tooth-colored composite and all-ceramic restorations.

Once rubber dam is placed, everyone on the dental team appreciates it, because working in an absolutely dry field is substantially easier. It is also more comfortable for the patient, who does not have to endure the dentist's constant struggle with cotton rolls, retractors, and aspirators to counteract the effects of saliva, blood, and swallowing.

Proven solution: Efficient use of rubber dam in the restoration of larger areas

This procedure is also divided into the process-planning stage and the application process itself, as in industrial production. The preparatory work is subdivided into long-term and short-term measures.

Long-term preparatory work

The medium-gauge dental dam should be bought as precut squares of 15 cm. Cutting rubber dam from a roll is too much bother (Figs 2-5a and 2-5b). The color chosen should depend on the planned treatment. The following choices can be recommended:

1. Endodontic treatment: dark blue or dark green rubber dam to contrast with the open tooth (Fig 2-6)
2. Resin composite restoration using a direct bonding technique: pink rubber dam, almost gingiva colored (Fig 2-7)

In procedures such as the latter, do not use intense colors such as dark blue or green, because the human eye is strongly influenced by these colors. To the eye, the original color changes instantly in a specific way when another color is held beside it. The eye judges a color largely by its surroundings. The red squares shown in Fig 2-8 are all printed in exactly the same shade of red, but they seem different, depending on the surface they are viewed against. The tone of the red square always shifts toward the complementary color of the base. This color contrast effect becomes particularly evident when a translucent paper or glassine paper is laid over it. The human eye perceives a single hue differently when it is combined with different colors, much like the same musical note can sound different when a chord shifts.

Therefore, in direct bonding, pink rubber dam should be used because it resembles the color of the gingiva and enables the clinician to see the colors in the customary way. A gingiva-red rubber dam would be desirable (Fig 2-9). An ivory-colored dam is too weak a contrast with the tooth and thus with the direct restorative materials. Gray rubber dam makes the tooth look too bright and is a rather dull working color (Fig 2-10).

For tooth-colored restorations placed with an indirect bonding technique, dark blue or dark green rubber dam is recommended to provide contrast to the tooth and materials. The rubber is stamped in red on the matte side and punched (Fig 2-11).

The biggest challenge, however, is the placement of a floss ligature around the tooth. The dental floss is looped around the tooth and the first reef knot is tied. As is the case in gift wrapping, the dentist will need someone else (in this case, the dental assistant) to hold a finger on the first knot while the second knot is tied. When that person removes the finger, the knot is tied but not tightened. A maneuver such as this is extremely difficult for distal molars, especially if the patient has difficulties opening his or her mouth wide enough.

This inevitably leads to the following questions: Can the ligatures be preknotted? If they can, what kind of knot could be used for that purpose? Two recommendable knots will be demonstrated using a length of sailing rope (Fig 2-12):

1. Half-hitch as a self-tightening sliding knot. A half-hitch is tied (Fig 2-13a) and the long end is passed through the loop. Voilà: the ligature is already prepared (Fig 2-13b).

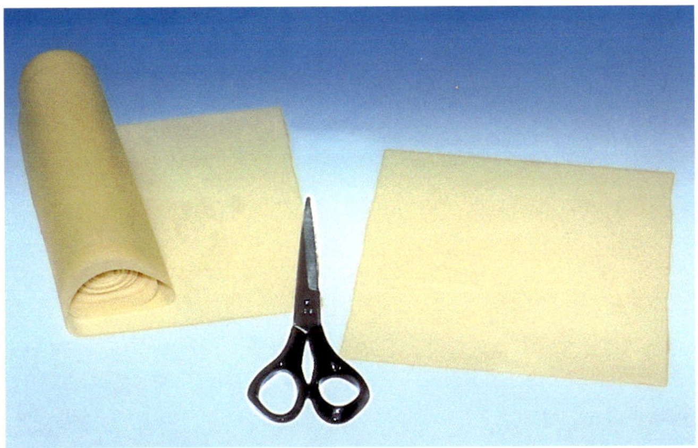

Fig 2-5a Rubber dam rolls are inefficient.

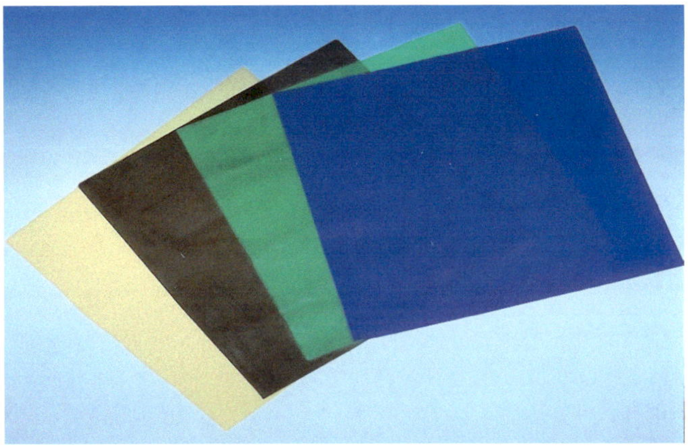

Fig 2-5b Precut square rubber dam sheets.

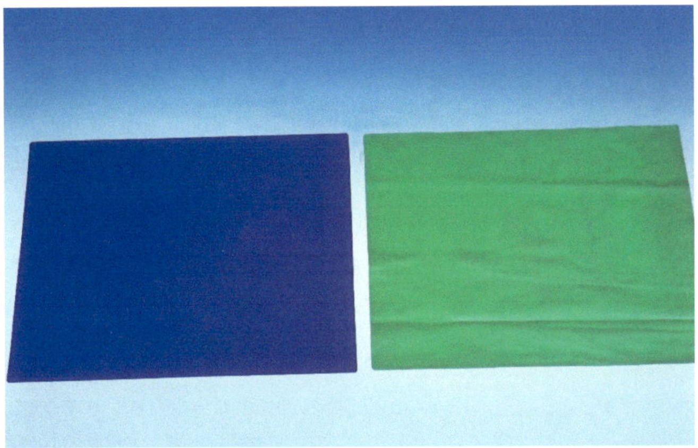

Fig 2-6 Precut rubber dam sheets in green and blue.

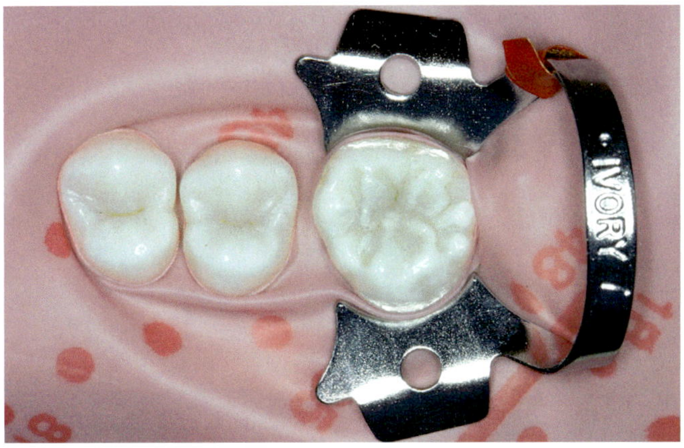

Fig 2-7 Pink rubber dam, placed for direct restoration.

Fig 2-8 *(left)* Relative color perception: Each red square is the same color.

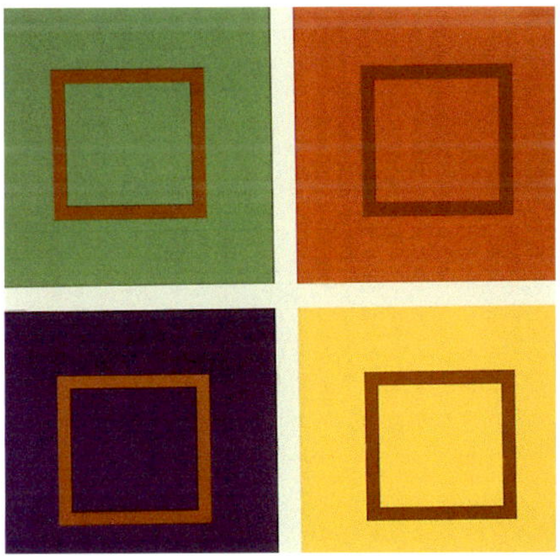

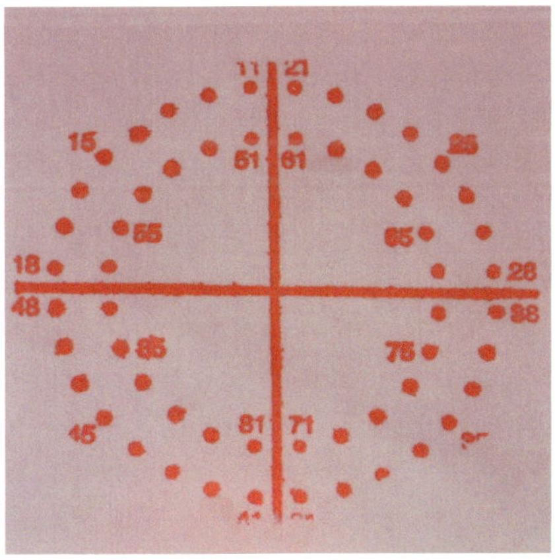

Fig 2-9 *(right)* Pink rubber dam sheet.

2. Half-hitch, double tied. The rope is laid out as a bend (Fig 2-14a), and the doubled end is tied as a half-hitch. This knot is also self-tightening (Fig 2-14b).

Waxed dental floss should be used to form floss ligatures. It has a better grip, and a second knot is rarely needed.

The preknotted ligatures are stored in a box until they are needed (Fig 2-15).

Short-term preparatory work (before the patient arrives)

The holes are punched in the required rubber dam sheet according to the treatment plan (Fig 2-16a). The appropriate clamp is selected from the set and tried on the cast. Only the tips of the clamp should rest against the tooth (Fig 2-16b).

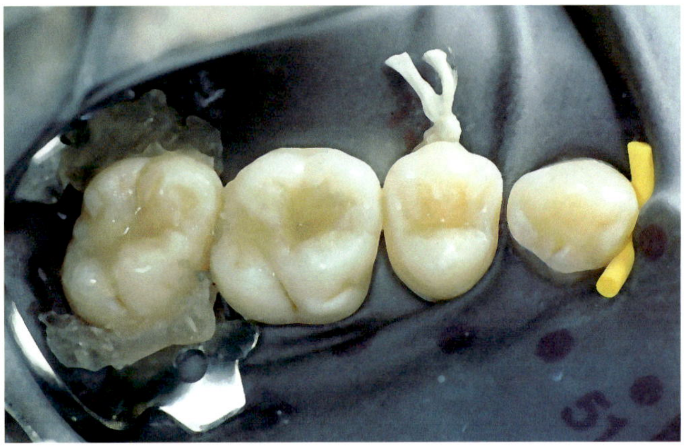

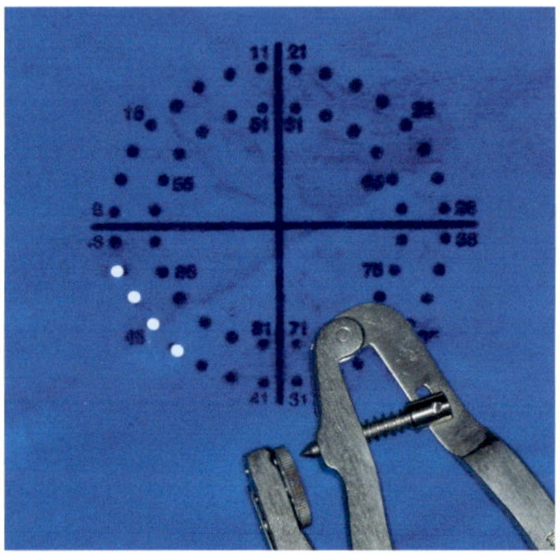

Fig 2-10 *(left)* Gray rubber dam, placed for direct restoration. The teeth look too bright.

Fig 2-11 *(right)* Blue rubber dam sheet, stamped red.

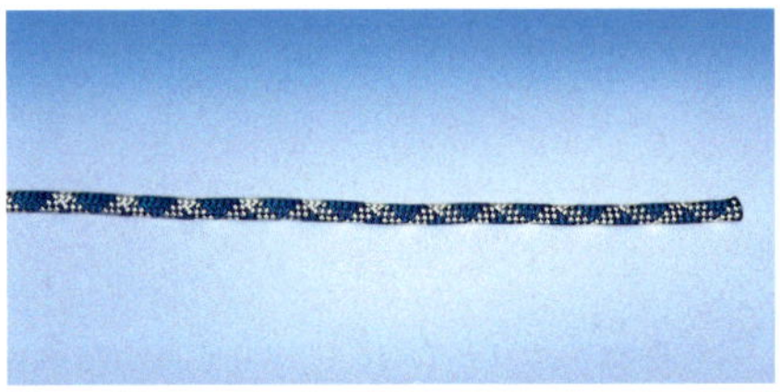

Fig 2-12 Sailing rope for the demonstration of floss ligatures.

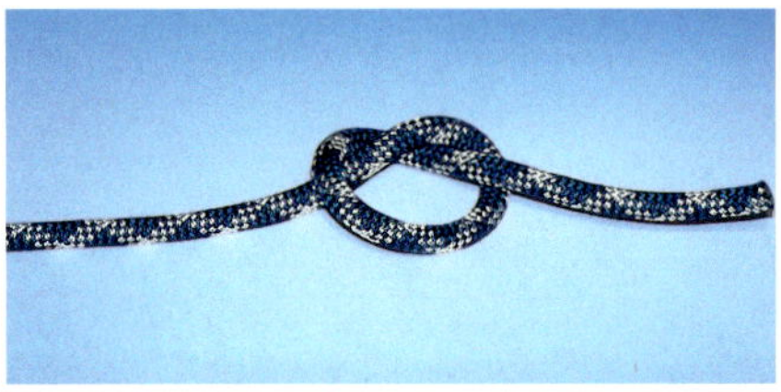

Fig 2-13a Half-hitch.

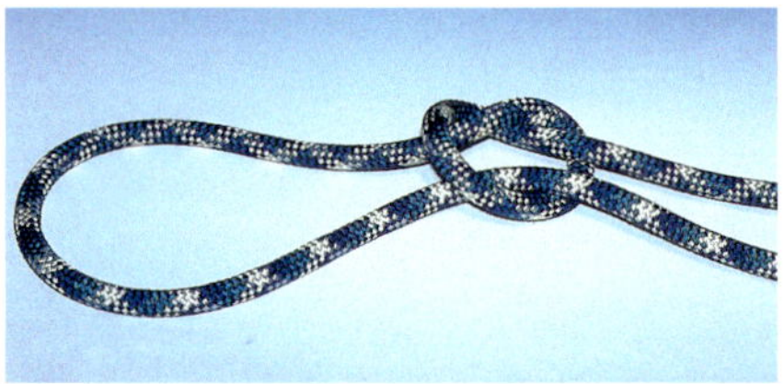

Fig 2-13b Finished sliding knot.

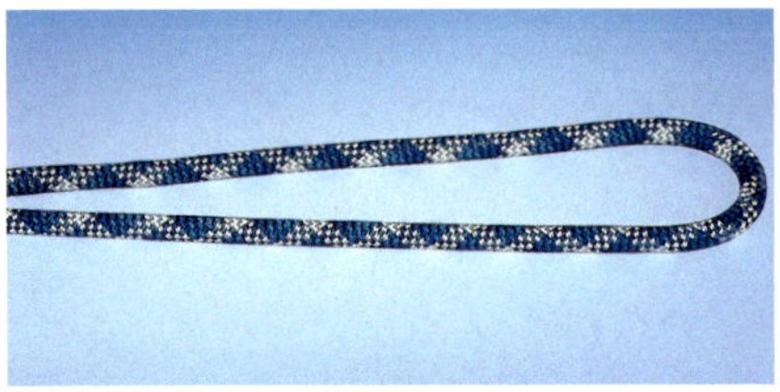

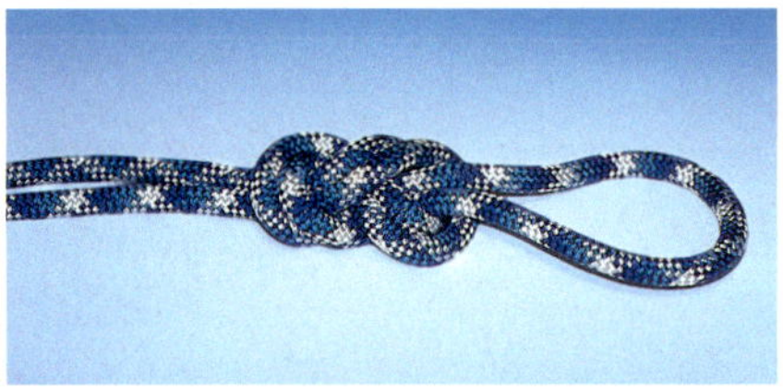

Fig 2-14a *(left)* Laid-out loop.

Fig 2-14b *(right)* Finished double tied knot.

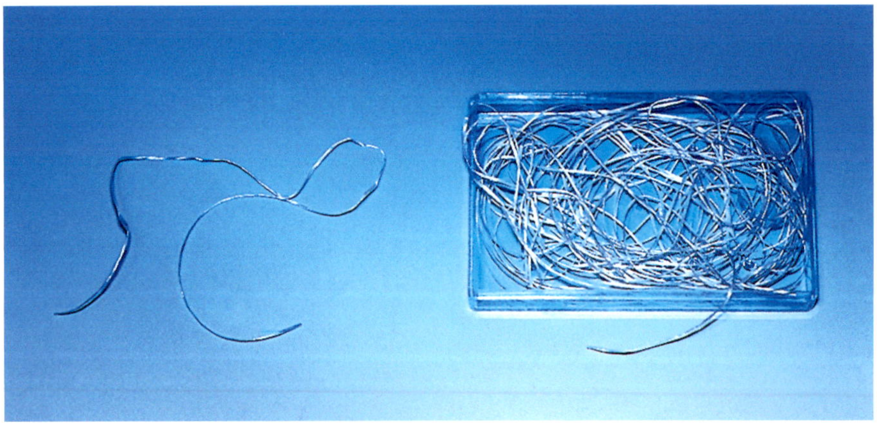

Fig 2-15 Preknotted ligatures of waxed dental floss.

The clamp is placed in the most distal hole; the rubber is stretched over the wings; and rubber dam sheet is loosely stretched over the metal frame (Fig 2-16c). After the clamp forceps are secured in the holes of the clamp (Fig 2-16d), the preparatory stage is finished.

Use of rubber dam in adhesive bonding of inlays in a larger area

Rubber dam set is held by the clamp forceps, and the clamp is placed over the most distal molar. The clamp forceps are removed carefully and the rubber is pushed off the wings with a spatula. It is a good idea to lift the clamp

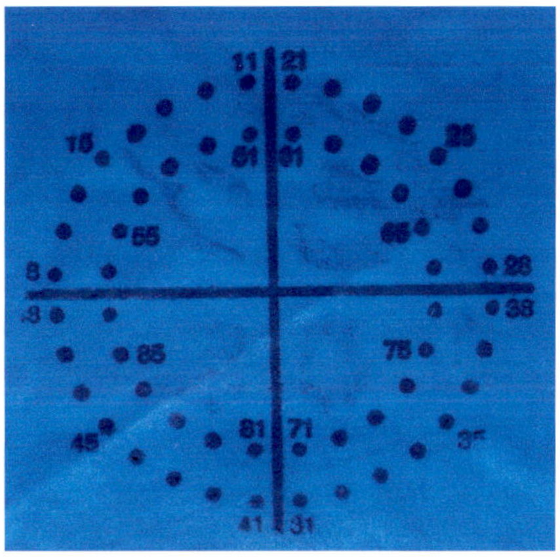

Fig 2-16a *(left)* Punched sheet with rubber dam punch.

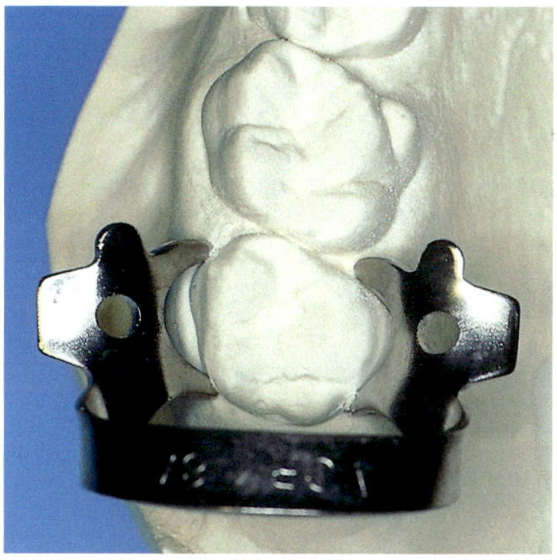

Fig 2-16b *(right)* Trying the clamp on the cast.

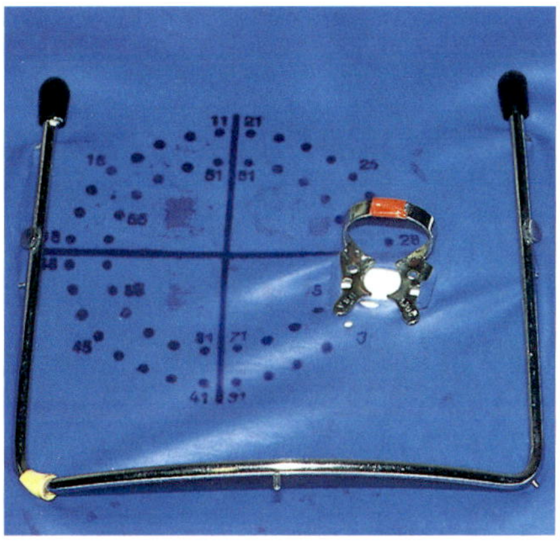

Fig 2-16c *(left)* Rubber dam sheet stretched over the frame with the clamp in place.

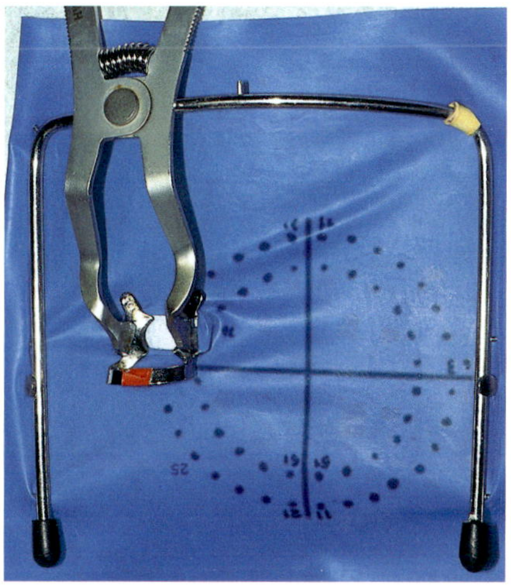

Fig 2-16d *(right)* Clamp forceps clamped on the prepared set.

again with the clamp forceps so that the rubber dam sheet can lie snug on the tooth under the clamp. The rubber dam sheet can then adapt itself to the tooth unhindered (Fig 2-17a). The rubber is adapted hole by hole, tooth by tooth, in a mesial direction (Fig 2-17b).

Rubber dam is secured in the premolar region but outside the working field. Either rubber cord such as Wedjets (Fig 2-17c) or an additional clamp can be used for this purpose. The rubber dam sheet has to be slipped through the interproximal contacts, which is not always quite so easy. Under no circumstances should the contacts be stripped or otherwise broadened (which would result in subsequent food impaction).

A double-layered piece of Glide floss is passed through the contact area and pulled through at one end (Fig 2-17d). If a double layer is used, the thread cannot get caught and can be easily removed. The Wedjets cord is stretched out, slipped through the interproximal contact, and released. The excess ends are cut off with a pair of scissors. The interproximal spaces are examined one by one to determine if the rubber dam sheet was placed correctly, ie, that all the preparation margins are freely accessible and visible and rubber dam is sealed.

If the preparation margin lies rather deep, it is wise to tie a ligature. A preknotted ligature is selected from the box and slid over the tooth. The assistant then adapts the ligature under the height of contour of the tooth with a spatula. The knot tightens itself. The ends are cut off, and the ligature is in place (Fig 2-17e).

With high papillae, sometimes rubber dam bulges upward and covers the interproximal margin of the preparation. In such cases, rubber dam can be moved to the correct position with the chip blower and spatula. It is essential that a ligature be placed afterward.

The dam should be stretched up the sides, creating a pouch that prevents liquids from flowing out and catching the restorations that are tried in with rubber dam (Fig 2-17f).

With rubber dam in place, total moisture control will be successful. Placement of rubber dam takes 3 to 4 minutes, which means that use of a rubber dam is economic

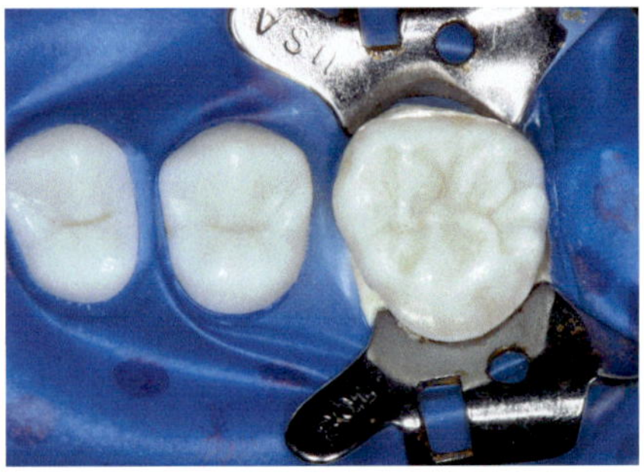

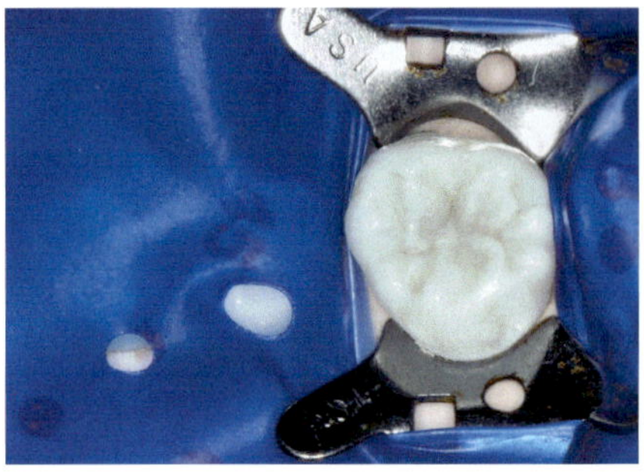

Fig 2-17a *(left)* Rubber dam set is adapted to the most distal tooth with the clamp.

Fig 2-17b *(right)* Rubber dam sheet is adapted tooth by tooth.

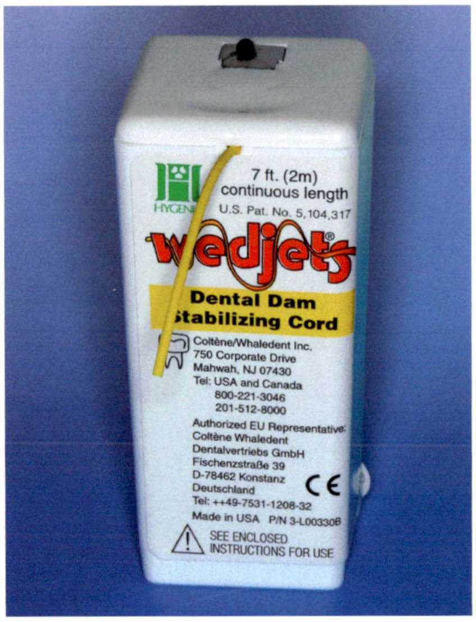

Fig 2-17c *(left)* Wedjets.

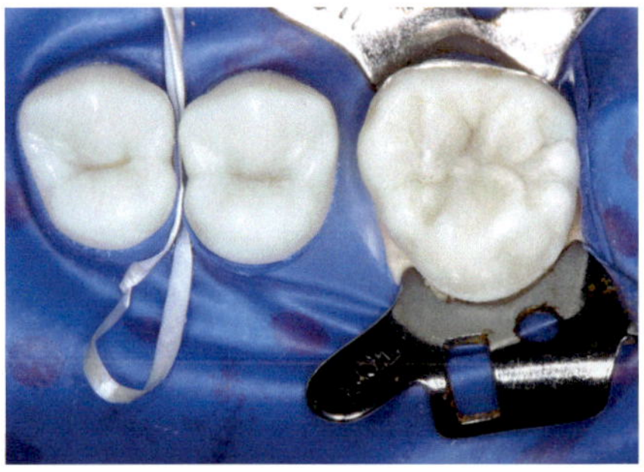

Fig 2-17d Glide floss loop in the interproximal space.

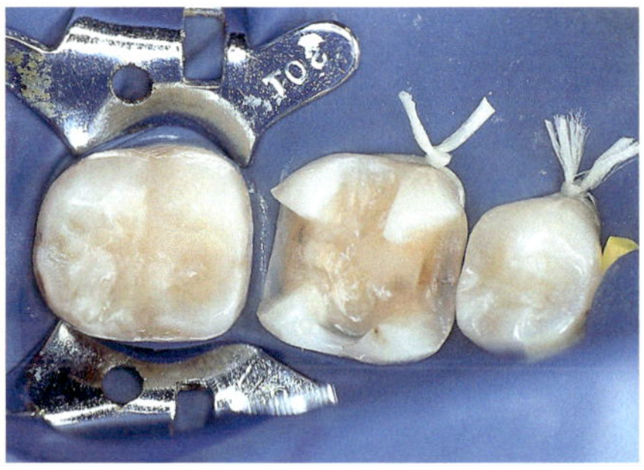

Fig 2-17e Quadrant after complete moisture control, ready for adhesive bonding.

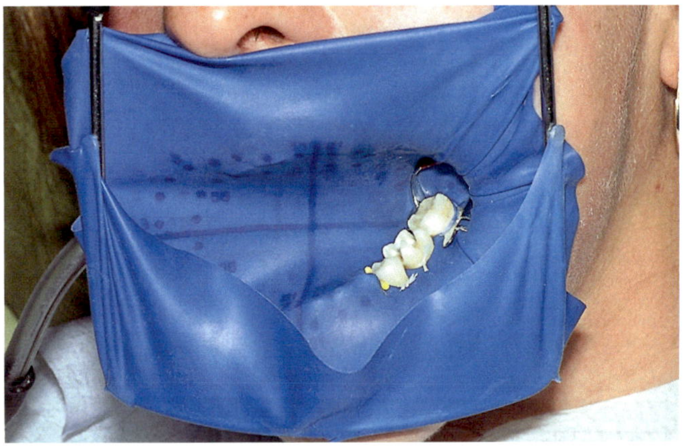

Fig 2-17f Rubber dam with safety pouch in place.

and efficient. Insertion of the all-ceramic restorations can begin.

Materials

Precut Hygenic rubber dam sheets (Coltène Whaledent); for patients with latex allergy, use the nonlatex Flexi Dam (Coltène Whaledent)
Rubber dam stamp (Hygenic, Coltène Whaledent)
Ivory rubber dam punch (Heraeus Kulzer)
Ash rubber dam clamps (Dentsply Ash)
Ivory clamp forceps (Heraeus Kulzer)
Frame Type Junior (Hygenic, Coltène Whaledent)
Wedjets (Hygenic, Coltène Whaledent)
Glide floss (Gore)
Waxed dental floss (Johnson & Johnson)

Class V Restorations

Common problem: Adhesion and duration of Class V restorations

In restorative dentistry today, it is still a challenge to create long-lasting restorations for cavity preparations in the gingival third of the tooth (Class V restorations; Figs 2-18a and 2-18b). Before any kind of treatment is initiated, the question of why and how the defect developed should be considered. Opinions on this issue seem to diverge vastly, but it is still important to summarize the current state of knowledge about the causes of cervical lesions:

1. Brushing technique. Horizontal brushing, especially with a toothbrush without rounded bristles or with hard bristles, causes a wedge-shaped lesion in the dentin of the cervical area of the tooth.
2. Functional overload. The enamel and dentin of the cervical area may chip off due to excessive pressure on a tooth, especially through flexure of a tooth in patients with bruxism.

Perhaps the combination of both these causes can increase the defect. Acidic foods and drinks can also contribute to the problem, while bacteria can cause the cervical lesions to become carious. Thus it is important to counteract the causes and to treat the defects.

Two main problems can affect treatment: flexure of the tooth and different adhesive properties (coronal with enamel, cervical with dentin). These are the biomechanical effects that make it so difficult to restore cavity preparations in the cervical areas of teeth.

All of the treatment options that involve restorations have minor or major disadvantages:

1. Cohesive gold foil restorations are very time consuming and costly. At the same time, they are the only kind of restoration that exhibits guaranteed longevity because of their adhesive yet flexible properties. Modern treatment methods, however, demand lower-cost alternatives, preferably with tooth-colored materials.
2. Glass-ionomer restorations show favorable adhesive properties, but the surface cannot really be permanently polished and is very susceptible to fracture.
3. With resin composite or compomer restorations, despite improved dentin-bonding agents and special lamination techniques, there is no way to ensure marginal integrity, especially cervically in the dentin. This is due to the fact that the adhesive forces are much stronger toward the coronal part of the tooth in enamel than they are in the cervical dentin. Moreover, the cervical margins have to be monitored regularly and resealed if necessary.
4. Sandwich technique restorations are too time consuming and do not provide better results. Moreover, they involve a certain risk: when you etch the glass-ionomer cement, the strong bonds with the resin composite lift the glass-ionomer cement from the dentin, which causes leakage.

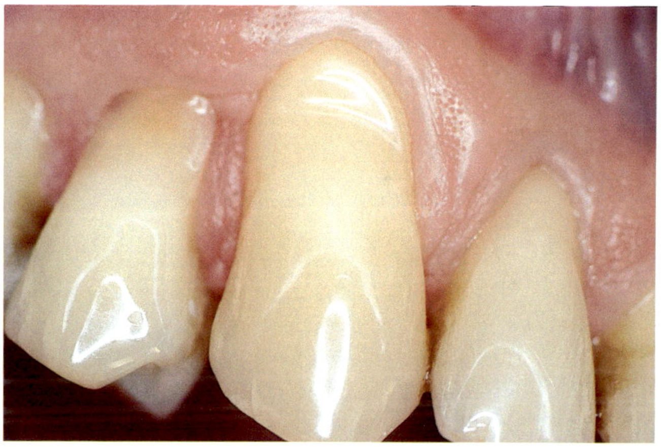

Fig 2-18a Multiple defects in the cervical area.

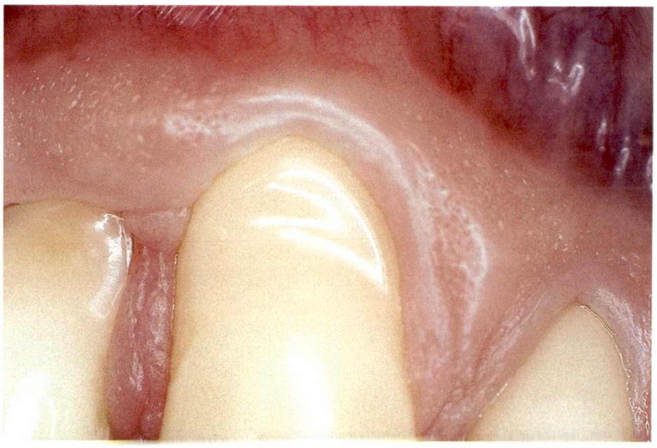

Fig 2-18b Cervical defect at the maxillary right canine.

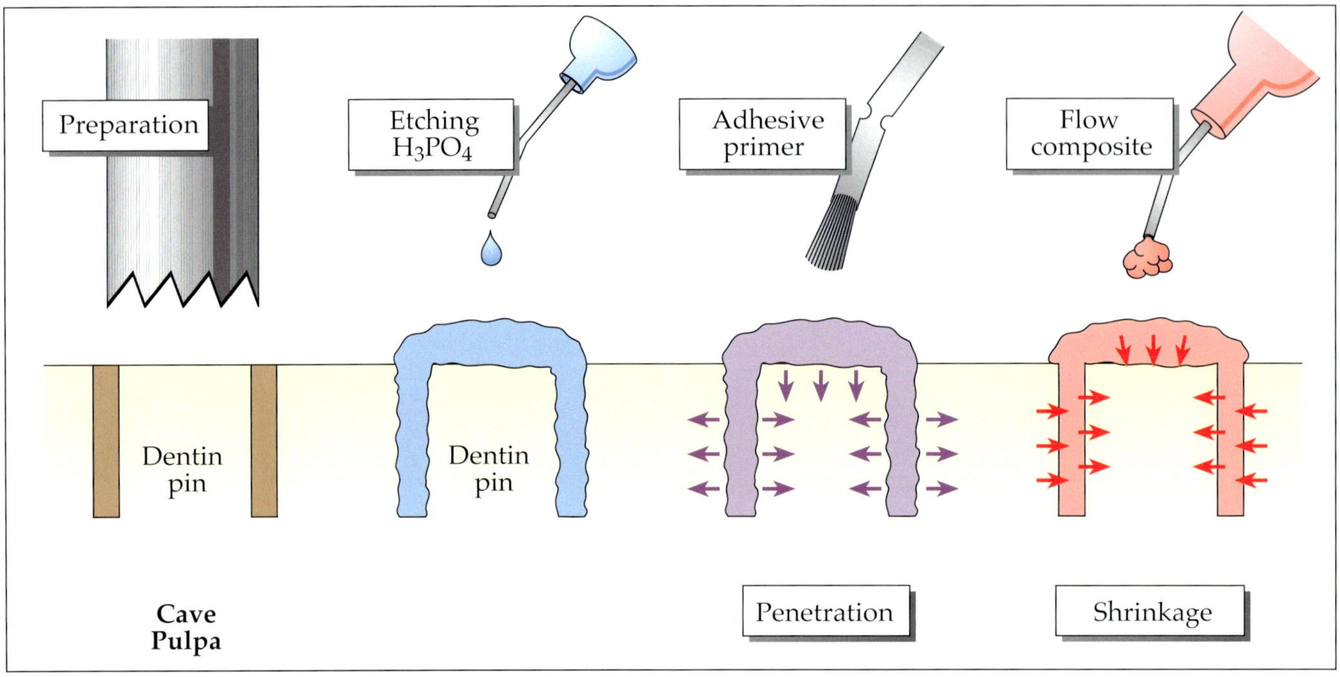

Fig 2-18c Restoration of Class V defects with the help of cut dentin pins.

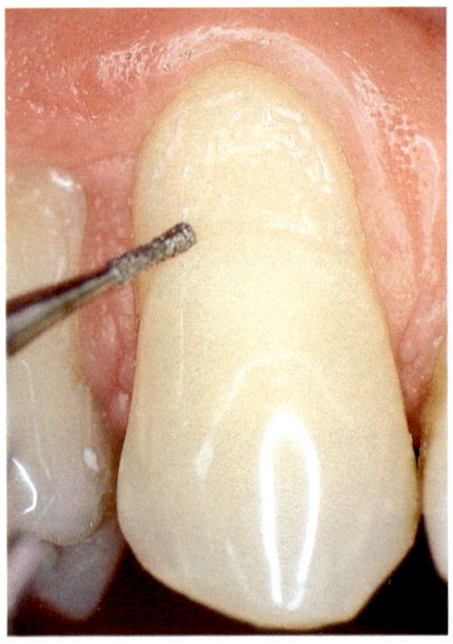

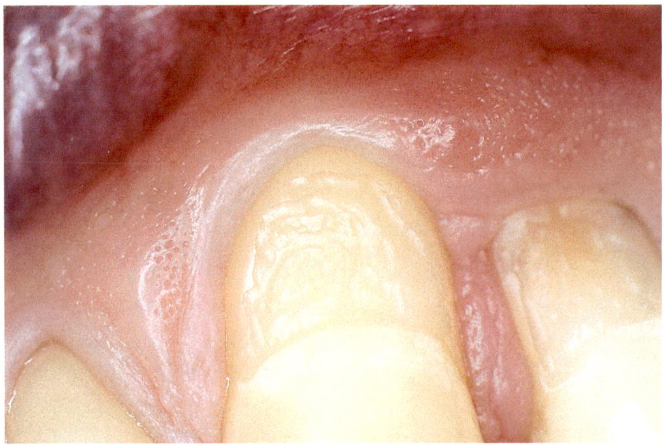

Fig 2-18d *(left)* Preparation of the cervical cavity.

Fig 2-18e *(right)* Finished preparation with undercuts and beveled enamel.

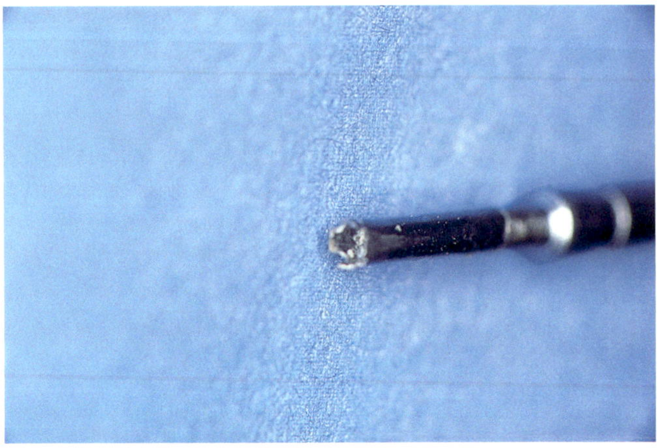

Fig 2-18f Trephine bur.

5. Resin composite restorations with additional retention have been tried, but the cervical insertion of pins has proven inadequate, hazardous to the pulp, and unattractive.

Proven solution: Class V restorations with trephined dentin pins

This method has proven in practice to be long lasting and esthetically satisfactory.

The step-by-step procedure is outlined in Fig 2-18c. The dentin is cleaned with an abrasive paste. A flat Class V cavity with a marginal undercut is prepared (Figs 2-18d and 2-18e). A trephine from the Masserann kit is used to cut the pins out of the dentin (Fig 2-18f). The direction of rotation must be changed to counterclockwise, as the trephines only cut when turning in this direction. Special care must be taken to avoid injuring the pulp—central bores must not be used (Fig 2-18g).

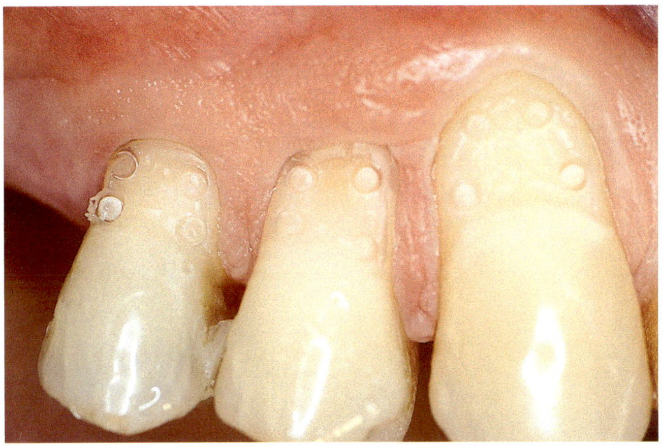

Fig 2-18g Preparation of the dentin pins.

Fig 2-18h *(left)* Etching the cavity with orthophosphoric acid.

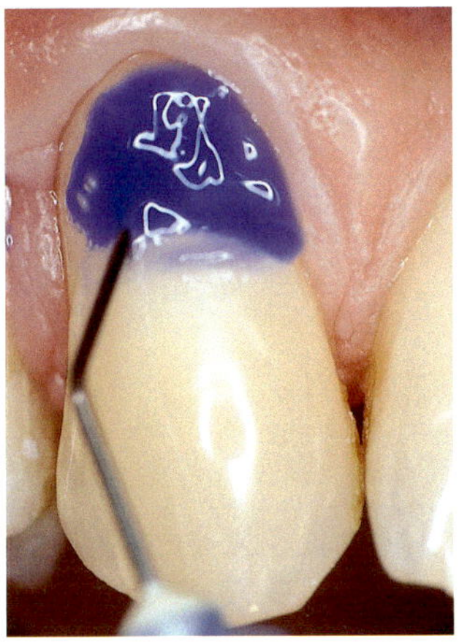

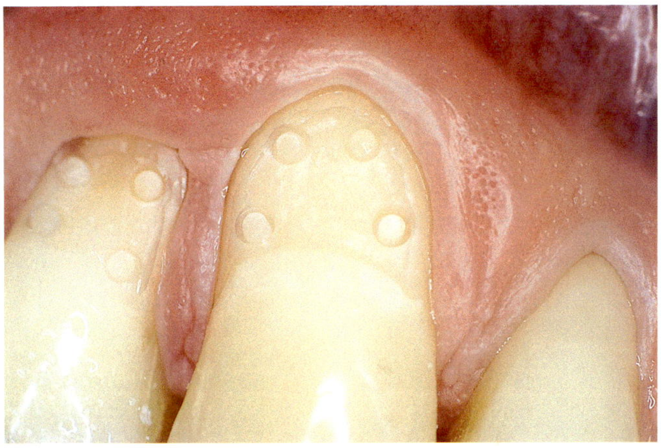

Fig 2-18i *(right)* Appearance after rinsing and thorough drying.

The dentin is etched with phosphoric acid for 10 seconds, rinsed, and dried (Figs 2-18h and 2-18i). Dentin adhesive is applied as described in the manufacturer's instructions and dried (Figs 2-18j and 2-18k). The first layer of flowable resin composite is massaged on the dentin with a brush and polymerized for a short time. A covering layer of viscous resin composite is applied and polymerized from multiple angles (Figs 2-18l to 2-18n). The restoration is finished and polished (Fig 2-18o). As a last step, fluoride is applied.

The occlusion and articulation are checked to eliminate possible functional interferences. The patient should also be informed about proper brushing techniques.

Discussion

Whether or not noncarious Class V lesions (such as the ones shown here) should be treated at all is the subject of some debate. In this case, the patient explicitly insisted on treatment, since he perceived these areas of his teeth as a conspicuous problem.

Another way of compensating for these defects in an esthetic manner is periodontal mucogingival surgery. An array of very successful methods are now available to conceal these recessions with soft tissue.

To the present day, the author has not yet come across any department of conservative dentistry in the German academic community that would be willing to evaluate the method shown, despite the fact that practitioners urgently need advances in Class V restorations and desire a scientific foundation for dealing with this critical challenge.

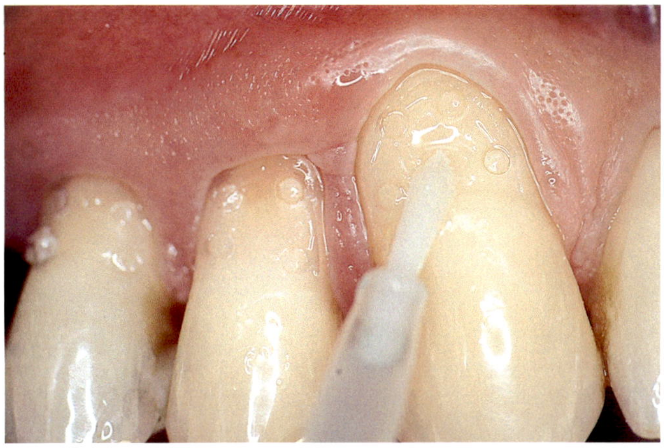

Fig 2-18j Application of the dentin bonding agent.

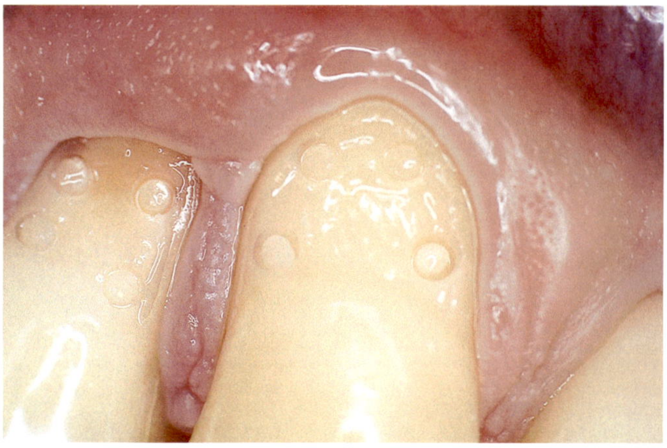

Fig 2-18k Appearance after polymerization of the adhesive.

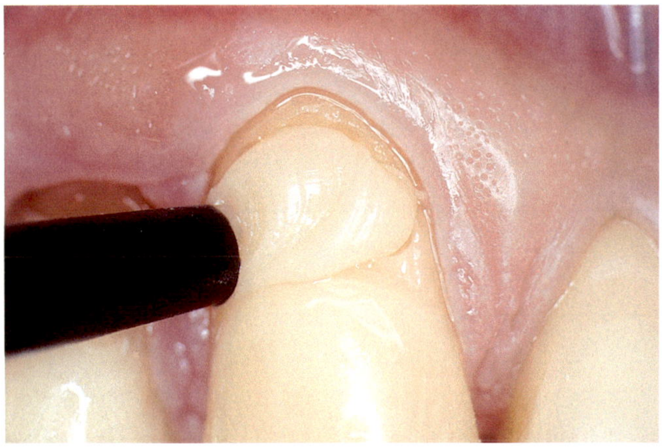

Fig 2-18l Application of the resin composite with an application syringe.

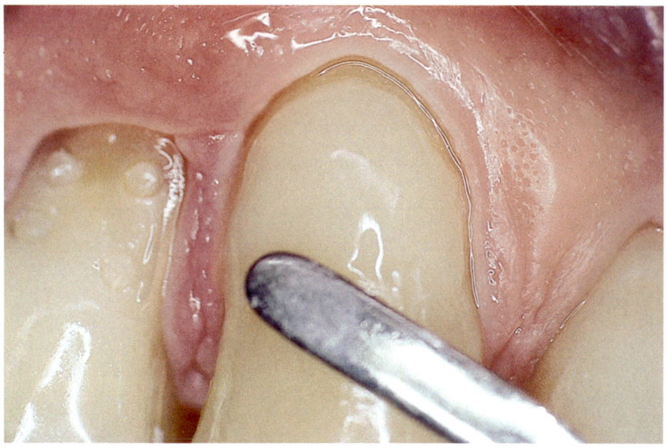

Fig 2-18m Formation of the resin composite restoration.

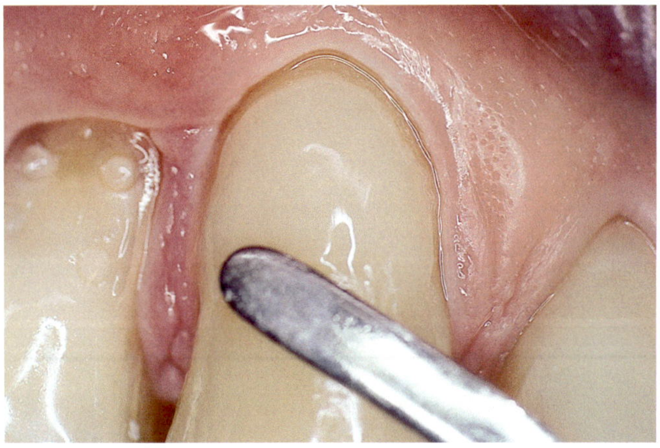

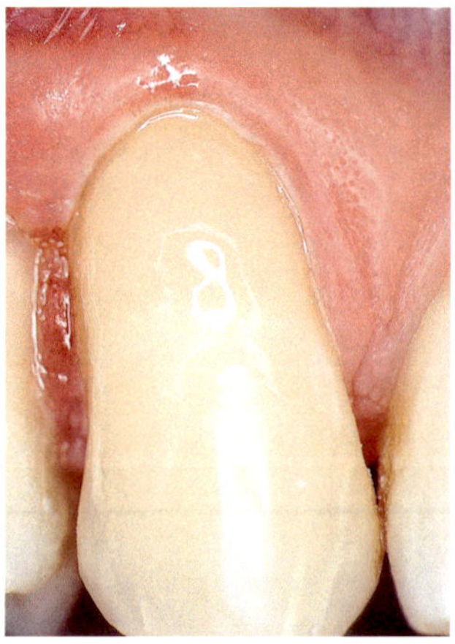

Fig 2-18n *(left)* Light-curing from multiple angles.

Fig 2-18o *(right)* Finished Class V restoration.

Materials

Trephine drills, sizes 13, 14, and 15 from the Masserann kit (Micro Mega), which can be resharpened with a separating disk (instructions provided in the kit)
Shorter trephines, especially designed to cut dentin pins, with a depth stop at 1.5 mm (soon available from Dentatus)
Ultra-Etch etchant gel, 35% orthophosphoric acid (Ultradent)
Excite dentin bonding agent (Ivoclar Vivadent)
Tetric Flow and Tetric resin composites (Ivoclar Vivadent)

Efficient Adhesive Bonding of Ceramic Inlays

Common problem: Adhesive bonding of ceramic inlays is too complicated and time consuming

Since 1985, the author has been treating patients with tooth-colored inlays for posterior teeth. At first, resin composite inlays made in the dental laboratory were used. Beginning in 1988, conventional feldspar porcelain inlays were used, and in 1990 leucite-reinforced ceramics were used, until a switch was made to copy-milled ceramic inlays. However, the problems always remained the same–adhesive bonding of ceramic inlays was too cumbersome and time consuming (Fig 2-19).

Because careful procedures were followed, it usually took us 30 minutes to place a ceramic inlay. Thus the restoration of an entire quadrant with four ceramic inlays required far more than 1 hour. Inlay after inlay was placed, finalized, and polished, one after another. If the fit, especially at the interproximal contact, was not minutely accurate, the inlay had to be ground in and adapted. The adhesive resin composite was too runny and formed messy, hardly visible overhangs that could only be removed through tedious effort. The large investment of time required meant that it was difficult to make and place ceramic inlays in posterior teeth in an economically efficient way.

If a process is cumbersome and complicated, it has to be integrated, simplified, and thoroughly prepared without affecting quality. If dentists follow this principle, they will find a solution to restorative difficulties.

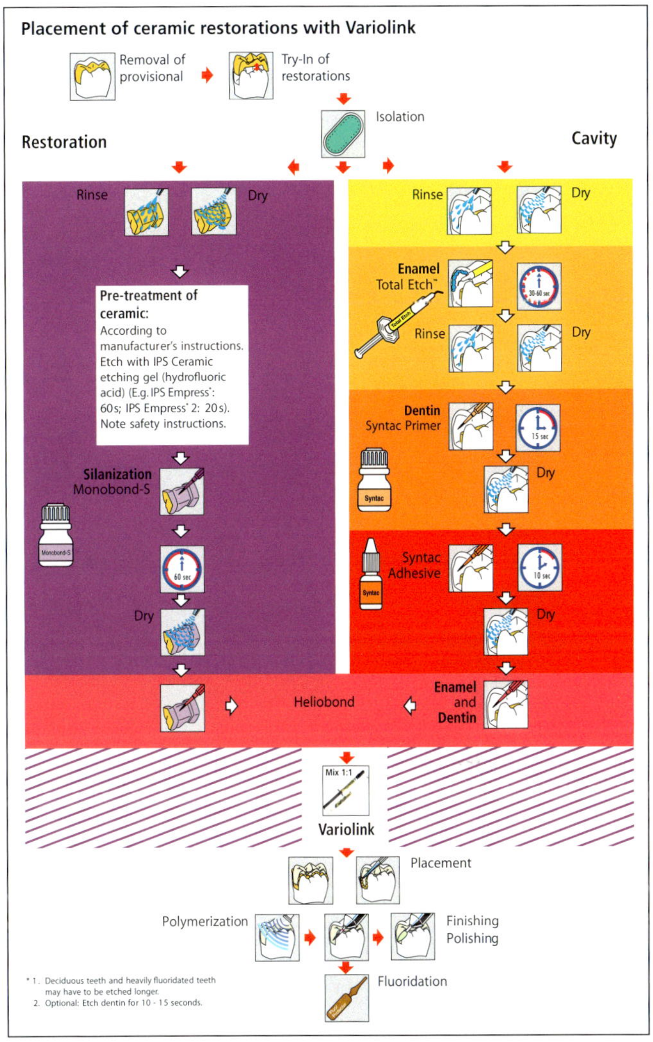

Fig 2-19 Flowchart of the steps in adhesive bonding. (Courtesy of Dr Jürg Kleinmann.)

Proven solution: Adhesive bonding with ultrasound

The act of streamlining a task but keeping the quality constant will be demonstrated through the restoration of an entire quadrant with ceramic inlays.

Preparation

The patient's teeth are prepared in compliance with the guidelines for the adhesive bonding of restorations. In this example, the following teeth are prepared: the mandibular left second premolar, first molar, and second molar. The conical, block-shaped preparations are carried out with a ceramic inlay preparation set and vertical diamond files and under visual control with the magnifying loupe (see chapter 3). All the margins and interior surfaces are defined and smooth. There are no chamfers. The proximal boxes should be prepared with the Sonicsys system to prevent the adjacent teeth from being damaged by a rotary instrument.

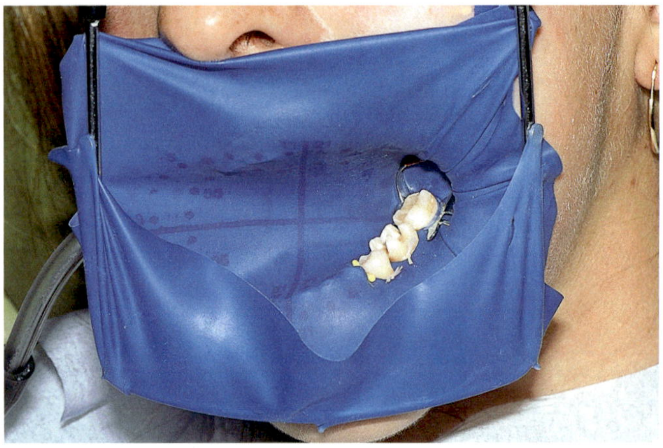

Fig 2-20a Rubber dam is in place.

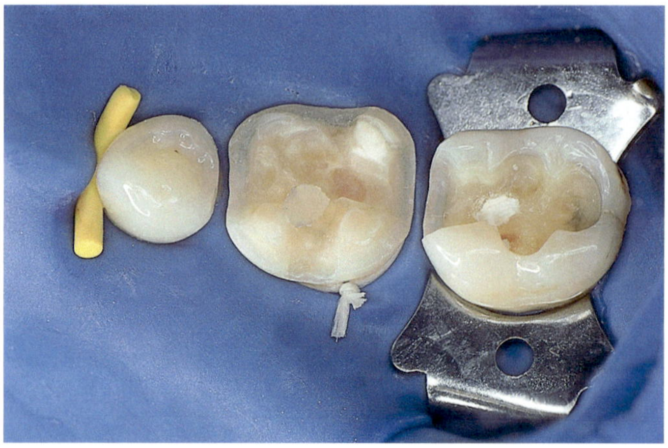

Fig 2-20b Total moisture control is achieved.

If they are part of the preparation, all cusps are prepared smooth and rounded. Retentive elements are not prepared, because they only create pressure on the teeth during try-in, cementation, and subsequently through occlusal stress. Enamel is prepared, where possible.

A base of dentin bonding agent and flowable tooth-colored resin composite is placed under the restoration to preserve enamel.

Provisional inlays

Dual-cured resin composite provisional restorations (Luxatemp Solar), made with the help of a vacuform matrix, are placed. They can be prefabricated at chairside with a fast deep-drawing process (Perfect-Plast Kit; see chapter 3).

The dual-cure resin composite cures chemically until it reaches a rubbery consistency. After contouring, it can be light-cured on the teeth until it has reached its final hardness. This eliminates polymerization in undercuts and the related problems.

The provisional restorations are cemented with a noneugenol temporary cement, preferably a dual-curing cement (eg, Provilink). In connection with full and partial crowns, we advise cementing the provisional restorations with carboxylate cement (Durelon) that is applied in a thinner layer toward the margins.

Preparatory stage

The patient arrives at the office for the appointment. The prepared teeth have a normal and positive response to the pulp test. Nerve block anesthesia should be used, because a lot of air blowing and irrigating are involved in adhesive bonding. The provisional restorations are removed and rubber dam is placed (as described earlier). The cavity preparations are mechanically cleaned with air abrasion and then chemically cleaned and disinfected with Tubulicid.

Total moisture control with rubber dam

Because adhesive bonding can only be successful in a dry environment, total moisture control with rubber dam is an absolute must. Efficient placement of rubber dam in a quadrant takes only 2 to 3 minutes, provided it was prepared beforehand and the team is trained accordingly (Figs 2-20a and 2-20b). Placement of rubber dam is also possible after the try-in but is preferable beforehand instead to prevent swallowing or aspiration.

Try-in

The ceramic inlays that the dental laboratory provided are examined on the uncut cast. The marginal fit, contact points, layering, and color have to be adequate (Fig 2-21a). The first inlay is removed from the cast with an adhesive-placing instrument (VivaStick) that is bent so that the inlay can be accessed mesially (Figs 2-21b to 2-21d). The inlay is covered with try-in paste (a tooth-colored, water-soluble glycerin) and carefully placed in the cavity in the direction of insertion (Figs 2-21e to 2-21g). The next inlay is placed in the same fashion.

After the excess material is removed, the inlays are checked for marginal integrity, shape, and color. The patient is asked if he or she is satisfied with the restora-

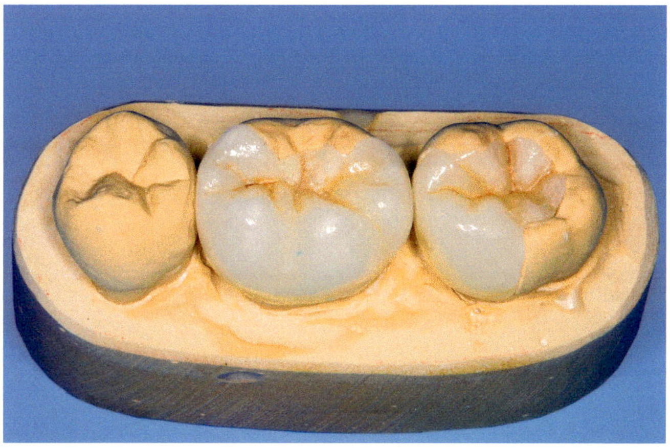

Fig 2-21a Ceramic inlays are tried on the uncut laboratory cast.

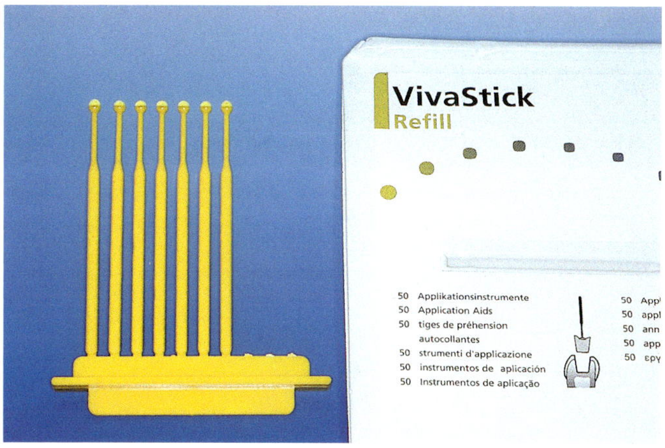

Fig 2-21b Adhesive sticks.

tions (Fig 2-21h). The color has to be exactly the right shade in the first place, because it is nearly impossible to correct the shade afterward with adhesive resin composite. The author strongly advises against painting the inlay to correct the color. The paint will be partially removed by occlusal grinding, which leads to unesthetic and uneven results.

The precision of the restorations is checked twice: once with a low-viscosity colored impression material, and once with a pressure spot test under the laboratory microscope (Figs 2-21i to 2-21n; see chapter 3). If the fit is accurate and the paths of insertion and the interproximal contacts are correct, under no circumstances should the occlusion be checked, because this may result in breaks.

If the try-in satisfies the patient, the dentist, and the dental technician, the inlays are removed, cleaned, and prepared for integration. After a try-in with silicone, sandblasting in the laboratory is imperative because the silicone oil can only be removed mechanically and not chemically (Fig 2-21o).

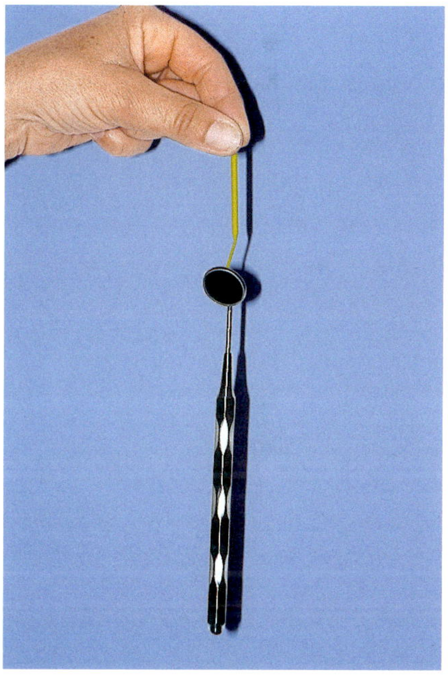

Fig 2-21c The adhesive strength is demonstrated with a dental mirror.

Adhesive bonding with ultrasound

The individual steps of adhesive bonding are carried out at the same time; ie, the cavities are simultaneously conditioned and prepared in the patient's mouth while the ceramic inlays are prepared at chairside (see the flowchart in Fig 2-19).

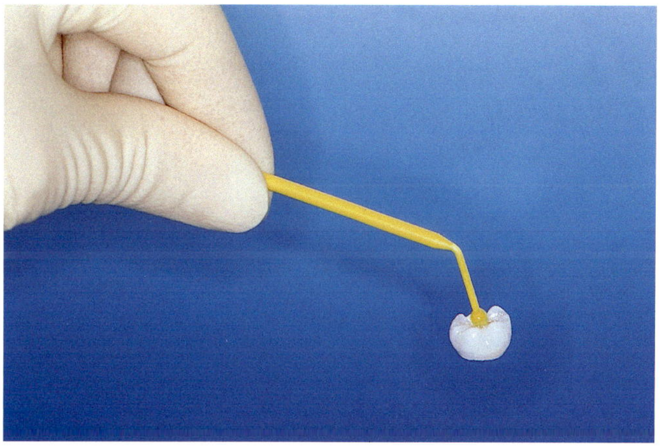

Fig 2-21d Handling of the ceramic inlay with the adhesive stick.

Preparation of the cavities

The cavities are cleaned mechanically with a polishing brush and pumice or by air abrasion. After irrigating and drying are completed, the teeth are etched in two steps. The enamel is etched for 30 seconds with 40% phosphoric acid gel (Figs 2-22a to 2-22h); after a 20-second pause, the dentin is etched for 10 seconds (Fig 2-22i). Etching the dentin longer than that can lead to postoperative sensitivity, which can be very unpleasant for both the patient and the dentist.

The cavities are irrigated for 15 seconds—for 5 seconds with a water jet only to prevent the acid gel from being spattered (Fig 2-22j) and then with water spray for 10 seconds but always into the direction of the large aspirator (Fig 2-22k). Then the cavities are gently dried (but not overdried) with the chip blower. It is very useful to blow the drops of water into a cotton roll held beside the cavities to keep the water from splashing onto rubber dam and to quicken drying (Fig 2-22l). Afterward, the etching pattern is checked (Fig 2-22m).

The dentin is conditioned with a two-bottle adhesive system, such as Syntac Classic (Figs 2-22n to 2-22p). There are many debates and claims and even more opinions about the countless one-bottle systems, with their diverse components and possible uses. "All in one" is a typical advertising phrase that is more or less code for, "This is a high-risk product that will not save you much time." The way things are developing, in the future someone is bound to claim that dentists can create sufficient

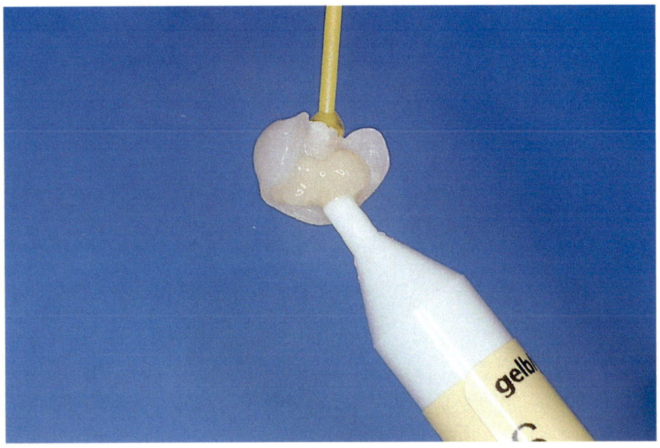

Fig 2-21e The try-in paste is applied to the ceramic inlay.

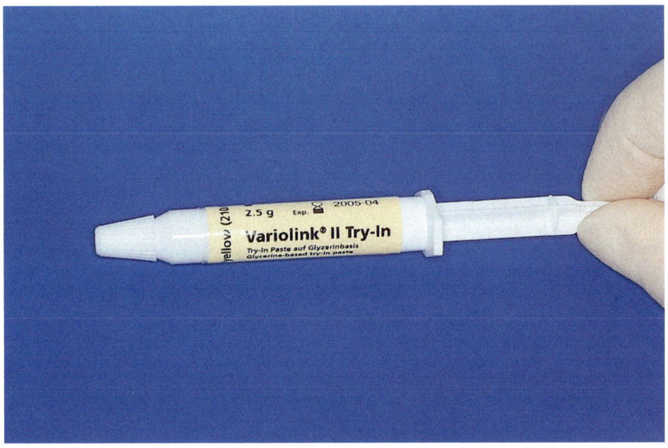

Fig 2-21f Try-in paste in the designated tooth color.

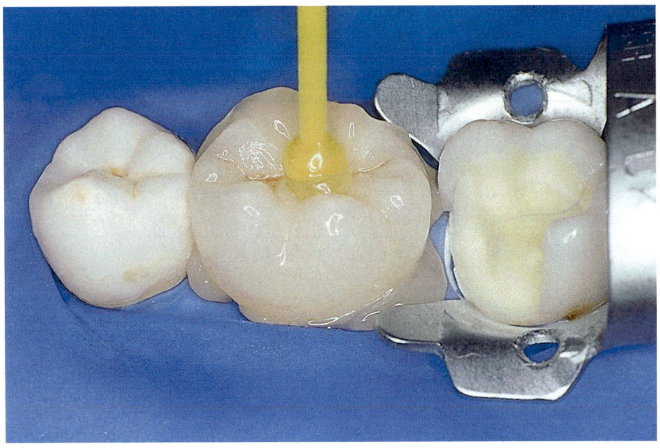

Fig 2-21g The ceramic inlay is tried in.

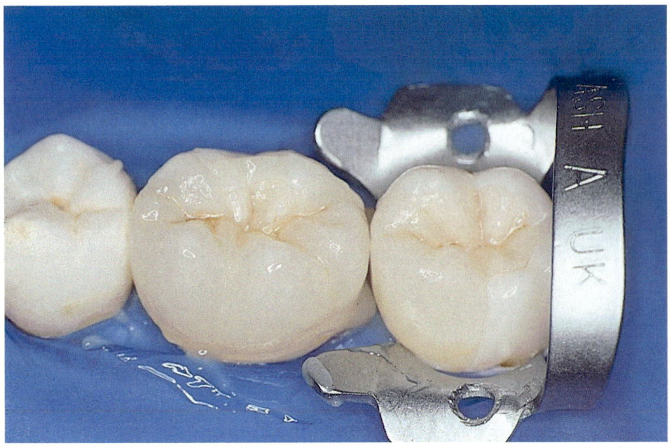

Fig 2-21h Both ceramic inlays are placed in the cavities for try-in.

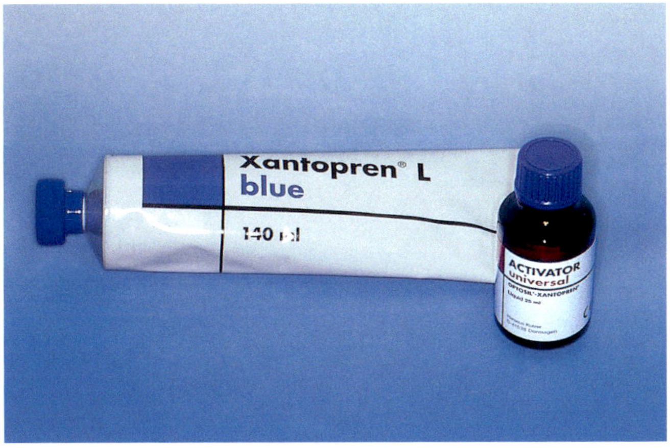

Fig 2-21i Brightly colored try-in silicone.

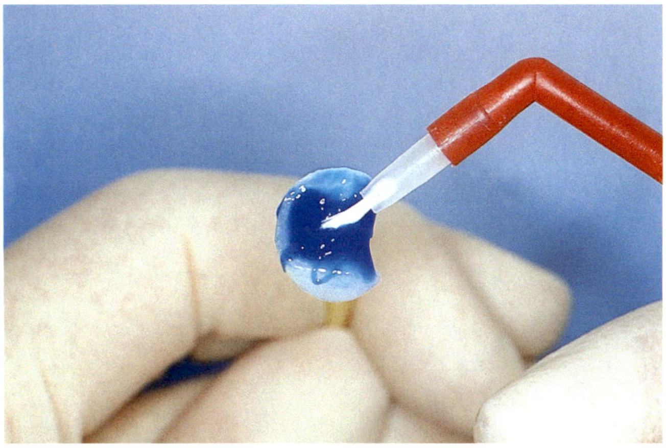

Fig 2-21j A fine layer of silicone is applied.

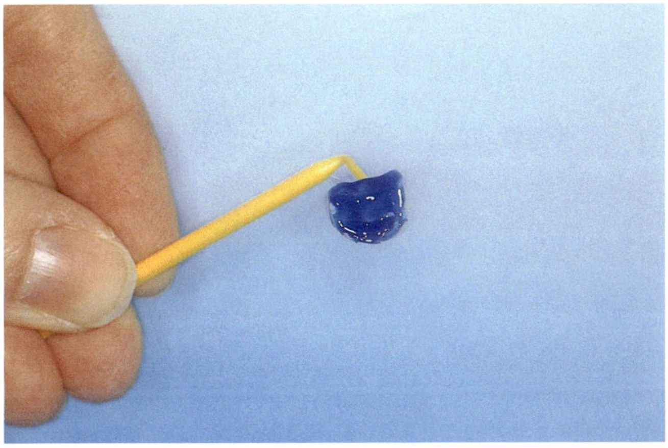

Fig 2-21k Inlay with the silicone applied on the adhesive stick.

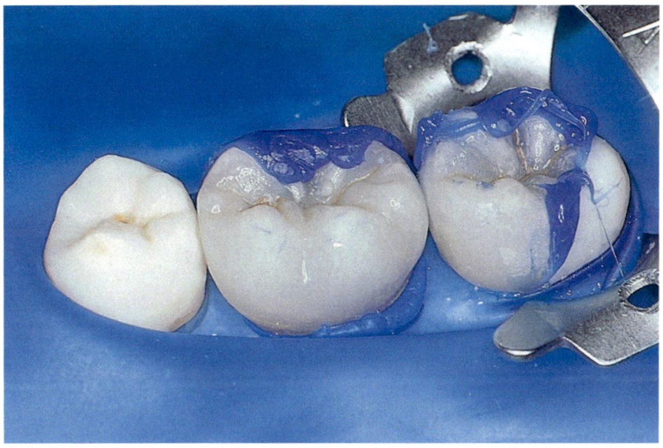

Fig 2-21l Both ceramic inlays are adapted by pressing gently.

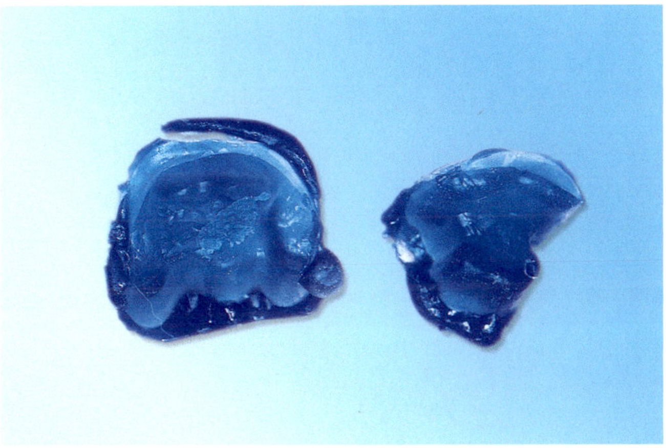

Fig 2-21m Pressure spot test (removed).

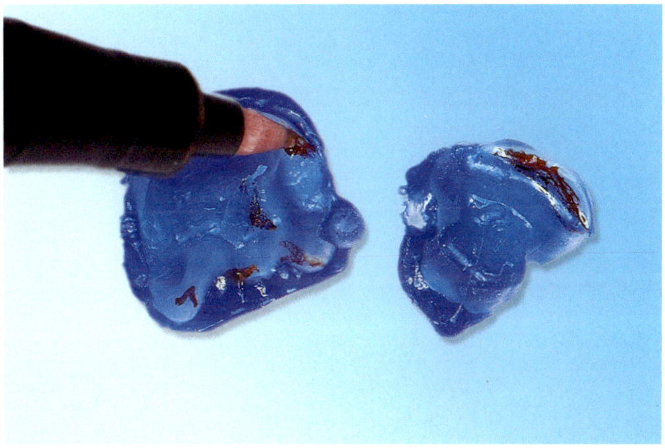

Fig 2-21n Pressure spot test (the primary contacts are marked with waterproof felt-tip pen).

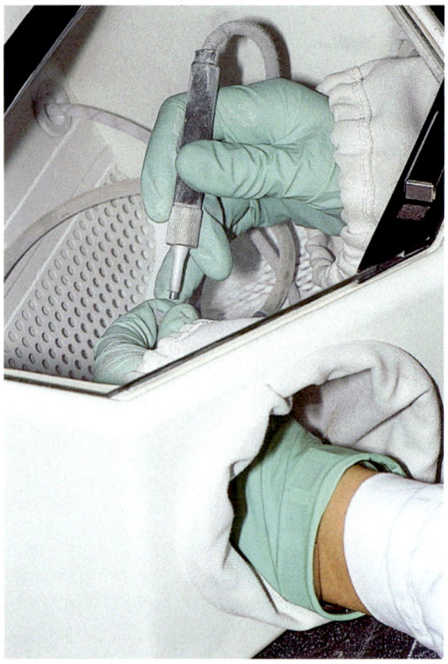

Fig 2-21o Sandblasting with 50-µm particles after the pressure spot test is absolutely essential.

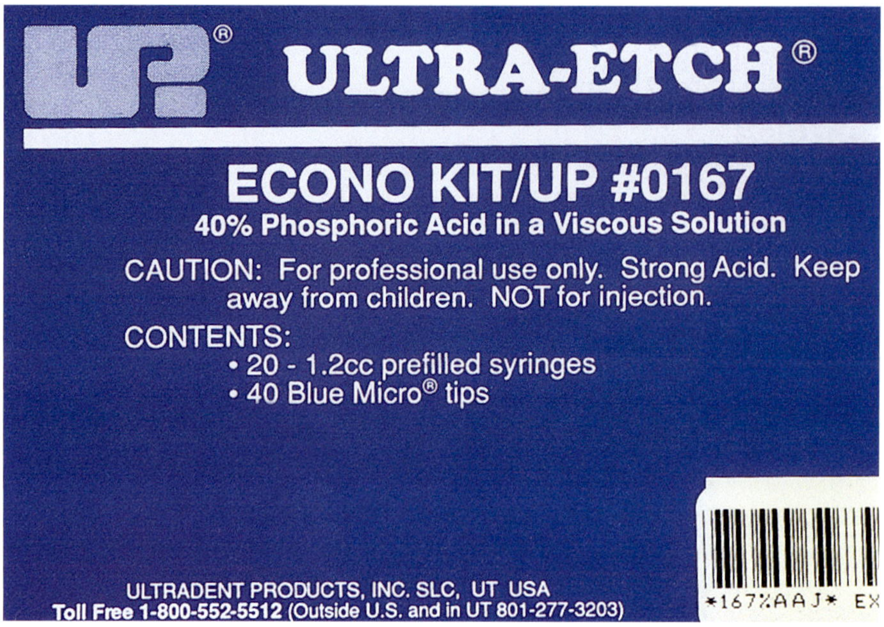

Fig 2-22a Phosphoric acid (40%).

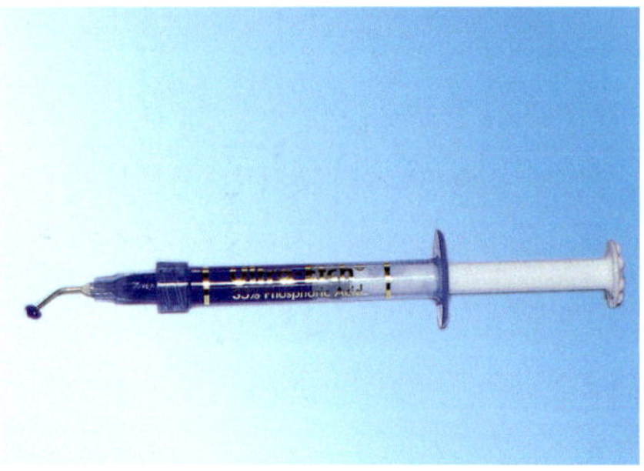

Fig 2-22b Application syringe.

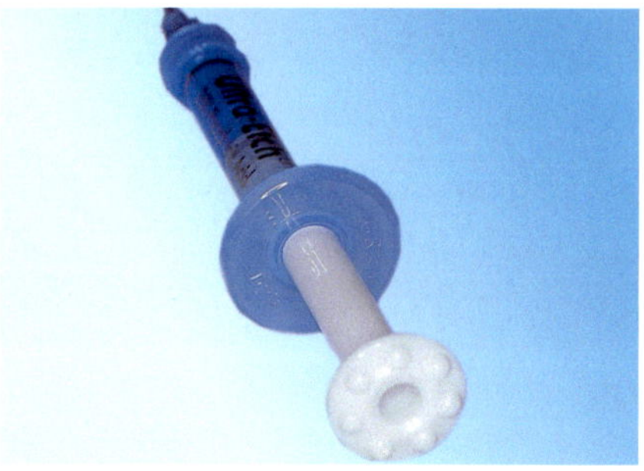

Fig 2-22c The circular grip makes the syringe keep rolling away.

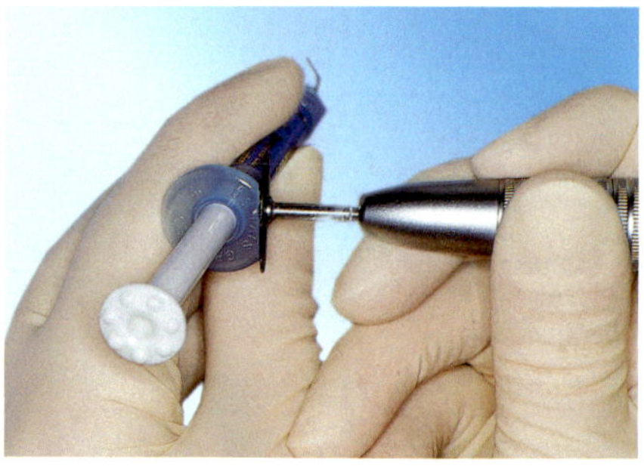

Fig 2-22d A separating disk can be used to create an edge for it to rest on.

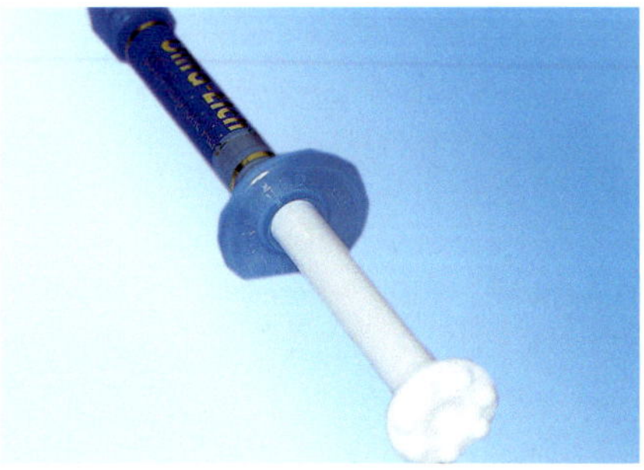

Fig 2-22e The syringe lies safely: The cannula is pointing upward.

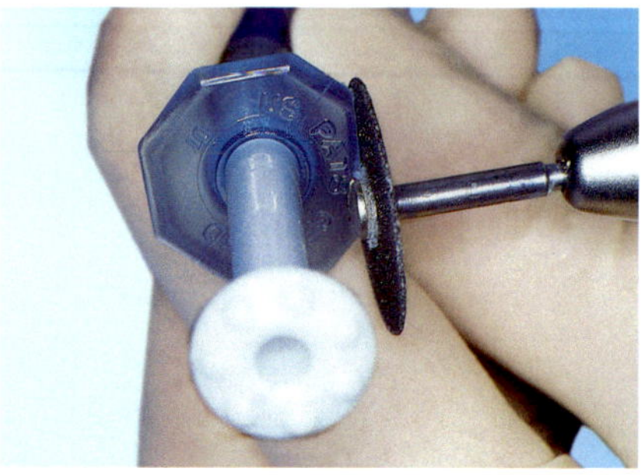

Fig 2-22f With the new octagon rests, an upright position of the cannula is still not ensured, so a defined rest is created with the separating disk.

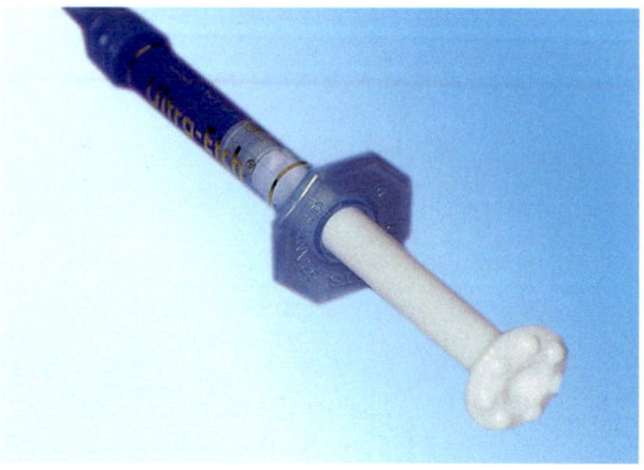

Fig 2-22g Application syringe with defined rest.

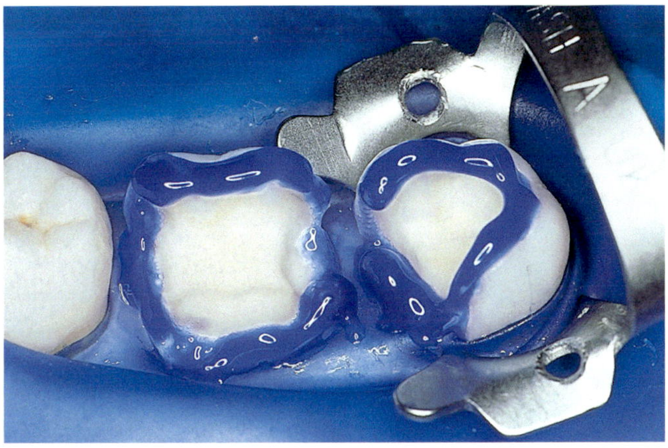

Fig 2-22h The enamel is etched for 30 seconds.

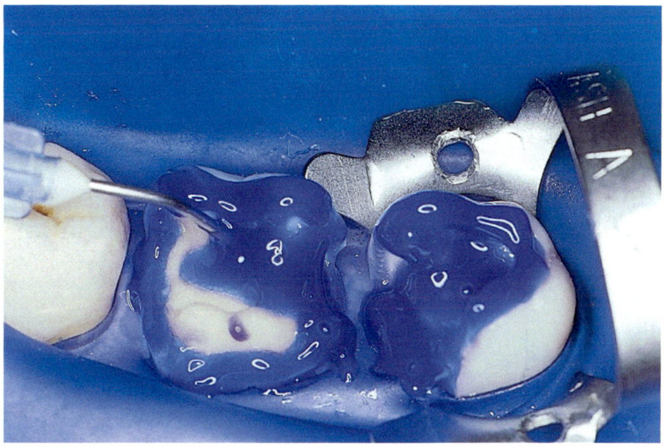

Fig 2-22i After a 20-second pause, the dentin is etched for 10 seconds.

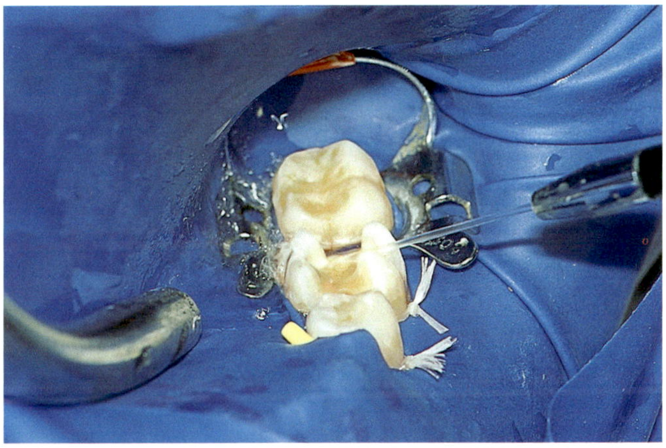

Fig 2-22j The acid is rinsed off with a water jet for 5 seconds.

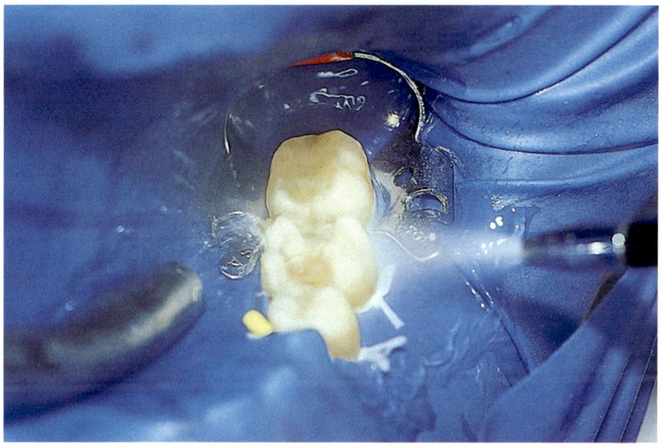

Fig 2-22k The acid is rinsed off with water spray for 10 seconds.

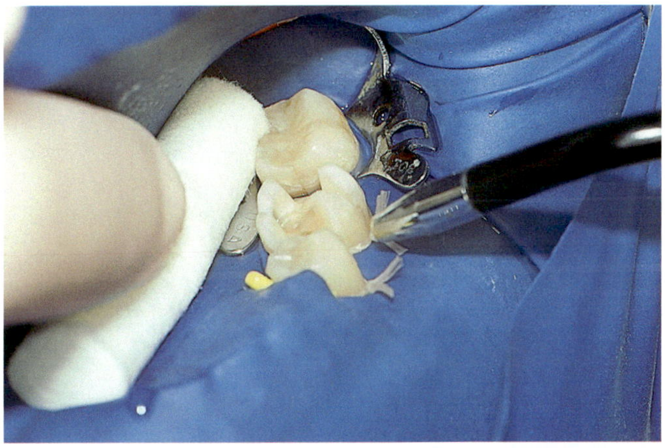

Fig 2-22l Drying is accomplished with the help of a cotton roll.

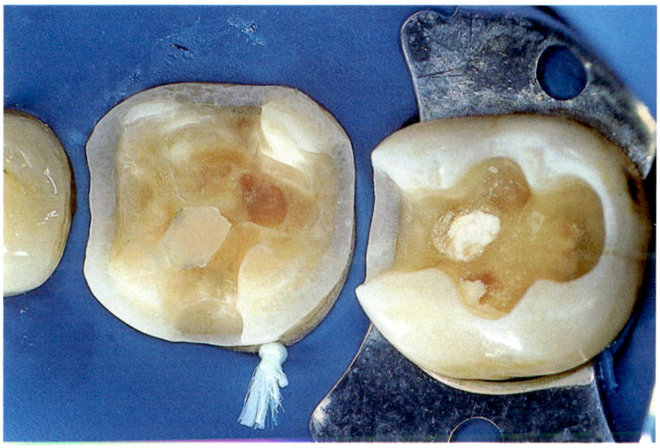

Fig 2-22m The etching pattern is checked.

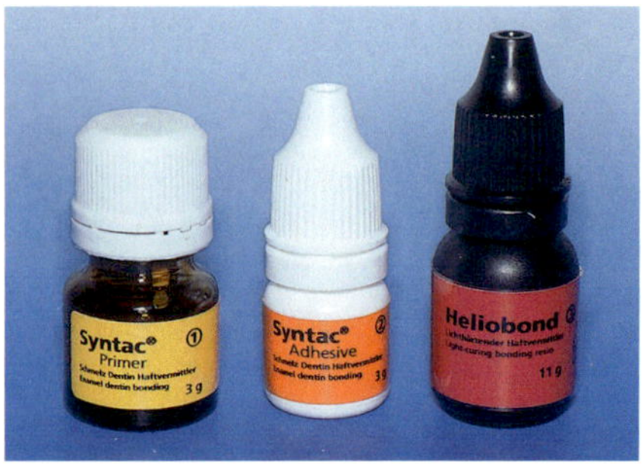

Fig 2-22n Primer, adhesive, and bonding resin.

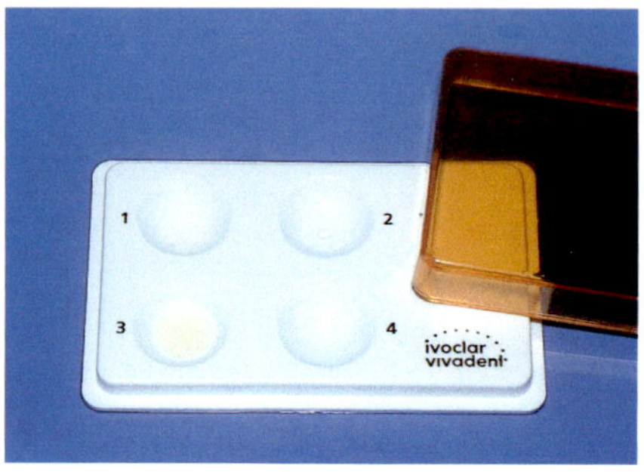

Fig 2-22o Palette with a light guard and numbered areas.

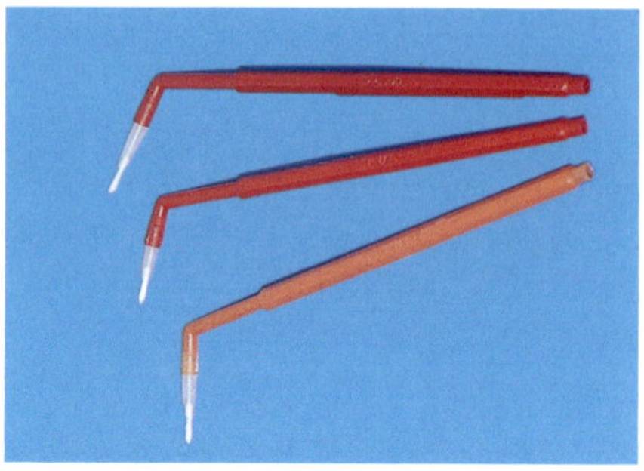

Fig 2-22p Disposable brushes with a color-coded sequence.

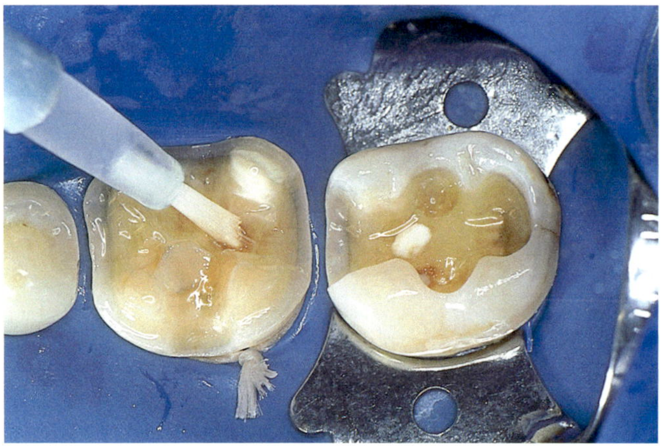

Fig 2-22q The primer is applied.

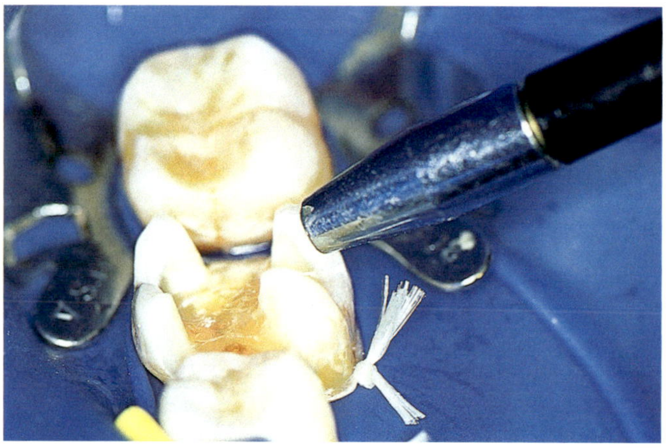

Fig 2-22r The primer is dried after 30 seconds.

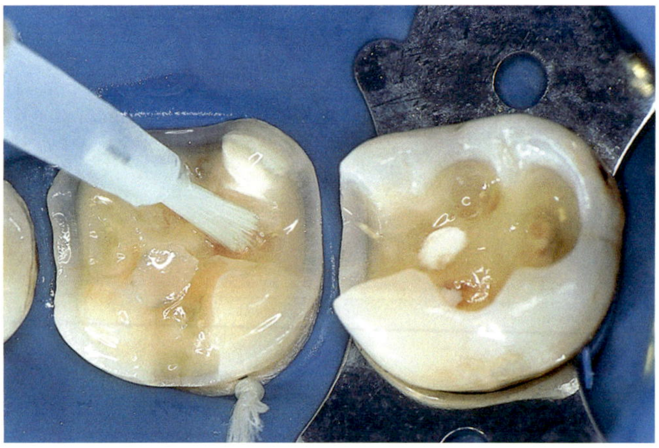

Fig 2-22s The adhesive is applied.

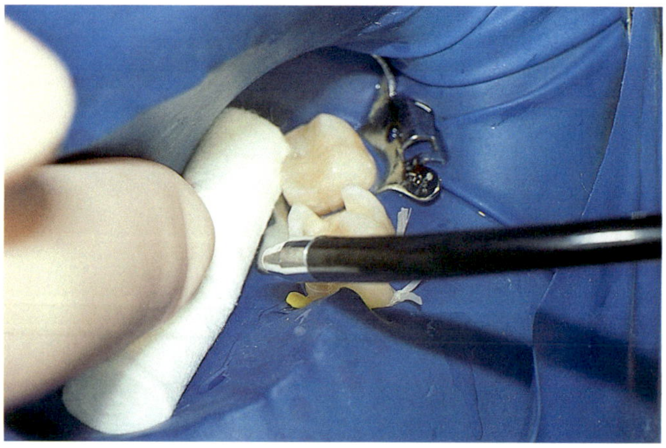

Fig 2-22t The adhesive is dried. A cotton roll can be useful.

adhesion just by showing the cavity the bottle! All-in-one systems are considered unreliable for indirect restorations and do not have a long shelf-life, a property the dentist is not able to judge well.

The primer from the first bottle is applied carefully with a brush and blown dry after 30 seconds (Figs 2-22q and 2-22r). As soon as the surface looks shiny, a thin layer of the adhesive bonding agent from the second bottle is

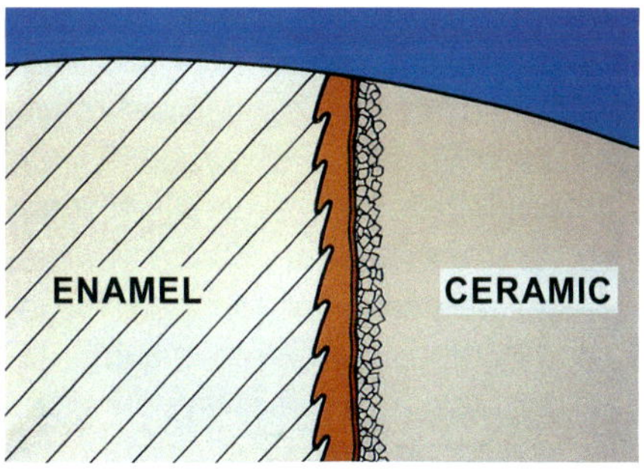

Fig 2-23a Enamel-ceramic interface.

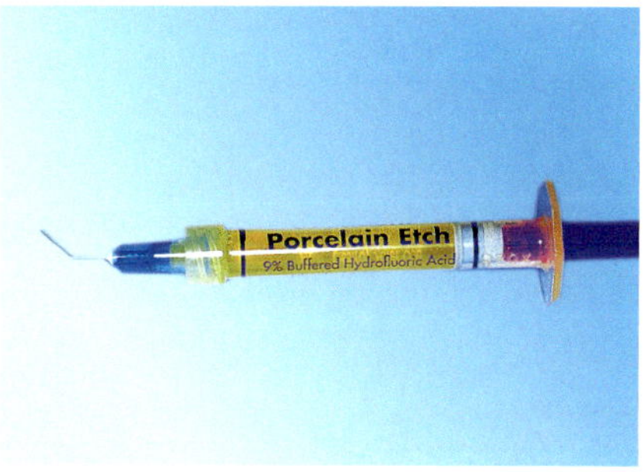

Fig 2-23b Application syringe.

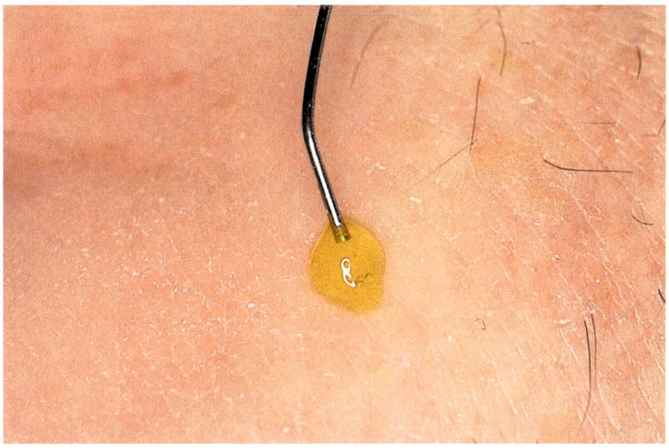

Fig 2-23c Skin test.

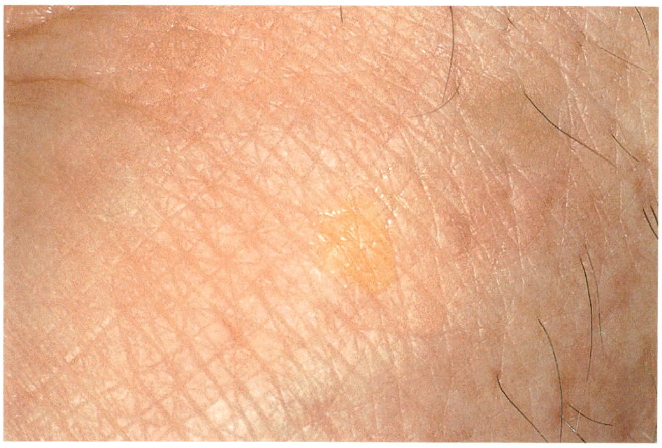

Fig 2-23d Discoloration is noticeable after 5 minutes, but there are no other effects on the skin.

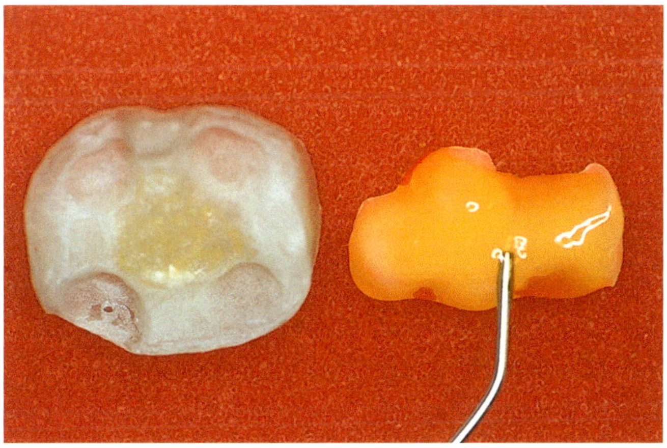

Fig 2-23e The base of the ceramic inlay is etched.

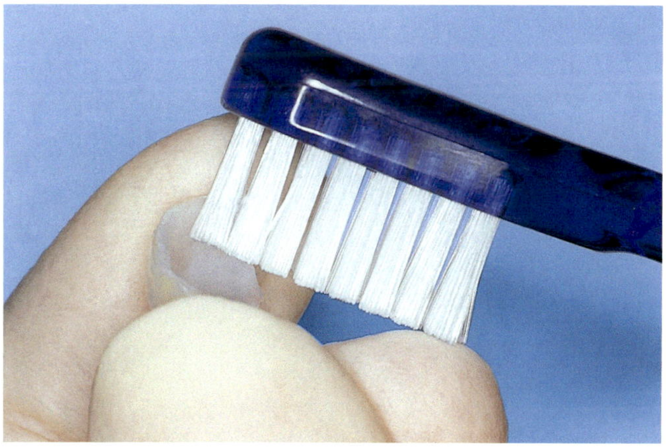

Fig 2-23f The inlay is brushed with a soft toothbrush with synthetic bristles.

carefully applied. The chip blower is used immediately to disperse the layer evenly and dry it (Figs 2-22s and 2-22t). The cavities are now prepared to receive the inlays.

Preparation of the ceramic inlays

The ceramic inlays are cleaned and dried after the try-in in the patient's mouth. They can then be conditioned (Fig 2-

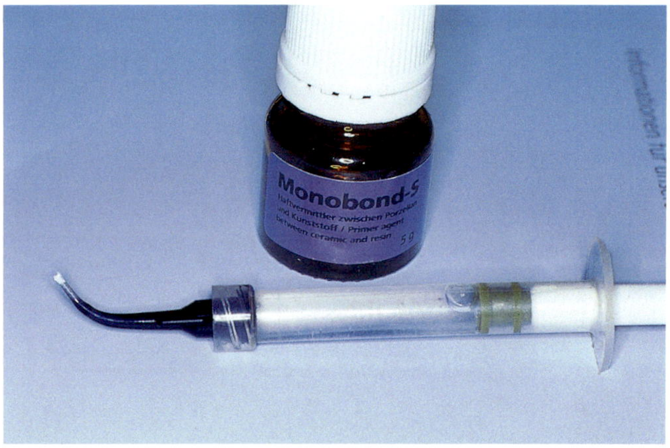

Fig 2-23g Silane with application syringe.

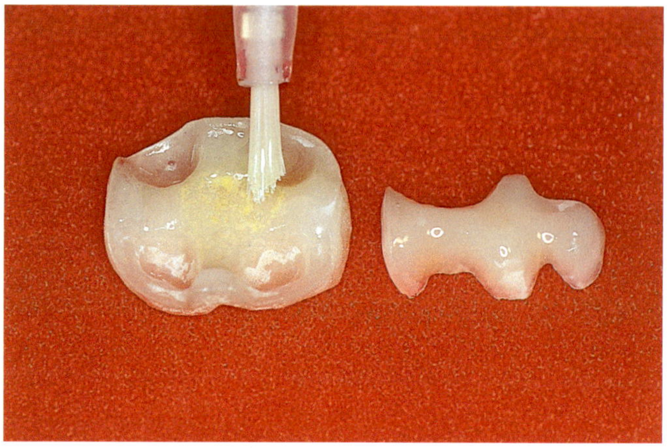

Fig 2-23h The silane is applied to the ceramic inlays.

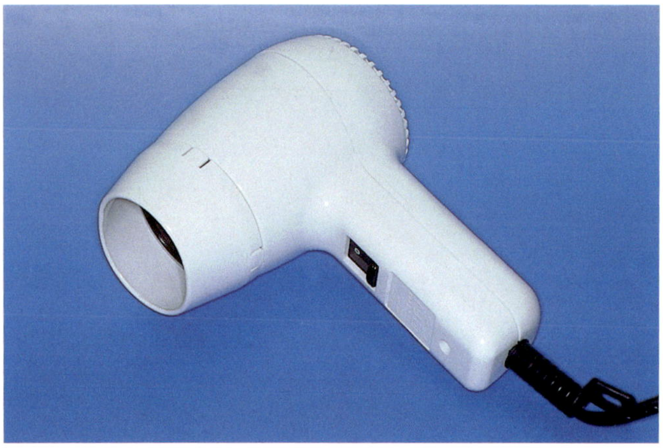

Fig 2-23i Small hairdryer.

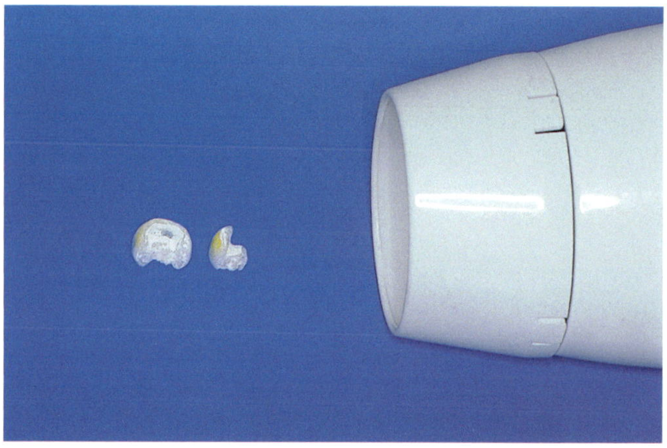

Fig 2-23j The inlays are dried and warmed with the hairdryer.

23a). Hydrofluoric acid (9.5%, Porcelain Etch) is applied to the undersurfaces of the inlays. The members of the dental team should wear eyewear to protect their eyes. Hydrofluoric acid gel has no effect on the skin but is extremely dangerous if it comes in contact with the mucous membranes (Figs 2-23b to 2-23e).

After 90 seconds, the hydrofluoric acid gel is rinsed off; care must be taken with ceramic sinks—a plastic cup should be used. The undersurfaces of the etched ceramic inlays are brushed with a soft toothbrush with synthetic bristles to remove any loose etching patterns that would negatively affect the adhesive bond (Fig 2-23f). The etching pattern is checked, and silane is applied to the etched surfaces with the application syringe (Figs 2-23g and 2-23h). After 1 minute, the silane is carefully blown and dried with warm air from a small hairdryer. The warm air is necessary to completely vaporize the solvent of the silane (Figs 2-23i and 2-23j). The ceramic inlays are ready to be placed.

Placement of the inlays with ultrasonic vibration

The inlays are placed following the principles of adhesive bonding, in this case with the Variolink System (Figs 2-24a and 2-24b).

A tough but workable dual-cure adhesive resin composite is mixed on a mixing pad (Variolink Ultra; Figs 2-24c and 2-24d). The cavities in the patient's mouth and the ceramic inlays in your hand are simultaneously dried and warmed with warm air. Warm and dry bonding surfaces hold much better than do surfaces that are only dried. While the ceramic inlays are brushed with bonding resin (Fig 2-24e), the cavities are lined with the highly viscous luting resin composite (Fig 2-24f). It is very important to have some excess material and to cover the margins thoroughly, because the adhesive resin composite—unlike cements with low viscosity that flow out toward the top—will only sag down into the cavities when the inlays are subsequently inserted with the help of ultrasound. (Some authors exclusively use light-curing resin composite. This is certainly worth discussing, although this author thinks that properly curing through all of the areas underneath the ceramic inlay can only be guaranteed with dual-curing resin composite.)

It is not necessary to brush the cavities with bonding resin. The ultrasonic vibration will wet the cavities adequately, although this step can be performed as well, if the dentist is concerned. The adhesive tip is used to hold the ceramic inlay, the first inlay is set on the appropriate tooth, and the inlay is placed with very little pressure onto the adhesive resin composite (Fig 2-24g). The ceramic inlay is vibrated into the cavity, with little pressure, through the help of the Sonocem ultrasonic tip (Fig 2-24h). The next inlay is placed in the same way.

The Sonocem tips can be obtained for all common piezo devices (Figs 2-24i to 2-24k). In the author's office, a threadcutter was used to adapt the tip for the air scaler in use. An ultrasonic scaler can also be insulated with a length of suction tube (Figs 2-24l to 2-24o) to prevent the

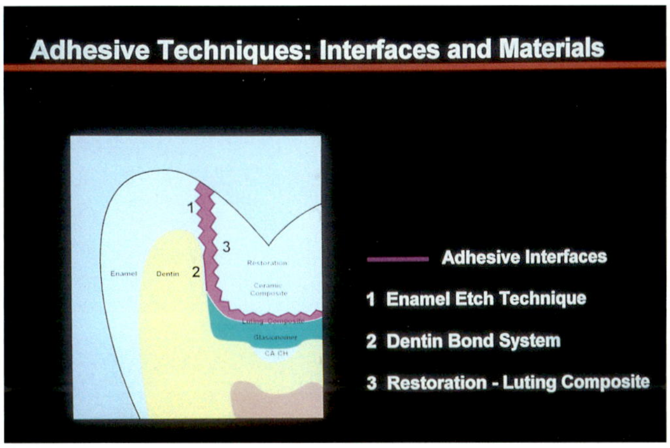

Fig 2-24a Interfaces in adhesive bonding.

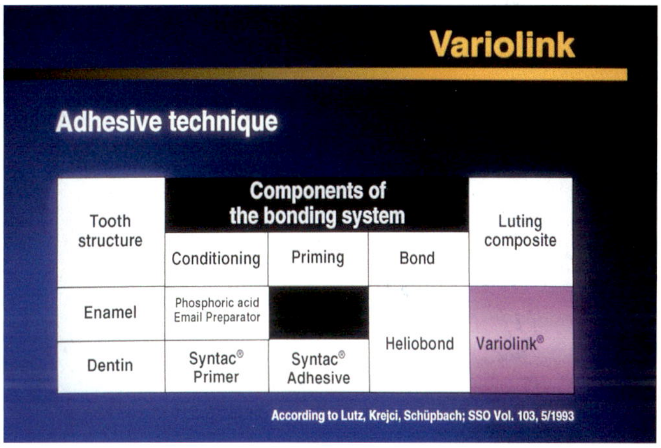

Tooth structure	Components of the bonding system			Luting composite
	Conditioning	Priming	Bond	
Enamel	Phosphoric acid Email Preparator		Heliobond	Variolink®
Dentin	Syntac® Primer	Syntac® Adhesive		

Fig 2-24b Interfaces and materials in adhesive bonding.

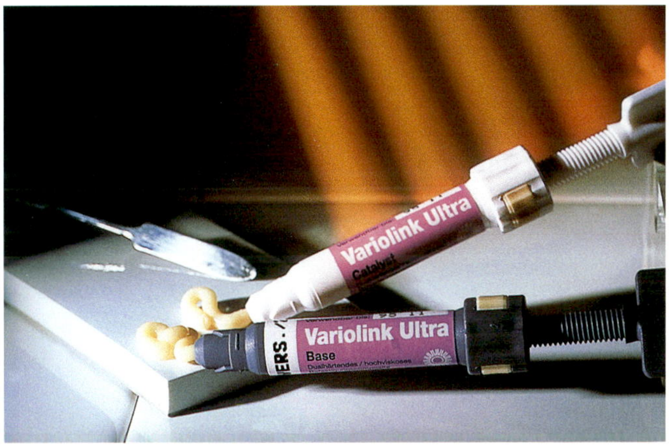

Fig 2-24c Highly viscous resin composite cement.

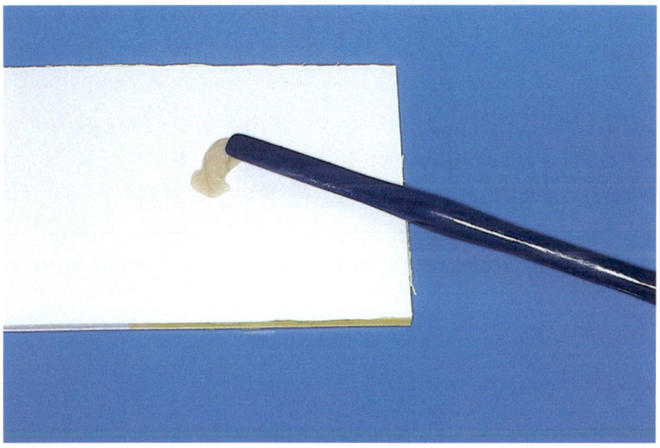

Fig 2-24d The resin composite cement is mixed.

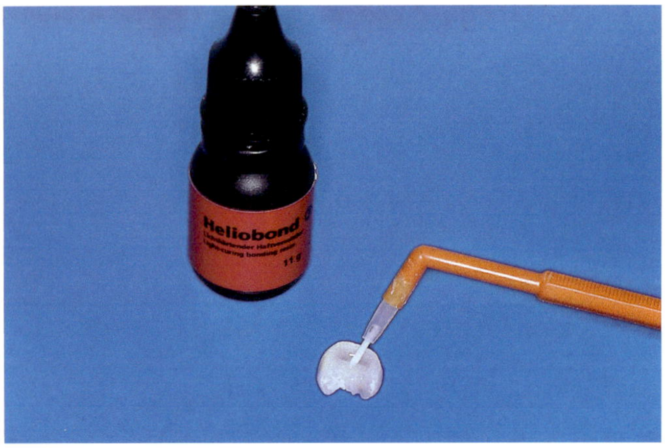

Fig 2-24e Inlay with bonding resin.

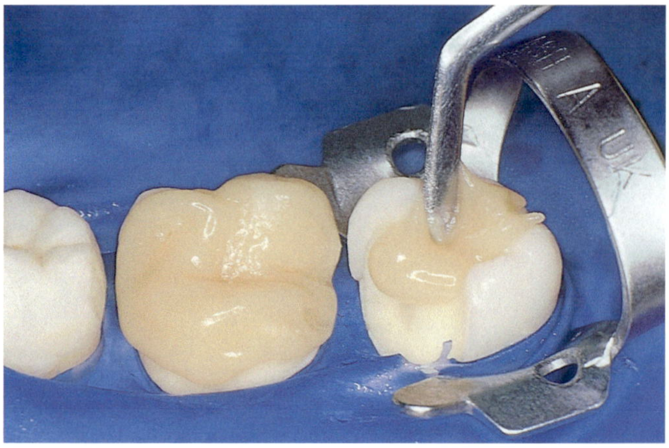

Fig 2-24f The cavities are lined with the strong resin composite cement.

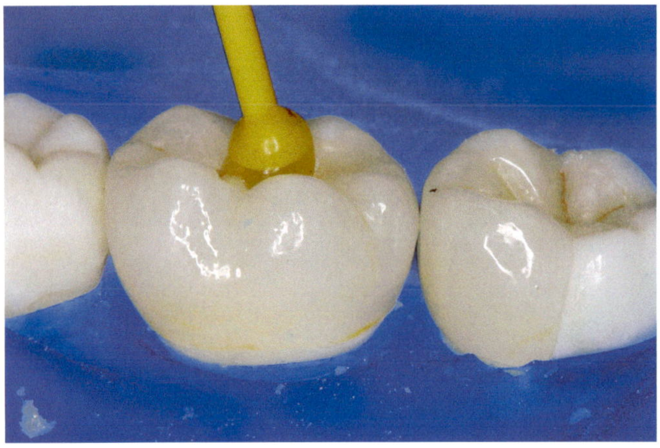

Fig 2-24g The ceramic inlays are placed in the cavities.

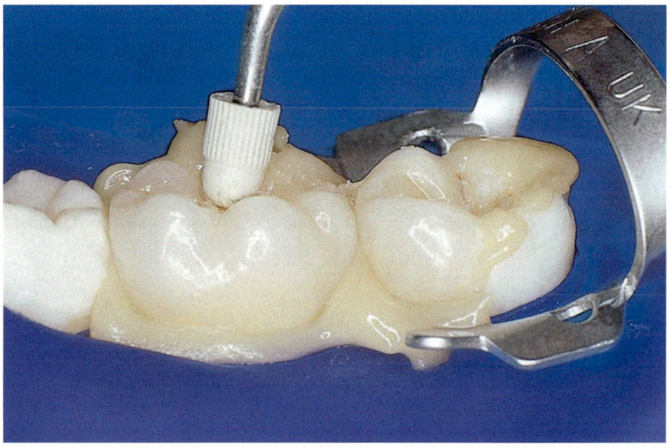

Fig 2-24h The ceramic inlays are vibrated in with the Sonocem tip.

metal from directly touching the ceramics when the inlays are vibrated into the cavities. This helps to avoid unattractive traces of metal abrasion.

After the inlay is carefully vibrated into the cavity (Fig 2-24p), the excess is removed with a scaler, spatula, and brush (Figs 2-24q to 2-24t). Then the inlay is vibrated in a second time (Fig 2-24u), and the accuracy of fit is checked.

Any excess material is removed with the brush. Then the ceramic inlays are fixed on the buccal side with the help of a curing light. The author uses a self-made aperture plate for curing to create a narrow beam (like in soldering) for not more than 10 seconds. Alternatively, a light tip could be used for fixation, although the light tends to diffuse despite being focused; this means the dosage of light cannot be measured as accurately as it can with the aperture plate (Figs 2-24v to 2-24z).

Fine cleaning is now begun. First, a length of Glide floss is run through the interproximal contacts (Figs 2-24aa and 2-24bb); then all excess resin composite is removed from the interproximal spaces with Super Floss (Figs 2-24cc and 2-24dd). A magnifying loupe is used to check whether all the excess material has been removed. To inhibit ambient oxygen and thus to prevent the margins from being cured insufficiently, glycerin gel is applied to all margins, including the interproximal space (Figs 2-

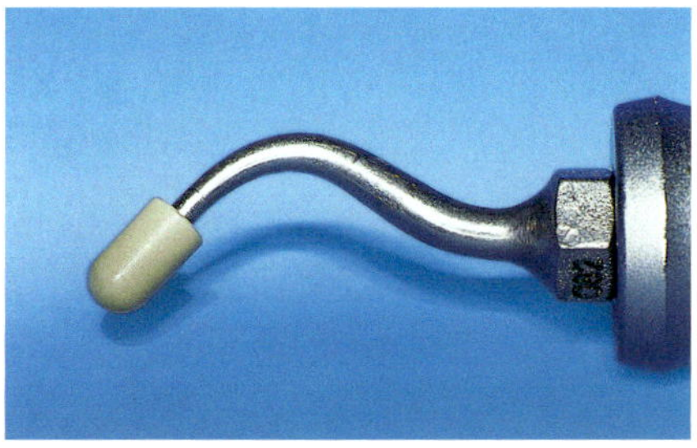

Fig 2-24i Sonocem tip.

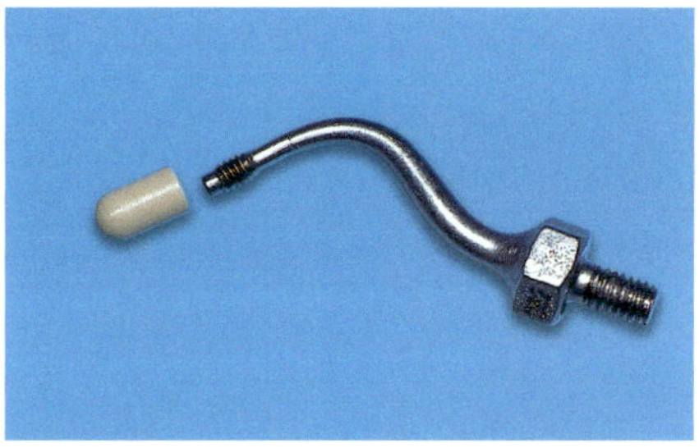

Fig 2-24j Sonocem tip with unscrewed Teflon tip.

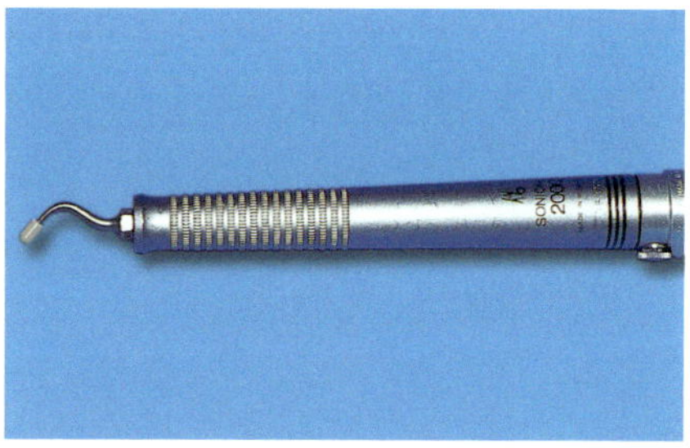

Fig 2-24k Air scaler with the Sonocem tip screwed in.

Fig 2-24l *(left)* Scaler tip.

Fig 2-24m *(right)* Length of suction tube cut to size.

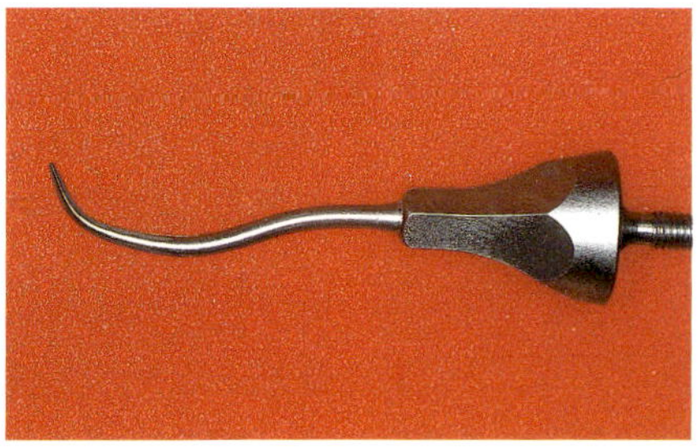

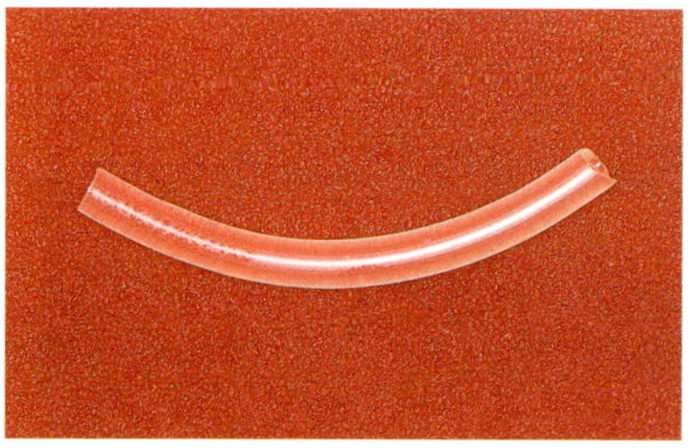

Fig 2-24n *(left)* Tube slid onto the scaler.

Fig 2-24o *(right)* The air scaler is prepared for vibrating the inlays into the cavities.

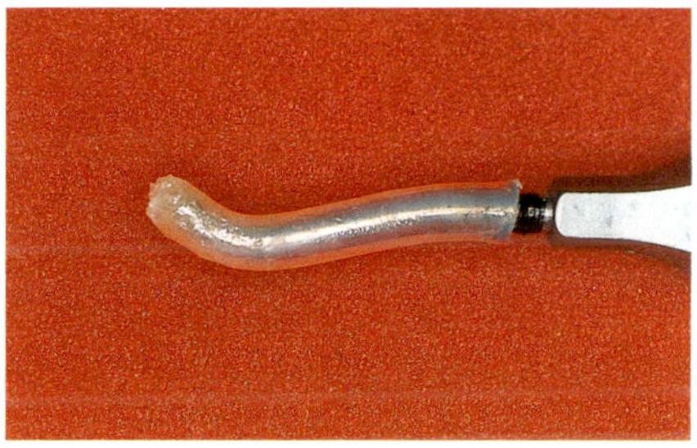

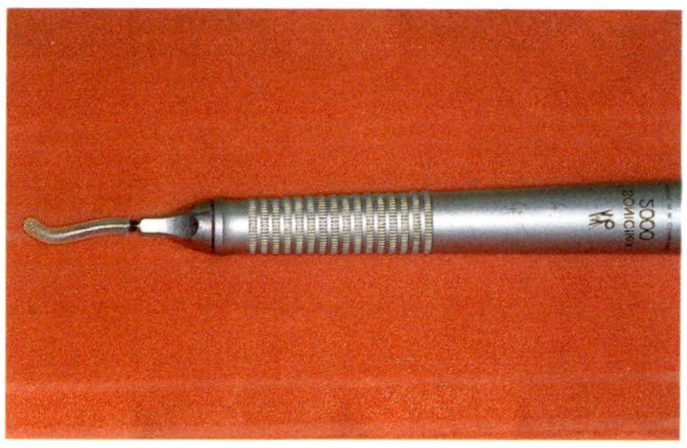

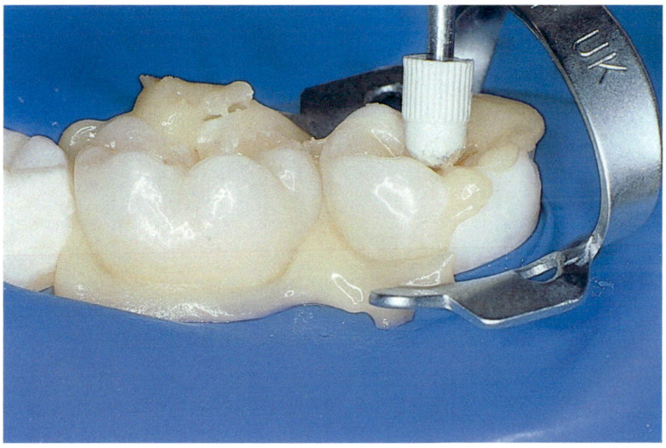

Fig 2-24p The inlays are vibrated into the cavities.

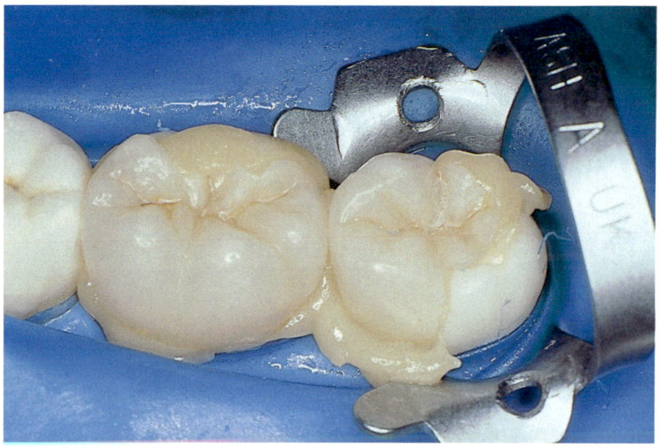

Fig 2-24q The excess cement runs off.

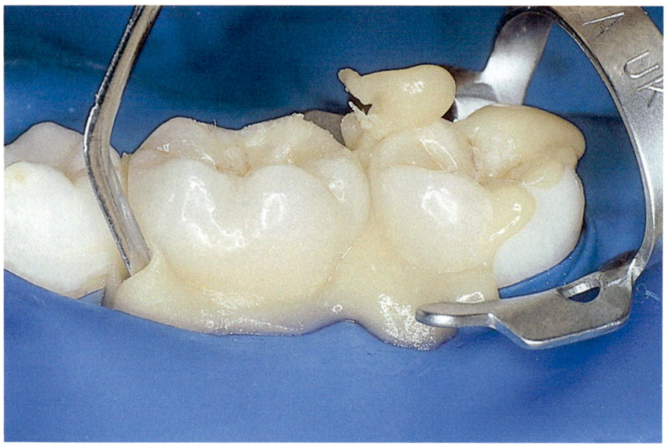

Fig 2-24r The excess is removed with the Heidemann spatula.

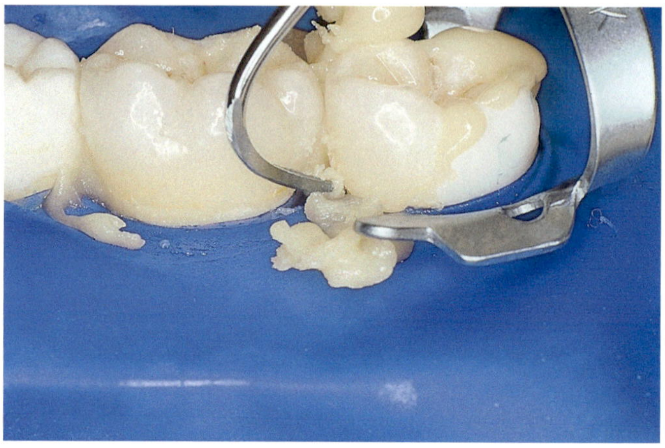

Fig 2-24s The excess is removed with a sickle-style cement remover.

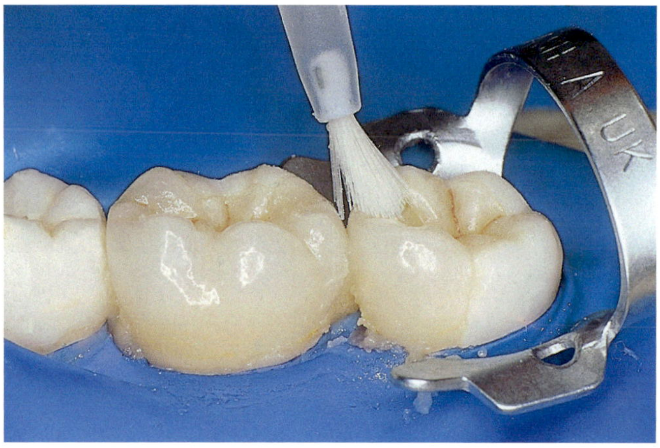

Fig 2-24t The excess is wiped off with the disposable brush.

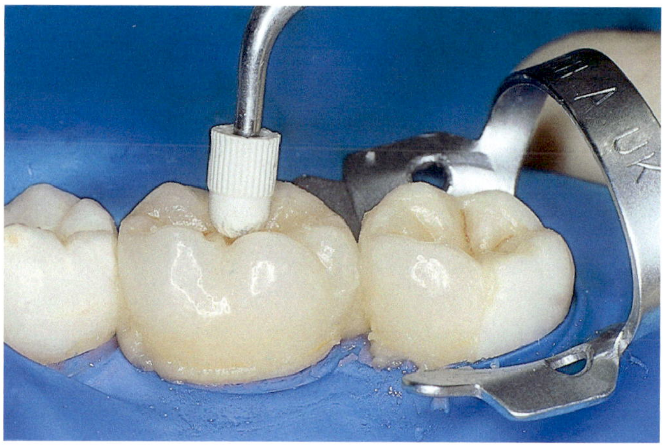

Fig 2-24u The inlays are vibrated again with the Sonocem tip.

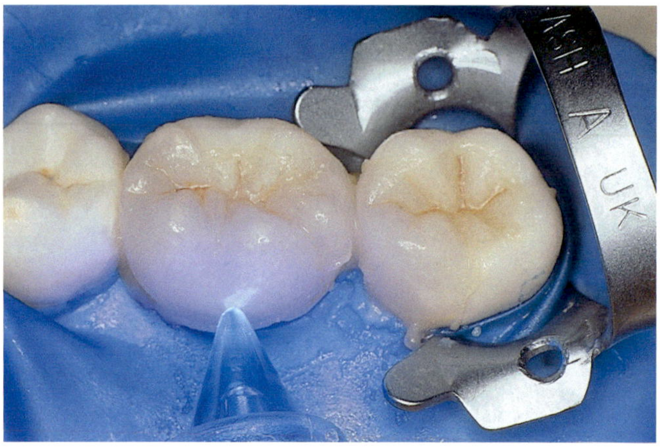

Fig 2-24v Punctiform fixation with the light tip at the mandibular left first molar.

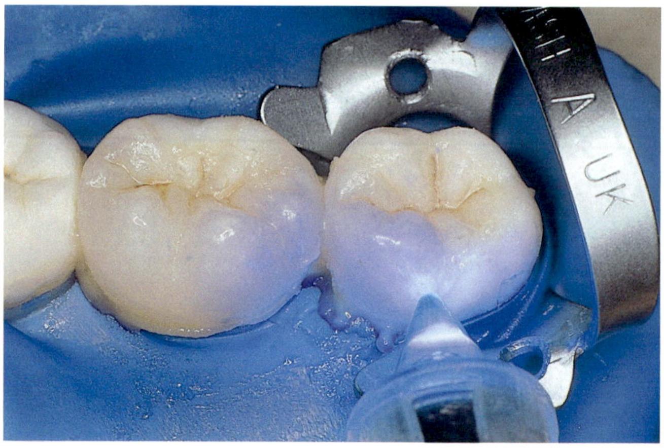

Fig 2-24w Punctiform fixation with the light tip at the mandibular left second molar (strong diffusion is visible in both figures).

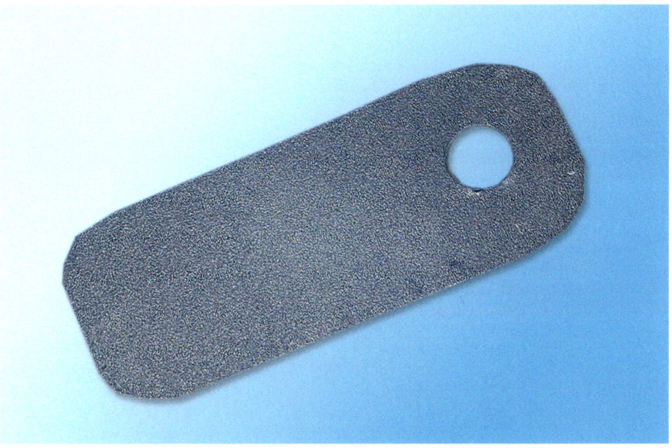

Fig 2-24x Self-made aperture plate. Opaque plastic film is cut to size and perforated with a paper-punch.

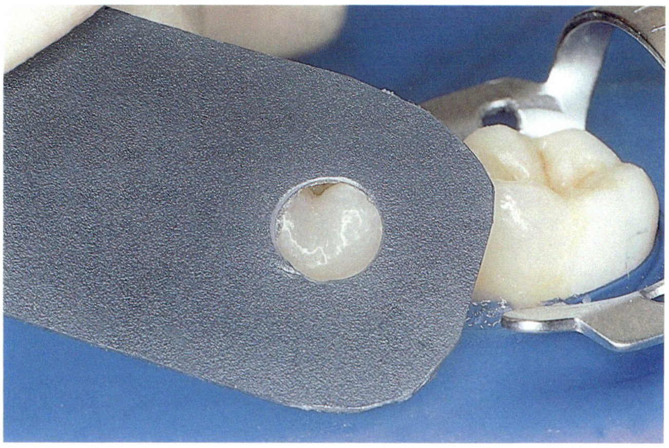

Fig 2-24y Aperture plate at the tooth.

24ee to 2-24gg). This helps to achieve significantly improved bonding margins. Final curing is initiated with two sufficiently strong curing lights (1,000 mW/cm^2) positioned opposite each other (Figs 2-24hh and 2-24ii).

All areas are polymerized from at least four positions for 40 seconds each. Rubber dam is removed, and the adhesively cemented ceramic inlays are finished with polishing disks and fine diamonds. The inlays are carefully ground to adjust the occlusion, and then all surfaces are thoroughly polished with very fine diamonds, rubber wheels, and Occlubrushes (Figs 2-24jj to 2-24mm). Fluoride is applied to the teeth to finish adhesive bonding (Fig 2-24nn).

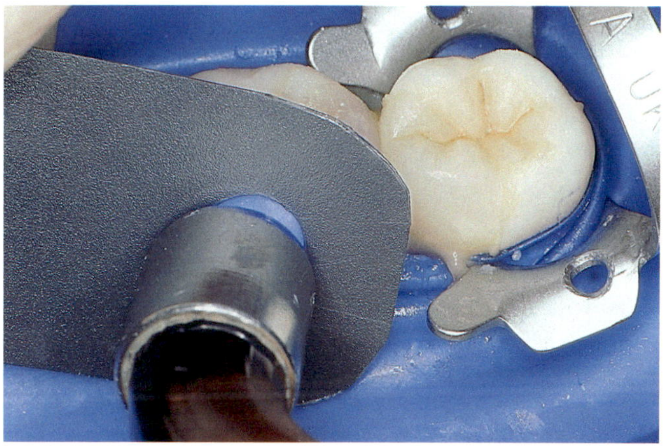

Fig 2-24z Fixation is accomplished with light passing through the aperture plate.

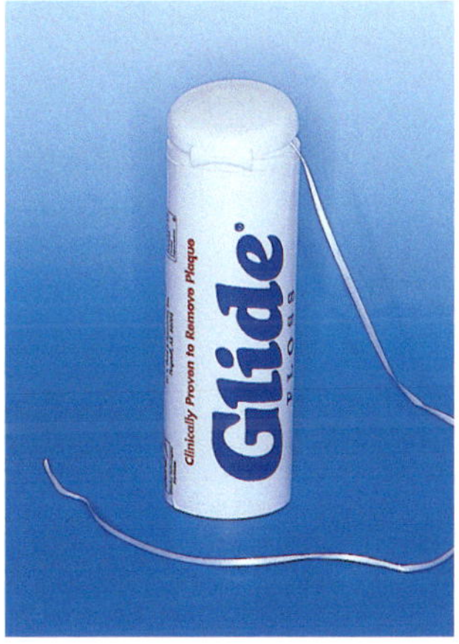

Fig 2-24aa Glide floss.

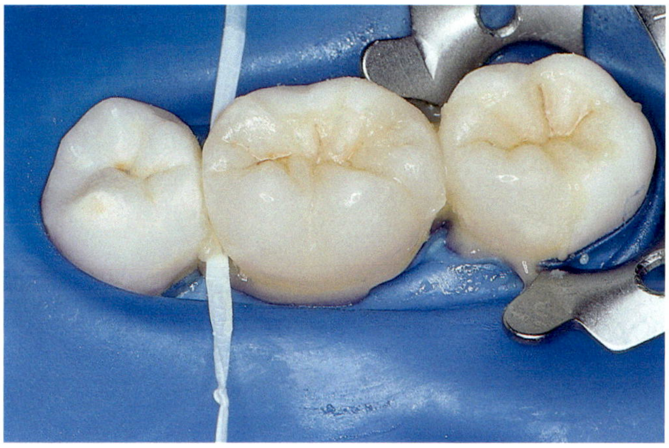

Fig 2-24bb The interproximal space is opened.

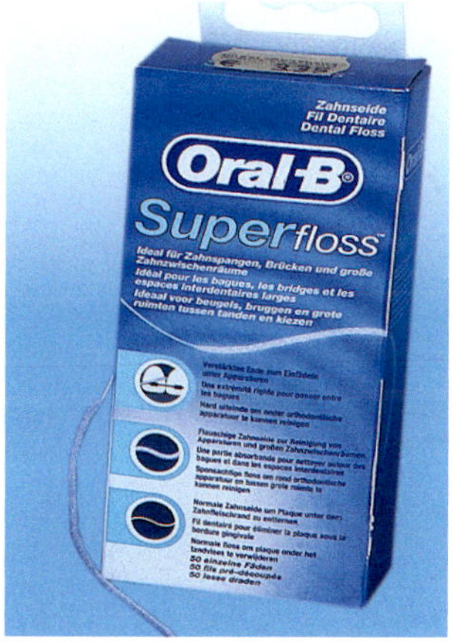

Fig 2-24cc Super Floss.

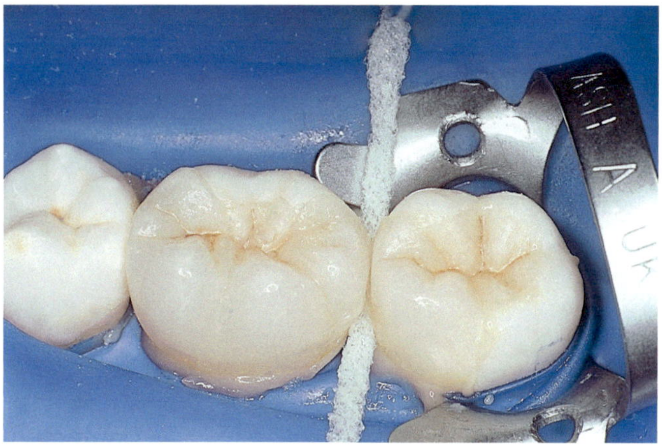

Fig 2-24dd The interproximal space is cleaned.

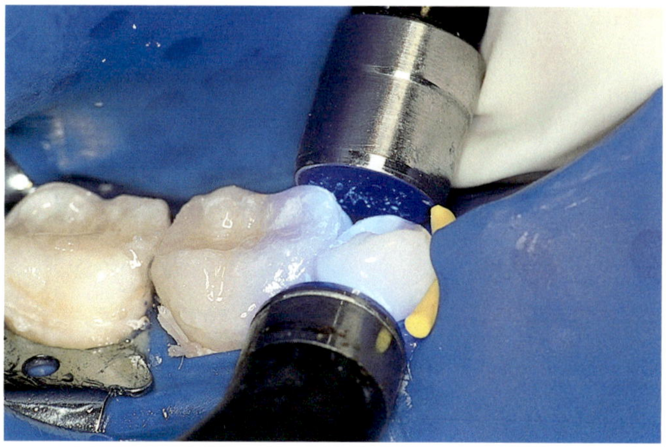

Fig 2-24ee Primary oxygen inhibition.

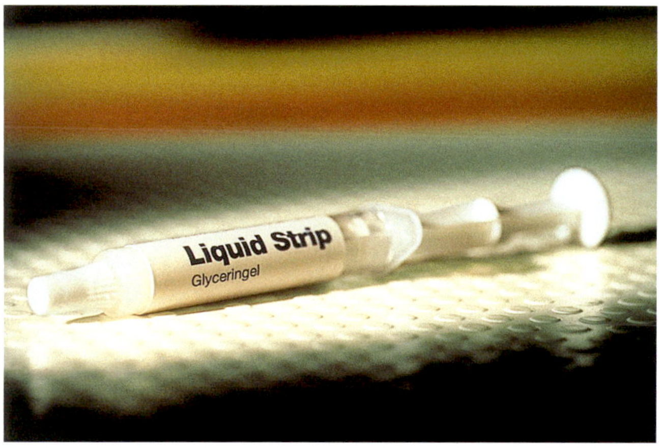

Fig 2-24ff Oxygen inhibitor gel.

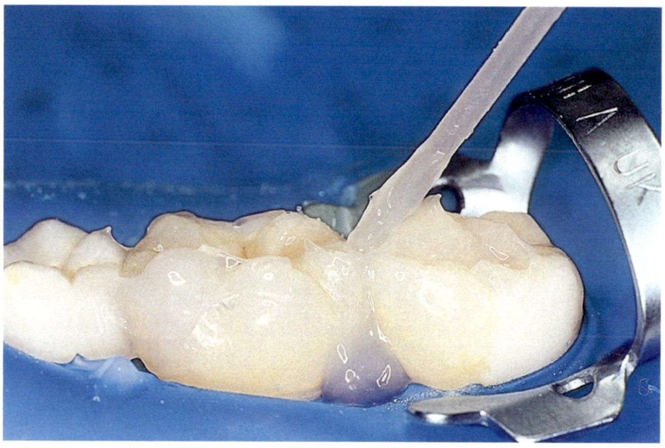

Fig 2-24gg The gel is applied carefully to all margins.

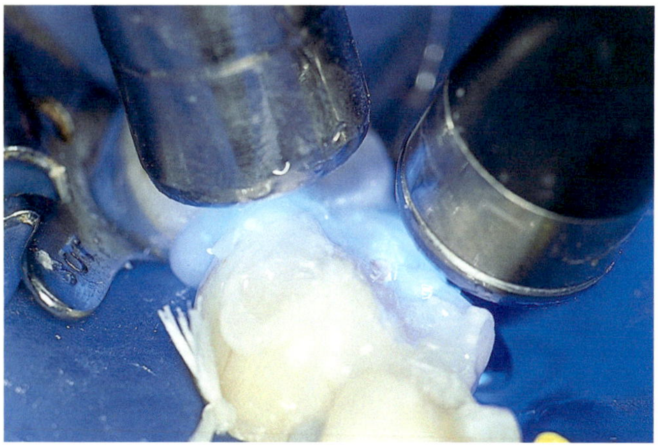

Fig 2-24hh Light curing with two light sources.

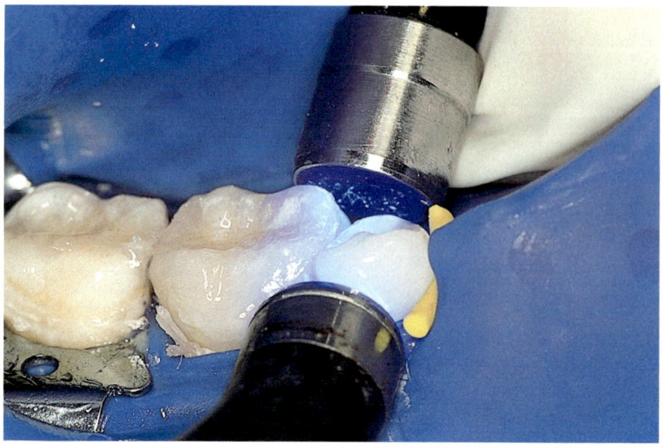

Fig 2-24ii Curing with two lights opposite each other to expose the entire tooth.

If any remaining edges can be felt in the interproximal space, they should be removed with the vertical diamond files (Profin system). If the fit is in doubt, a single-tooth radiograph should be taken (Fig 2-24oo).

The final check is carried out with a fine probe and a magnifying loupe. If an interproximal space is closed up, it can be reopened with the Proxo Planer, used with tilting movements. This should be done, however, only after the adhesive resin composite has been completely cured (Figs 2-24pp and 2-24qq). However, if the procedure described is used, such problems will rarely arise.

Over the course of the past 13 years, the author has adhesively cemented more than 1,000 ceramic restorations as described, and only a very few have had to be replaced. Of course these successful numbers are also based on the patients' good dental hygiene and on supervision and follow-up by the dentist and the hygienist.

The final images show the successful restoration with the adhesively bonded ceramic inlays (Figs 2-24rr to 2-24uu).

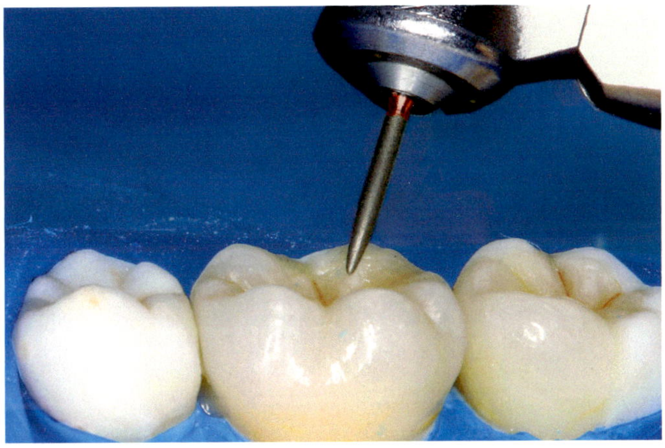
Fig 2-24jj Finishing with a fine diamond (red).

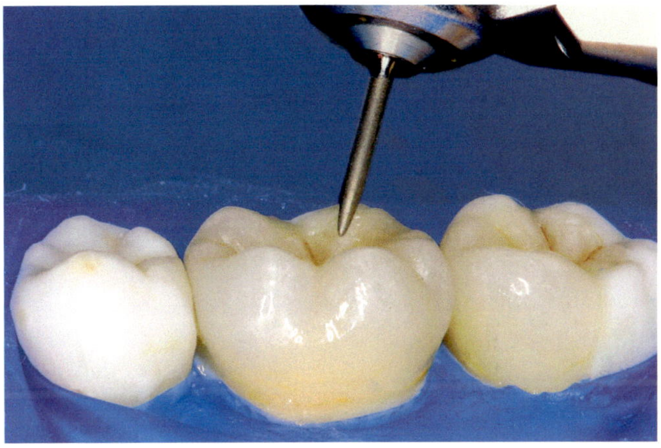
Fig 2-24kk Finishing with a fine diamond (yellow).

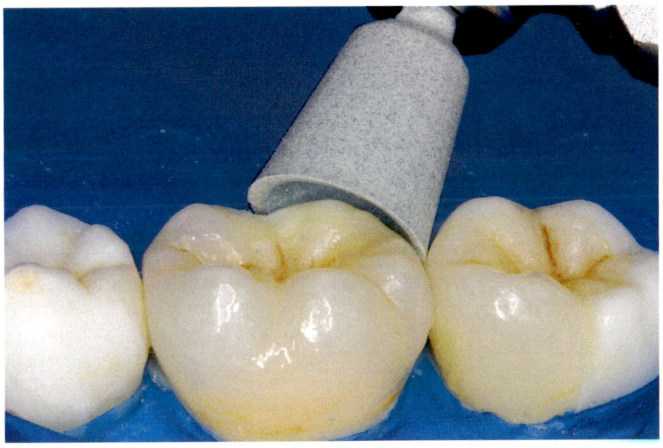
Fig 2-24ll Initial polishing with coarse polishing cups.

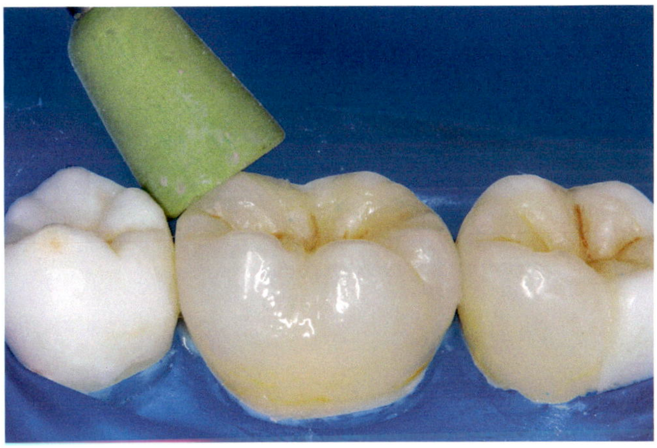
Fig 2-24mm Polishing with fine polishing cups.

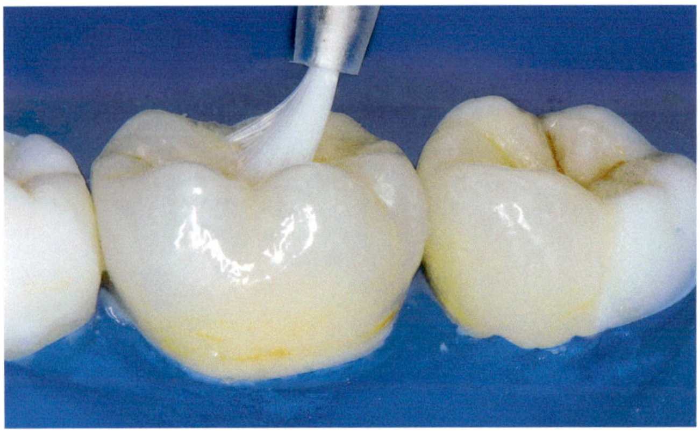

Fig 2-24nn Final application of fluoride.

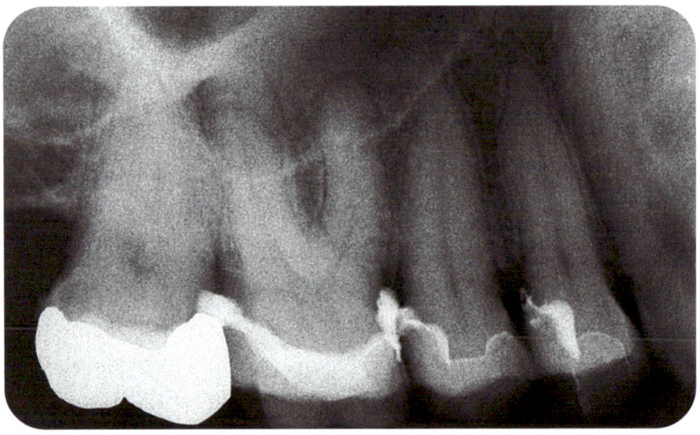

Fig 2-24oo Insufficient cleaning. There is an overhanging excess of resin composite cement.

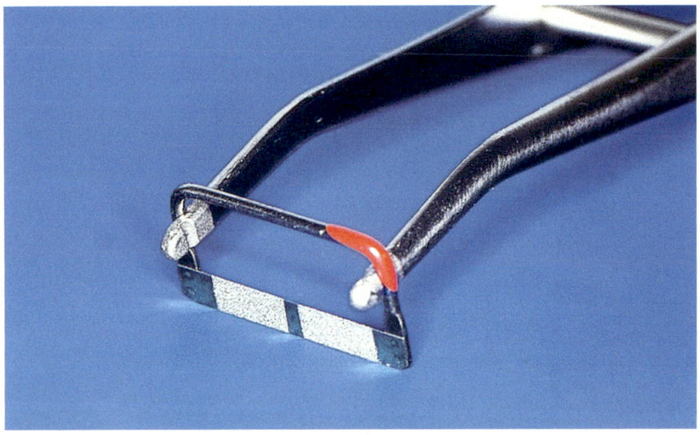

Fig 2-24pp Proxo Planer.

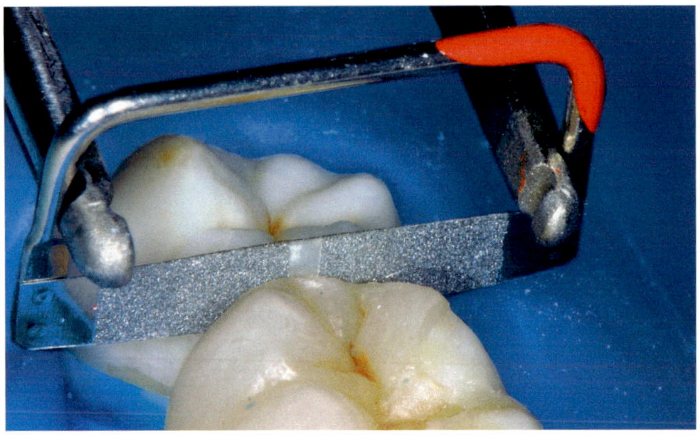

Fig 2-24qq The interproximal contact is opened with the Proxo Planer.

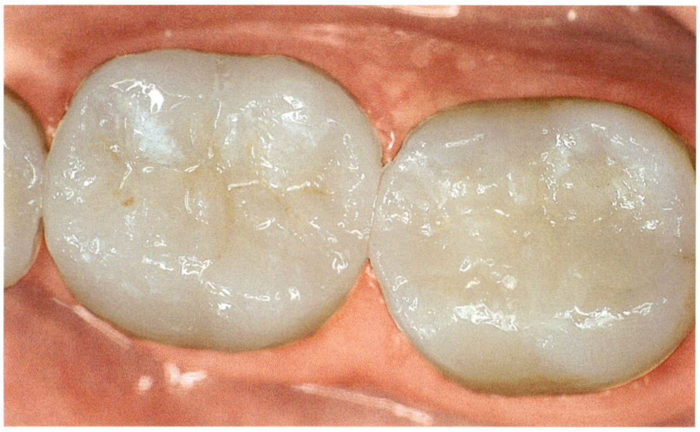

Fig 2-24rr Adhesive bonding is finished.

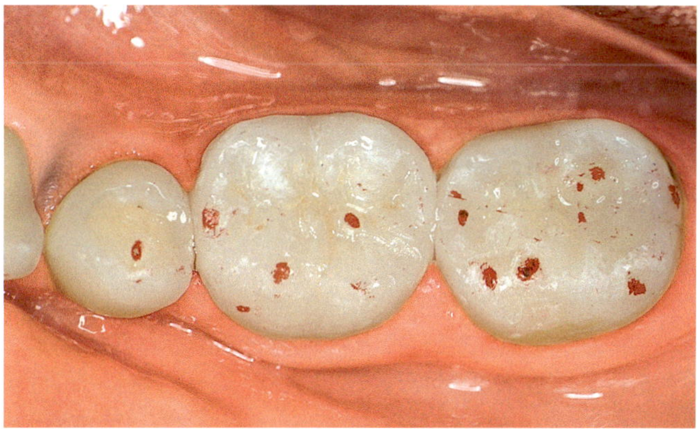

Fig 2-24ss The occlusion is assessed.

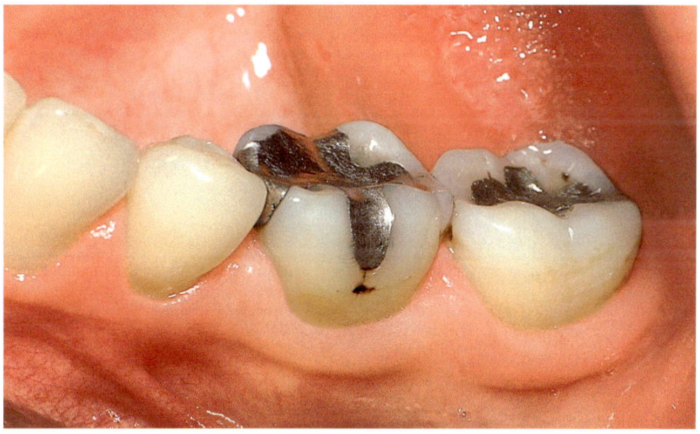

Fig 2-24tt Before restoration with ceramic inlays.

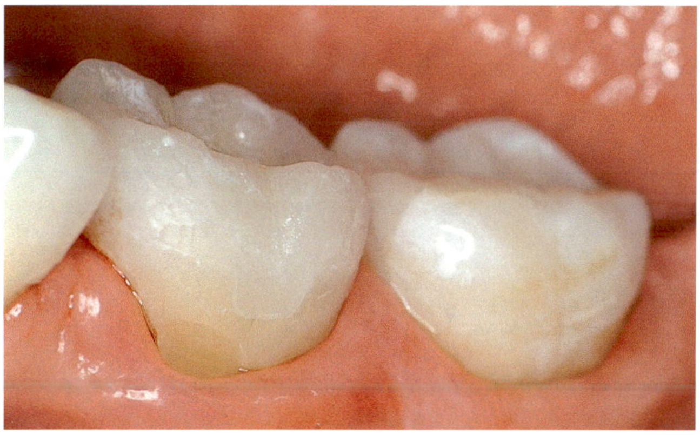

Fig 2-24uu After restoration with ceramic inlays

Materials

Tubulicid (Global Dental)
Ceramic inlays made from Empress pressed ceramics (Ivoclar Vivadent). There are a variety of high-quality inlay ceramics by other manufacturers;however, much more care should be taken with conventional feldspathic porcelain inlays.
Adhesive system (Ivoclar Vivadent): Syntac Classic dentin adhesive; Variolink Ultra adhesive cement; Liquid Strip glycerin gel for oxygen inhibition; and Fluor Protector for fluoridation. There are, of course, good systems produced by other companies, but the dentist should always stick to one chemically uniform system.
Etching and silanization products (Ultradent): Ultra-Etch for enamel and dentin; Porcelain Etch for ceramics; Silane for silanization; Ultrapak retraction cords; and Astringedent hemostat.
Provisional restorations: Perfect-Plast Kit for fast deep-drawing (Hager & Werken); Luxatemp Solar resin composite (Zenith); Durelon temporary luting cement (3M ESPE); Provilink temporary luting cement (Ivoclar Vivadent).
Preparation: Ceramic inlay kit 4263 (Brasseler); contra-angle for vertical files with a scope of 0.4 mm (W & H or Dentatus); Profin Directional System vertical files (Dentatus); Sonicsys system (KaVo).
Magnifying loupe, x6 (Eickhorst, Heine, Orascoptic, or Zeiss).
VivaStick placing instrument (Ivoclar Vivadent).
Xantopren blue (Heraeus Kulzer) or any other dark-colored A-silicone for the pressure spot test for ceramic restorations.
Try-in paste (Ivoclar Vivadent).
Moisture control: tearproof Keydent rubber dam sheet (American Dental); rubber dam clamps; Wedjets (Coltène Whaledent); and rubber dam stamp (Hygenic, Coltène Whaledent).
Sonocem ultrasound tip for common piezo systems (Sirona).
Aperture plate, cut out of dark plastic film and perforated with a hole punch.
Astralis 10 curing light (Ivoclar Vivadent). Very good curing lights are available from various producers. The light power density should be 1,000 mW/cm^2. Recently, LED curing lights with sufficient strength have been developed (eg, Bluephase, Ivoclar Vivadent).
Glide floss (Gore) and Super Floss (Oral-B).
Proxo Planer interproximal file system (Intensiv) for opening the contact points.
As a general rule, the dentist should always follow the manufacturer's current instructions for use.

Diastema Closure with a Matrix System and Resin Composite

Common problem: An anterior space troubles the patient

A woman paid a visit to the dental office after years of being troubled by an anterior diastema between the lateral and central incisors. She told us that she hardly ever dared to smile because of the ugly space. Her former dentist, who had placed the anterior crowns on both maxillary central incisors a few years previously, reportedly claimed that there was nothing that could be done about the situation and she had to live with it (Figs 2-25a to 2-25c).

After careful examination, the author discussed an esthetic solution to her problem and gave her a cost estimate. The suggested treatment included veneers on the maxillary lateral incisors and all-ceramic crowns on the central incisors to correct the displaced midline and allow for esthetic positioning of the incisors.

Because the patient did not have the financial means to permit this esthetically optimum solution, the following question arose: How could the space be closed in a reliable way?

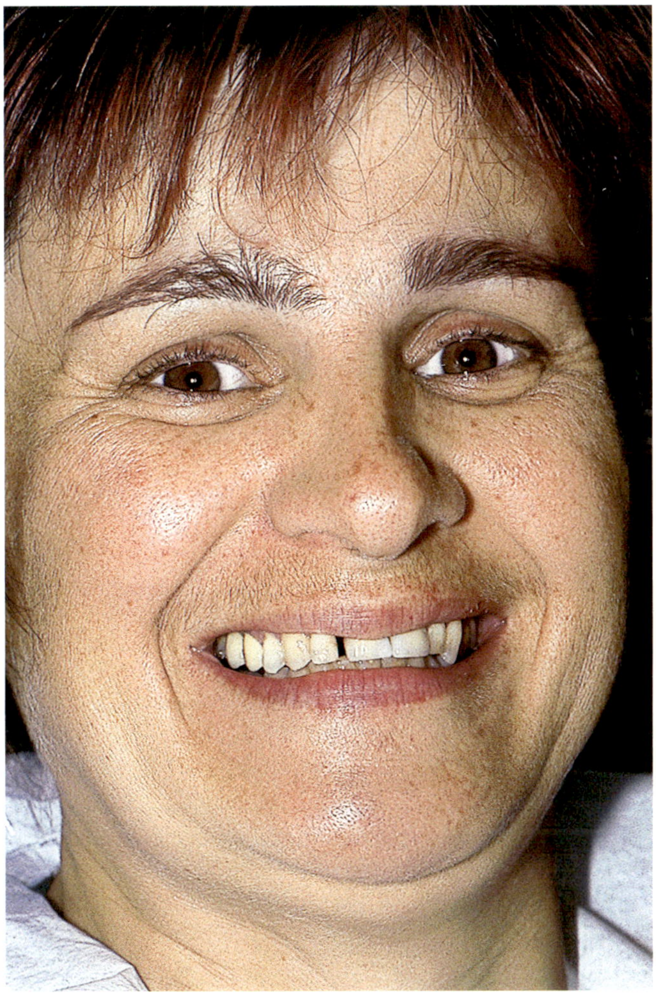

Fig 2-25a The patient is showing her anterior space with a pained smile.

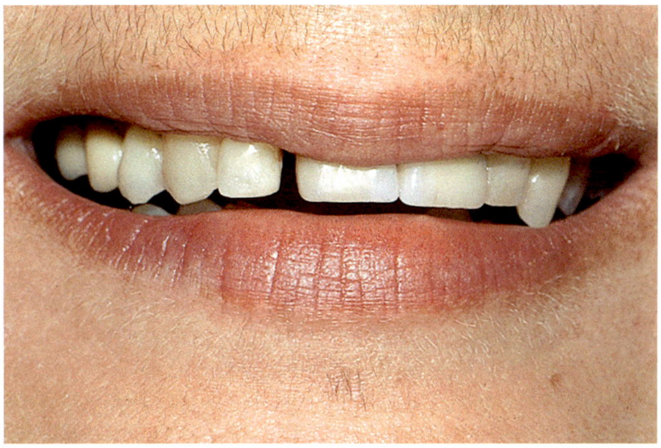

Fig 2-25b The bothersome gap is visible when she smiles.

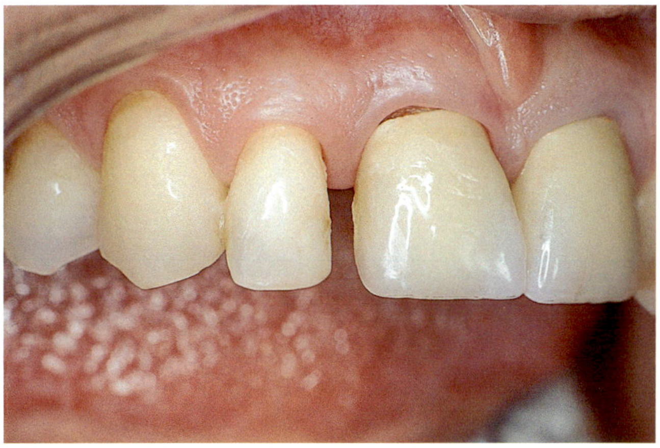

Fig 2-25c There is a space between the maxillary right central and lateral incisors.

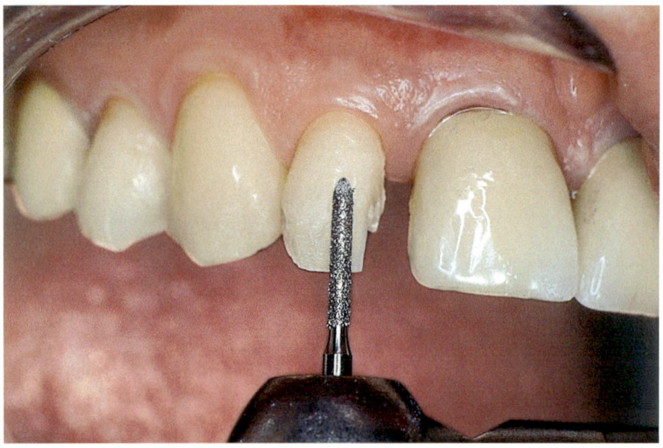

Fig 2-25d The restoration is prepared, somewhat below the gingiva in the proximal area.

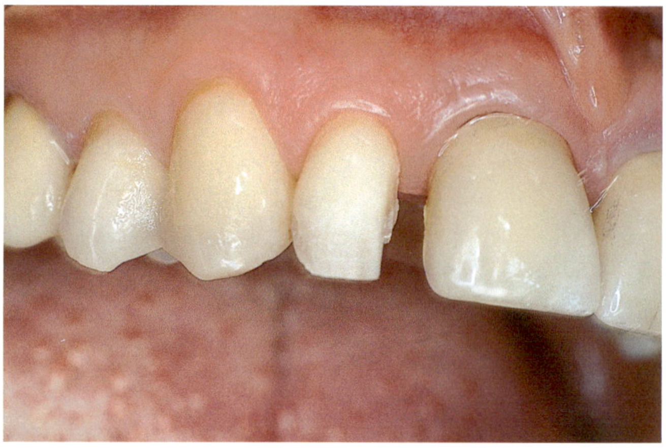

Fig 2-25e Finished preparation.

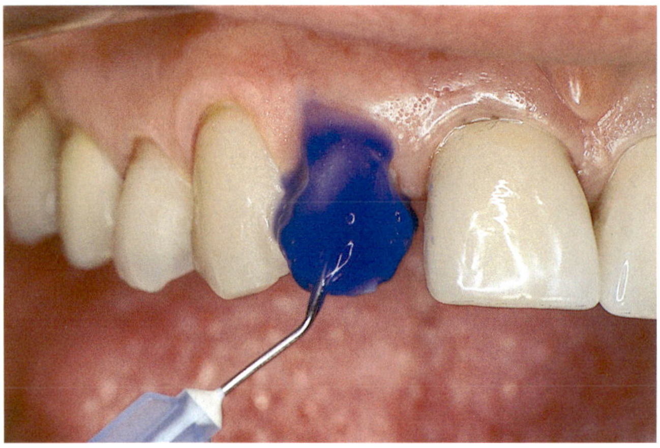

Fig 2-25f The prepared surfaces are etched.

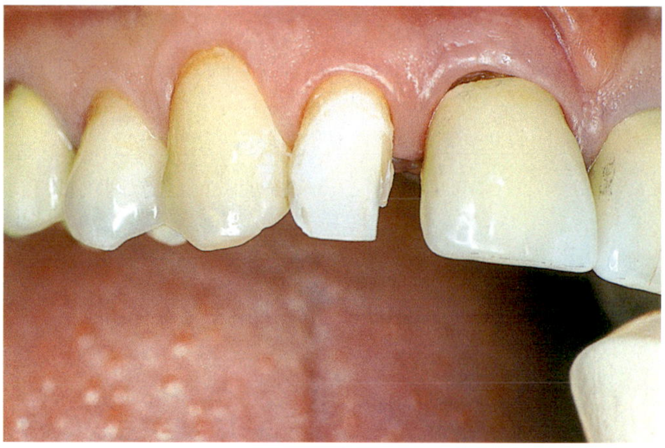

Fig 2-25g The etched surfaces are checked after irrigation and drying.

Proven solution: Space closure with a matrix system and resin composite

Spaces such as these can be closed with direct resin composite restorations, as is often done in orthodontics. The results are esthetically acceptable for a longer period. However, the clinician cannot work freehand to close a space—the result would be neither durable nor esthetically pleasing. Contouring of the margins in the cervical regions is especially hard to achieve satisfactorily. In most cases, the margin of the restoration will be incomplete or will protrude.

In the mid-1980s, Paul Belvedere designed an entirely new matrix system, known as Contour Strip, which is suitable for the following indications in the resin composite technique: Class V restorations; broadening teeth; direct veneers; and repairing cervical facings.

The only reason the Contour Strip had such difficulty becoming established was that nobody ever seemed to have read the instructions for use—which were by no means complicated and even had illustrations. The result was that the Contour Strip was completely misused, which caused an excellent matrix system to fall into oblivion.

The Contour Strip has two particularly noteworthy features: perfect marginal integrity (centrally, in the cervical area, and in the interproximal space) and total moisture control in the adhesive working area.

So there is hope for this patient. With the help of the Contour Strip and resin composite, the space between the maxillary right central and lateral incisors can be closed reliably.

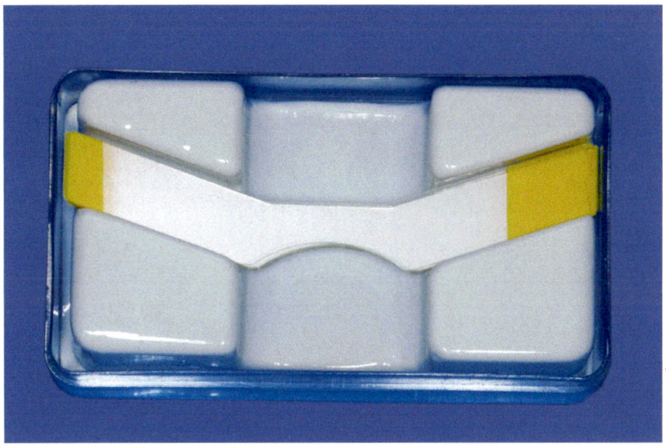

Fig 2-25h Contour Strip: a sophisticated matrix.

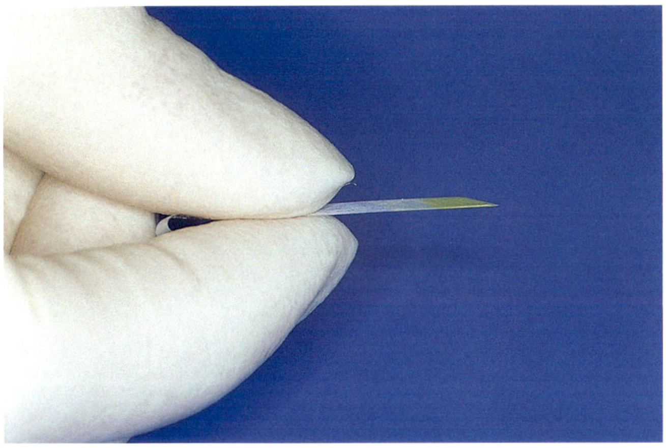

Fig 2-25i The strip is rolled between two fingers with gentle pressure. It should not be bent.

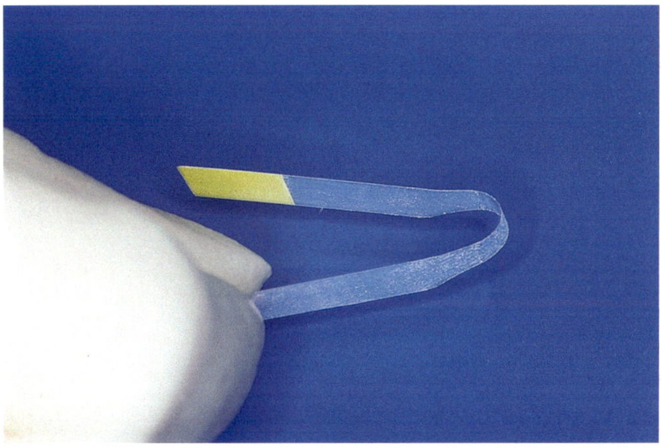

Fig 2-25j The strip has the desired shape.

Step-by-step technique

The mesial restoration was removed from the lateral incisor and a cavity for a direct veneer was prepared with a mesial extension toward the central incisor. The proximal area somewhat below the gingiva and the entire labial surface centrally were prepared with chamfers with a torpedo diamond bur (Figs 2-25d and 2-25e). The prepared surfaces were etched for 30 seconds with phosphoric acid gel, irrigated, and dried (Figs 2-25f and 2-25g).

A Contour Strip was removed from its pack (Fig 2-25h). The different sections of the Strip are visible in the figure: a straight upper part, a curved cervical part, and proximocervical wings.

The Contour Strip was held between two fingers and rolled with gentle pressure to give it a curvature that corresponded to that of the tooth (Figs 2-25i and 2-25j). The proximocervical wings were bent toward the inside with pointed flat-nose pliers (Figs 2-25k and 2-25l). To create a concave curvature for the cervical area of the tooth, the grip of a probe was used to make the matrix bulge out (Figs 2-25m and 2-25n).

The shaped strip was dried with the chip blower and adapted to the tooth, slipping the cervical part underneath the gingiva (Figs 2-25o and 2-25p). A cannula was attached to the bottle that contains the bonding agent; this enabled application of a thin layer of bonding agent to the outside of the strip (Fig 2-25q). The bonding agent was polymerized immediately with a curing light (Fig 2-25r). This fastened the strip along the gingiva at the cervix and created a tight seal. The effect of the bonding agent to the gingiva corresponds to that of adhesive tape.

Because the tooth was to be broadened to close the space, the strip was glued proximally to the distal surface

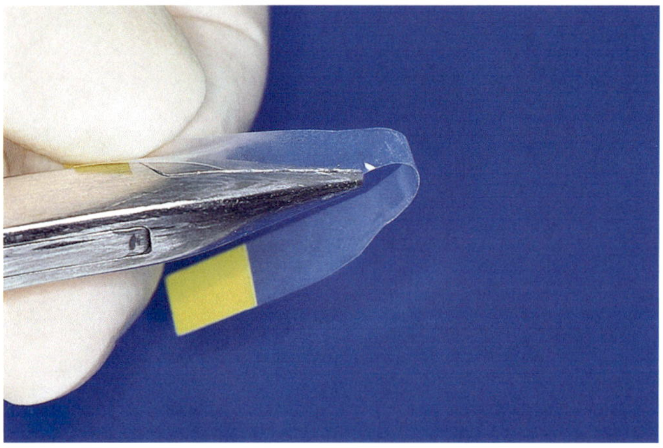

Fig 2-25k The proximocervical wings are bent with pointed flat-nose pliers.

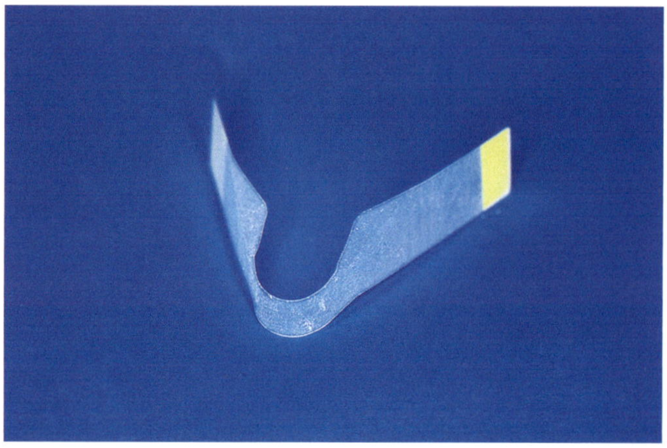

Fig 2-25l The strip is shaped so it adapts cervically.

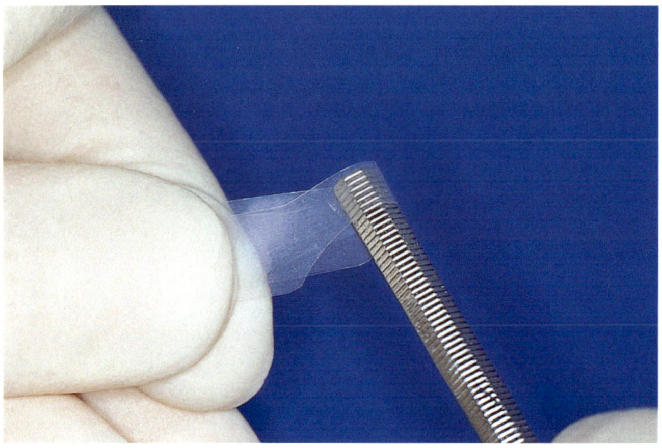

Fig 2-25m The strip is given a concave shape with the grip of a probe.

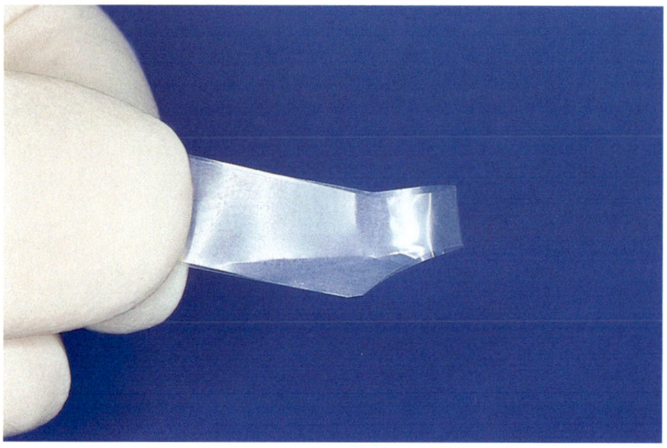

Fig 2-25n Correctly shaped strip.

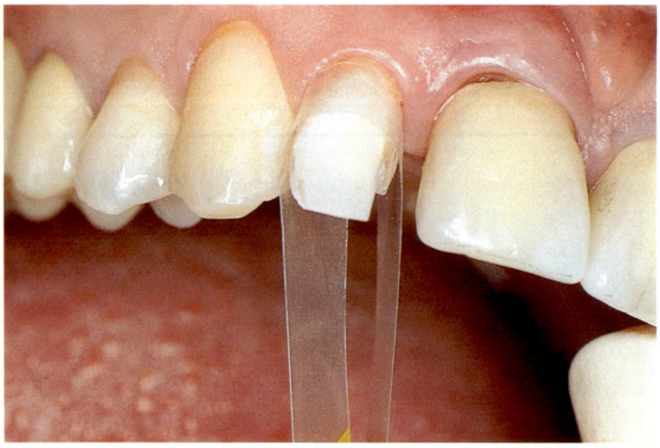

Fig 2-25o The strip is placed under the gingiva and adapted to the lateral incisor.

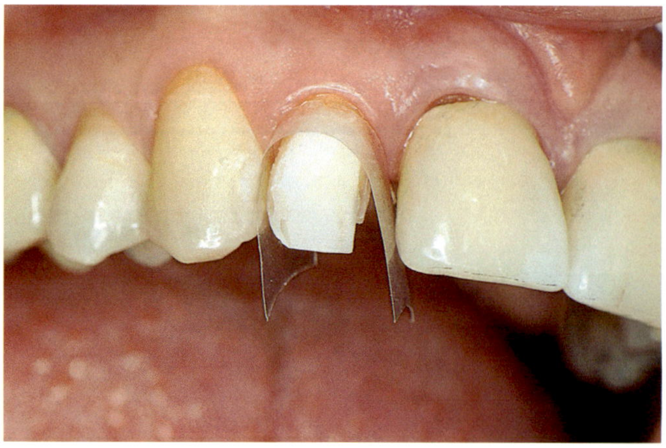

Fig 2-25p The ends that were sticking out palatally are cut off.

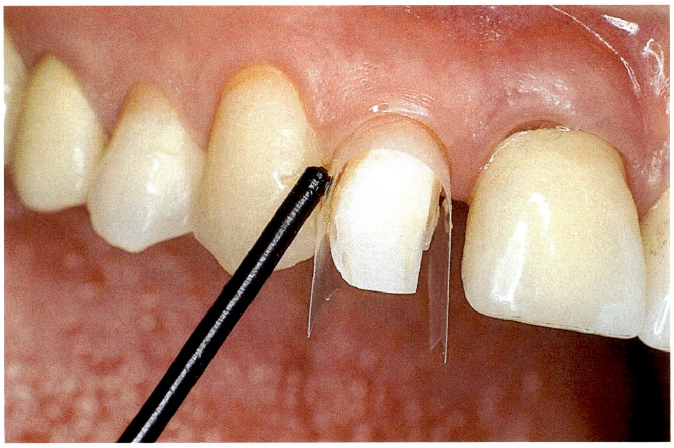

Fig 2-25q The bonding agent is applied on the outside with a cannula.

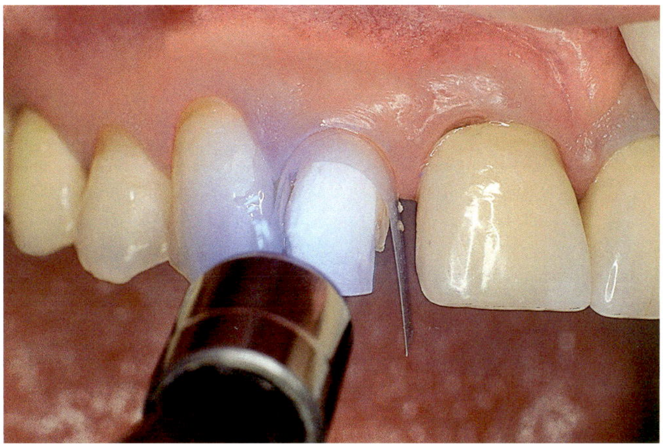

Fig 2-25r Immediate curing is performed with a curing light.

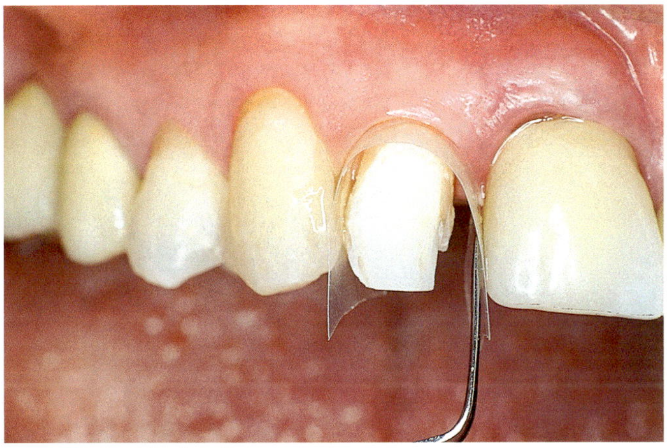

Fig 2-25s The matrix is adapted to the adjacent central incisor with a spatula.

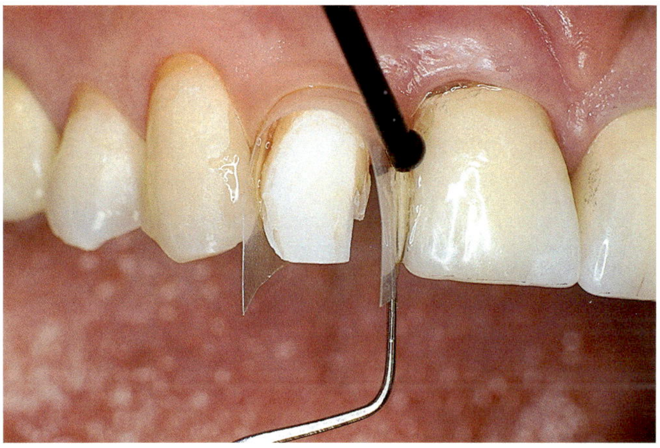

Fig 2-25t The matrix is bonded to the adjacent central incisor.

of the central incisor with the bonding agent (Figs 2-25s and 2-25t). The entire prepared and etched surface was covered with a thin layer of bonding agent and precured (Fig 2-25u). The opaque dentin shade A3.5 was syringed into the proximal area and shaped carefully with a flat, narrow watercolor brush (Figs 2-25v and 2-25w). Two lights were used to cure from the palatal and labial angles simultaneously. This saved time and ensured thorough curing throughout the material (Fig 2-25x).

The cover layer, enamel shade D3, was applied, shaped with the brush, and cured (Figs 2-25y to 2-25aa). The bonding material on the outside of the matrix was removed with a sickle-style cement remover (Fig 2-25bb). Then the Contour Strip was removed as a whole with pointed flat-nose pliers (Figs 2-25cc and 2-25dd).

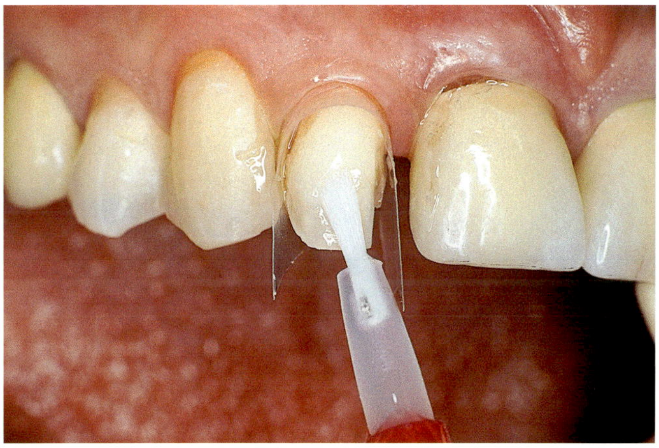

Fig 2-25u A thin layer of bonding agent is applied to the surface and cured.

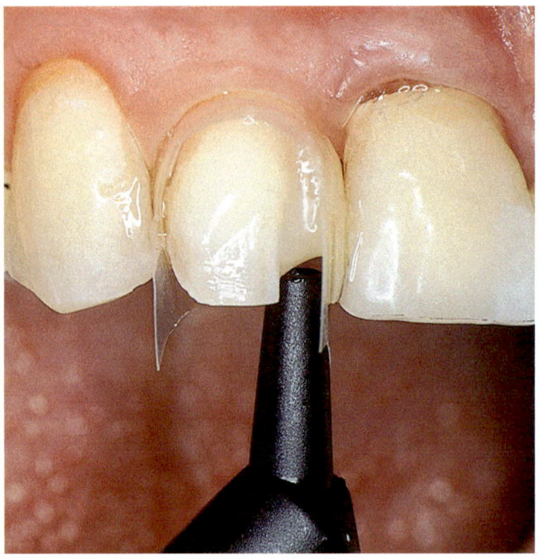

Fig 2-25v The dentin resin composite shade A3.5 is applied with a syringe.

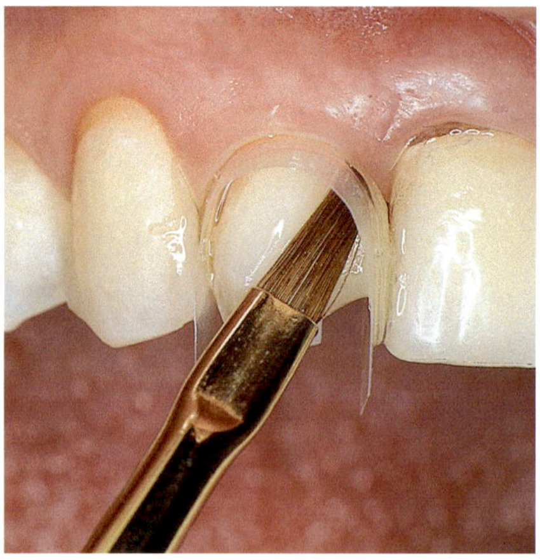

Fig 2-25w The resin composite is carefully shaped with a watercolor brush.

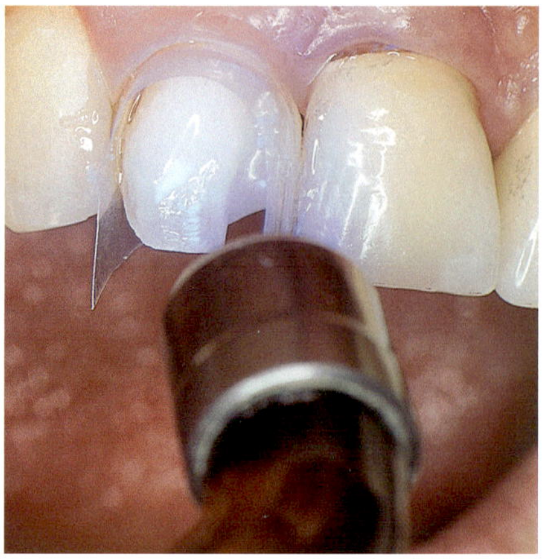

Fig 2-25x Palatal and labial polymerization is performed simultaneously with two lights.

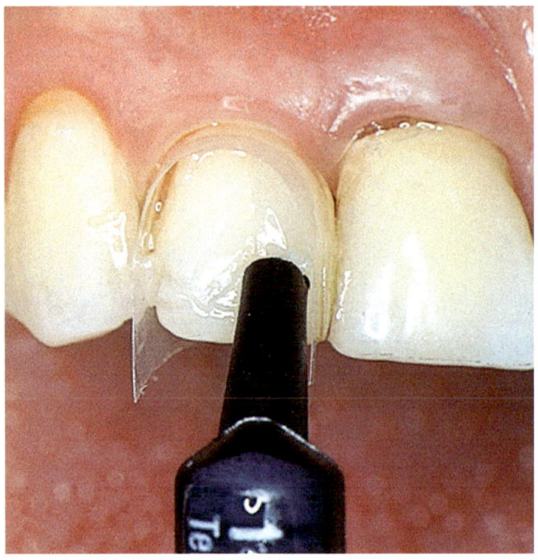

Fig 2-25y The enamel shade D3 is applied.

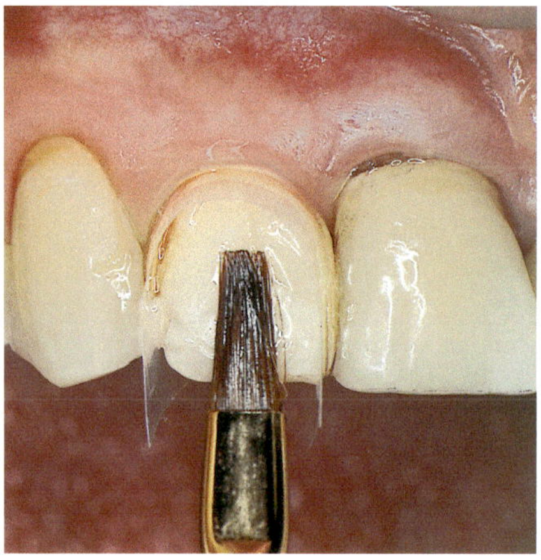

Fig 2-25z The restoration is contoured with the brush.

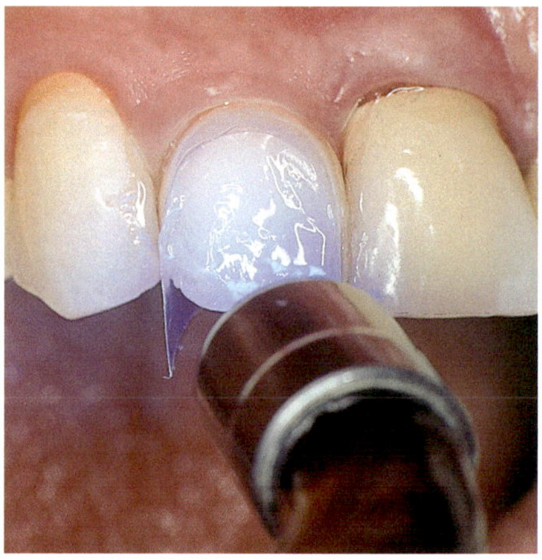

Fig 2-25aa Final curing.

The restoration was ready to be esthetically contoured. A dark or black background was used to aid contouring. A template was cut from black acrylic resin and carefully polished. The black background template is used for oral photography and for esthetic grinding. In this patient, the template was placed directly behind the maxillary incisors (Figs 2-25ee to 2-25gg).

The restoration in the lateral incisor was contoured and polished with a fine diamond against the dark background. A dark aspirator was used to allow total concentration on the contour of the tooth. The restoration was polished first with a coarse and then with a fine rubber polishing point, and the finishing was completed with a brush filled with polishing paste (Figs 2-25hh to 2-25kk).

The finished restoration was esthetically pleasing compared with the initial situation (Figs 2-25ll and 2-25mm). The patient was happy and marveled at the results (Figs 2-25nn and 2-25oo). With a confident smile she left the office contentedly (Figs 2-25pp and 2-25qq). When her budget allows, she plans to have all-ceramic restorations placed for her maxillary incisors. This will allow an esthetic design of the entire anterior region.

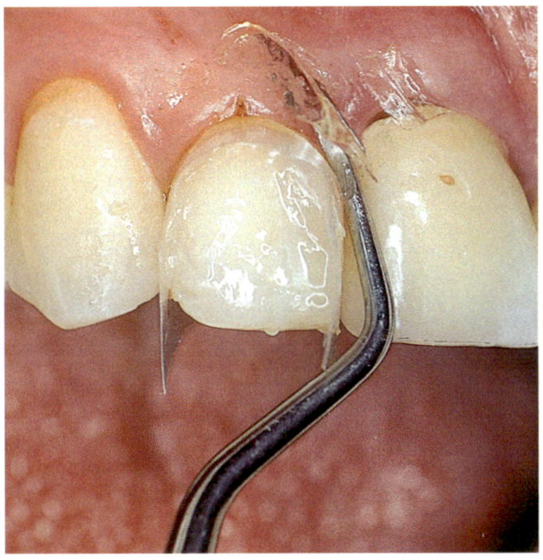

Fig 2-25bb Excess bonding resin is removed with a sickle-shaped cement remover.

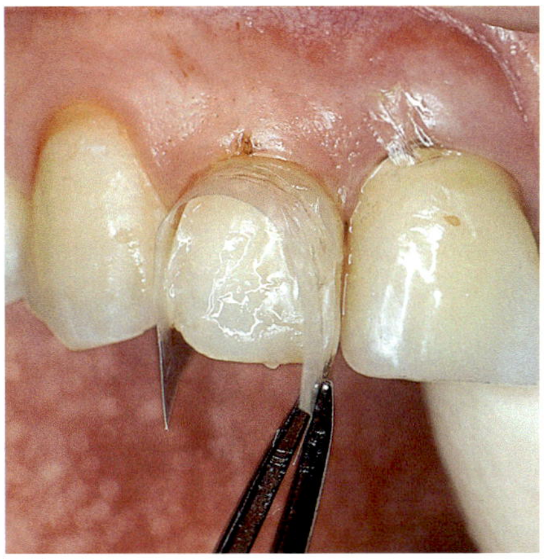

Fig 2-25cc The strip is gripped with pliers.

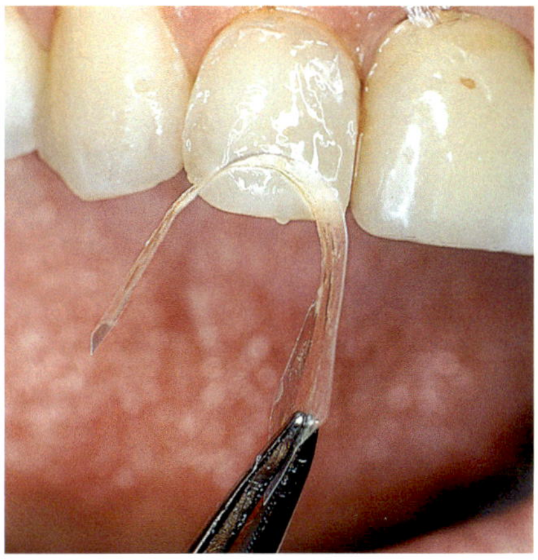

Fig 2-25dd The strip is removed with pliers.

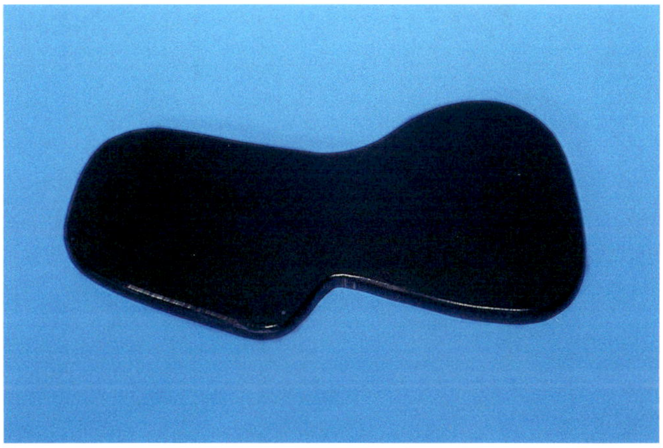

Fig 2-25ee Black acrylic resin background template.

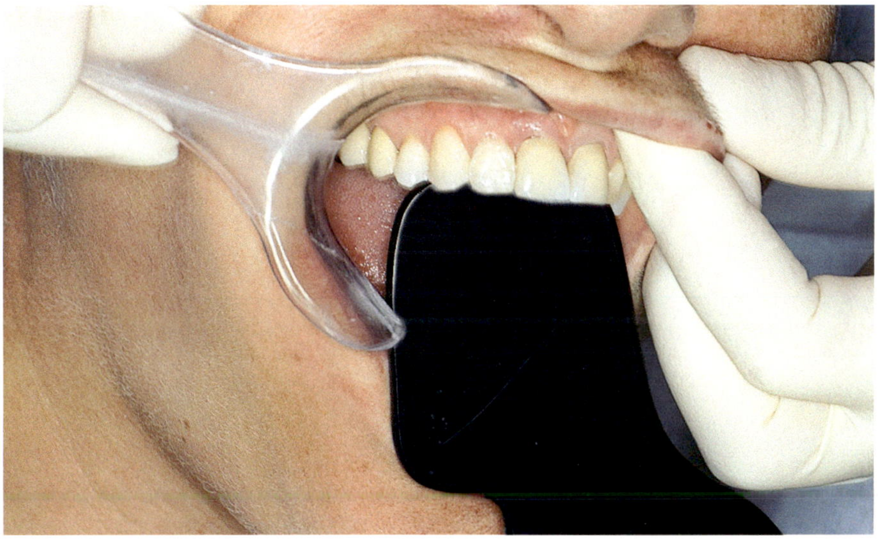

Fig 2-25ff The template is placed orally behind the maxillary incisors.

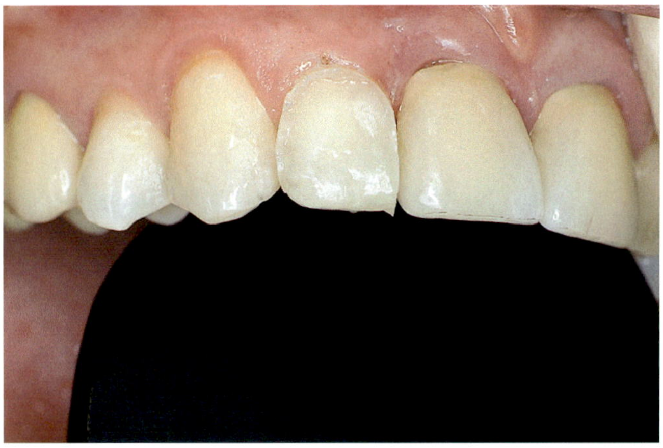

Fig 2-25gg Esthetic adaptation by grinding is easy against the black background.

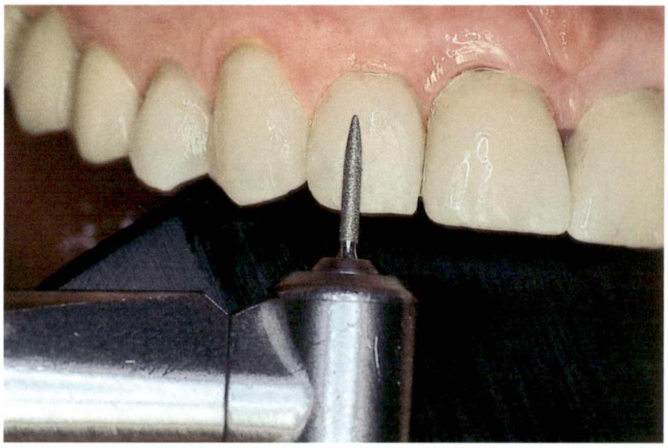

Fig 2-25hh The restoration is contoured with a fine flame-shaped diamond.

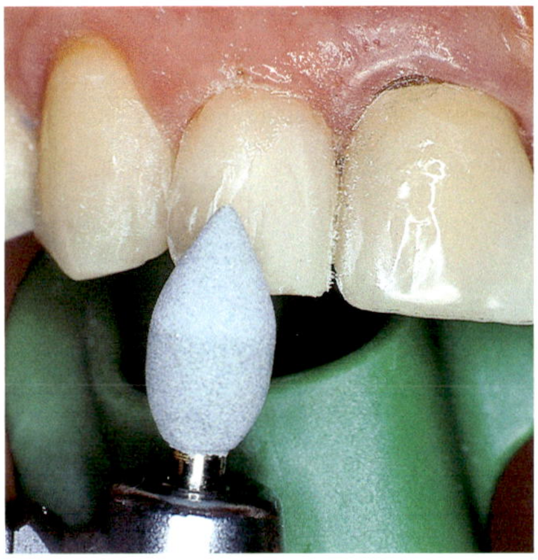

Fig 2-25ii Initial polishing is carried out with a coarse polishing point.

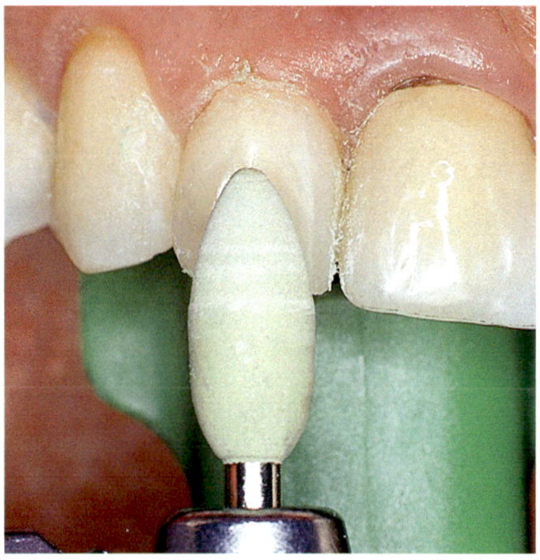

Fig 2-25jj Fine polishing is performed with a fine polishing point.

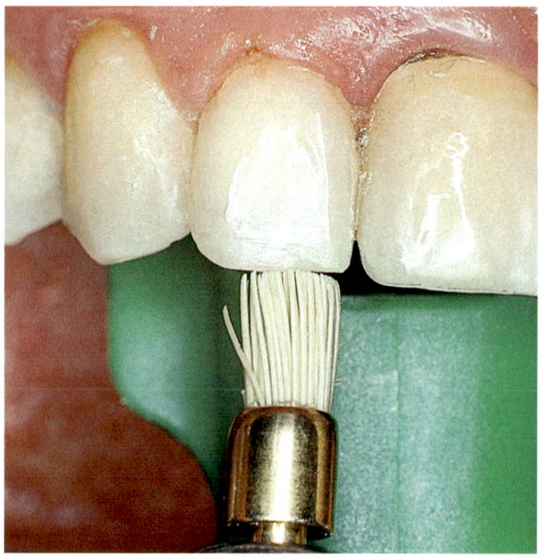

Fig 2-25kk Final finishing is performed with the Occlubrush.

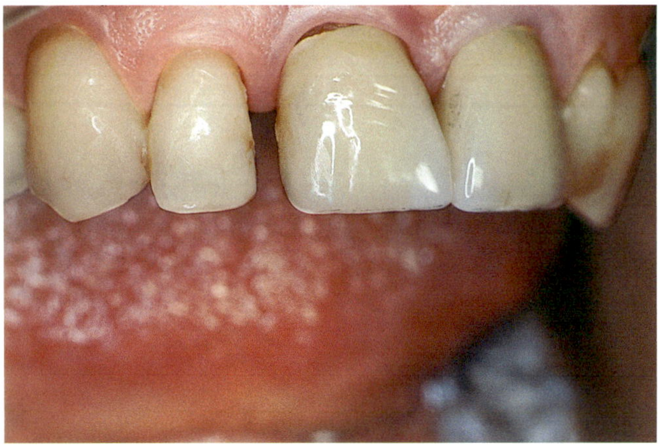

Fig 2-25ll Pretreatment appearance.

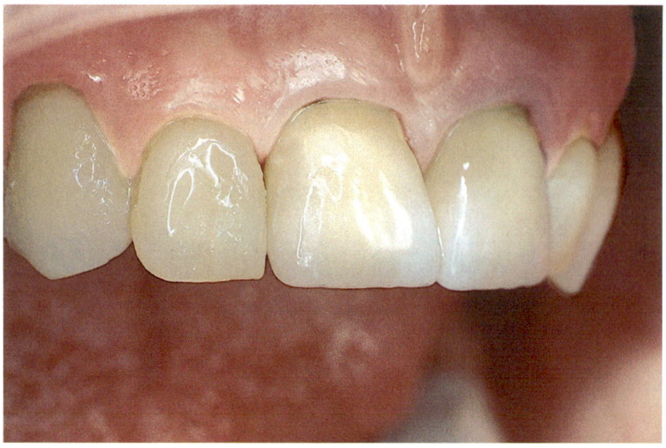

Fig 2-25mm Posttreatment appearance.

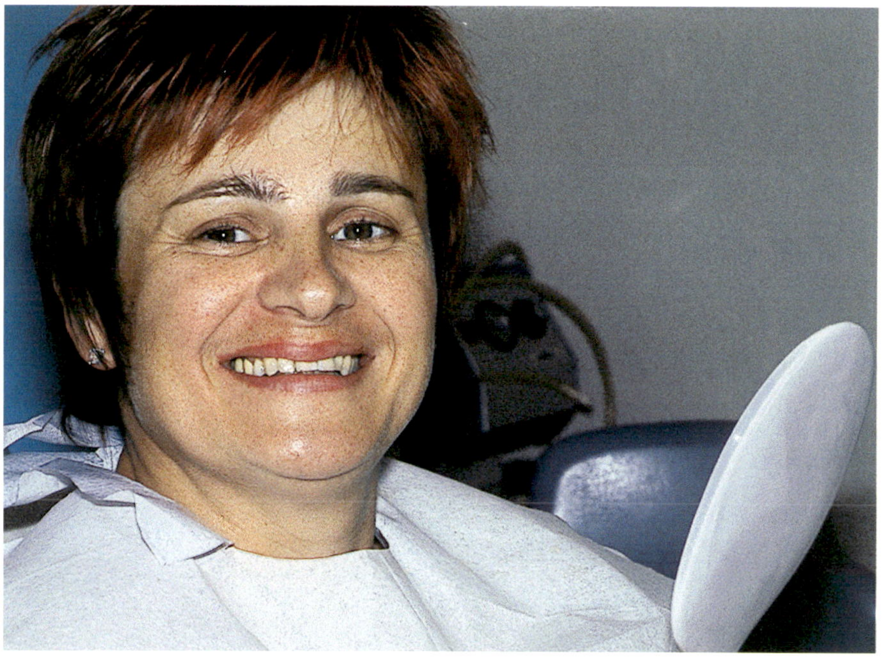

Fig 2-25nn The patient is satisfied.

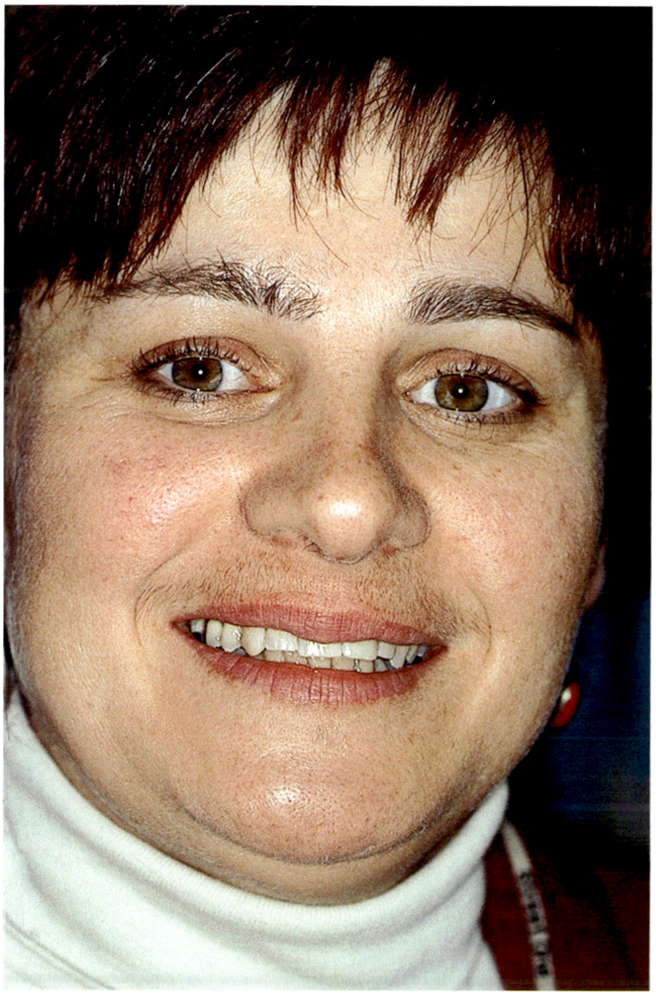

Fig 2-25pp She exhibits a confident smile after the restoration.

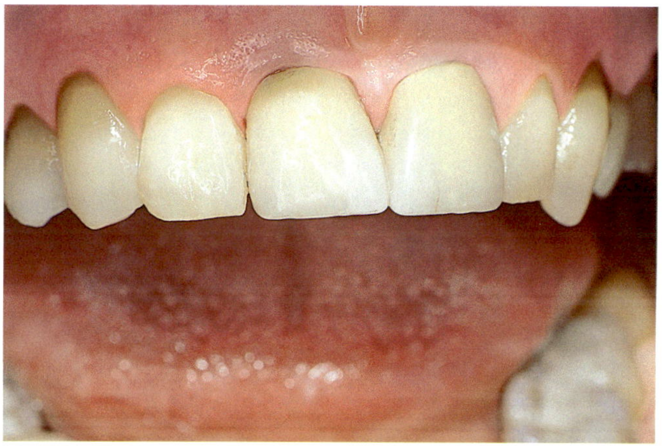

Fig 2-25oo Close-up view of the results.

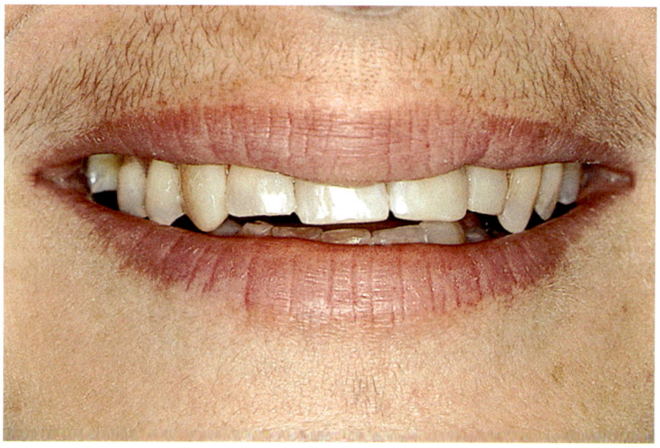

Fig 2-25qq The space has disappeared.

Materials

Contour Strip (Ivoclar Vivadent), stiff strips only, not the ones from the roll, which are too soft
Ultra-Etch phosphoric acid gel (Ultradent)

Tetric and Heliobond composite system (Ivoclar Vivadent)
Narrow watercolor brush (from an art supply store)
Rubber polishing points, gray and green (Ivoclar Vivadent)
Occlubrush polishing brush (Kerr Dental)
Black acrylic template (handmade)

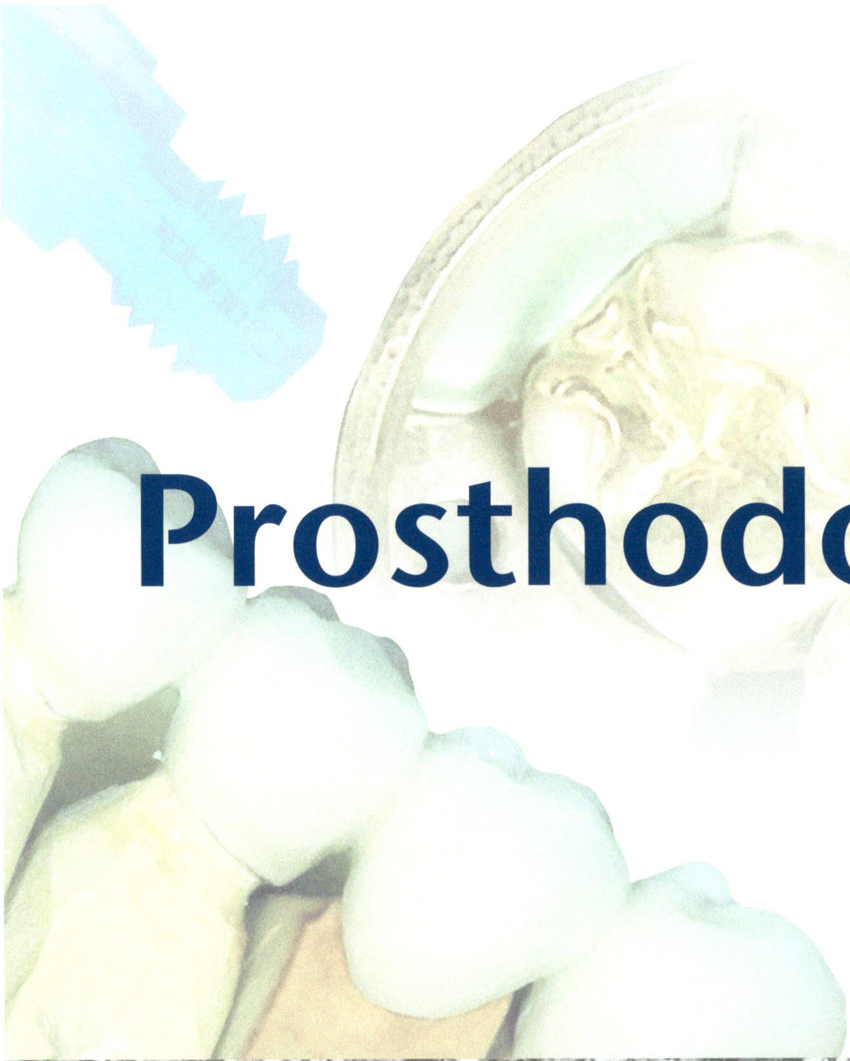

3

Prosthodontics

3

Benefits of the Magnifying Loupe

Systematic Workflow in the Dental Laboratory and Office

Conventional Cementation

Adhesive Inlay/Onlay Supported Fixed Partial Dentures

Accurate Provisional Fixed Partial Dentures

Expedient Placement of Complete Dentures

Causes of Bruxism

Fabrication of Centric Splints With Anterior Guidance

Diagnostic Measures in Implant Prosthodontics

Benefits of the Magnifying Loupe

Common problem: Improving precision in dentistry

Knowledge has increased enormously in all areas of dentistry, thus raising the demand for greater precision in a dentist's daily work:

1. In conservative dentistry, the detection of tiny caries lesions, the minimally invasive treatment of caries, the application of fissure sealant, and ultrasonic preparation have all become increasingly important (Figs 3-1 and 3-2).
2. Prosthetic dentistry postulates that the marginal gaps be less than 50 μm (Fig 3-3) to prevent colonization by microbes. Thus a high degree of precision is necessary for preparation and impression taking (Figs 3-4 to 3-6).
3. In periodontal surgery, sutures of 6-0 to 9-0 are used to allow for irritation-free, fast, and scar-free wound healing.
4. Restorations should have invisible margins, especially in the anterior region.
5. In endodontics, finding accessory canals is impossible without magnification.
6. In oral surgery, long-term success of an apicoectomy can only be ensured when the apex is optically magnified during the procedure.
7. The precision of selective grinding to adjust the dental occlusion is largely dependent on a magnified view.

In short: Seeing is believing—you can only be sure of what you can see!

Proven solution: Magnification with a loupe

By using a magnifying loupe or surgical loupe, a dentist can avoid many of the aforementioned problems (Figs 3-7 and 3-8). This section will discuss the demands a magnifying loupe has to meet and other considerations for buying a magnifying loupe.

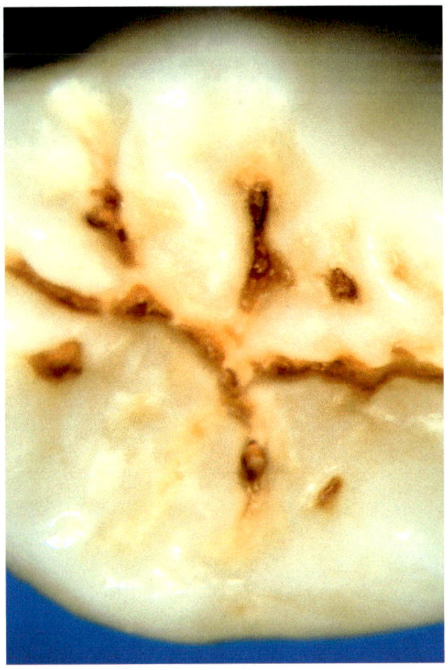

Fig 3-1 Fissure caries.

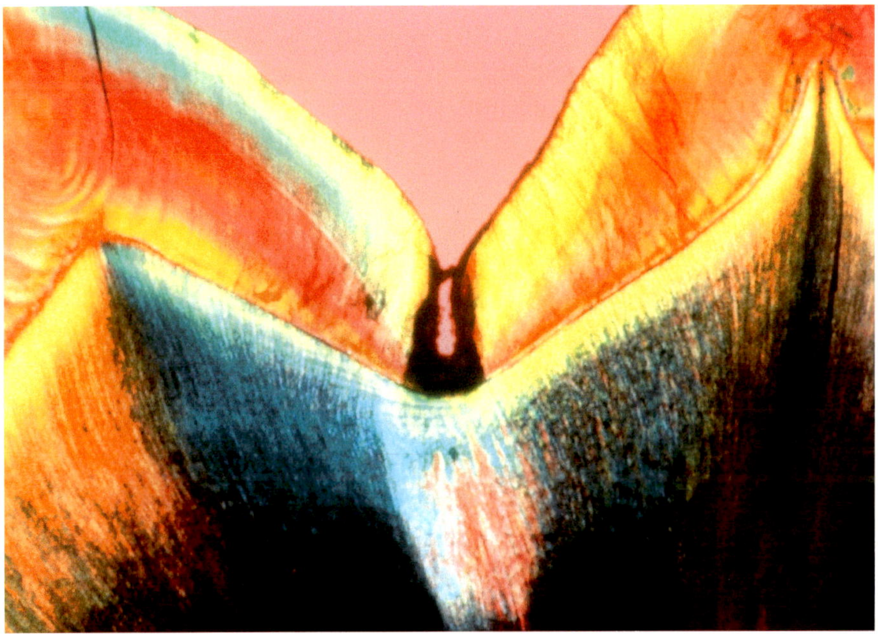

Fig 3-2 Fissure caries in a polarization image. (From Heinrich-Weltzien et al.[1] Reprinted with permission.)

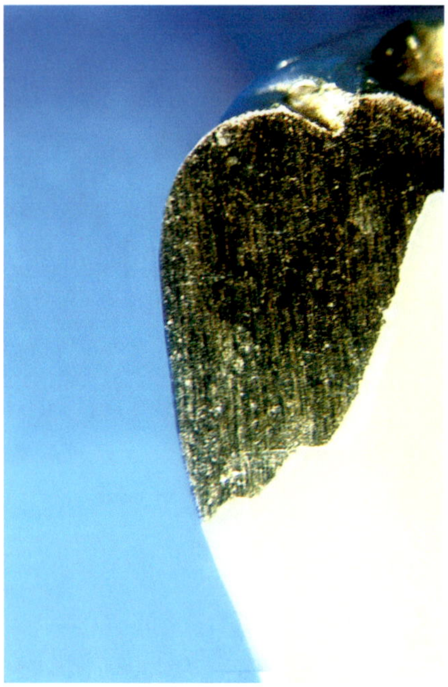

Fig 3-3 Cross section of a posterior tooth with a partial gold crown.

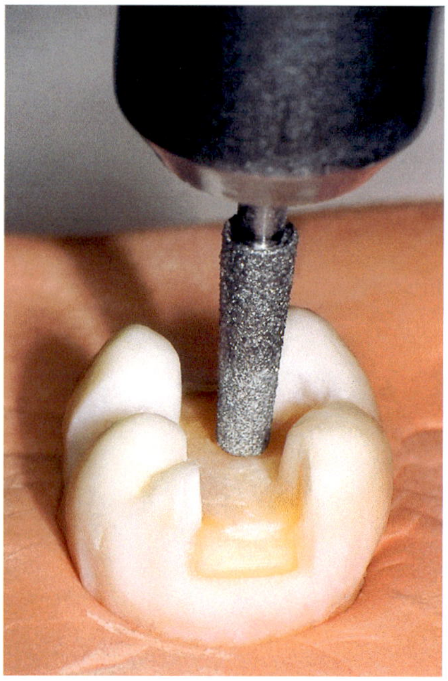

Fig 3-4 Mock preparation with an extracted tooth.

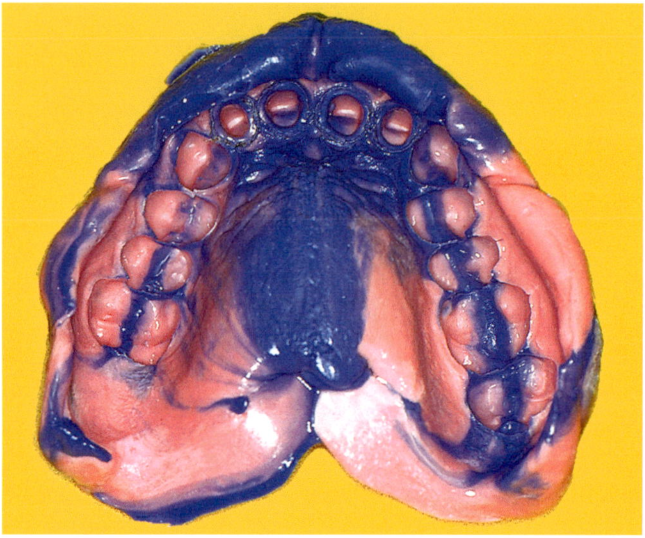

Fig 3-5 Polyether impression.

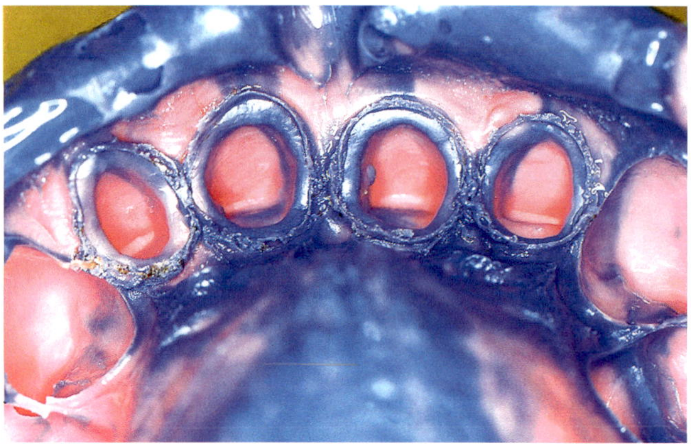

Fig 3-6 Polyether impression as viewed through the magnifying loupe.

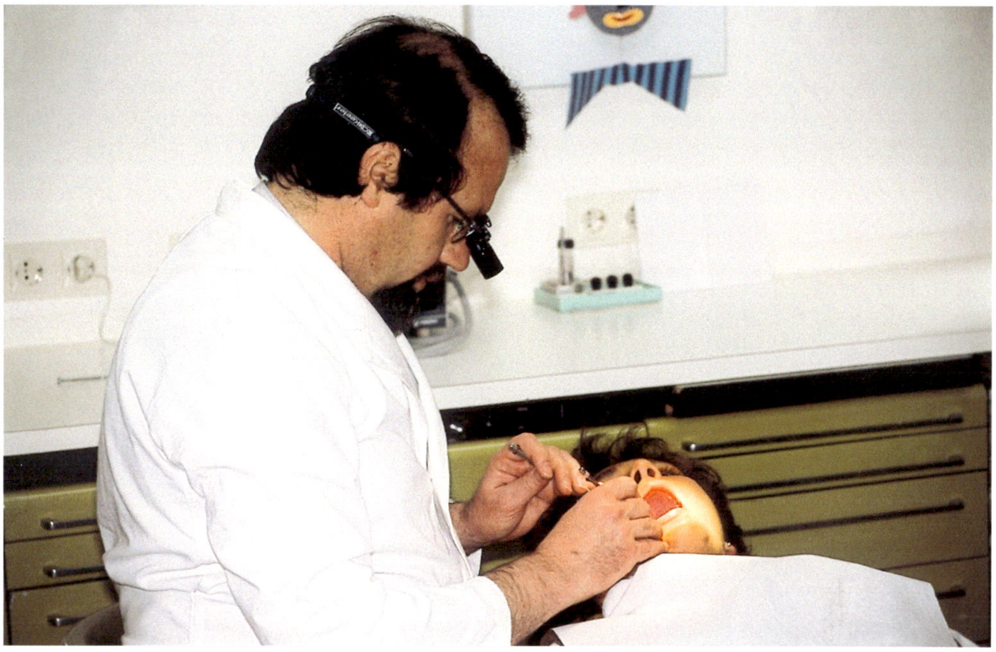

Fig 3-7 The author during a preparation with the magnifying loupe.

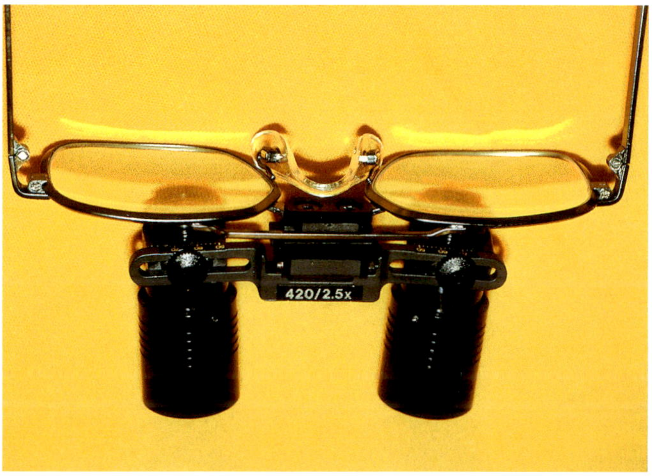

Fig 3-8 *(left)* Magnifying loupe (3x magnification).

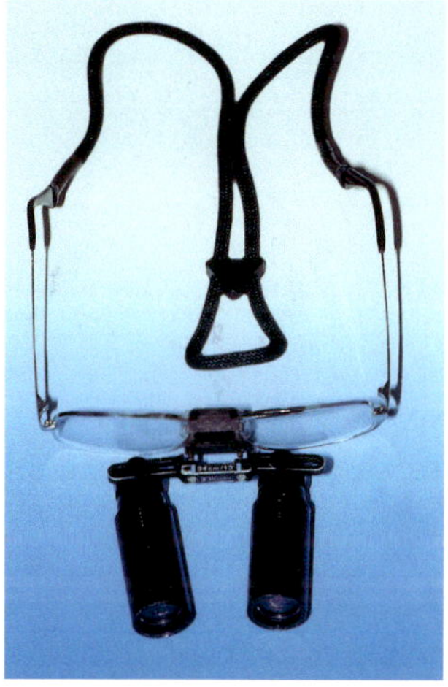

Fig 3-9 *(right)* Magnifying loupe (6x magnification) with a comfortable headband.

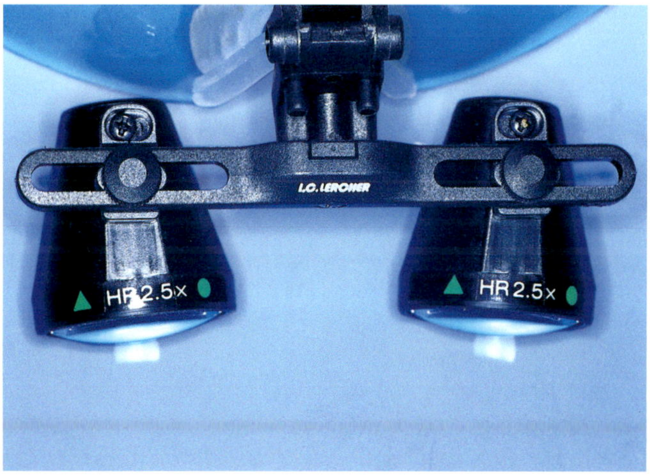

Fig 3-10 *(left)* Magnifying loupe (3x magnification) with wide-angle lenses.

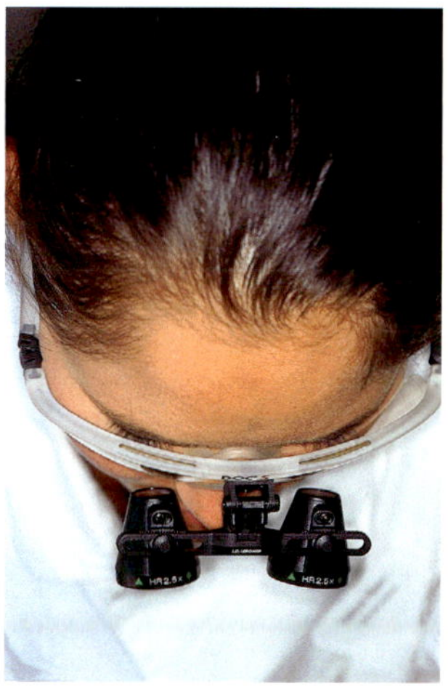

Fig 3-11 *(right)* Magnifying loupe (3x magnification) with elastic temple pieces.

Comfortable fit

The magnifying loupe should not be too heavy, should have an elastic strap to relieve the neck, and should offer a comfortable nose pad (Fig 3-9).

Magnification

Beginners should work with 2.5x to 3.0x magnification (Figs 3-10 and 3-11), and advanced users should use 3.0x to 6.0x magnification (Fig 3-12). In keeping with the laws of optics, stronger magnifications cause the depth of focus to significantly decrease; above all, this makes prismatic lenses so heavy that wearing such a magnifying loupe can hardly be called comfortable.

When using a strong magnification, the dentist must slow the working speed (as in slow motion) to enable constant control of his or her actions in the field of vision.

Wide-angle lenses

To facilitate working with magnification, the magnifying loupe should feature a wide-angle or panoramic lens.

Working distance

The working distance with a magnifying loupe is measured from the surface of the eye to the object. The standard values in occupational physiology for Germany are defined by the University of Darmstadt. The values are currently set at 32 to 35 cm from the eye to an object (Fig 3-13). This distance, however, is strongly dependent on individual physical proportions. There are people with a proportionally long upper body and long arms, who are "tall" when seated and others who have the same body height but have a shorter upper body and shorter arms. Therefore the working distance should be individually tested and determined.

Interpupillary distance

For stereoscopic vision, it is important that the individual images from the left and right eyes are both correctly aligned. It is useful to have the interpupillary distances measured by an ophthalmologist or optometrist, because they tend to be asymmetric. Most magnifying loupes have a horizontal bar with a millimeter scale to allow adjustment of the distance to the determined value. The dentist should check this preadjusted setting individually for both eyes and readjust. Then the stereoscopic vision is tested with both eyes. The clinician should look at a cross against a bright background to adjust the image.

Inclination

The magnifying loupe should allow the inclination of the telescopes to be adjusted to the posture of the head. When the upper body is in an upright position, the head should be slightly and comfortably bent (see Figs 3-7 and 3-13).

Dentists and dental assistants frequently contract musculoskeletal conditions that can be prevented if enough attention is paid to the angle of inclination, the working distance, and the position of the patient. Clinicians tend to adopt a bent posture to gain a better view. This constant isometric muscle contraction in an unphysiologic body posture inevitably leads to orthopedic problems.

If the working distance and the inclination are correctly adjusted from a physiologic point of view, this will ensure a physically relaxed vision in an upright posture.

Illumination

The operating light at the dental chair often does not permit direct and shadow-free illumination of the working field. The following light sources provide alternative options: cold light source attached to a headgear, connected to a stationary generator via a fiber-optic cord; cold light source attached to the magnifying loupe, connected to a stationary main adapter via a power cord; and cold light source attached to the magnifying loupe, connected to a battery pack worn on the dentist's body via a power cord.

Halogen lamps, diodes, and xenon lamps can be used as a light source. The illuminating light should not be excessively bright, because this would result in a counterproductive dazzling effect, which especially affects the ability to see color. In dentistry, an intensity of 10,000 to 15,000 lux is sufficient.

Hygiene

The magnifying loupe should have a protective lens (like the ones used for reflex cameras) that can be placed in front of the telescopes to protect their sensitive surfaces.

Unfortunately, to date, only one manufacturer offers this feature. In addition, it would be desirable to have waterproof optical systems so that the magnifying loupe could regularly be subjected to ultrasonic cleaning. Examination of a magnifying loupe after a difficult preparation shows why this would be absolutely essential.

Training schedule

Many dentists borrow a loupe to test it and immediately start using it for tooth preparations. They then get a headache and experience vertigo, which leads them to believe that working with a magnifying loupe is not quite up their alley. Use of strong magnification, however, is a process that requires adaptation, and it takes between 1 and 3 weeks of gradual acclimatization, depending on the magnification. The point is not about vision alone; the dentist must relearn the proprioception of his or her movements in the magnified working field.
Therefore, the following training schedule is recommended:

1. Contouring of provisional restorations outside the patient's mouth, that is, marking of the margin of preparation with a fine pencil and subsequent performance of accurate contouring (Fig 3-14)
2. Root planing and curettage in periodontal treatment (Fig 3-15)
3. Contouring and finishing of resin composite restorations (Fig 3-16)
4. Selective occlusal grinding (Fig 3-17)
5. Oral surgery with 6-0 to 9-0 sutures
6. Examination of tooth preparations for restorations
7. Preparation of restorations (Fig 3-18)

Selection of a magnifying loupe

For a dentist who is lay person in optical matters, the author recommends the following buying guide:

1. Lens quality: The clinician should take a square sheet of graph paper (10 cm^2) along when planning to buy a magnifying loupe. The lenses can be considered good if the squares are still visible and there are no distorted figures toward the edges of the sheet when it is viewed through the magnifying loupe (Fig 3-19).
2. Comfort: The magnifying loupe should be worn for a couple of minutes. The wearer should look at different objects and ask: Is the nose pad comfortable? Does the headband pinch? (It shouldn't!) Is the weight of the magnifying loupe acceptable?
3. Posture: Are the angle of inclination and the working distance correct? Is it possible to sit relaxed in an upright position and still see well in all of the working field?

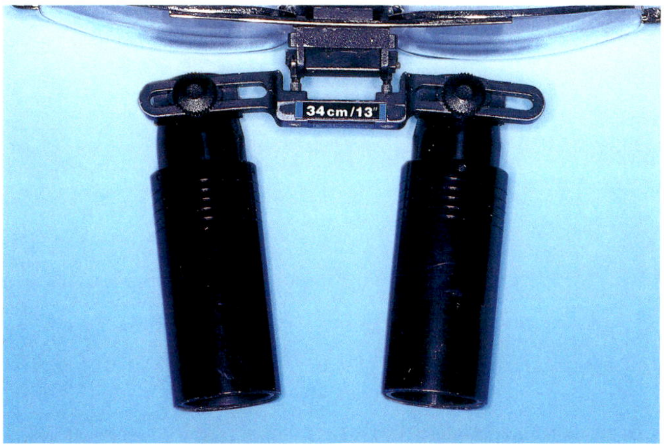

Fig 3-12 Magnifying loupe (6x magnification) with heavy lenses.

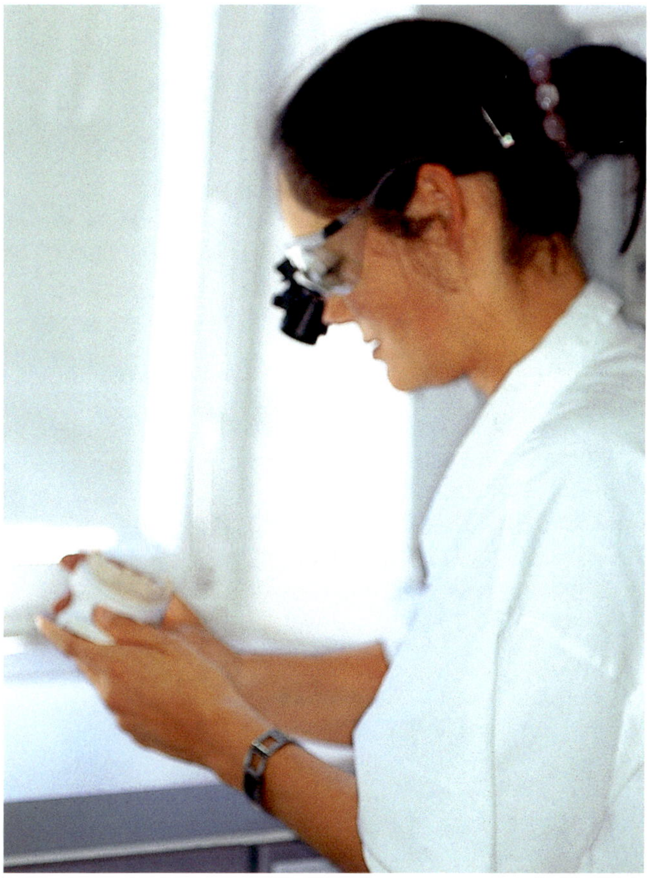

Fig 3-13 Working distance in a relaxed posture.

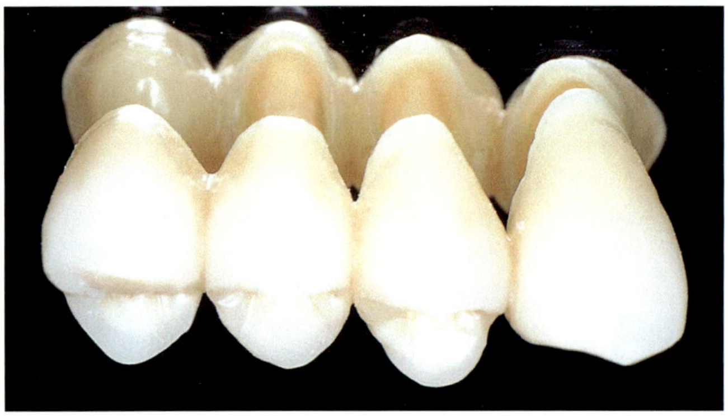

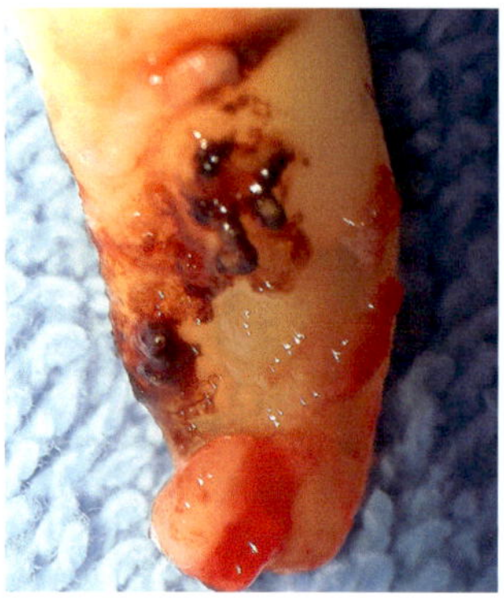

Fig 3-14 *(left)* Finished provisional restoration.

Fig 3-15 *(right)* Extracted tooth after closed curettage and extraction.

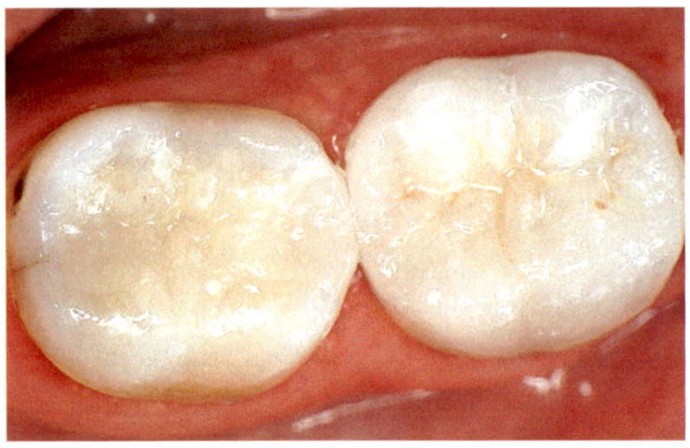

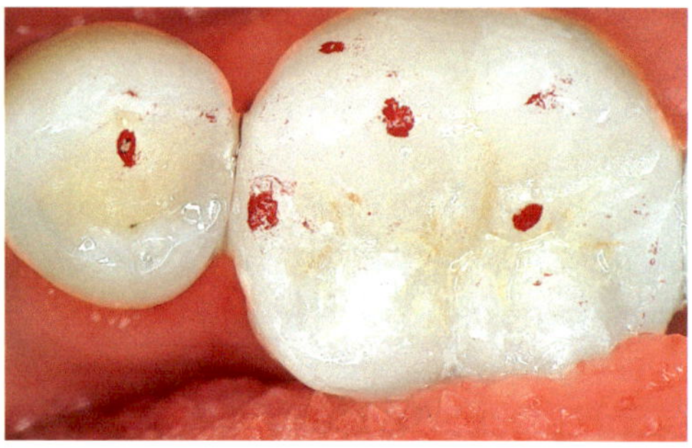

Fig 3-16 *(left)* Polished restorations in posterior teeth.

Fig 3-17 *(right)* Selective grinding of the occlusion with use of the magnifying loupe.

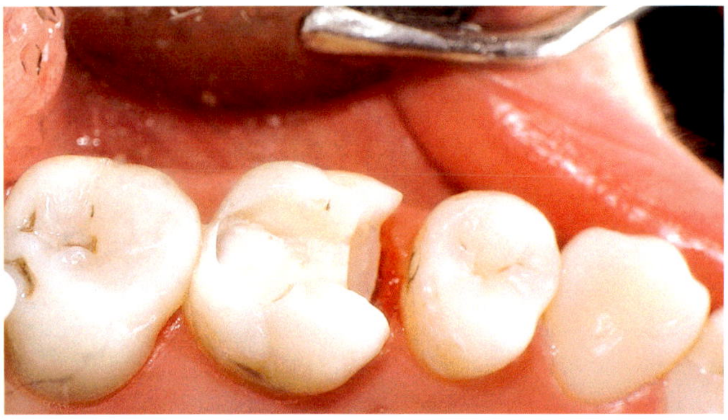

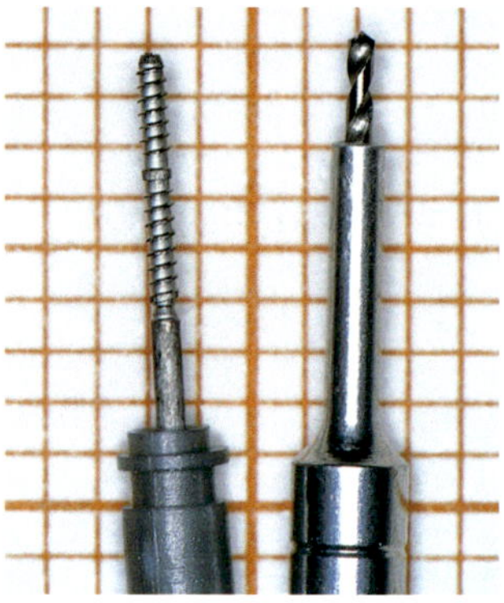

Fig 3-18 *(left)* Preparation of a ceramic inlay.

Fig 3-19 *(right)* Testing the vision with a magnifying loupe (view of posts on graph paper). The optical system works well.

4. Illumination: Are all the working fields well illuminated? Is the technical equipment manageable?

Conclusion

In the opinion of the author, the magnifying loupe is the single most important tool for the dentist in modern dentistry. It permits vision into ranges that the eye cannot normally perceive, thus allowing previously unheard of precision. In many fields of dentistry, clinicians can now achieve long-term success for the benefit of patients to a degree that was once unthinkable.

Materials

A magnifying loupe can be purchased from an optometrist and the following companies, among others: Zeiss, Orascoptic, Heine, and Eickhorst. The aforementioned companies offer detailed consultation and the opportunity to borrow the loupes and equipment to test them in the office.

Systematic Workflow in the Dental Laboratory and Office

Common problem: Maintenance of precision between the dental office and the dental laboratory

The preparation was good, impression taking was successful, the dental technician produced a crown, and fitted it onto the cast. Then the crown was cemented, and suddenly the problems arose: The crown was too high and had to be ground to size. A lack of marginal integrity is clearly visible (Fig 3-20).

What went wrong with the fabrication method from the preparation to cementation? Where did the problem develop? Was it the preparation, the impression, the stone cast, the casting, a lack of attention, a mistake by the dental technician, the cement, or the dentist's own error that caused the problem?

Proven solution: A systematic workflow from the dental office to the laboratory

Every step, from tooth preparation to cementation, should be performed with continuously high precision. Furthermore, all of the general steps involved in each process have to be regularly reevaluated by the dentist and the dental technician for other options with regard to the materials and methods employed. If something goes wrong, there is no point in assigning blame to an individual. Instead, the clinician should examine every aspect of the process when seeking the cause of the failure and focus on opportunities for improvement.

When the stereomicroscope found its way into the dental laboratory at the beginning of the 1980s, the question arose as to what degree of precision could be achieved with it (Fig 3-21). Research by Reinhard Marxkors at the University of Münster in 1976 revealed crown margins to have an average gap of 0.46 mm at collar crowns and 0.22 mm at cast crowns. To prevent the crown margin from being colonized by bacteria, it was postulated that the microleakage should not exceed 0.03 mm.

This goal was thought to be unachievable at the time. However, this limitation was changed by the introduction of the stereomicroscope, which is one of the most important tools of the dental technician. It now is an integral part of the dental laboratory, although it used to be employed only for grinding diamonds, checking computer chips, precision mechanics, and watchmaking (Fig 3-22).

The most important features for a dental laboratory stereomicroscope are listed in brief:

1. Type: The microscope should be a binocular stereomicroscope with reflected light illumination (Fig 3-23).

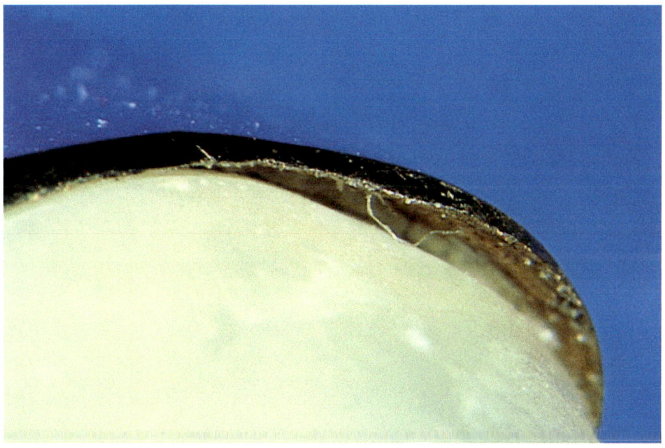

Fig 3-20 Crown margin with a large gap.

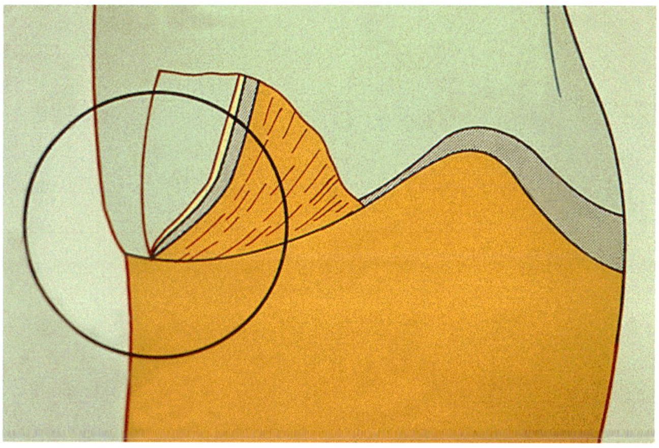

Fig 3-21 The crown margin—a problematic zone.

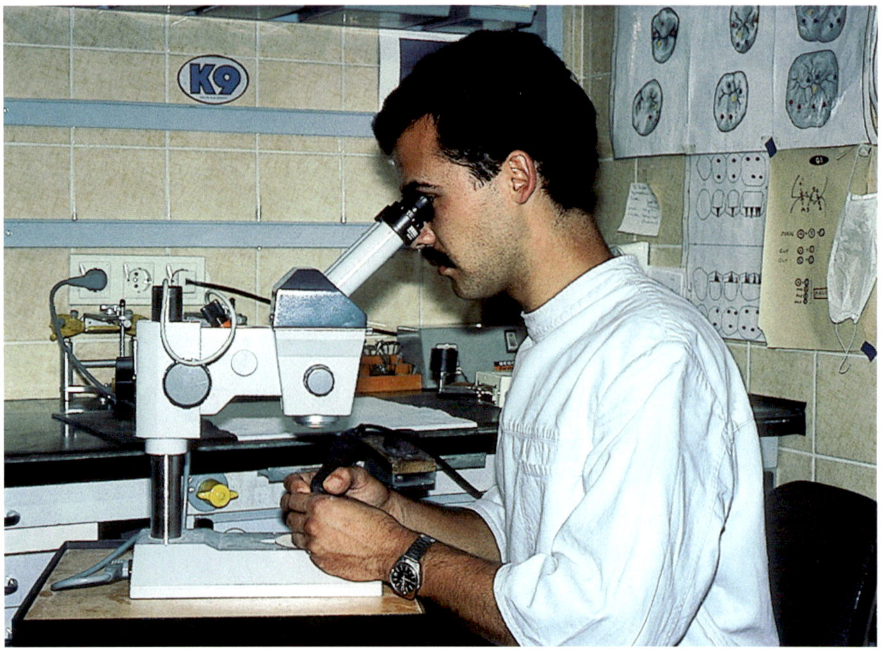

Fig 3-22 The stereomicroscope is an important tool in the dental laboratory.

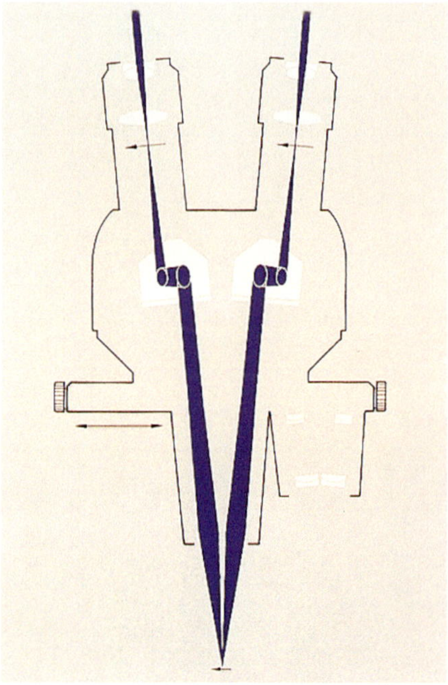

Fig 3-23 Optical path in a stereomicroscope.

2. Magnification: The technician should use 10x magnification for regular work and 30x magnification to check that work. It is important to proceed gradually and consistently: The technician should start by using the stereomicroscope only to check work and then over time learn to perform all work with it. After 4 weeks, a dental technician should feel comfortable enough to do everything with a stereomicroscope.
3. Wide-angle optical system: Wide-angle eyepieces enlarge the working field under the stereomicroscope exponentially.
4. Ergonomics: To allow the technician to have a physiologically correct posture when working with the stereomicroscope, the device should be tilted toward the technician. This can be accomplished either by laying a wedge underneath the stereomicroscope or by adapting it in the working area with the help of a swivel arm.
5. Lens quality: Testing with graph paper is a good way to judge the quality of the lens. If all the squares at the edge of the field of vision actually appear square, the lenses can be considered good.
6. Manufacturers: Good stereomicroscopes are available from Zeiss, Leica, Eickhorst, and Renfert.
7. Photo and video adapter: A photo and video adapter (C-mount) is useful for documentation and for training courses.
8. Illumination: Stereomicroscopes normally have a built-in illumination system that provides enough light. For photography and training courses, illumination with an additional cold light source is recommended.

Step-by-step procedure for systematic workflow

The teeth are prepared with the help of a magnifying loupe (see previous section). The impression is examined under the stereomicroscope (Fig 3-24a). A die stone (eg, Moldasynt)—previously weighed using a tensometer—and the appropriate amount of liquid are mixed under vacuum and filled in the impression on a laboratory vibrator (Figs 3-24b to 3-24d). The working cast is checked with a stereomicroscope (Figs 3-24e and 3-24f).

The margin of the preparation is marked with a pencil, and the mark is fixed with cyanoacrylate (Figs 3-24g and 3-24h). A layer of varnish is applied as a placeholder (Fig 3-24i). The cast crown is waxed up (Figs 3-24j to 3-24l). The waxed-up crown is carefully lifted to avoid damage to the margins (Fig 3-24m). The sprue pin is fixed (Fig 3-24n), and the crown is invested. After the unfinished castings are examined, the sprue button and the casting beads are removed (Figs 3-24o to 3-24q).

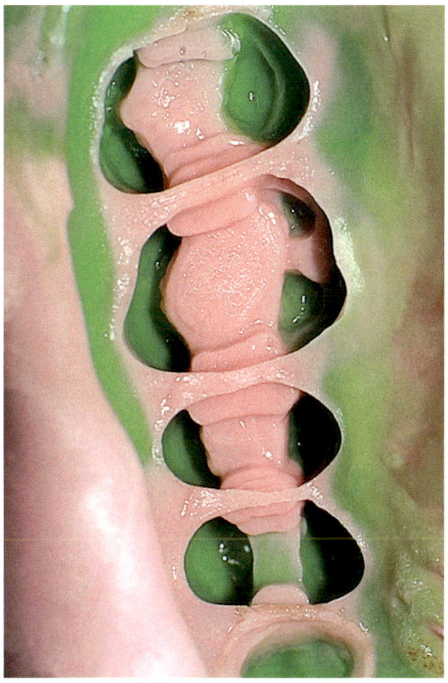

Fig 3-24a *(left)* The hydrocolloid impression is checked for completeness.

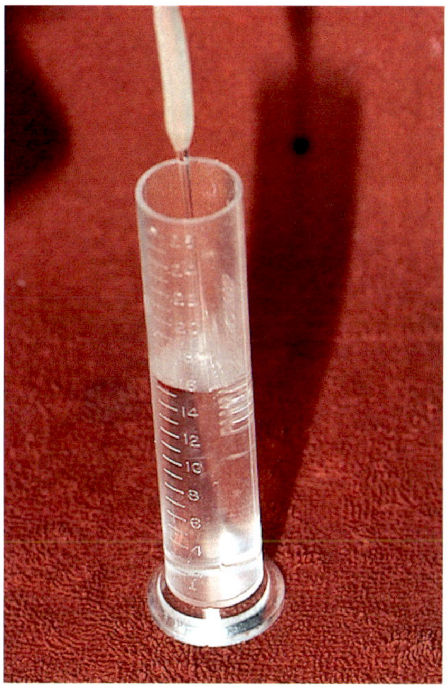

Fig 3-24b *(right)* The liquid is measured in the measuring vial.

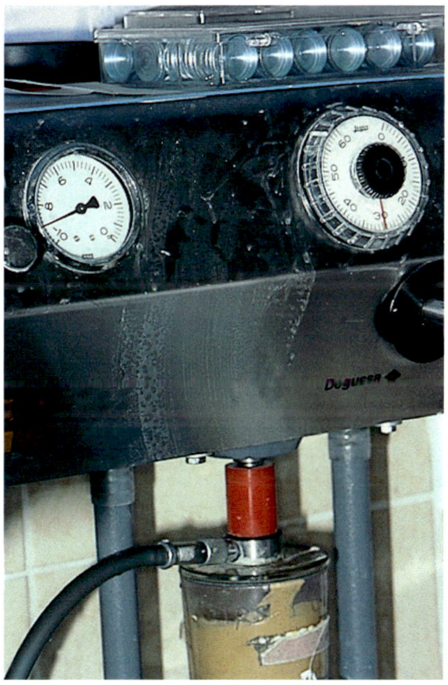

Fig 3-24c *(left)* The die stone is mixed under vacuum.

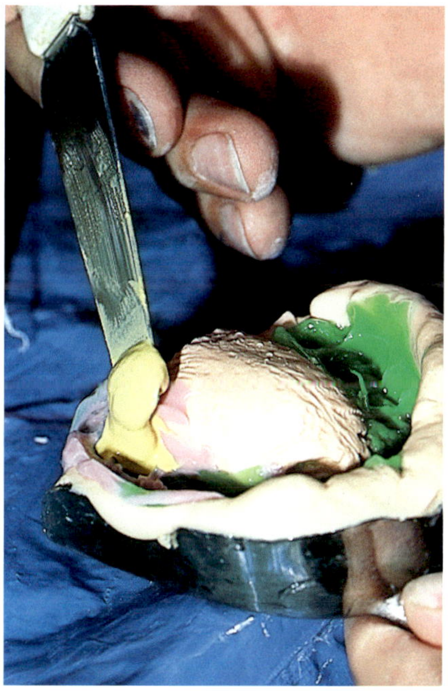

Fig 3-24d *(right)* The impression is filled with the die stone on a laboratory vibrator.

The crown is adapted to the die with the help of a thick, water-soluble felt-tip pen; the technician can reactivate the markings after each try-in by breathing on them (Figs 3-24r and 3-24s). The red primary contacts are removed with a sharp bud bur (Fig 3-24t). The try-in is repeated until the crown sits neatly on the die without any pressure. If pressure is applied, this will cause abrasion of the die stone and create a fit that seems to be very accurate—much more so than it actually will be in the patient's mouth. The crown is finished and polished (Fig 3-24u).

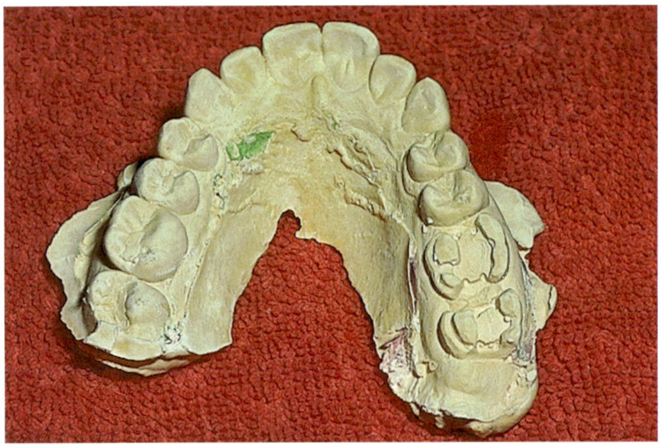

Fig 3-24e The cast is removed from the impression.

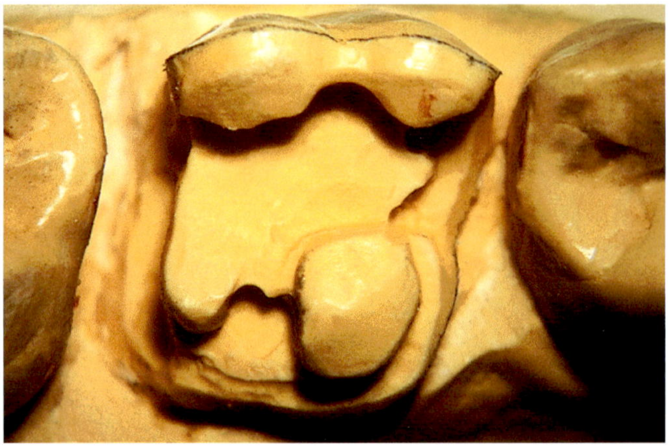

Fig 3-24f The die is examined under the stereomicroscope.

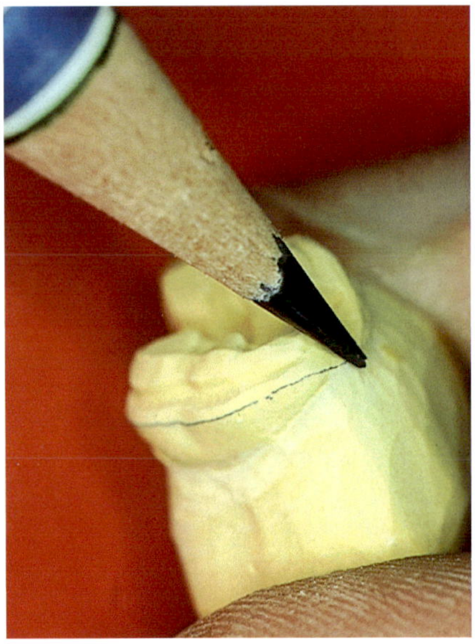

Fig 3-24g The preparation margin is marked in pencil.

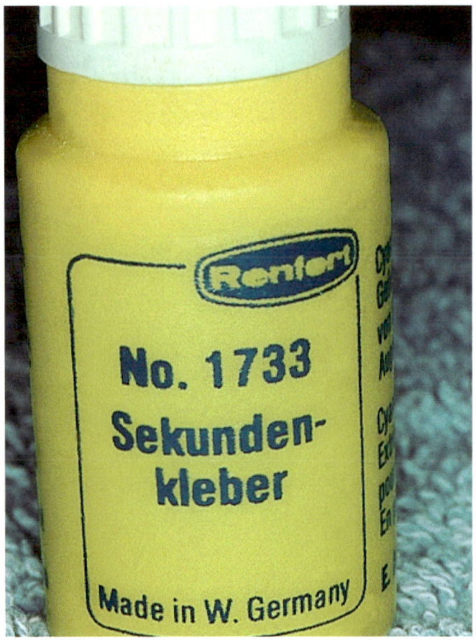

Fig 3-24h Liquid cyanoacrylate is used to fix the penciled preparation margin on the die.

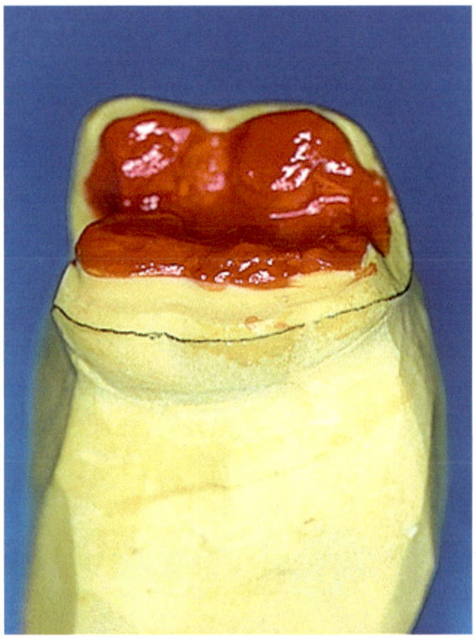

Fig 3-24i A layer of varnish is applied to the die as a placeholder to simulate the thickness of the cement.

Common problem: Transferring the precision achieved in the dental laboratory to the restorations on the tooth

The restoration on the working cast has a precision of 0.02 mm with respect to marginal integrity. Can this precision be transferred to the tooth? The key is to continue with the systematic workflow.

Proven solution: A systematic workflow from the laboratory to the dentist's office

A pressure spot test is performed in several steps. The crown is adapted in the patient's mouth with the help of a thixotropic opaque silicone (thixotropic means that the silicone becomes less viscous when pressure is applied to it) for the pressure spot test. A small amount of pressure spot indicator is mixed and applied to the crown (Fig 3-25a). The crown is pressed on the tooth with an inlay setter and allowed to cure (Fig 3-25b).

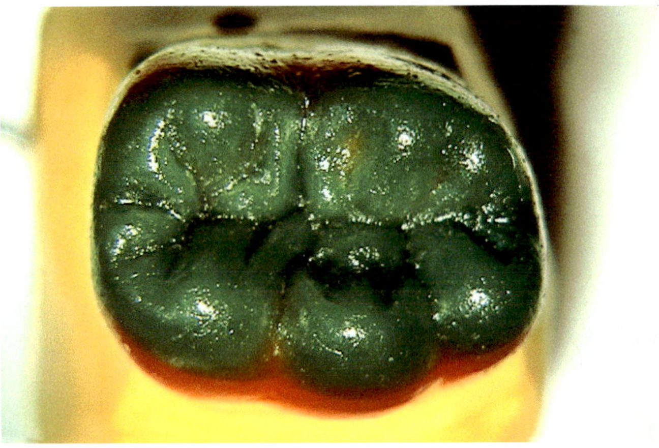

Fig 3-24j Occlusal view of the finished waxup.

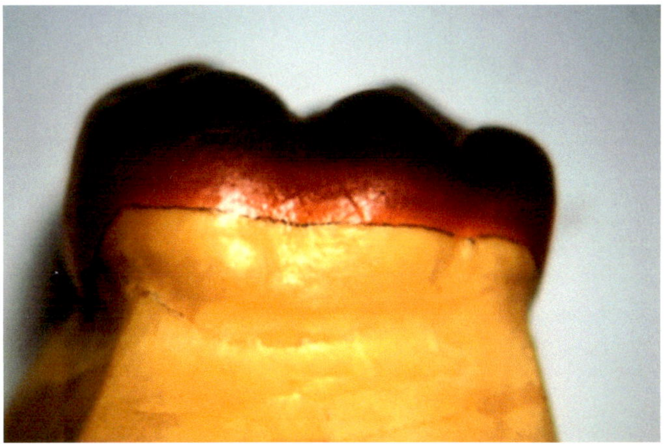

Fig 3-24k Buccal view of the finished waxup.

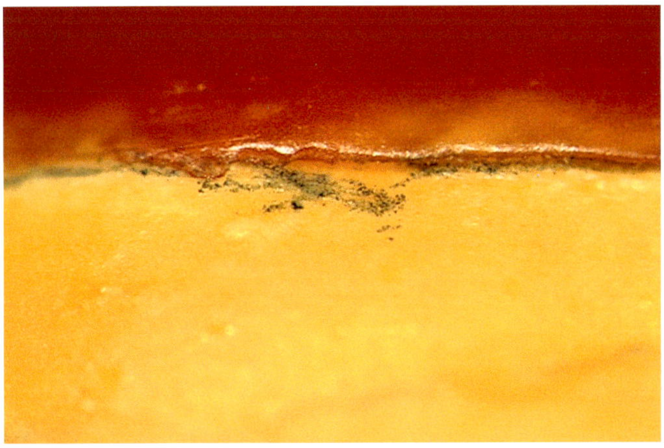

Fig 3-24l The waxed-up crown margin is shown at 50x original magnification.

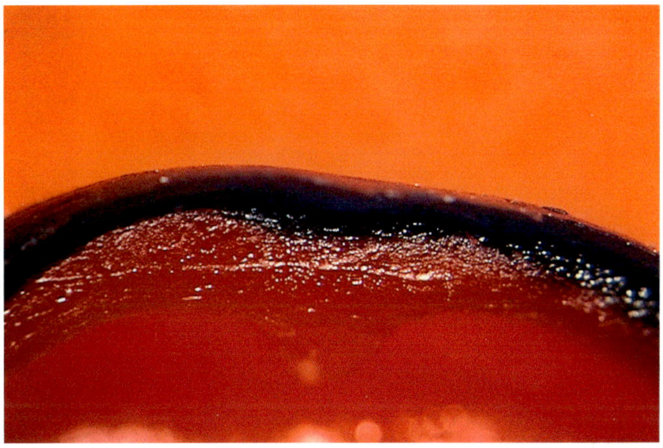

Fig 3-24m The margin of the crown is shown after the waxed-up crown has been lifted off.

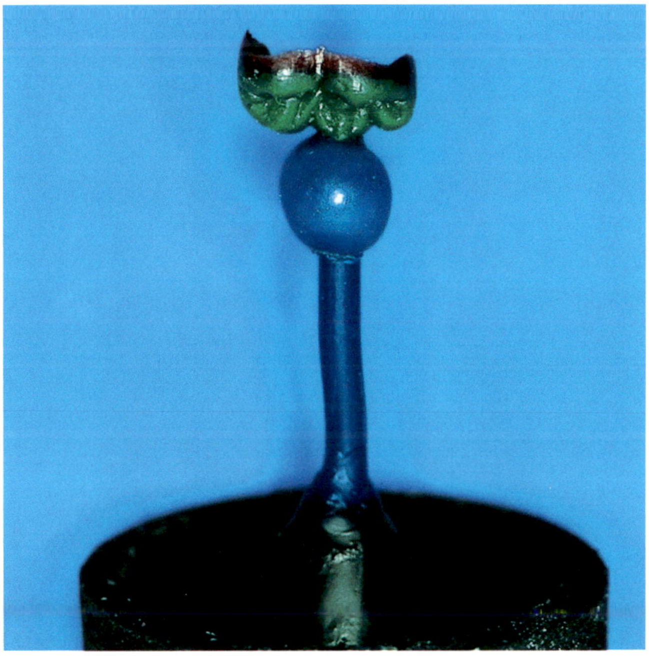

Fig 3-24n The partial crown is on the sprue pin, ready to be put in place.

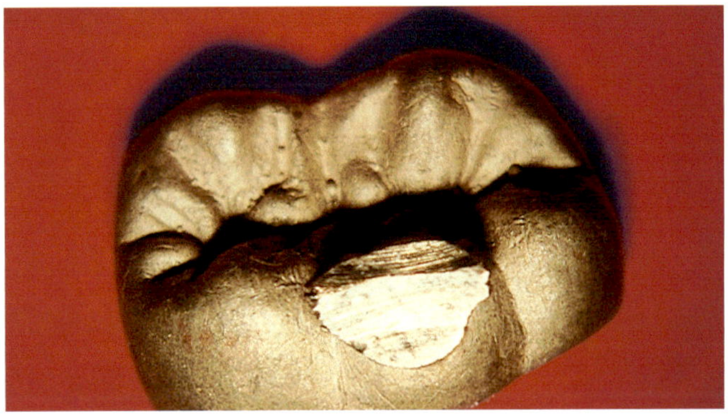

Fig 3-24o The unfinished casting is shown after the sprue pin has been removed.

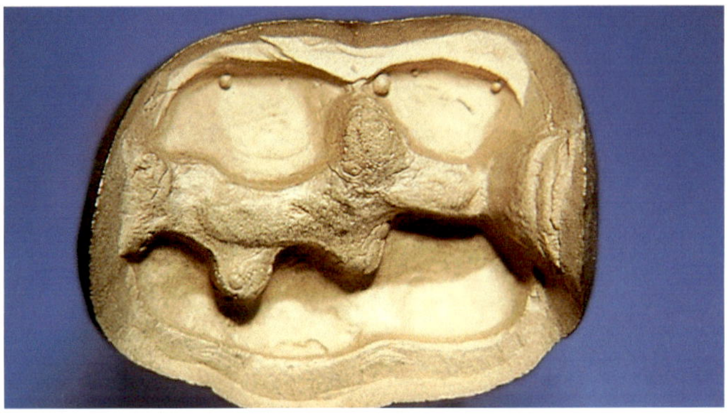

Fig 3-24p The bottom of the unfinished casting is examined.

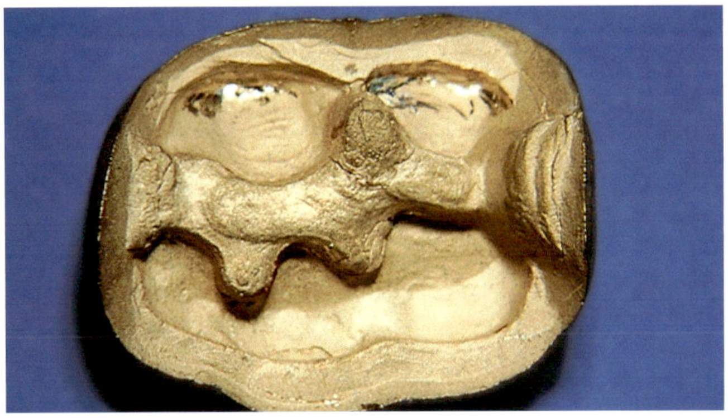

Fig 3-24q The bottom of the unfinished casting is shown after the casting beads have been removed.

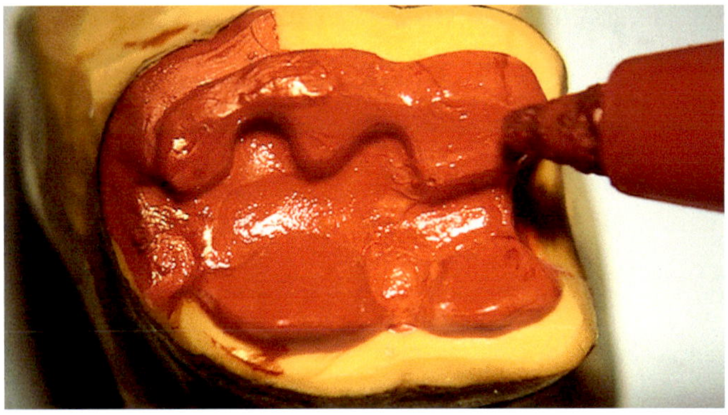

Fig 3-24r The die is marked with a water-soluble felt-tip pen.

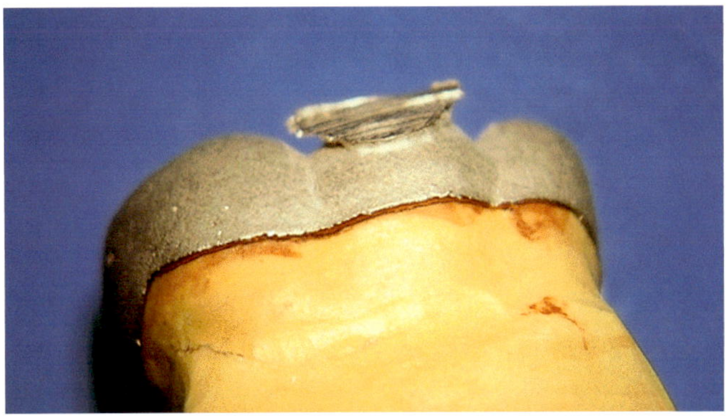

Fig 3-24s The unfinished casting is adapted to the marked die with minimal pressure.

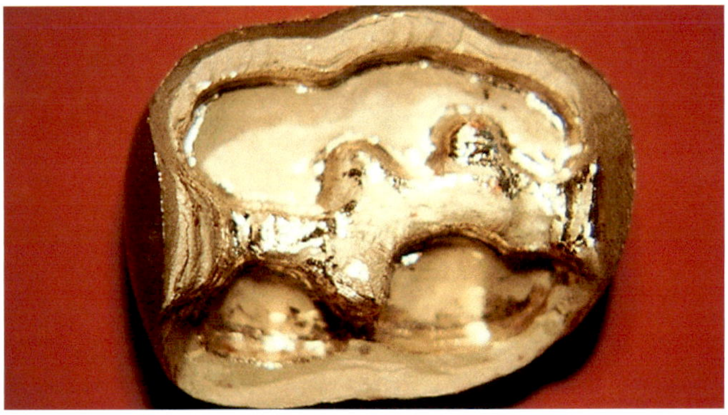

Fig 3-24t Internal marks reveal the primary contacts.

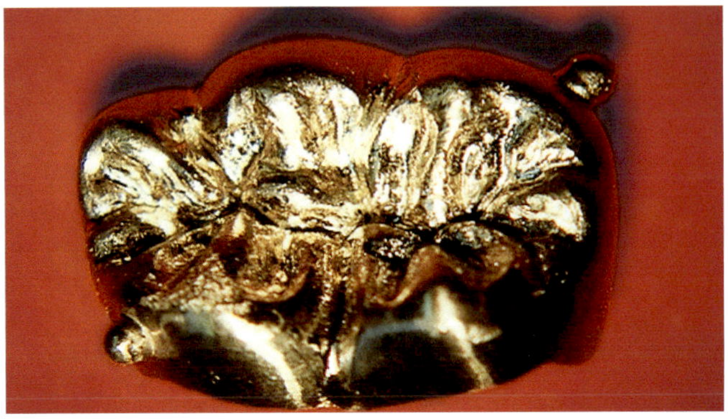

Fig 3-24u Finished partial crown.

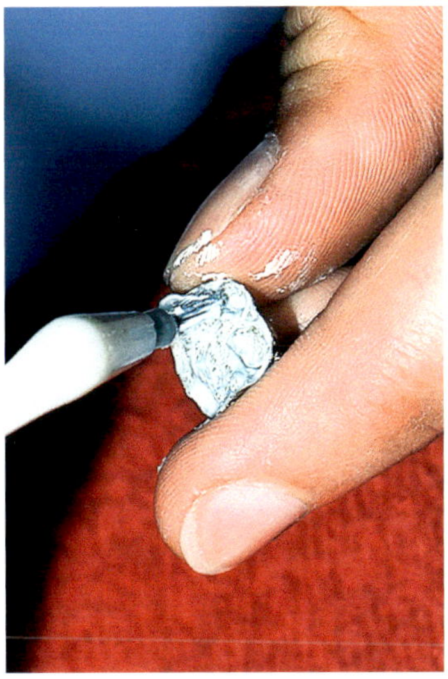

Fig 3-25a The silicone for the pressure spot test is brushed into the partial crown.

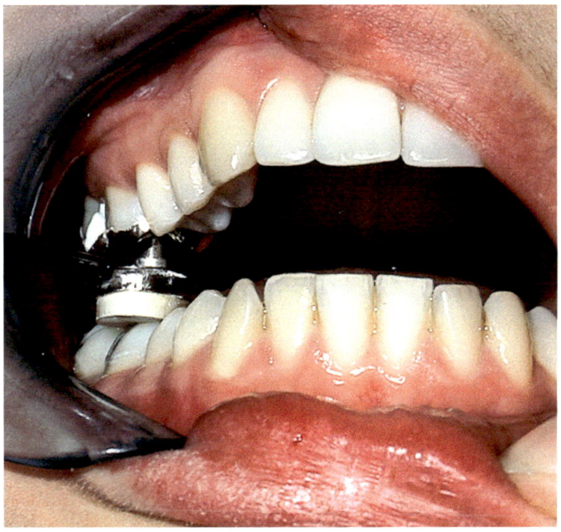

Fig 3-25b The partial crown is adapted to the tooth with an inlay setter.

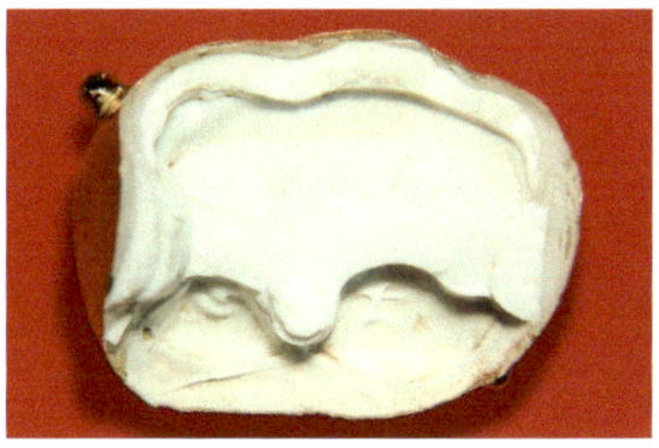

Fig 3-25c First spot test.

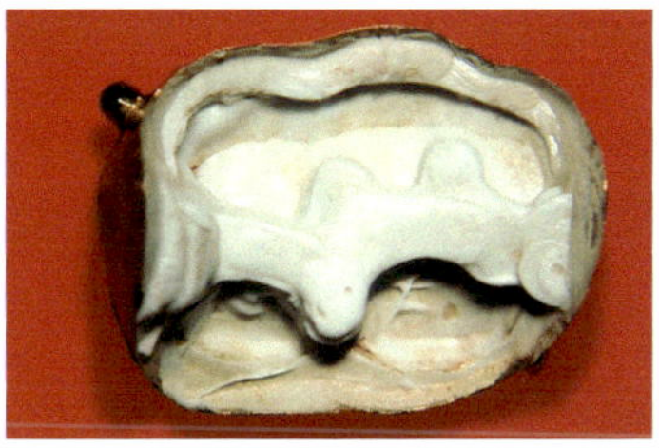

Fig 3-25d Final spot test.

Fig 3-25e *(left)* The partial crown is brushed with cement.

Fig 3-25f *(right)* The prepared tooth is brushed with cement.

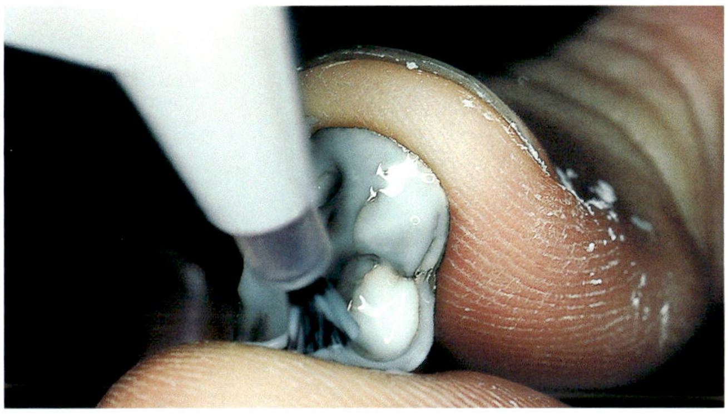

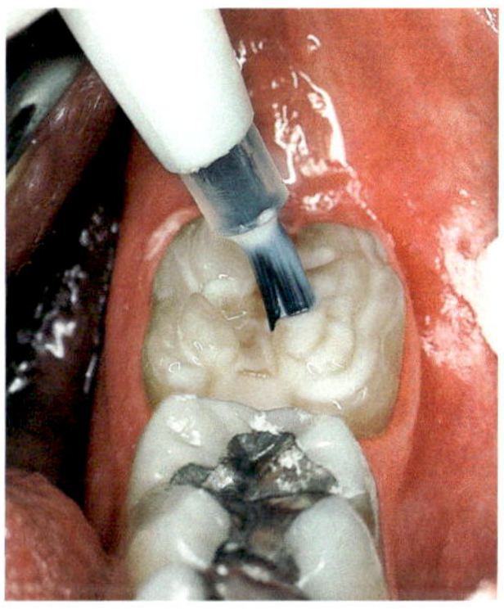

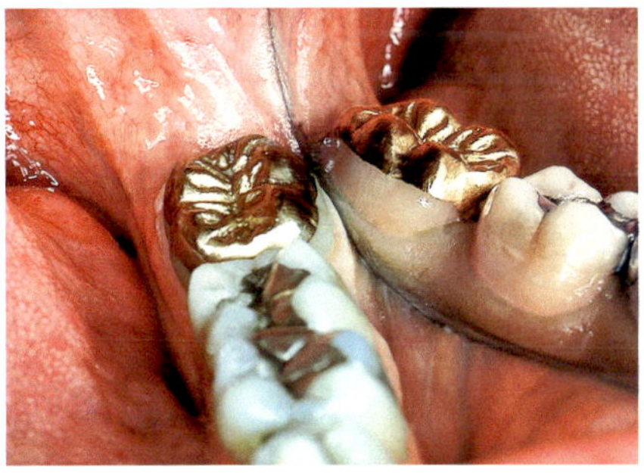

Fig 3-25g Permanently cemented partial crown.

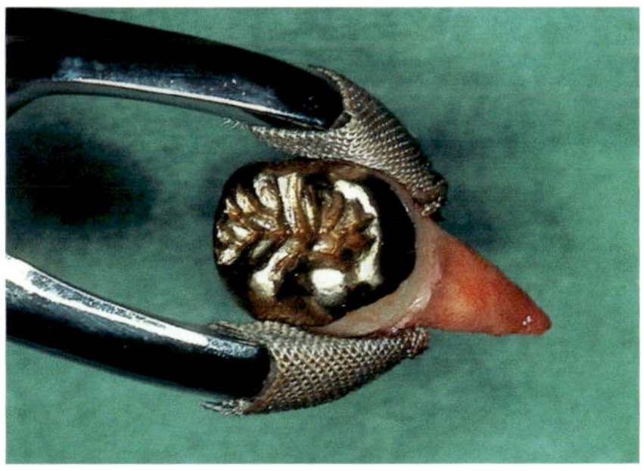

Fig 3-25h The tooth with the partial crown has been extracted.

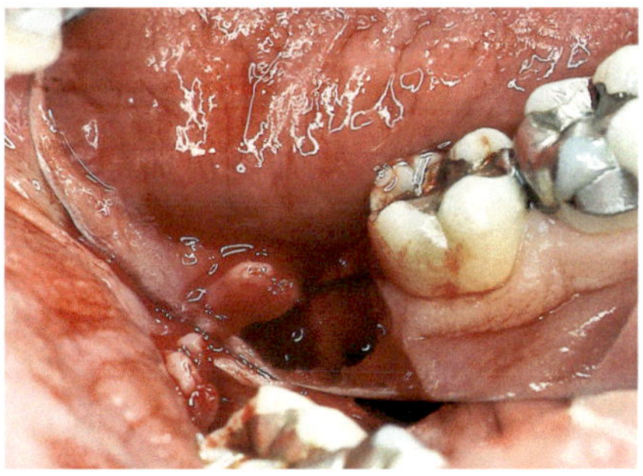

Fig 3-25i Extraction site.

After the silicone is cured, the crown is removed and the primary contacts are highlighted with a waterproof felt-tip pen under the stereomicroscope (Fig 3-25c). The silicone film is removed, and the marked primary contacts are ground with a bud bur. Pressure spot testing is repeated until the silicone layer becomes transparent in the marginal area (Fig 3-25d). Measurements with a stereomicroscope revealed the thickness of the silicone layer to be approximately 0.020 mm.

Glass-ionomer cement should be used, because this material allows a film thickness of approximately 0.010 to 0.015 mm. The crown and the tooth preparation are

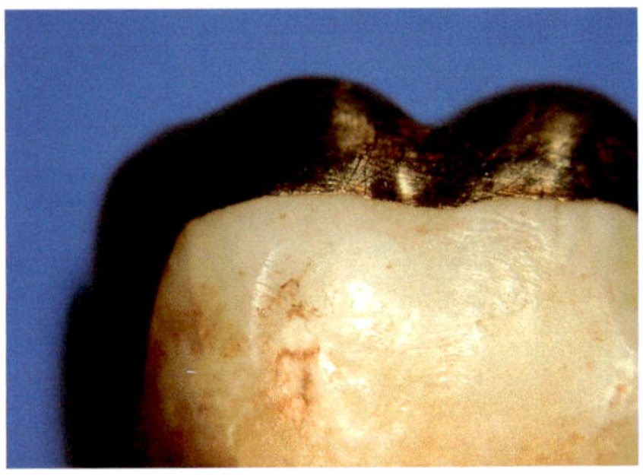

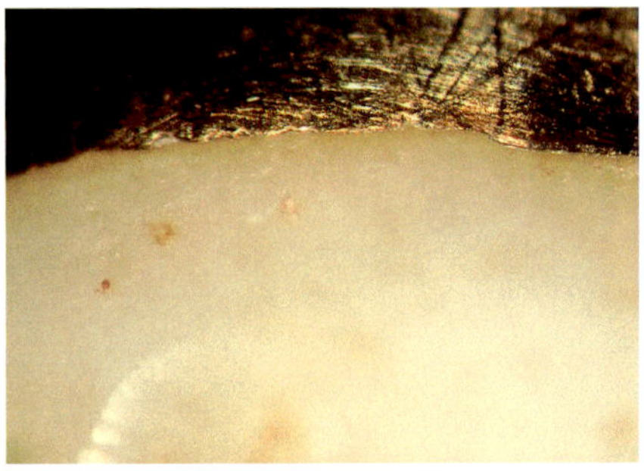

Fig 3-25j *(left)* Buccal crown margin at 10x original magnification.

Fig 3-25k *(right)* Buccal crown margin at 50x original magnification.

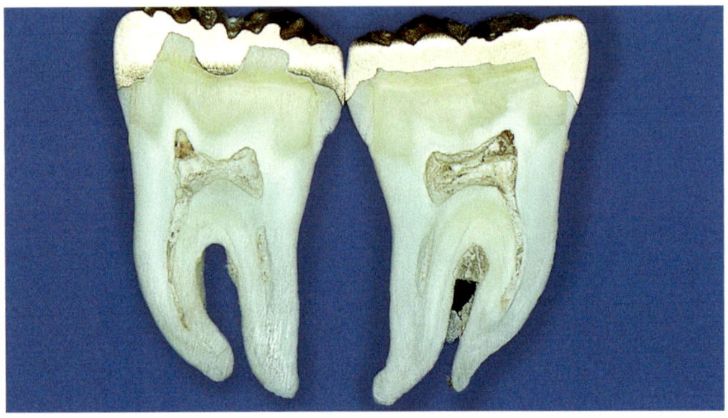

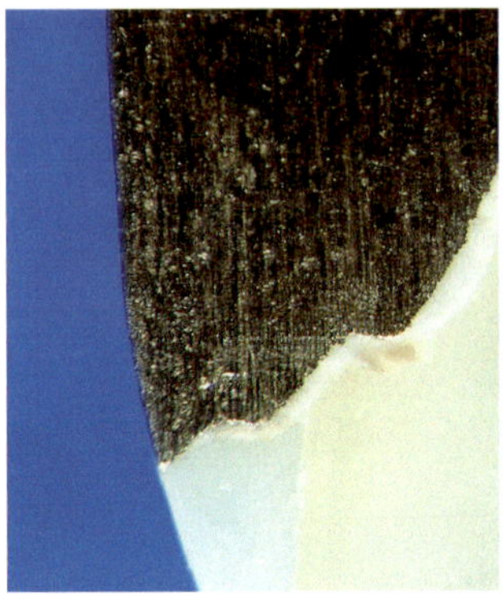

Fig 3-25l *(left)* Cross section of the extracted partial crown.

Fig 3-24m *(right)* Margin of the partial crown at 50x original magnification.

brushed with the cement (Figs 3-25e and 3-25f). It is important not to fill the crown entirely with the cement; this would result in an overflow and an inaccurately placed crown, which in turn would lead to a raised bite. A final inspection is performed (Fig 3-25g).

In 1982, Dr Klaus Lehman from Marburg University made a wager about a partial crown placed by the author on a mandibular left third molar that was going to be extracted anyway. The wager was about whether cementation would allow a marginal fit of less than 0.050 mm in the patient's mouth. The crown remained in situ for 4 weeks. Then the tooth was extracted very carefully (Figs 3-25h to 3-25k) and cut into plates to allow evaluation of the marginal integrity in several zones (Figs 3-25l and 3-25m). The following values were measured: mesial margins, 0.031 and 0.018 mm; distal margins, 0.040 and 0.030 mm; and buccolingual margins, 0.033, 0.044, and 0.032 mm. This single experiment—for which the author would like to thank Dr Lehmann sincerely—provided so much insight that nowadays it is possible to almost constantly achieve results of 0.030 mm, thanks to improvements in materials and methods. This degree of marginal integrity was questioned by Dr Carlo Marinello, who was still at the University of Zurich at that time. The tooth with the partial crown was measured a second time, with the same results.

Materials

Cyanoacrylate (Renfert) PSI silicone for pressure spot testing (Coltène Whaledent)
Ketac-Cem luting cement (3M ESPE)
Moldasynt synthetic stone (Heraeus Kulzer)
Vario microscope (Zeiss)

Conventional Cementation

Common problem: Errors in cementation with conventional cements

Problems can arise during cementation of cast restorations such as inlays, onlays, partial crowns, or full crowns. These problems can lead to undesirable microleakage or even to an incorrect position of the cast restoration. In such cases, any one of the following factors may have contributed to the situation:

1. The cement was mixed by hand and a homogenous mix was not achieved.
2. The cement had already begun to set during cementation.
3. The cast restoration was placed in an incorrect position (leakage).
4. The cast restoration (especially in the case of crowns) was completely filled with cement and does not fit on the abutment tooth correctly (raised occlusion).
5. The abutment teeth could not be kept dry enough (the cement was washed away).

Proven solution: Efficient cementation with the brushing technique, encapsulated cement, and first-aid tape

For conventional cementation, the dentist can choose from among several kinds of cements, whose properties are listed in Table 3-1. The values are averages taken from various scientific evaluations that can help the clinician to choose the appropriate cement for conventional cementation.

Since 1980, the author has cemented all cast restorations conventionally with glass-ionomer materials (see also the previous section about precision in the laboratory and dental office). The following criteria speak in favor of glass-ionomer cements:

1. They are high-quality cements when mixed in a capsule within 10 seconds.
2. They have low film thickness.
3. They provide good tensile and compressive strengths.
4. They allow efficient cementation in a short amount of time.
5. They release fluoride.

Preparation of the abutment teeth

The abutment teeth are cleaned with Tubulicid, a substance that contains ethylenediaminetetraacetic acid, and dried by the first assistant with the help of cotton rolls. For deeper cavities, dry retraction cords should be placed.

Absorbent sponges such as Sugi are inserted in the interproximal spaces. The Sugi sponge is made of pressed cellulose and can absorb up to 10 times its volume in water. By expanding, the sponge keeps itself in position and thus constitutes an ideal means to keep interproximal spaces dry.

Table 3-1 Properties of cements used in conventional cementation

	Glass-ionomer	Zinc phosphate	Carboxylate	Resin composite
Setting time	3.5 min	9 min	4 min	3 min
pH	6	< 3	6	7
Film thickness	15 mm	22 mm	13 mm	10 mm
Water solubility	0.25%	0.2%	0.2%	0.07%
Tensile strength	16 psi	10 psi	1.7 psi	6.8 psi
Compressive strength	17 psi	10.8 psi	12.3 psi	40 psi
Mixing	In capsules in a machine	By hand	By hand	By hand
Moisture control	Cotton rolls	Cotton rolls	Cotton rolls	Rubber dam

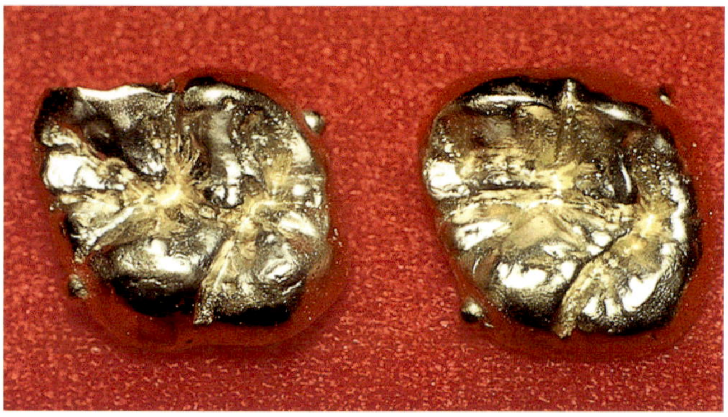

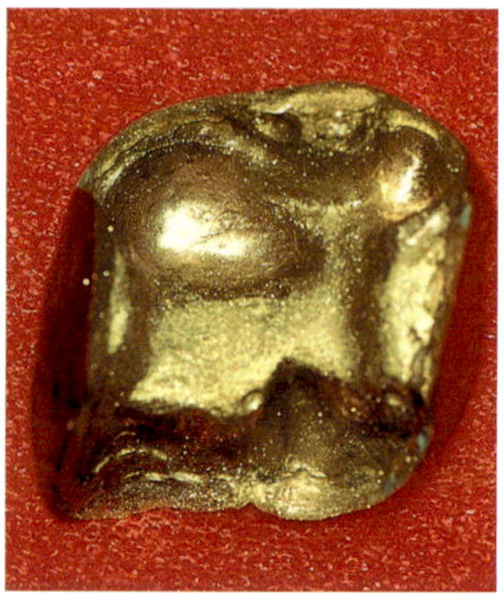

Fig 3-26a *(left)* Partial gold crowns for the maxillary left first and second molars at try-in.

Fig 3-26b *(right)* Partial gold crown for the first molar after sandblasting.

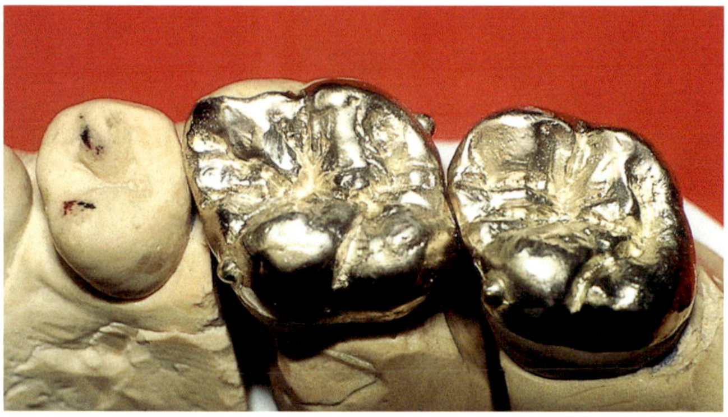

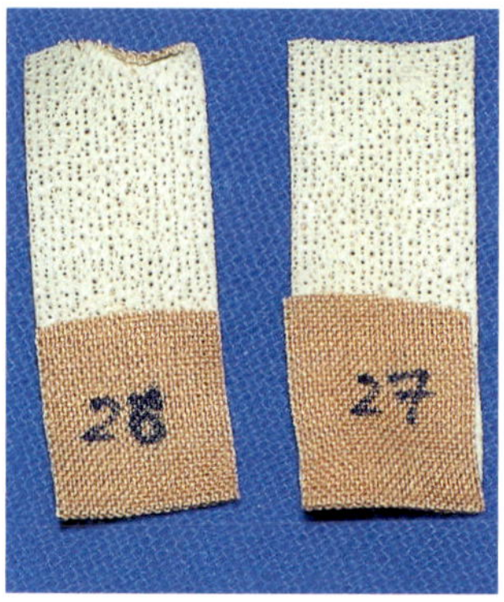

Fig 3-26c *(left)* Partial crowns placed back on the laboratory cast after the try-in.

Fig 3-26d *(right)* Prepared first-aid tape.

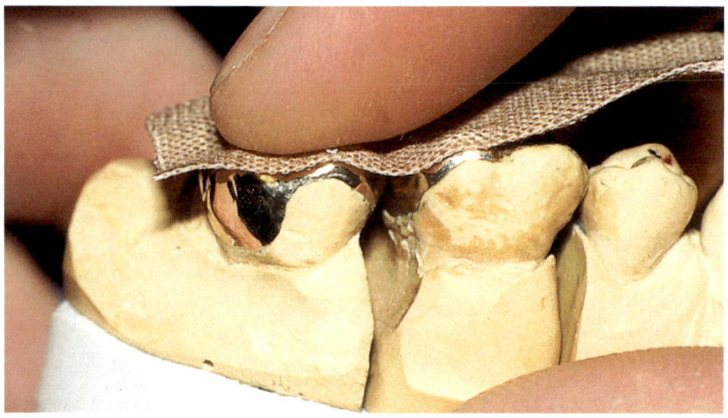

Fig 3-26e The first-aid tape is adapted carefully onto the partial gold crown.

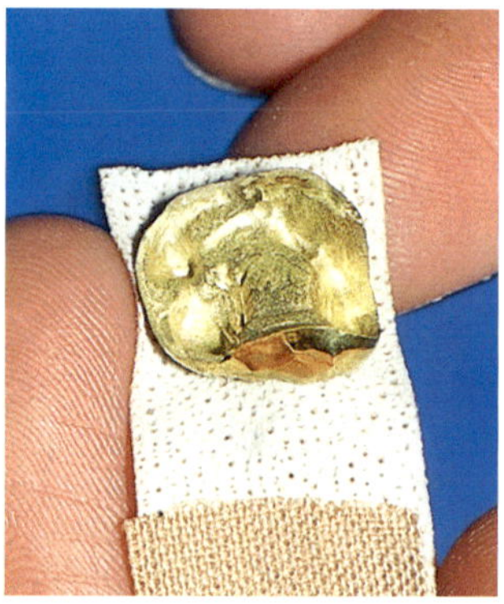

Fig 3-26f The partial gold crown is removed with the help of the first-aid tape.

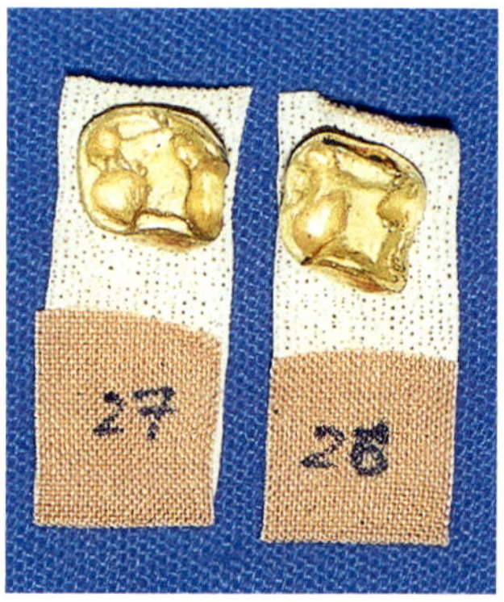

Fig 3-26g The partial gold crowns for the maxillary left first and second molars are ready for cementation.

Preparation of the cast restorations

After a pressure spot test with silicone, the cast restorations (Fig 3-26a) are sandblasted carefully (50-μm sandblasting medium) by the second assistant. It is important not to damage the margins when they are sandblasted (Fig 3-26b). Then the restorations are cleaned with alcohol and dried carefully. The cast restorations are repositioned correctly on the laboratory cast (Fig 3-26c).

For the taping technique, approximately 4 cm of first-aid tape is cut from a roll and folded over at one end to create a 1-cm long "handle." The number of the tooth is written on the handle with a felt-tip pen (Fig 3-26d). The cast restorations are removed from the cast with the first-aid tape, beginning on the mesial side, and kept ready for cementation (Figs 3-26e to 3-26g).

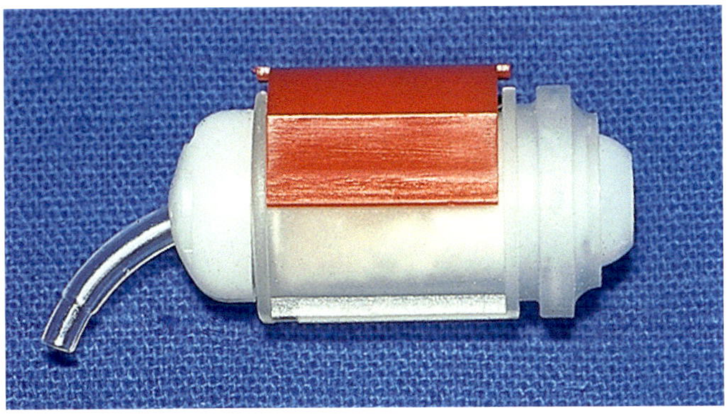

Fig 3-26h MaxiCap with glass-ionomer cement.

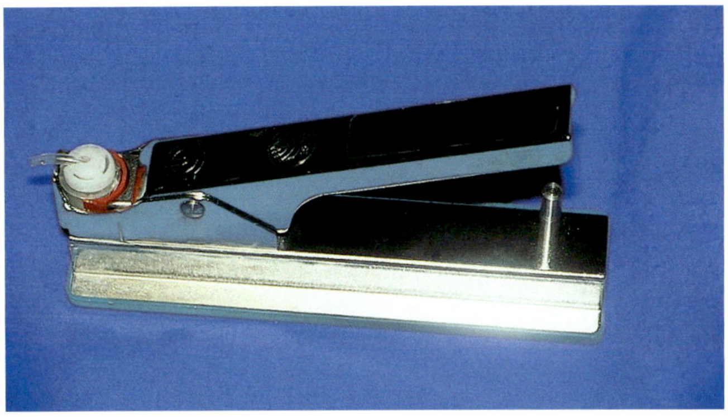

Fig 3-26i The MaxiCap is activated for 3 seconds.

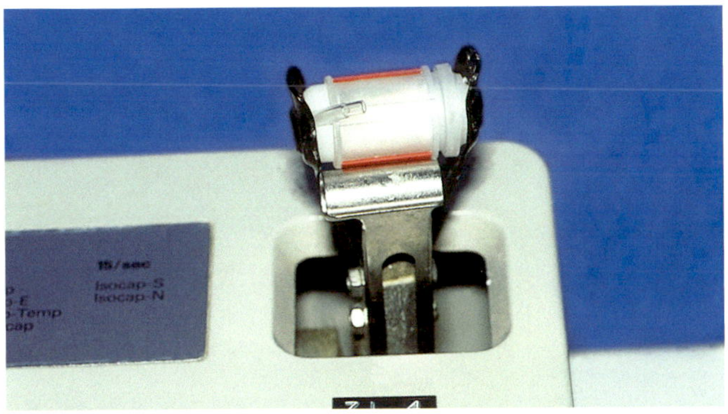

Fig 3-26j The cement is mixed in the capsule mixer for 10 seconds.

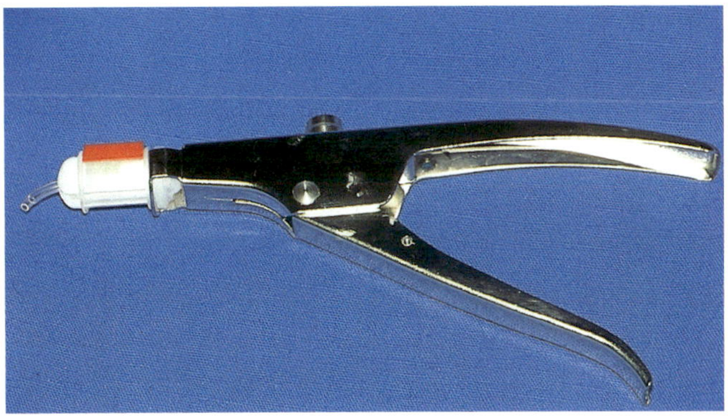

Fig 3-26k The MaxiCap is inserted in the application syringe.

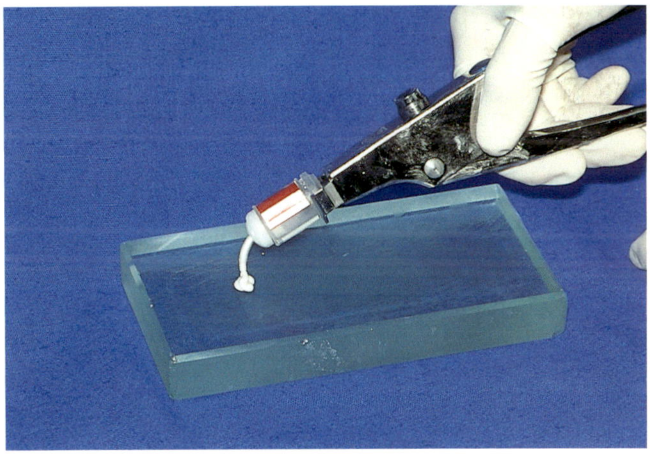

Fig 3-26l The glass-ionomer cement is applied to a cooled glass slab.

Mixing of the cement

The cement capsule is activated in the activator for 3 seconds and mixed in a capsule mixer for 10 seconds (Figs 3-26h to 3-26j). Then the cement is pressed on a cooled glass slab (Figs 3-26k and 3-26l).

Cementation

The cement is picked up from the glass slab with a disposable brush, and the cavity preparations are brushed carefully with the cement (Fig 3-26m). In the meantime, the second assistant brushes cement on the cast restorations that are stuck to the first-aid tape (Fig 3-26n).

The clinician takes the prepared cast restorations from the assistant and applies them, beginning with the distal-

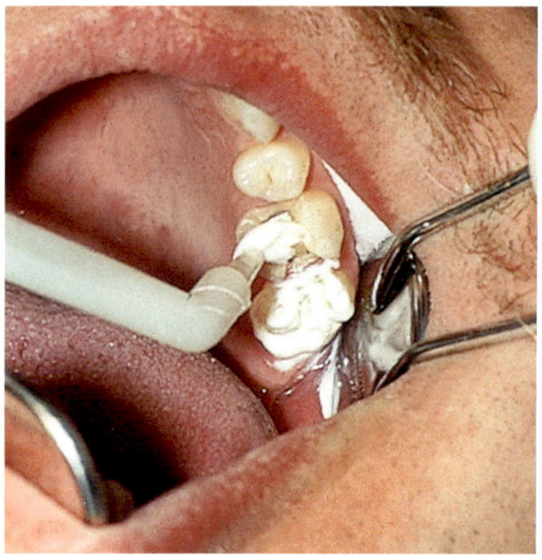

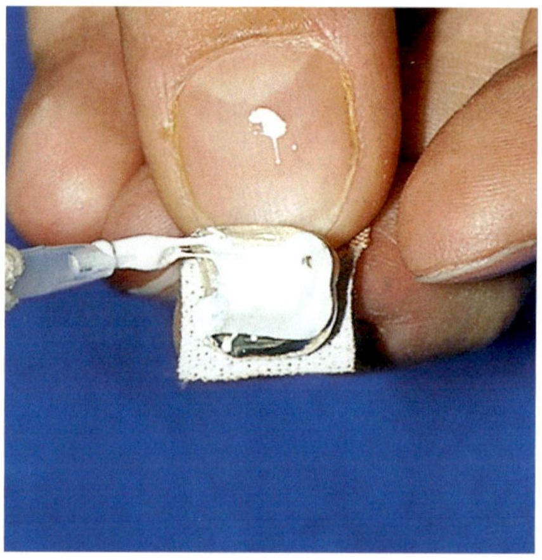

Fig 3-26m The cavity preparations are carefully brushed with the help of a disposable brush.

Fig 3-26n The partial gold crowns are brushed just as carefully.

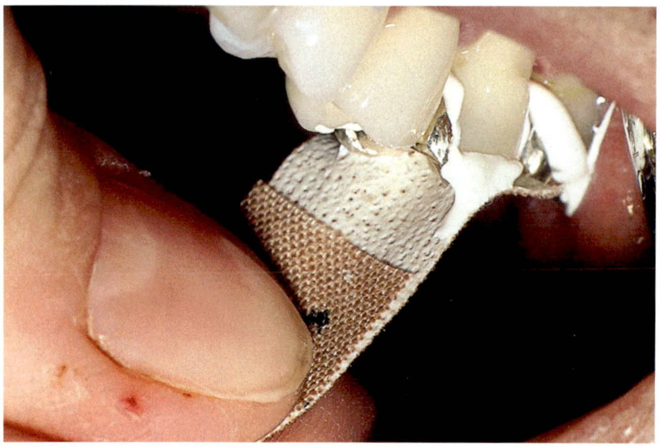

Fig 3-26o The partial gold crowns are placed on the first-aid tape, one after another.

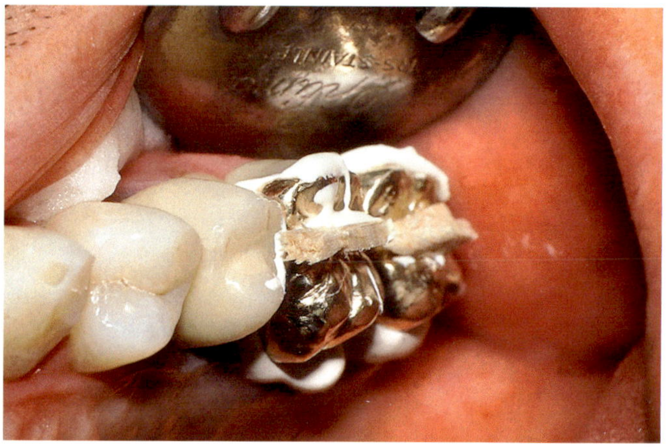

Fig 3-26p Balsa wood wedges are inserted in the central fossae to create occlusal stability.

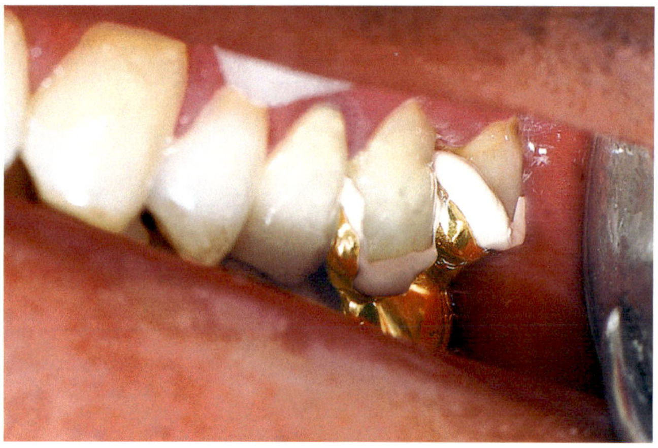

Fig 3-26q While the cement is setting, the partial crowns are kept in situ by the constant pressure of the patient's bite.

most tooth and moving forward mesially (Fig 3-26o). The first-aid tape is removed while the restorations are held in place with a pair of tweezers. The restorations that were placed in the cavities are vibrated into position with an ultrasonic tip.

To secure the position of the restorations, small balsa wood wedges are dipped in cement and placed in the central fossae of the restorations (Fig 3-26p). The patient is instructed to bite down with medium pressure (Fig 3-26q).

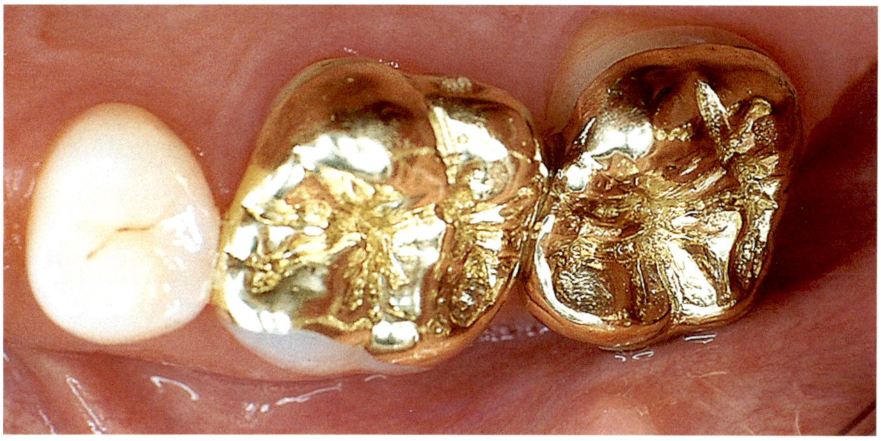

Fig 3-26r Cemented crowns.

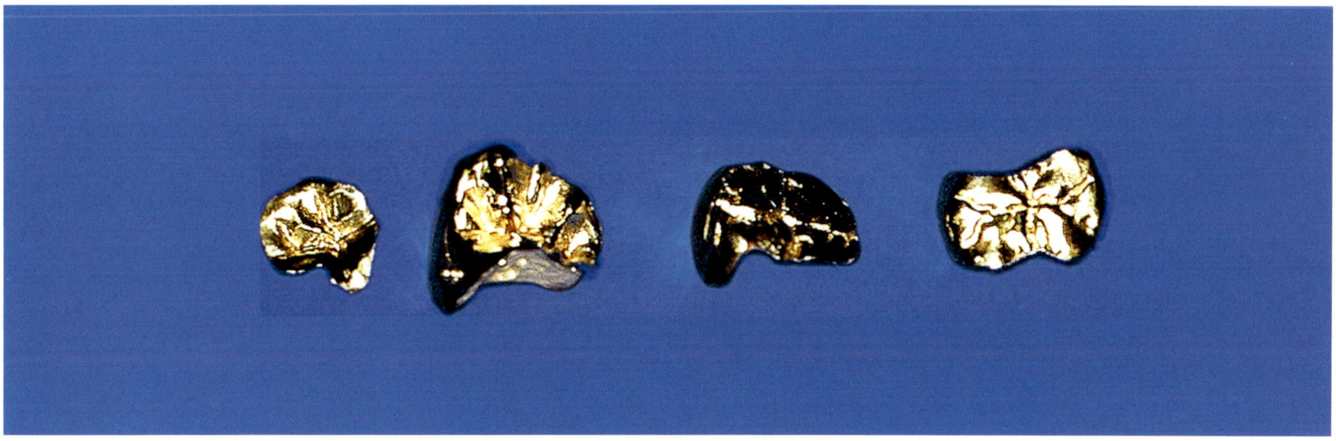

Fig 3-27a Tiny cast gold restorations that are difficult to place.

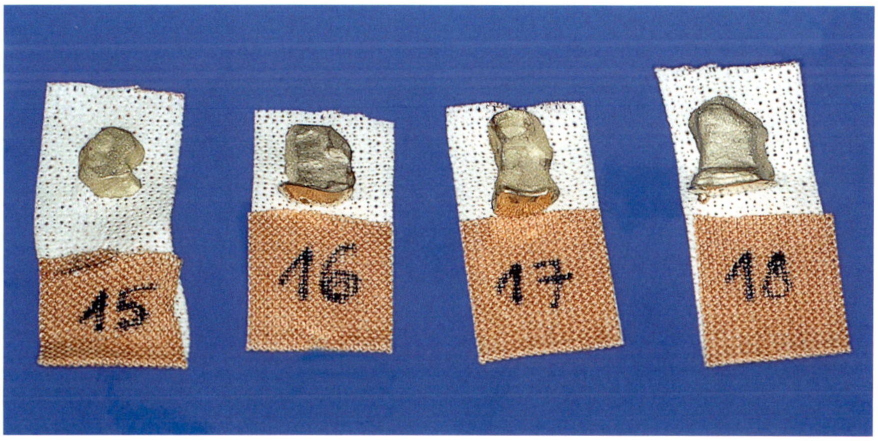

Fig 3-27b Everything is easier with the restorations adapted and aligned on the tape.

Removal of excess cement

Two minutes after all restorations have been placed, the first excess cement is removed from the buccal surfaces while the patient's teeth are closed. After 3 minutes, the patient is asked to open the mouth, and the remaining excess cement is removed with the help of sickles, floss, and knots. Cementation is finished with an occlusal examination and adjustment, and the patient is instructed about necessary dental hygiene (Fig 3-26r).

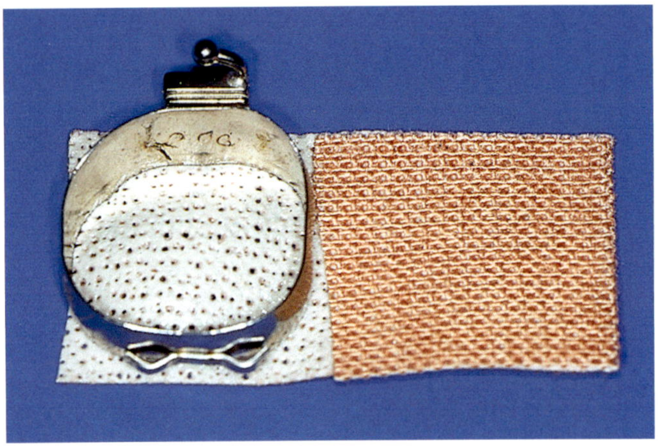

Fig 3-28 Origins of the method: orthodontic molar band stuck to first-aid tape.

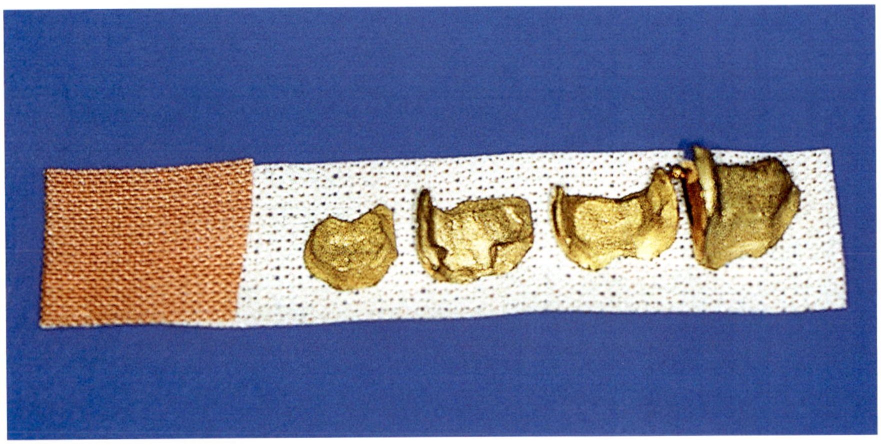

Fig 3-29 Just like the little tailor in the fairy tale: four at one blow.

Active cementing (as proposed by colleagues such as Tucker, Thomas, and Gutowski) has actually become obsolete since the introduction of the microscopic working technique in the dental laboratory. This is due to the fact that margins in easily accessible areas can hardly be improved anymore, and this method does not offer any improvement in inaccessible areas, in interproximal spaces, where improvement would be most needed.

Use of first-aid tape to place restorations is very useful, especially with small cast restorations that are hard to place (Fig 3-27a and 3-27b). This technique has been borrowed from orthodontists, who place orthodontic bands accurately on molars with the help of first-aid tape (Fig 3-28).

In prosthetic dentistry, some rather bold clinicians try to cement an entire quadrant with one length of tape in one pass. This approach seems similar to that of the brave little tailor from the fairy tale—but perhaps they are successful with it after all (Fig 3-29).

Materials

Ketac-Cem as a MaxiCap (3M ESPE)
Sugi pressed cellulose for keeping the interproximal spaces dry (Kettenbach)
Tubulicid (Global Dental)
Leukoplast first-aid tape (BSN Medical)
Sonocem ultrasonic tip for common piezo systems as designed by Dr Noack (Sirona)
Ultrapak retraction cords (Ultradent)

Adhesive Inlay/Onlay Supported Fixed Partial Dentures

Common problem: Designing an adhesive inlay/onlay–supported fixed partial denture for a patient with metal allergies

A young patient (Fig 3-30a) had a space in the maxillary right quadrant. The maxillary right first molar was missing; the second molar was elongated and was out of occlusion with the opposing teeth (Fig 3-30b). The patient presented the results of an allergy test that indicated that he had allergic reactions to many metals and alloys used in prosthetic dentistry. It was important to respect his request for a metal-free restoration.

Two questions immediately come to mind in such a case:

1. Would it be consistent with good clinical practice to place a fixed partial denture with full crowns on the two noncarious teeth that are virtually free of restorations? In recent years dentistry has moved away from very invasive techniques in favor of minimally invasive techniques. The goal of preserving tooth structure (particularly the enamel) can be achieved with increasing efficiency, thanks to adhesive bonding and new ceramic and resin composite materials.

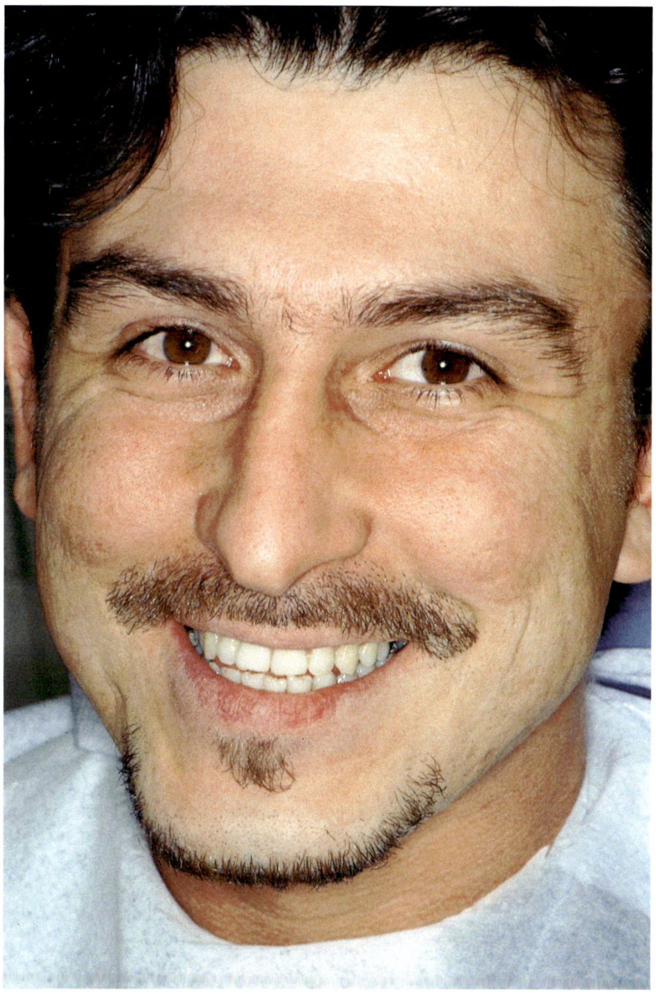

Fig 3-30a Patient who is missing his maxillary right first molar.

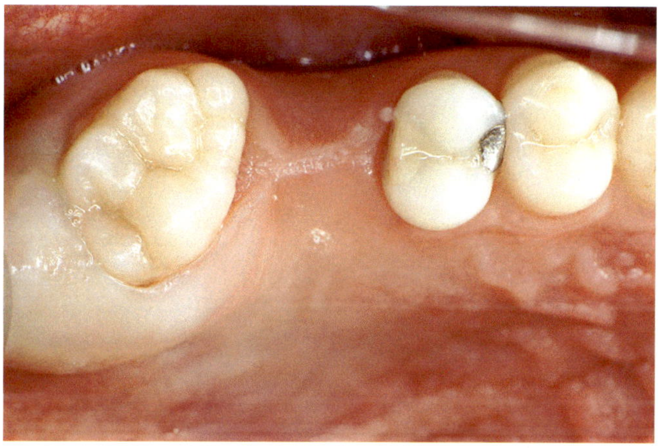

Fig 3-30b Posterior space that will be closed with a metal-free fixed partial denture.

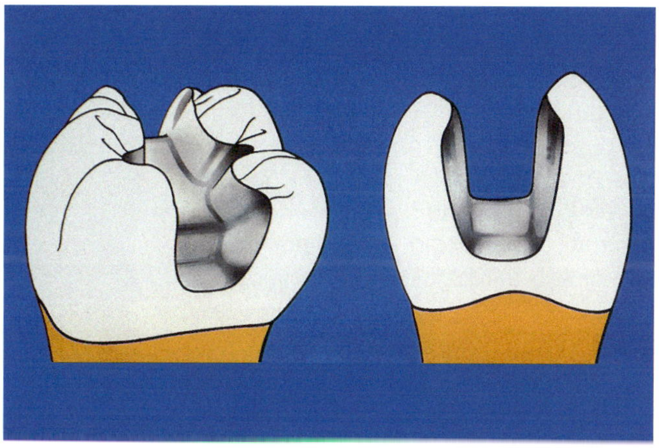

Fig 3-30c Box preparation with smooth surfaces.

2. Are there any metal-free materials available that are suitable for creating and placing a combined inlay/onlay-supported fixed partial denture? All-ceramic materials still pose a risk when they are used as a material for full crowns as part of bridgework in the posterior region, and they are certainly not suitable as an inlay/onlay fixed partial denture material if long-term success is the goal. What other options does the dentist have?

Proven solution: Fabrication of a metal-free inlay/onlay fixed partial denture of fiber-reinforced material

Different fiber-reinforced resin composite materials provide the opportunity to design tooth-colored, metal-free, and durable adhesive inlay fixed partial dentures. The author has been working with the Targis/Vectris system since 1996. The possible applications for this system are discussed and presented in detail in another text.[2] This technique will be demonstrated step by step through the example of this young patient.

Preparation

The inlay was prepared following the standard guidelines for the preparation of ceramic inlays (Fig 3-30c). A block-shaped preparation was created; only small retentive elements were prepared because an adhesive cementation technique was to be used. There were no corners; there were smooth, wavy contours in the preparation. No chamfers were created.

There was minimal abrasion (1.5 mm) in the area of fissures and at the margins. The preparation was open proximally 60 to 90 degrees. A base was placed to support and block out the enamel necessary for adhesive bonding, because the best possible adhesive bond can only come from bonding to enamel. With modern adhesive technology (with a total-etch/total-bond technique), pulpal protection in the classic sense is required only in exceptional cases.
The following instruments are recommended for the preparation:

1. Ceramic inlay preparation set 4263 with rounded, slightly conical burs of different lengths, diameters, and grit sizes (Fig 3-30d)
2. Oscillating files with an EVA head or with the special handpieces for oscillating file systems with a scope of 0.4 mm, especially designed for this preparation technique (Fig 3-30e)
3. Oscillating files such as Profin, Proxoshape (Fig 3-30f), or those manufactured by Brasseler, in various shapes and grit sizes

Only oscillating files allow the dentist to prepare smooth surfaces in box preparations and to bevel the enamel prisms. This technique is an invaluable advantage in preparing adhesive restorations and should be practiced on extracted teeth several times (Figs 3-30g and 3-30h).

For this patient, a preparation for a mesio-occlusodistal inlay was created in the maxillary right second premolar and a preparation for an onlay was created on the second molar in accordance with the treatment plan to bridge the gap at the first molar with an inlay/onlay-supported fixed partial denture (Figs 3-30i and 3-30j). When the boxes on the second premolar were prepared, both healthy enamel and secondary caries were encountered (Fig 3-30k). In such a case, if the caries were removed without due care, the proximal enamel would break off, thus shifting the preparation margin into dentin.

Without any doubt, the bonding strength between adhesive cementing materials and dentin is significantly lower. Therefore every little bit of enamel, however small, must be preserved and reinforced with a reconstructive base. To prevent the precious enamel from breaking off during the excavation of caries, the enamel was supported with an interproximal wedge (Fig 3-30l). Another possible alternative is to place a circular metal matrix as support.

The carious tooth structure was removed with a slowly rotating bud bur (Fig 3-30m). The preparation was examined to confirm whether the caries had been entirely removed. This task can be accomplished with a probe or with a caries detector. The total-etch/total-bond technique (Figs 3-30n and 3-30o) was used to apply a flowable compomer to the proximal enamel walls and to the noncarious dentin.

The final step was to finish the preparation. The same diamond shapes used for the preparation, but with a finer grain, should be used for finishing. Afterward the inner walls are smoothed with an oscillating diamond file (Figs 3-30p to 3-30s).

A retraction cord was placed at the second molar and then a final inspection was made with the help of a magnifying loupe (Figs 3-30t and 3-30u).

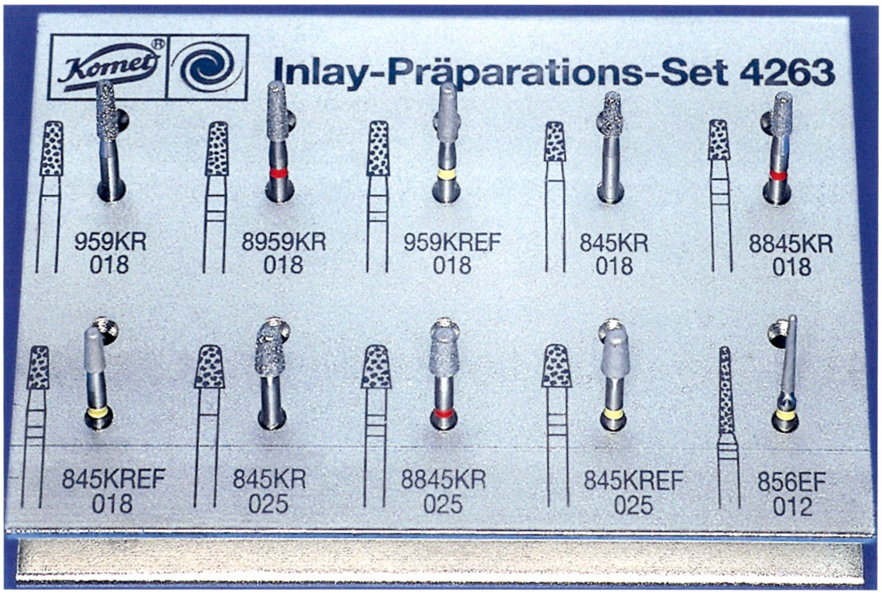

Fig 3-30d Preparation kit for ceramic inlays.

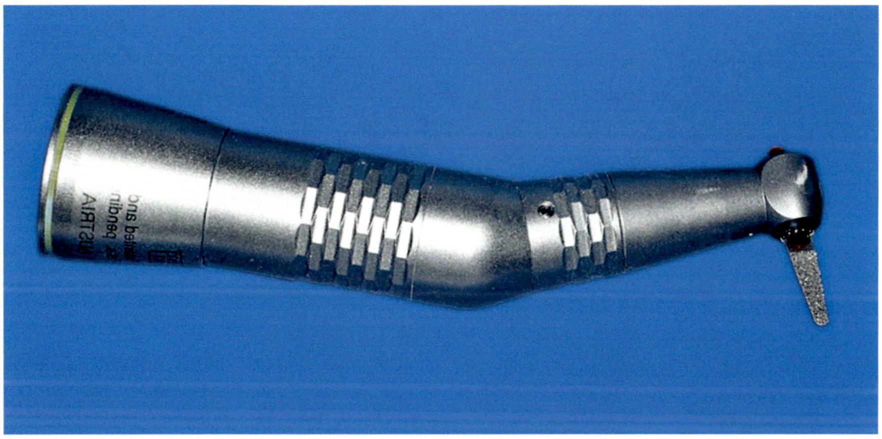

Fig 3-30e Contra-angle handpiece for oscillating files.

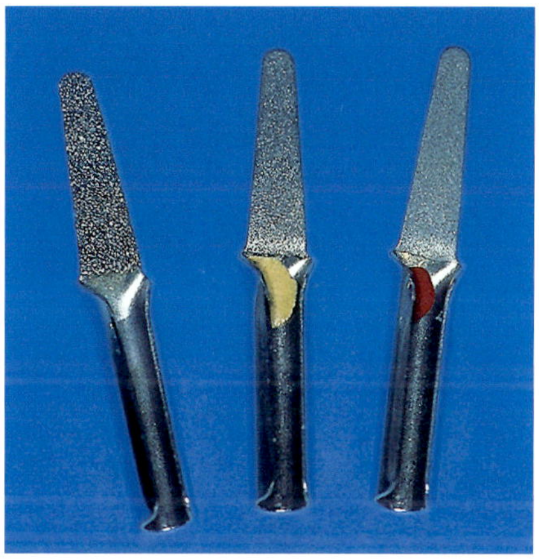

Fig 3-30f Proxoshape file kit.

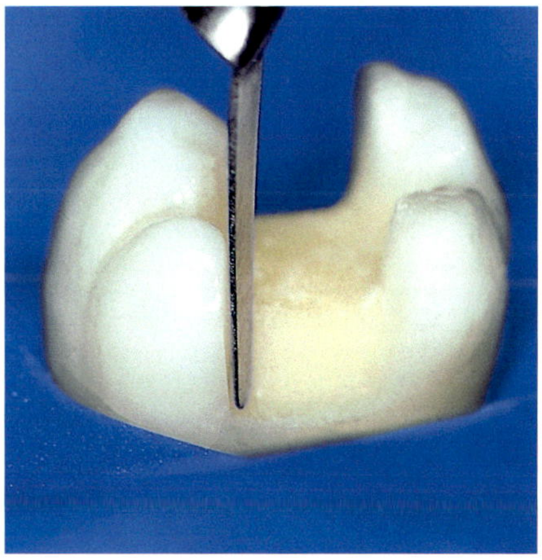

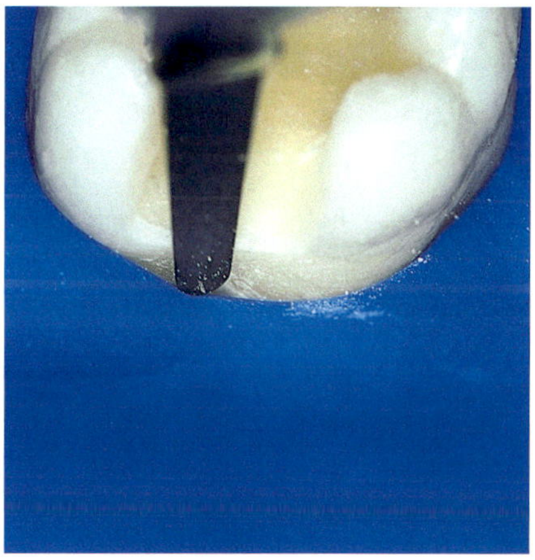

Fig 3-30g *(left)* Use of oscillating files to smooth the interior surfaces.

Fig 3-30h *(right)* Use of oscillating files to debur the enamel margins.

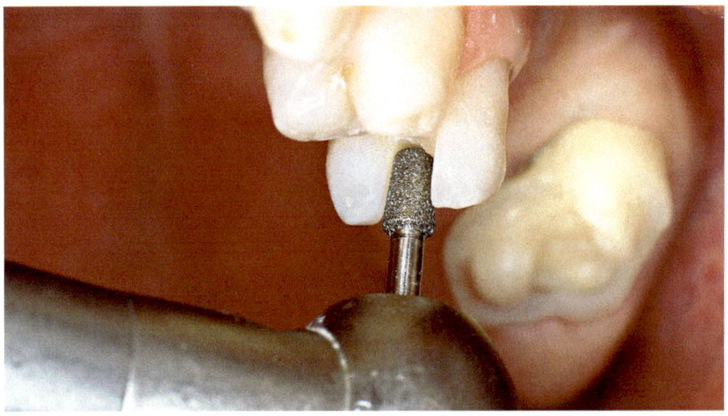

Fig 3-30i Mesio-occlusodistal inlay preparation at the maxillary right second premolar.

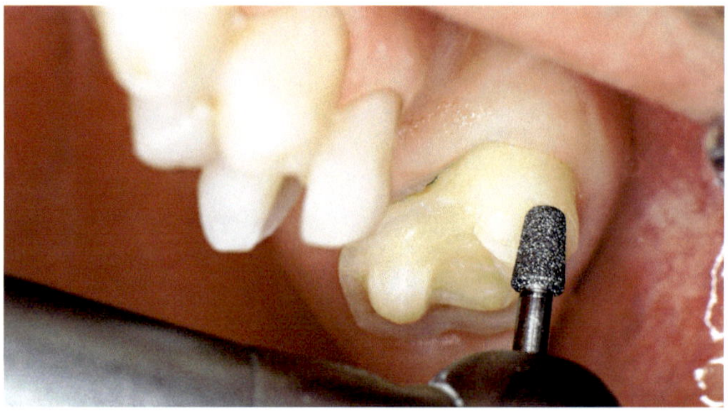

Fig 3-30j Onlay preparation at the maxillary right second molar.

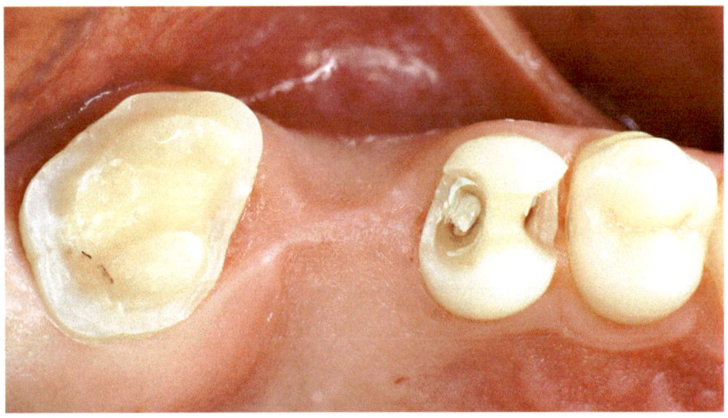

Fig 3-30k Secondary caries is clearly visible in the mesial and distal regions of the second premolar.

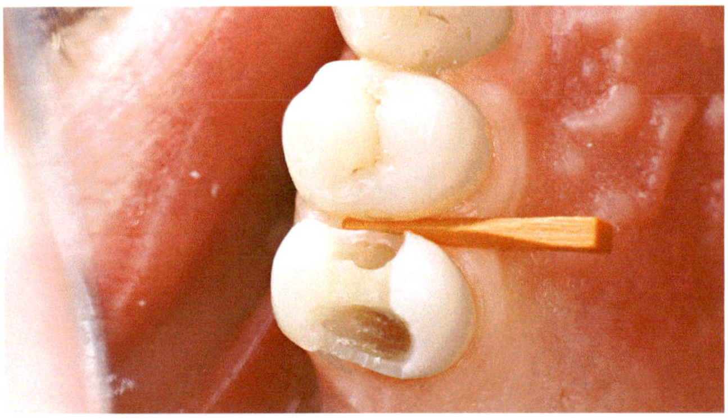

Fig 3-30l Before the caries is excavated, an interproximal wedge is inserted to preserve the cervical marginal crest of the tooth.

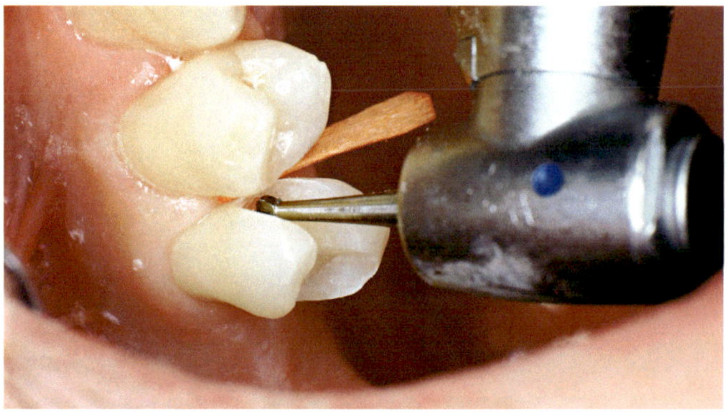

Fig 3-30m The caries is carefully excavated.

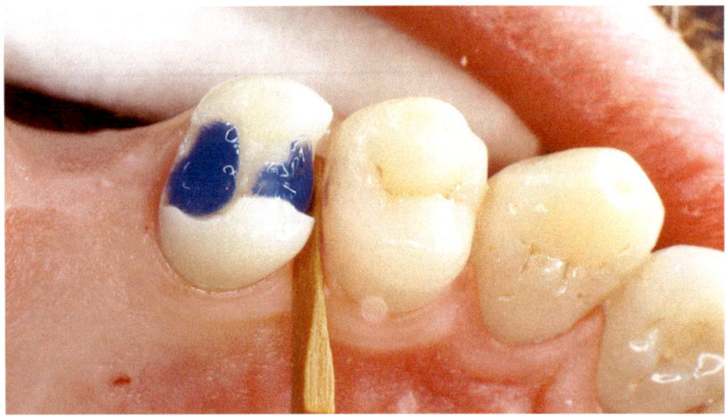

Fig 3-30n The proximal lesions are etched with orthophosphoric acid gel.

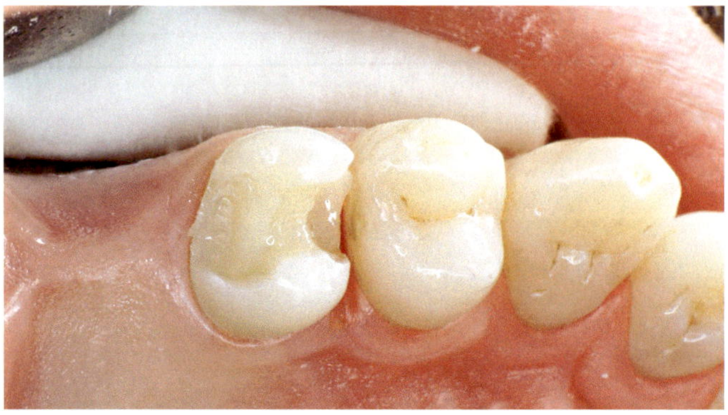

Fig 3-30o The cavities are restored with a low-viscosity, light-curing compomer and the total-etch/total-bond technique.

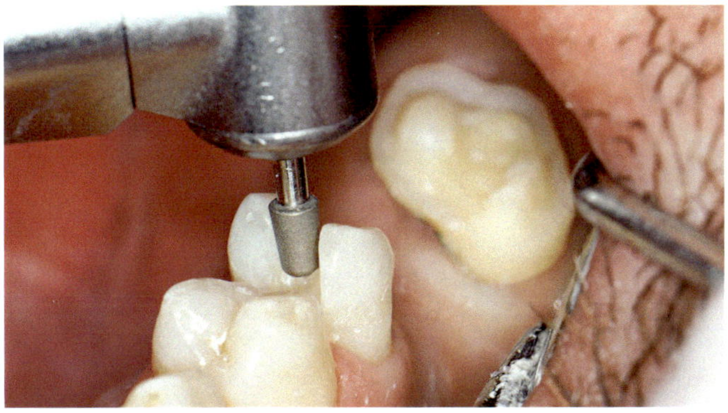

Fig 3-30p The cavity preparation at the second premolar is finished with a fine diamond.

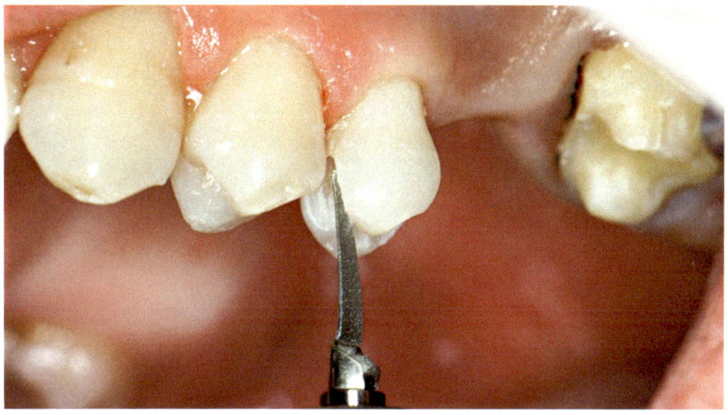

Fig 3-30q The cavity at the second premolar is smoothed with an oscillating file.

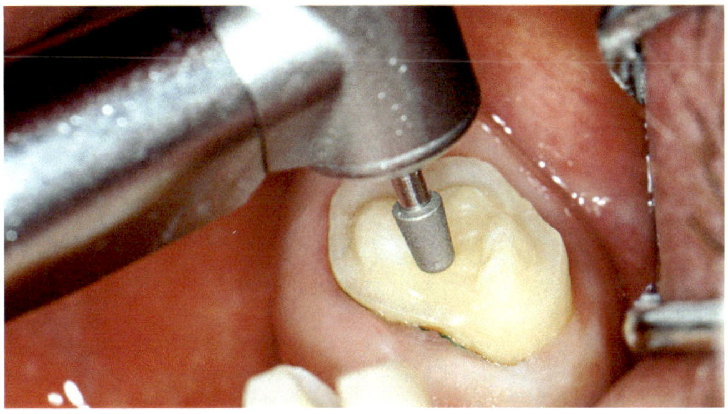

Fig 3-30r The preparation at the second molar is finished with a fine diamond.

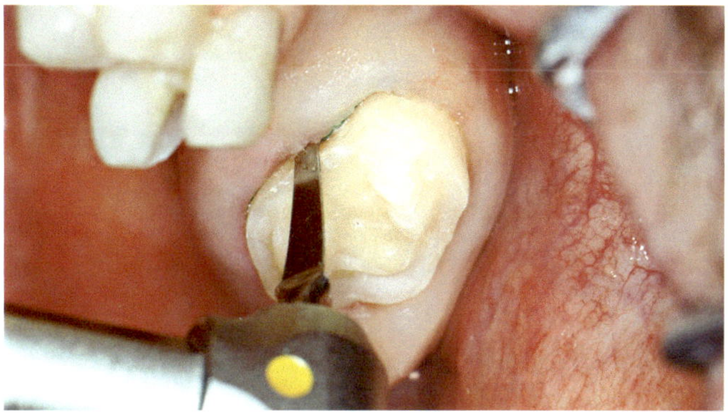

Fig 3-30s The marginal enamel at the second molar is deburred with an oscillating file.

Fig 3-30t *(left)* The retraction cord is placed.

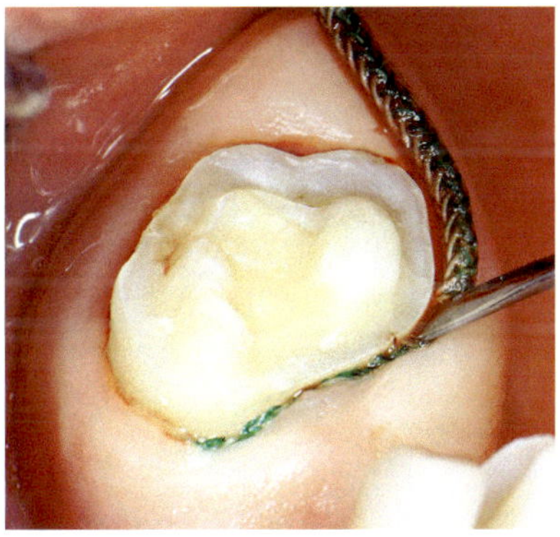

Fig 3-30u *(right)* The finished preparation has clearly visible preparation margins.

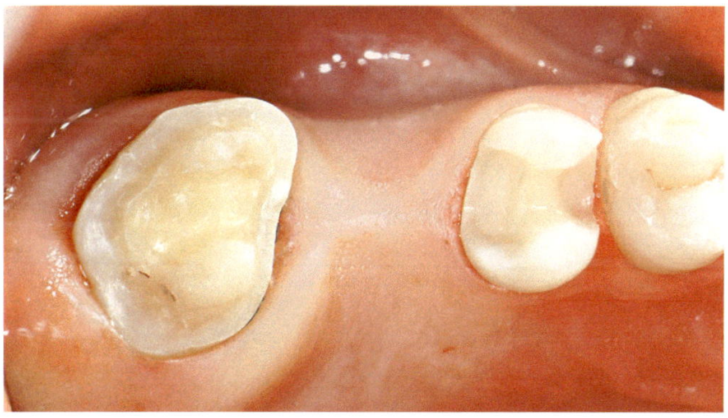

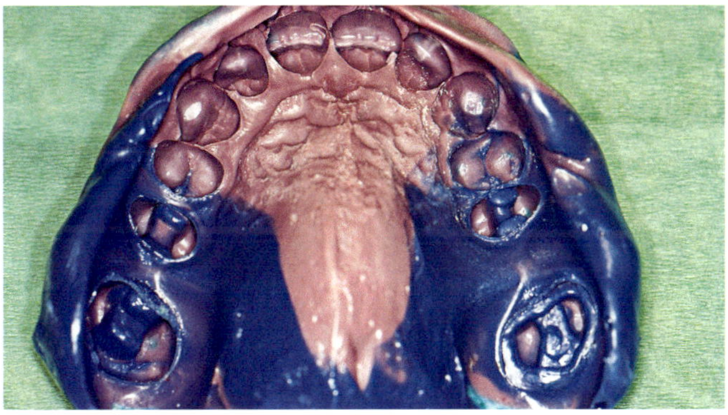

Fig 3-30v Polyether impression with the custom tray.

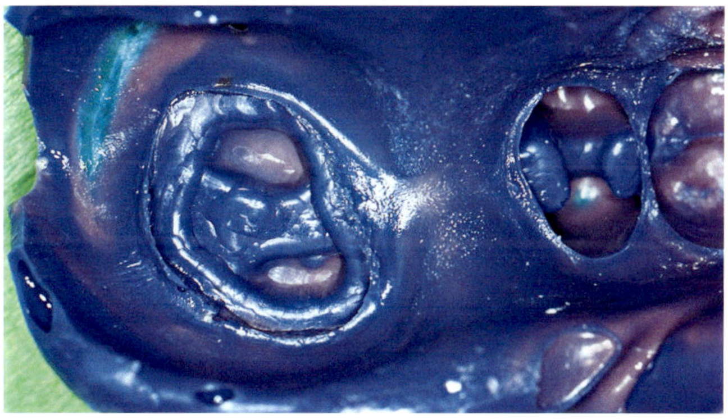

Fig 3-30w All the preparation margins are visible on the impression in a magnified view.

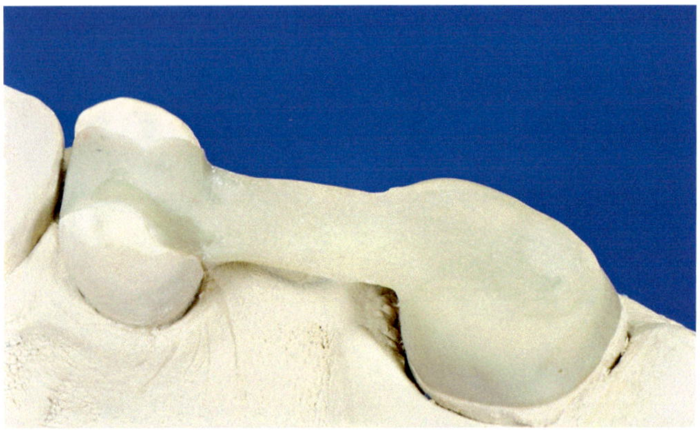

Fig 3-30x The fiber framework is on the cast, still oversized.

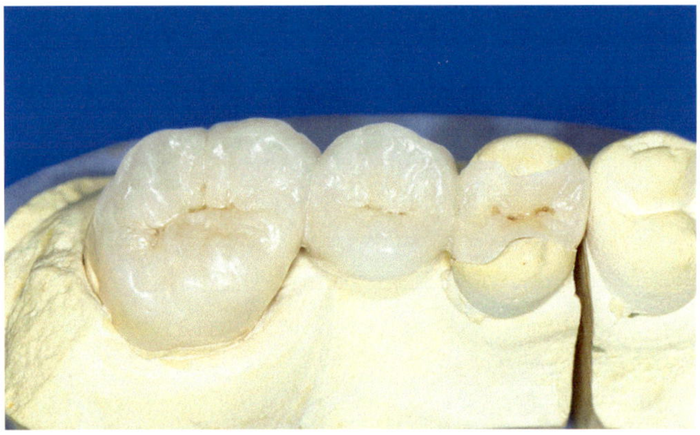

Fig 3-30y The finished inlay/onlay fixed partial denture has been completed by the laboratory.

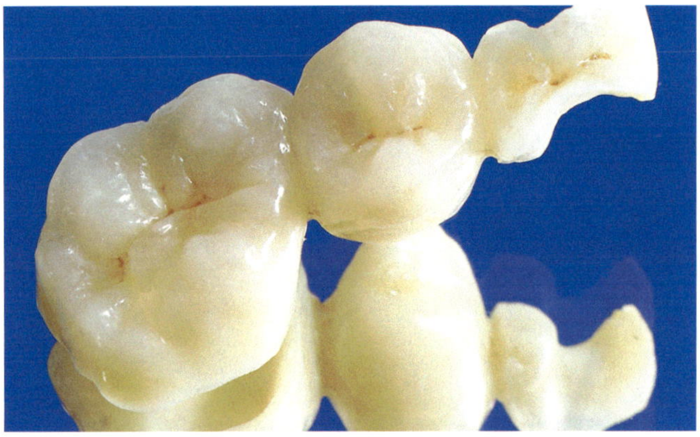

Fig 3-30z The sandblasted and silanized undersurface of the fixed partial denture.

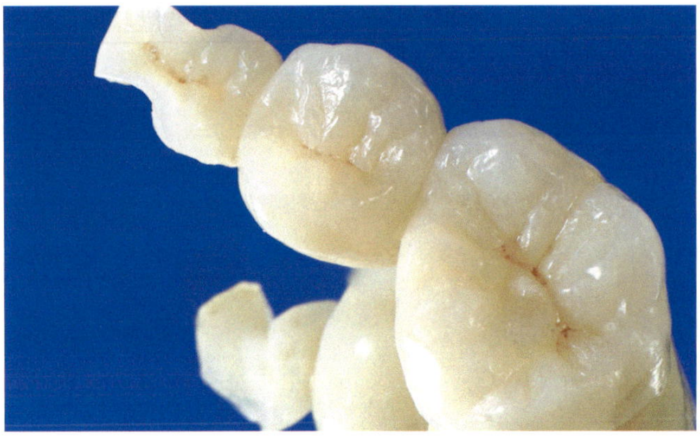

Fig 3-30aa The inlay/onlay fixed partial denture is ready for adhesive cementation.

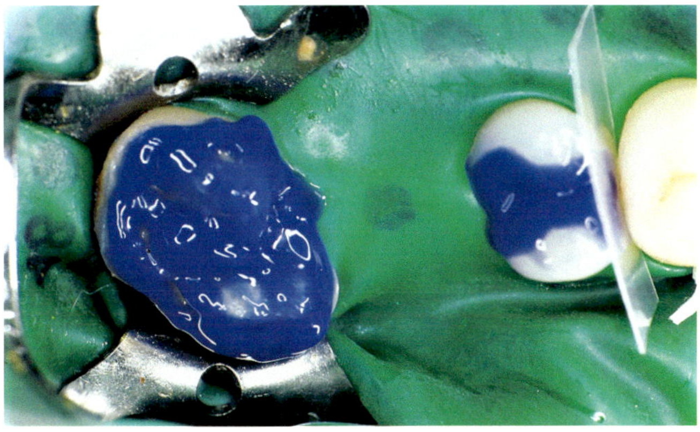

Fig 3-30bb After the enamel is etched for 20 seconds, the dentin is etched for 10 seconds.

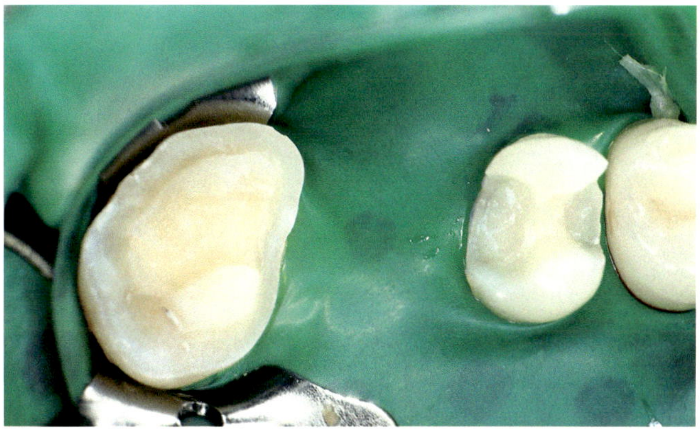

Fig 3-30cc The etching pattern is checked.

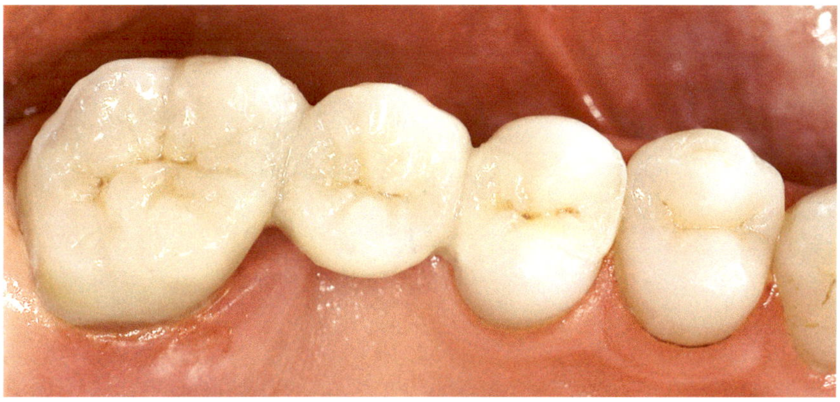

Fig 3-30dd Cemented fixed partial denture. The result is functionally and esthetically pleasing.

Impressions

The impression was taken with the help of an automatic mixing unit and a dual impression technique with a custom tray and polyether (Figs 3-30v and 3-30w).

Laboratory work

The laboratory procedures were carried out as specified by the manufacturer in the instructions for use of the fiber-reinforced resin composite materials (Targis and Vectris). The fixed partial denture framework had to be produced from glass material under light, pressure, and vacuum in a light unit and had to be significantly reduced to create enough space for the facing (Fig 3-30x). After facing and polishing, the laboratory work was complete, and the fixed partial denture was returned to the dentist's office (Fig 3-30y).

Adhesive cementation

After the try-in with silicone (see chapter 2) the undersurface was sandblasted and silanized. Unlike ceramics, these materials cannot be etched (Fig 3-30z).

When the inlay/onlay fixed partial denture was ready to be cemented (Fig 3-30aa), rubber dam was placed and the enamel and dentin were etched (Fig 3-30bb). After the etching pattern was inspected (Fig 3-30cd), the fixed partial denture was cemented with a dual-cure luting cement of medium viscosity exactly as specified in the instructions for use. The prosthesis was light-cured, finished, and polished (Fig 3-30dd).

The fixed partial denture was placed in summer 1996 and remains unaltered in situ. Repolishing was not necessary. The patient felt happy with the restoration. As an additional positive side effect, the restored teeth are not at all sensitive to hot and cold as they would have been with a metal inlay fixed partial denture. The allergist also approved of the procedure.

Conclusion

All in all, fiber-reinforced resin composite technology has not lived up to the promises its developers have made, especially when it comes to full crowns. Use of these materials for fixed partial dentures with full crowns is not recommended—they are only suitable as long-term provisional restorations. However, for indications such as the combined inlay/onlay-supported fixed partial denture, core buildups with fiber-reinforced posts, periodontal splinting, and orthodontic retainers, fiber-reinforced resin composites have become an integral part of daily dental work; furthermore, for these indications, they are also very successful over a longer term.

Materials

Komet 4263 ceramic inlay preparation set (Brasseler)
Contra-angle for vertical files with a scope of 0.4 mm (W&H or Dentatus)
Diamond-coated oscillating files (Dentatus)
Compoglass base liner compomer (Ivoclar Vivadent)
Ultrapak retraction cords (Ultradent)
Polyether mixed in a Pentamix unit (3M ESPE)
Targis/Vectris system (now Adoro/Vectris, Ivoclar Vivadent); alternatively, the Everstick system (Sticktech)
Variolink II luting cement (Ivoclar Vivadent)

Accurate Provisional Fixed Partial Dentures

Common problem: Fabrication of a provisional fixed partial denture with an accurate fit

In many dental offices, the fabrication of provisional fixed partial dentures with an exact fit is very often overlooked or outright ignored (Fig 3-31). There still are dentists who do not place any provisional restorations at all until the permanent restoration is ready to be placed. However, in the absence of an accurate provisional restoration, the following problems can arise, making placement of a permanent restoration very difficult, if not impossible:

1. If the prepared abutment teeth are not protected, pulpitis can ensue, which may provoke thermal sensitivity or may even require endodontic treatment.
2. If the abutment teeth are not appropriately splinted, they may migrate or tilt, thus making it very difficult or even impossible to place the permanent fixed partial denture.
3. Inadequate occlusion or lack of occlusion in the provisional restoration can result in the overeruption of abutment teeth. The provisional restorations often tend to break at primary contacts.
4. Poor marginal integrity of a provisional restoration very often gives rise to ingrowth of gingival tissues, necessitating periodontal surgery.
5. Inadequate contacts with the residual teeth can result in food impaction which in turn may cause gingivitis, gingival retraction, or even periodontal resorption.

Many dentists treat provisional restorations as a "poor cousin," mainly for the following reasons:

1. Too little time is scheduled for the fabrication of provisional restorations.
2. The dentist is not appropriately prepared.
3. The materials used are inadequate.
4. Mistakes in cementation cause the provisional restorations to break or dislodge.

So is it possible to make provisional restorations with an accurate fit, good occlusion, favorable esthetics, and proper cementation so that the permanent fixed restoration can be placed without difficulty?

Proven solution: Fabrication of provisional resin composite fixed partial dentures made with a vacuform template

Preparation

The following procedures can be employed to design a provisional fixed partial denture:

Pontic area cut out from a previously made impression

The use of alginate is completely obsolete, because remaking the provisional restorations is almost impossible if the provisional restorations are lost. The use of silicone is better, but often leads to a raised bite. Moreover, silicone often has voids that require repair. After all of the abutment teeth have been prepared, the provisional restoration can accidentally be misplaced, which would mean that a new provisional fixed partial denture has to be made immediately.

Matrix technique

Laboratory-fabricated vacuum-formed templates have many advantages, especially for long-term provisional restorations, but they involve additional laboratory work, more time, and higher costs. Fast deep-drawing at chairside allows the fabrication of a matrix on an existing cast in only a few minutes; this means little expenditure of time, lower costs, and easy processing with good results.

Direct-indirect technique

With this semidirect method, the surface of a provisional fixed partial denture (ie, the enamel portion of the bridgework) is created in the laboratory. The provisional fixed partial denture is then relined directly in the patient's mouth, thus creating the dentin portion of the provisional restoration. This is an excellent but elaborate and costly method that leads to very good results for long-term provisional restorations when high standards for function and esthetics are required.

Laboratory technique

A provisional restoration that is made completely in the laboratory is the optimum treatment but very expensive. Moreover it requires a direct interim provisional restoration. This method, however, is absolutely recommended

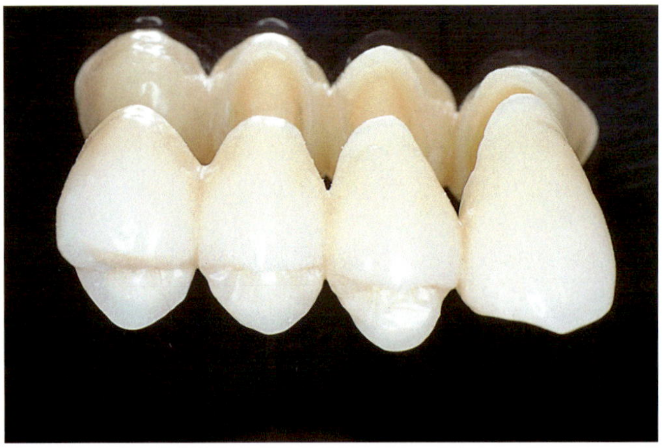

Fig 3-31 Perfect provisional fixed partial denture.

for cases involving changes in occlusal relationships, bite raising, esthetic mucogingival surgery, and for testing of materials, function, and esthetics.

The materials listed in Table 3-2 are available for the fabrication of direct provisional restorations. (These materials are just the ones that have proven useful in the author's practice, so this list is not exhaustive.)

For everyday restorative dentistry, the fast deep-drawing method is the procedure of choice with respect to precision, esthetics, and function. However, the permanent restoration has to be fitted within a few weeks.

Fast deep-drawing with the Perfect-Plast Kit

The spray in the Perfect-Plast Kit is used to isolate the existing cast (a master cast, possibly with a wax-up pontic or otherwise improved with regard to function and shape) in the region of the fixed partial denture (Figs 3-32a and 3-32b). The putty silicone is kneaded until it is soft, so that it can be used to press the plastic film onto the cast.

The plastic film is mounted in the frame and softened over the flame of a gas burner until it is soft and translucent (Fig 3-32c). Then the soft film is held over the cast and adapted to the cast, using the putty silicone as a stamp (Figs 3-32d and 3-32e). After approximately 1 minute, the matrix is removed and cut to size with a pair of scissors (Figs 3-32f and 3-32g). This concludes the preparatory steps.

After the preparation (Fig 3-32h), the matrix is tried in and adapted. The provisional resin composite material is pressed into the ready-cut provisional restoration matrix (Fig 3-32i) from the double-cartridge with a mixing tip (Fig 3-32j). It is necessary to ensure that there are no pockets of air (Fig 3-32k) . Then the matrix is pressed on the prepared abutments (Fig 3-32l). While the material is still curing, the matrix is removed from the mouth, and the cast blank is removed from the matrix. The excess resin composite is trimmed off with a pair of scissors (Figs 3-32m to 3-32o). The provisional fixed partial denture is seated back on the abutment teeth to avoid distortion through polymerization shrinkage.

If light-curing materials are used, the provisional restoration should be precured in the patient's mouth from the occlusal side only. The provisional fixed partial denture is removed; after the half-cured margins are trimmed with a pair of scissors, the provisional restoration is put back in the patient's mouth and cured from all sides. The provisional restoration is placed in a curing unit for final polymerization.

If dual-cure provisional resin composite is used, the provisional restoration remains in the patient's mouth until the dual-cure stage. Afterward, the provisional restoration is removed, trimmed with a pair of scissors, seated back in the patient's mouth, and cured gradually. Provisional restorations should *never* be polymerized outside the patient's mouth. Finally, the provisional restoration is placed in a curing unit for final polymerization.

Under the magnification of a magnifying loupe or a stereomicroscope, the preparation margins are marked

	Self-curing polymethylmethacrylate*	Self-curing provisional resin composite	Dual-cure provisional resin composite
Products	Dentacolor Cronsin Tab 2000	Protemp 3 Luxatemp Tempofit	Luxatemp Automix Solar
Characteristics months	Slow-curing (caution: undercuts) Color-stable; characterization colors available Can remain in situ for up to 9 months	Fast-curing (caution: undercuts) Color-stable; characterization colors available Can remain in situ for up to 2 months	Dual-curing; excellent for inlays, onlays, and partial crowns Color stable for 4 weeks (undercuts are not a problem) Can remain in situ for up to 4

*Producing only warmth, but no heat.

Table 3-2 Provisional crown and fixed partial denture materials for direct restorations

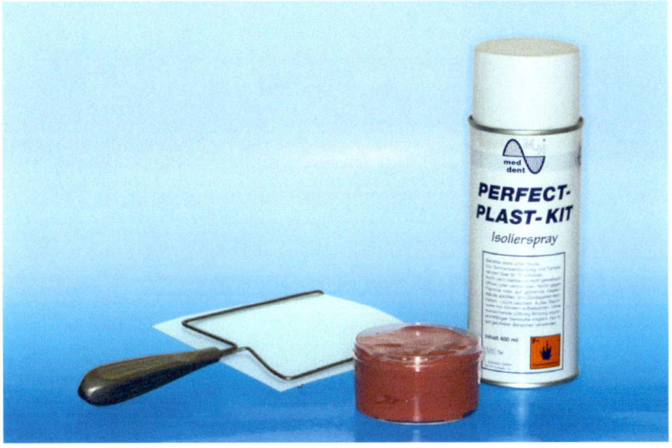

Fig 3-32a Matrix kit for fast deep-drawing.

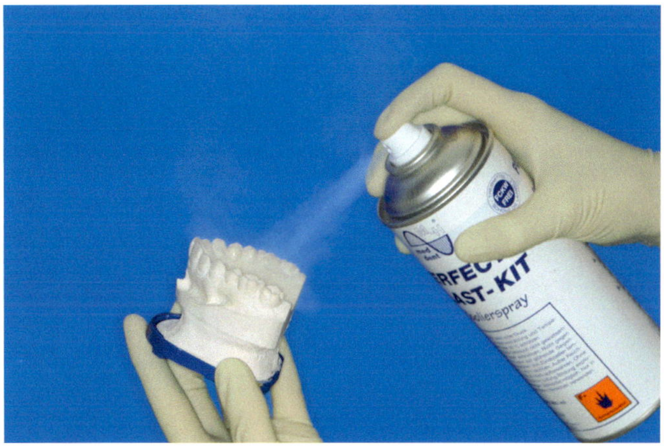

Fig 3-32b The master cast is isolated with spray.

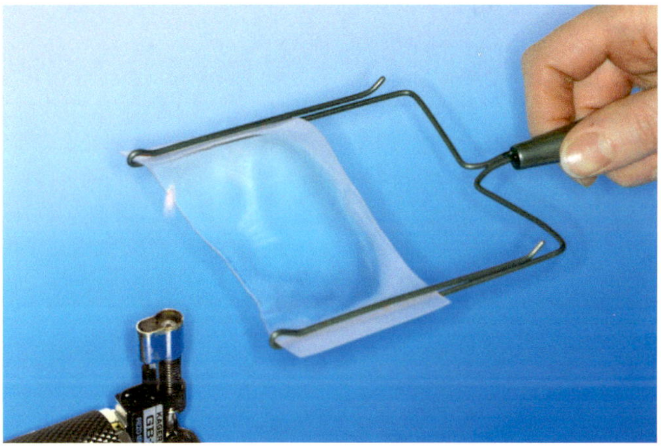

Fig 3-32c The plastic film is softened in the frame over the flame.

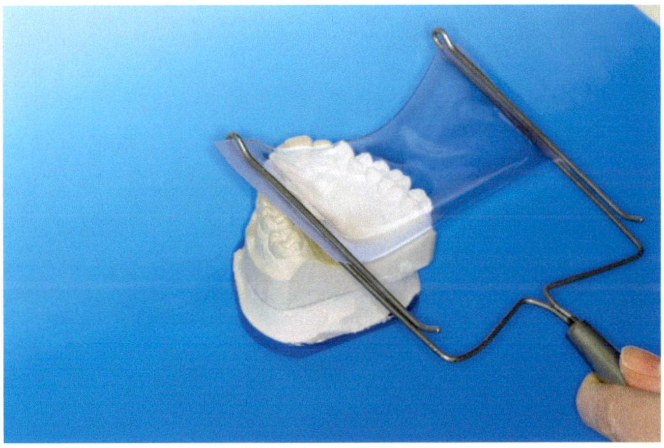

Fig 3-32d The soft film is placed over the dental arch.

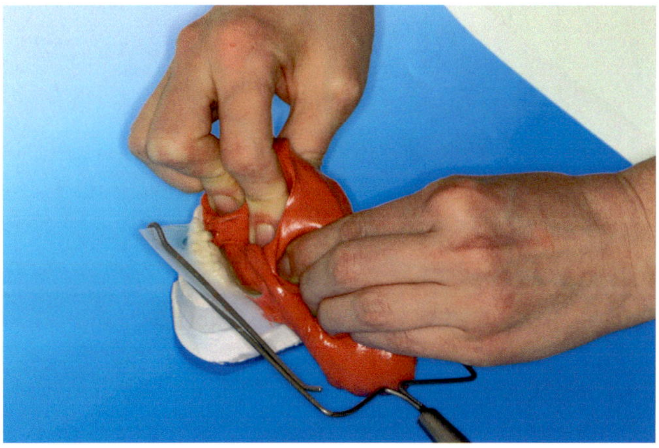

Fig 3-32e The soft film is adapted to the cast using the silicone putty as a stamp.

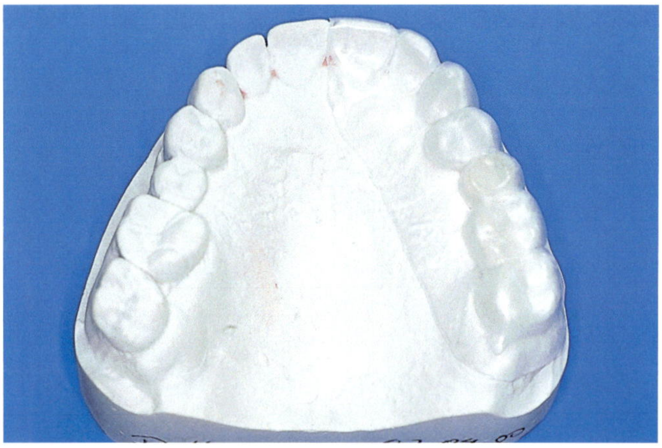

Fig 3-32f Hardened matrix.

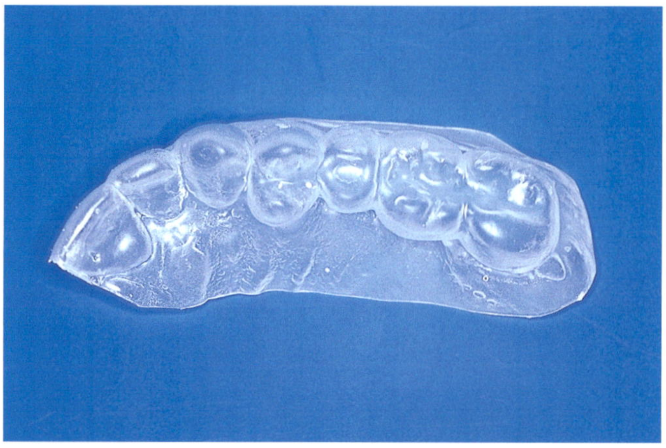

Fig 3-32g The matrix has been trimmed with scissors.

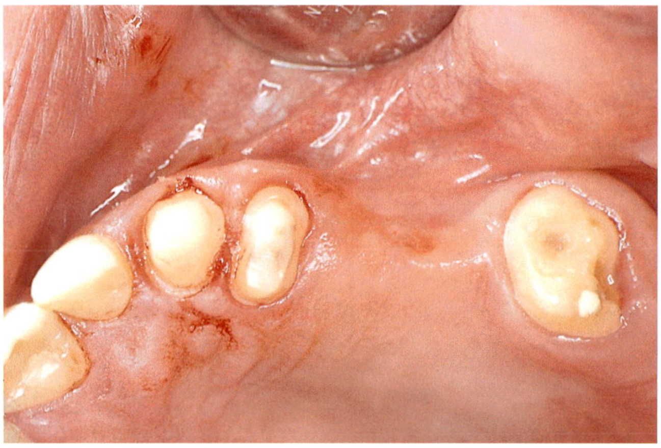

Fig 3-32h The abutment teeth are prepared for the posterior fixed partial denture.

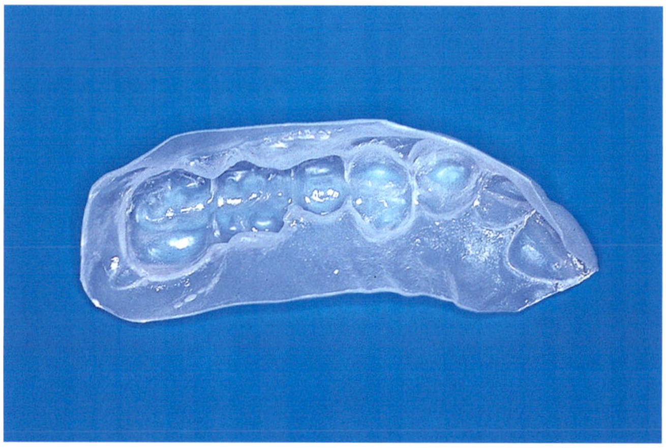

Fig 3-32i Underside of the finished matrix.

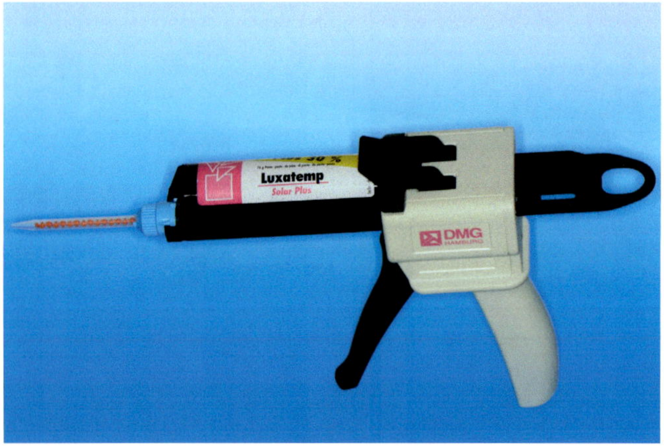

Fig 3-32j Provisional resin composite in the automix gun dispenser.

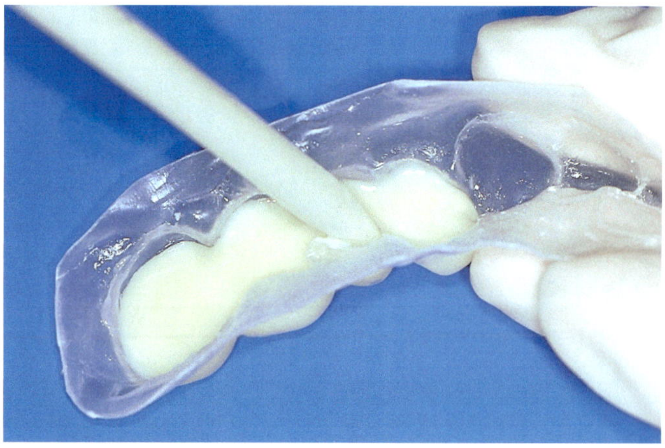

Fig 3-32k The matrix is carefully filled with resin composite.

with a fine pencil (Fig 3-32p), and then the restoration is finished with fine burs and points (Figs 3-32q and 3-32r). The occlusion is corrected with selective grinding, the interproximal contacts are checked, and the embrasure spaces are finished (Figs 3-32s and 3-32t). The embrasures and fissures can subsequently be characterized with resin composite stains. Then the final polishing is performed (Fig 3-32u).

Before the fixed partial denture is cemented, a desensitizer should be applied (eg, Gluma). The author recom-

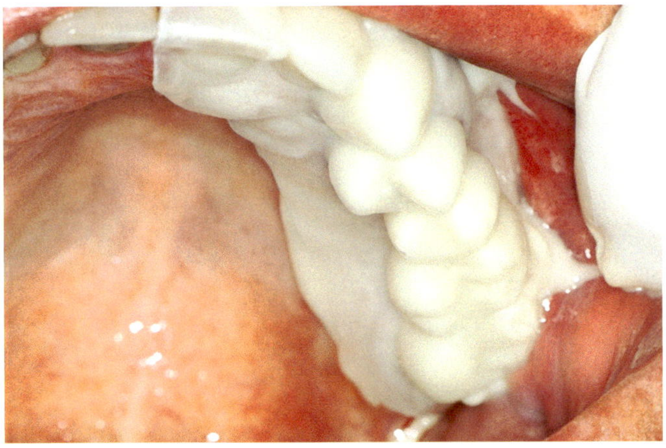

Fig 3-32l The provisional fixed partial denture is polymerized on the abutments in the patient's mouth.

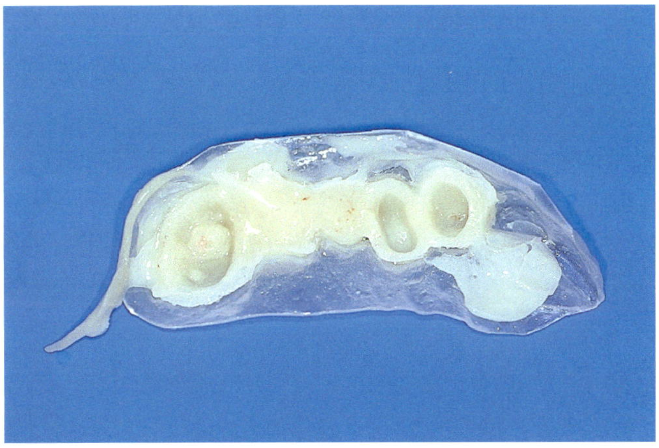

Fig 3-32m Matrix after removal.

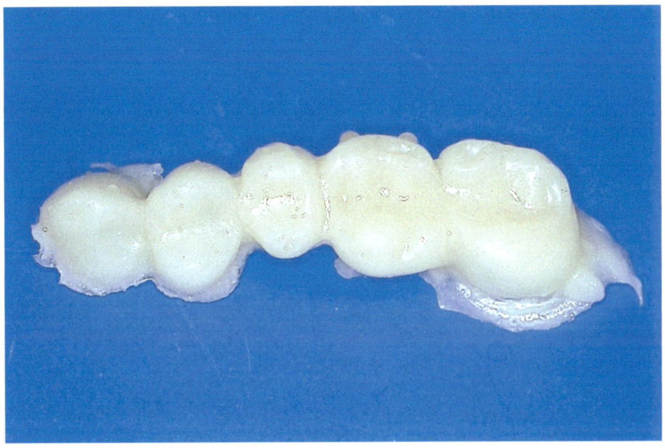

Fig 3-32n The provisional fixed partial denture is removed from the matrix.

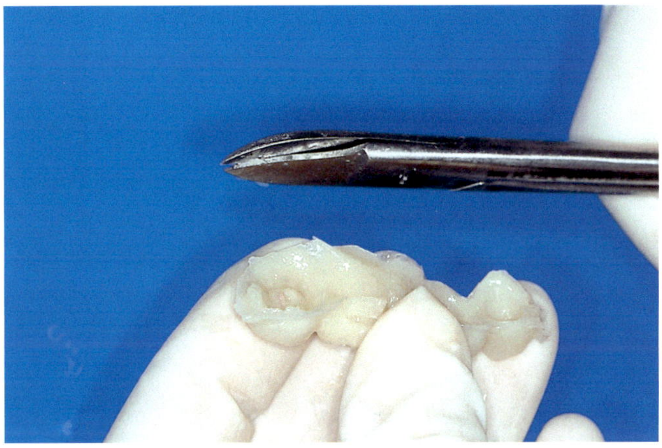

Fig 3-32o The cast blank is trimmed with scissors.

Fig 3-32p *(left)* The preparation margins are marked with a fine pencil.

Fig 3-32q *(right)* Grinding and polishing instruments for finishing the restoration: *(back row, left to right)* finishing bur with staggered teeth, carborundum stone (mounted), abrasive disk for the interproximal spaces, and mounted sandpaper disk; *(front row, left to right)* two kinds of rubber points and a polishing brush.

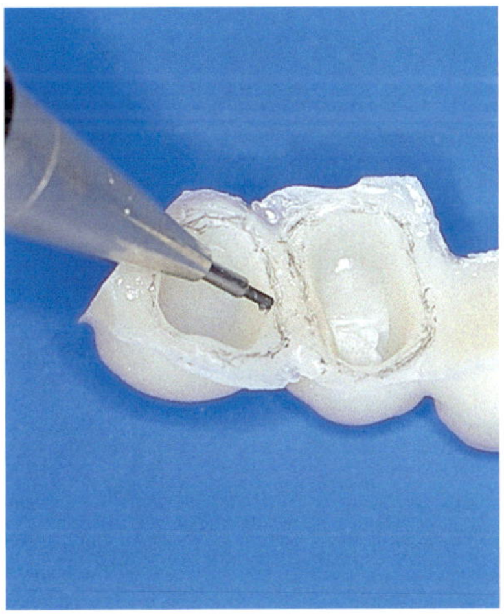

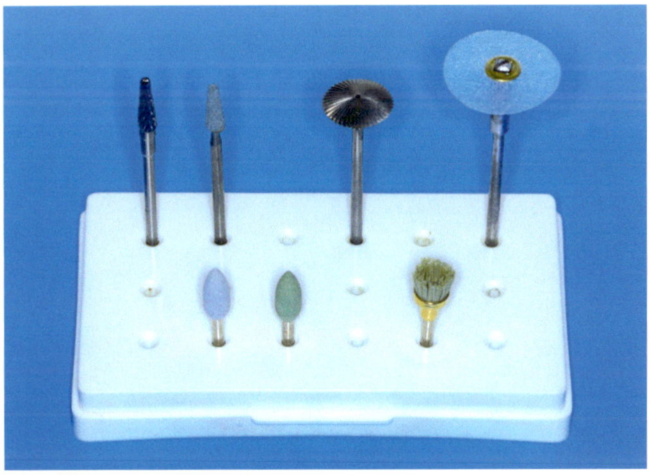

mends carboxylate cement for cementation, although the crowns should be covered with only a thin layer. Carboxylate cement (eg, Durelon) seals tightly and prevents the provisional restorations from dislodging while they are still needed. The material is somewhat difficult to remove, but with a crown and fixed partial denture remover (such as the Coronaflex; see chapter 1) removal can be accomplished almost effortlessly (Figs 3-32v and 3-32w).

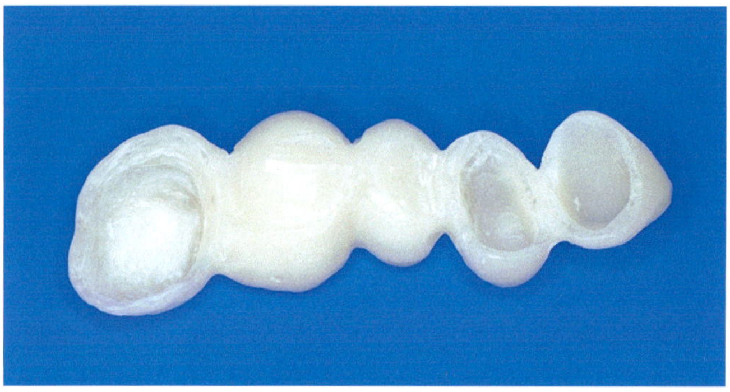

Fig 3-32r Provisional restoration after cervical finishing.

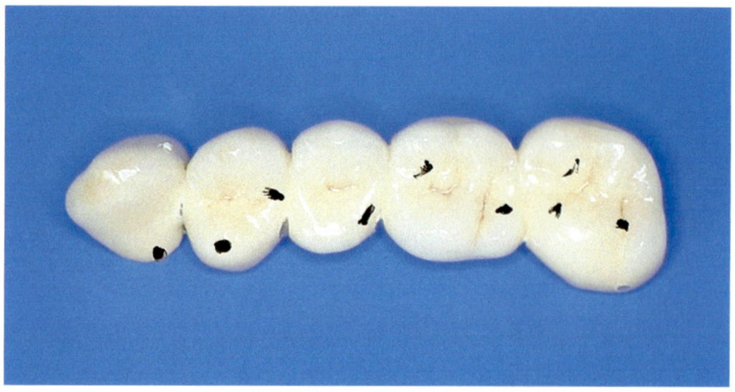

Fig 3-32s Occlusal adjustment is accomplished through grinding after the restoration is marked with articulating paper.

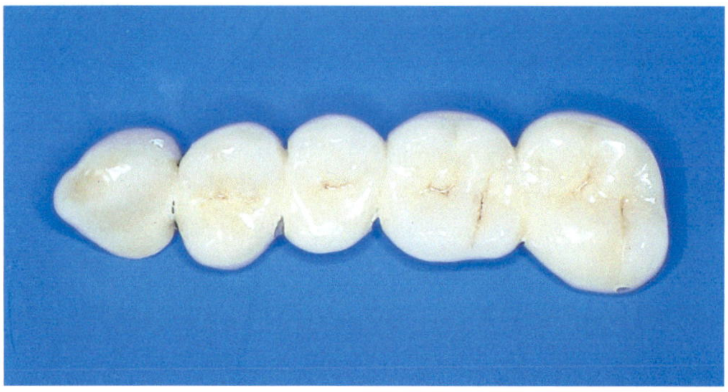

Fig 3-32t Occlusal view of the polished and characterized provisional fixed partial denture.

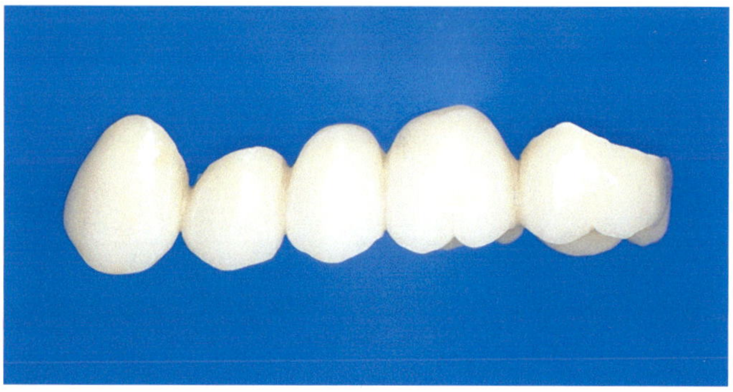

Fig 3-32u Buccal view.

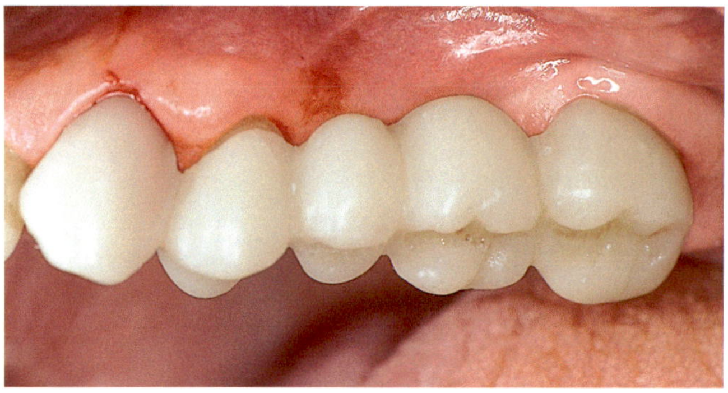

Fig 3-32v Buccal view of the cemented provisional fixed partial denture.

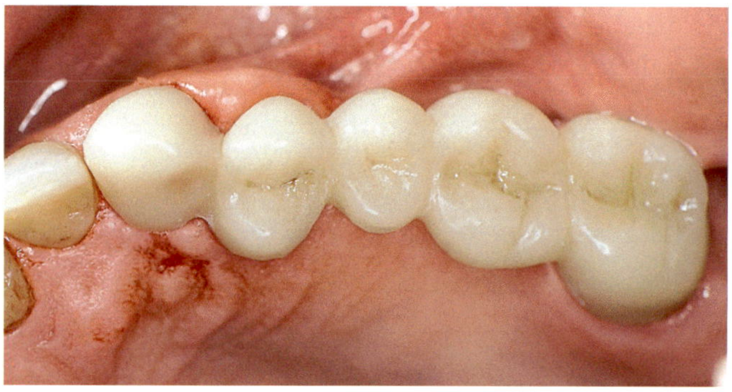

Fig 3-32w Occlusal view.

Materials

Perfect-Plast Kit for fast deep-drawing (Hager and Werken)
Provisional crown and bridge materials: Dentacolor (Heraeus Kulzer); Cronsin (Merz Dental); Protemp 3 (3M ESPE); Luxatemp Automix and Luxatemp Automix Solar (Zenith);
Tab 2000 (Kerr Dental); Tempofit (Detax)
Fine mechanical pencil (available at stationery shops)
Magnifying loupe/stereomicroscope (available at specialized shops)
Burs, points, disks (Brasseler)
Polishing paste for Targis/Vectris (now Adoro/Vectris, Ivoclar Vivadent)
Polishing brush (Kerr/Hawe)
Hanel articulating paper (Coltène Whaledent)
Durelon temporary cement for crowns and fixed partial dentures (3M ESPE); Provilink light-curing cement for inlays, onlays, and partial crowns (Vivadent)
Coronaflex crown and bridge remover (KaVo)
Gluma for isolating the tooth preparation (Heraeus Kulzer)

Expedient Placement of Complete Dentures

Common problem: Unwieldy and inefficient techniques for fabrication of complete dentures

For decades now, techniques for planning and fabricating complete dentures have been taught and demonstrated at dental schools in the exact same way with virtually no modifications. Does time stand still in the dental schools? Has the profession not learned more in the meantime? Have there not been any further developments?

Why are dentists always so frustrated when they are faced with the task of making a complete denture? The following is a brief history of complete dentures. When the systematic design of complete dentures was introduced by Alfred Gysi, the following traditional treatment steps emerged:

1. Completion of a master impression of the edentulous jaw
2. Creation of a temporary base for the functional impression in the laboratory
3. Completion of a functional impression
4. Fabrication of the master cast in the laboratory mounted with the wax rims
5. Preparation of a centric relation record with baseplates, measuring tools, and central bearing device 6. Selection of the tooth colors and shapes
7. Mounting of the casts on the articulator and arrangement of the artificial teeth on a wax baseplate in the laboratory
8. Try-in of the waxup
9. Completion in the laboratory
10. Placement of the complete denture
11. Final examination of the denture, removal of pressure points, and adjustment of the occlusion

The average treatment time for this procedure, from completion of the first impression to placement of the denture, is 3 weeks.

Arne Lauritzen and Axel Gutowski introduced new precision and occlusion into the process of making of complete dentures. Precision always involves a great expenditure of time, especially for complete dentures, and this is reflected in higher costs. From that point onward, however, patients received complete dentures held in place by suction in a precise occlusal position, which was an enormous improvement. With the growing success in implant dentistry, it became possible to treat cases that would have been considered hopeless before. Nowadays heroic surgical procedures—most of which were seldom successful—such as vestibuloplasty, lowering the floor of the mouth, or separating the mandibular ligaments, are only necessary in very rare cases.

The overall number of patients requiring complete dentures has been continuously decreasing since systematic prophylactic measures were introduced in dental offices and patients began accepting these measures as a motivation to try to keep their teeth. This is a great success for dentistry.

However, whenever a complete denture has to be made, the question is always the same: Are there any ways to make the procedure more efficient while maintaining quality?

Proven solution: Systematic integration of individual steps into more comprehensive steps

A case report will be used to describe the possibilities for organization in the office and laboratory.

A new complete maxillary denture was to be made for a 65-year-old woman (Figs 3-33a to 3-33d). She had a mandibular implant-supported telescopic denture (Figs 3-33e and 3-33f).

First day, in the morning

Chairside work

The margins that seal the denture to the gingiva, the palatal seal, and the occlusion of the existing complete denture were checked (Figs 3-33g and 3-33h). In addition, the denture-bearing area was examined to ensure that it did not show any pressure points (Figs 3-33i and 3-33j).

The existing margins that sealed the denture were ground slightly and the undercuts were significantly ground out (Fig 3-33k). The base was rechecked in the

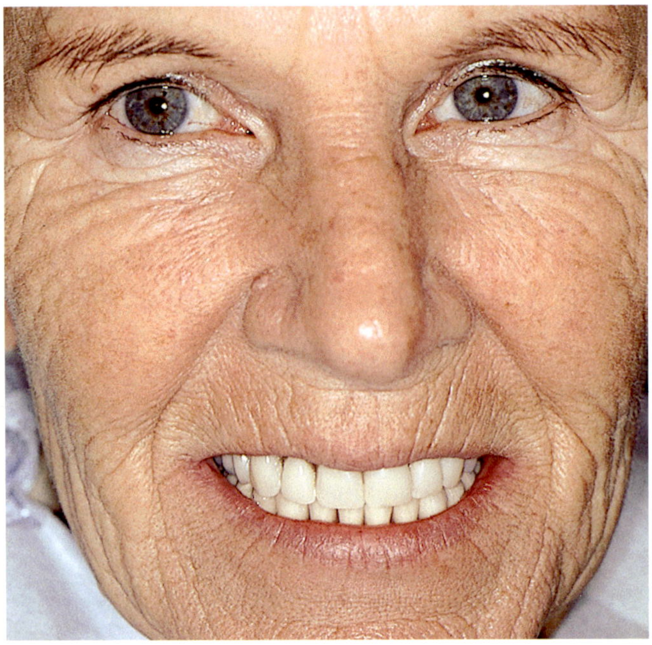

Fig 3-33a Patient in need of a new maxillary complete denture.

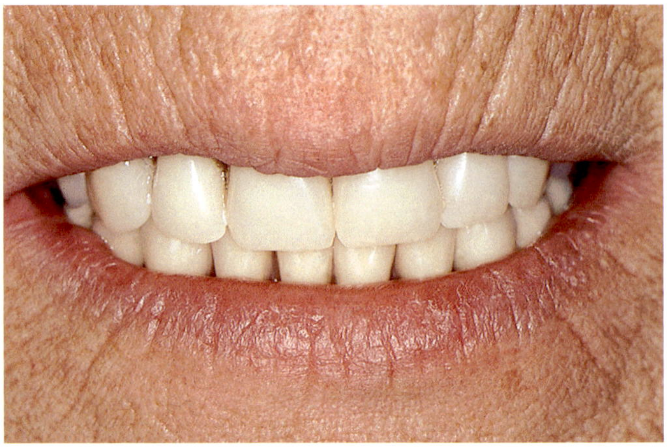

Fig 3-33b Patient's lip line.

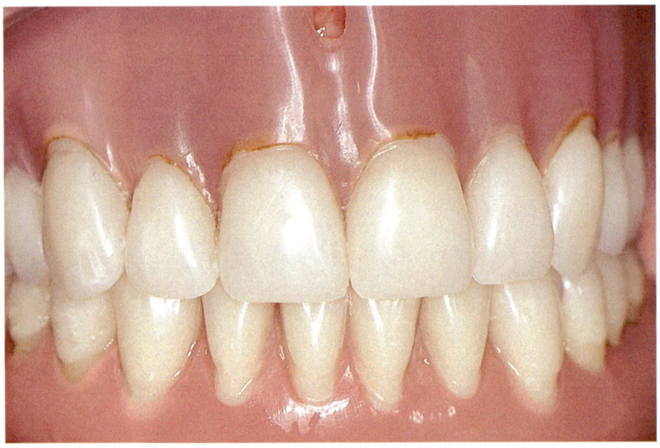

Fig 3-33c Patient's existing complete maxillary and mandibular dentures.

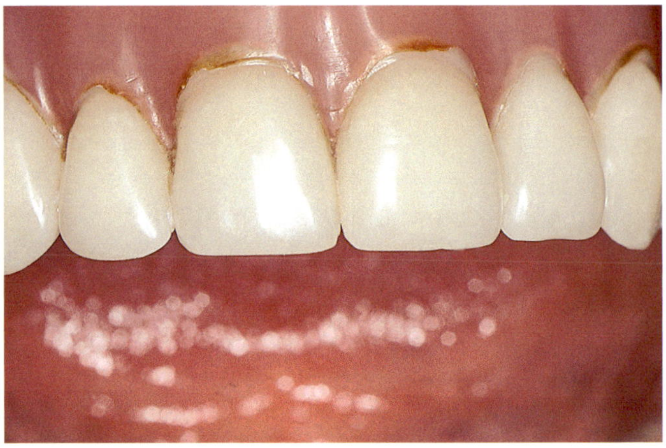

Fig 3-33d The existing maxillary denture has to be remade.

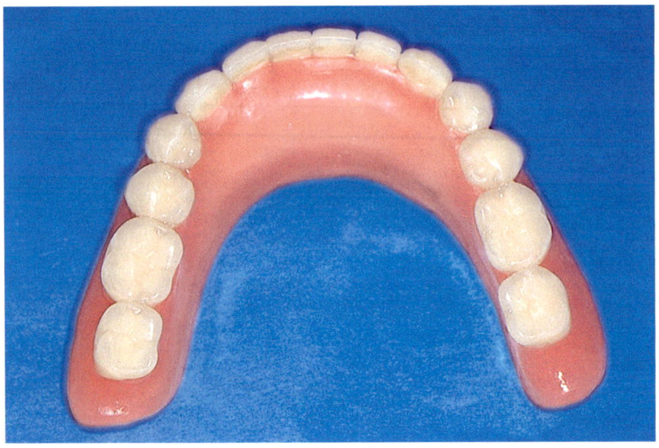

Fig 3-33e Complete mandibular denture.

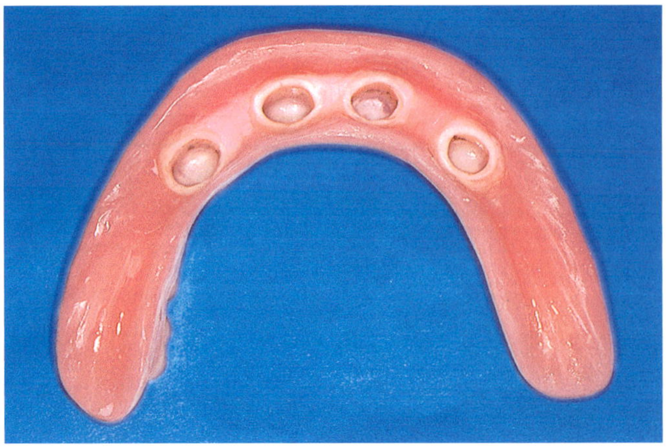

Fig 3-33f View of the Targis/Vectris telescopes.

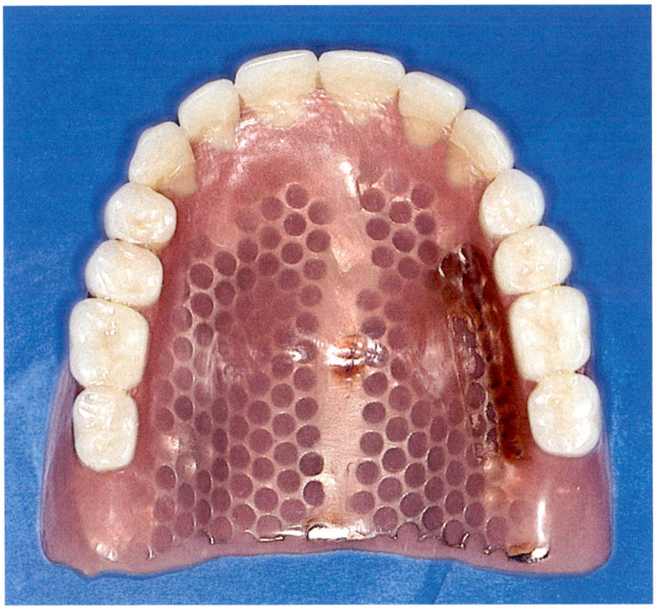

Fig 3-33g Maxillary denture with an integrated metal base.

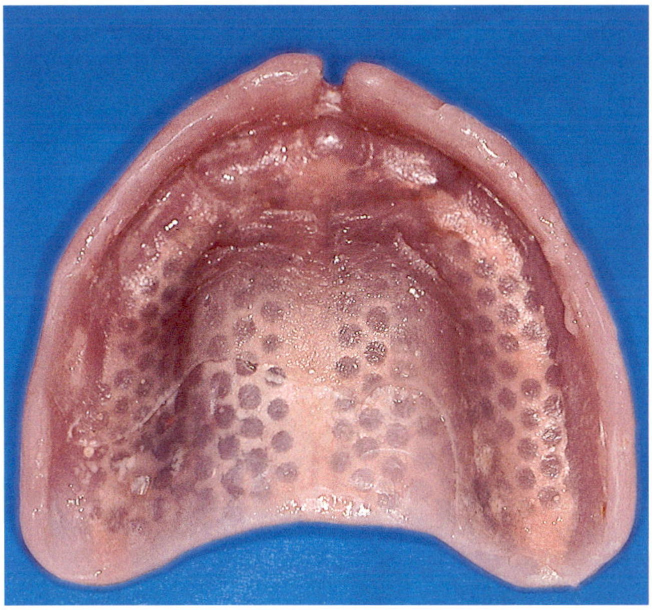

Fig 3-33h Palatal side of the denture.

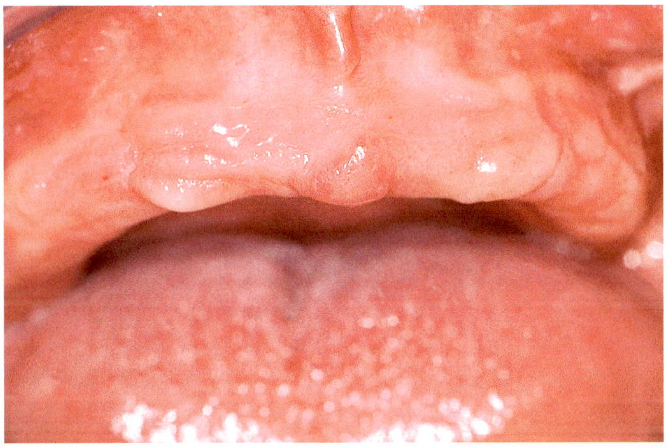

Fig 3-33i State of the maxillary alveolar ridge.

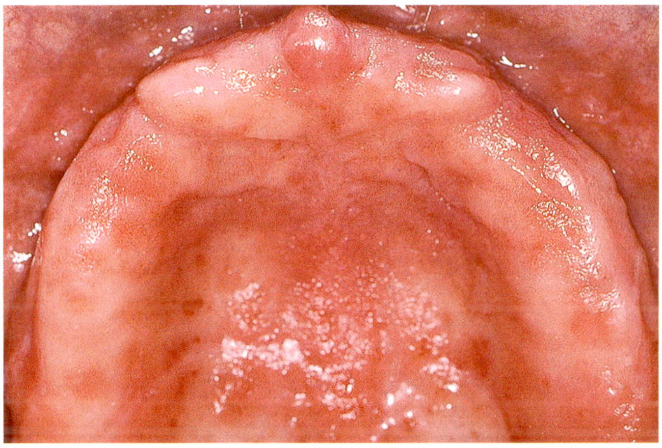

Fig 3-33j Occlusal view of the alveolar ridge.

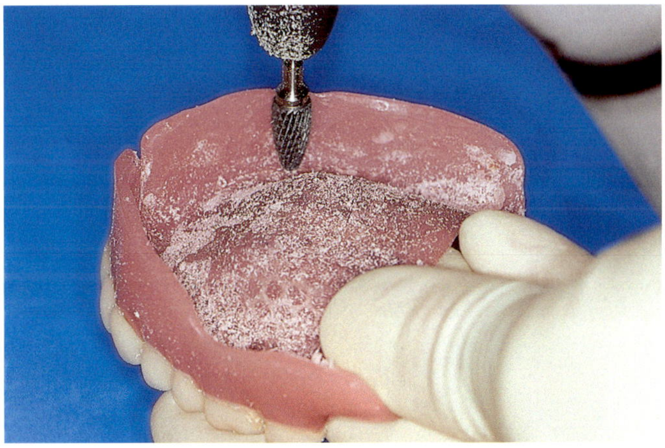

Fig 3-33k The margins that seal the denture and the undercuts are reduced.

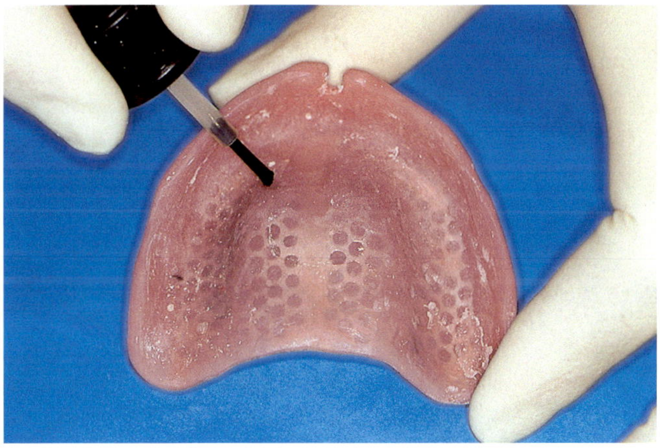

Fig 3-33l The silicone adhesive is applied.

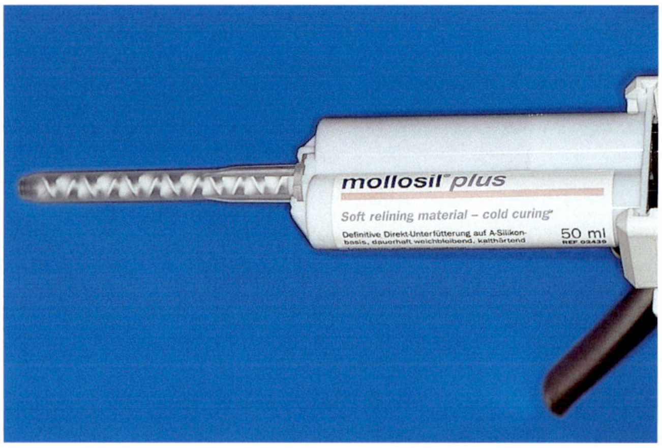

Fig 3-33m Double cartridge dispenser with the silicone liner.

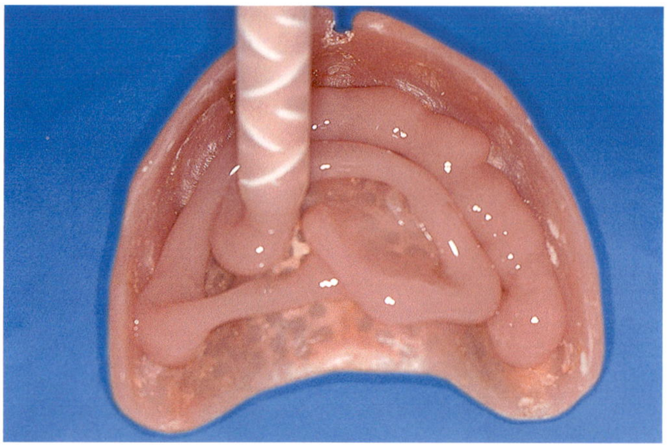

Fig 3-33n The silicone liner is applied.

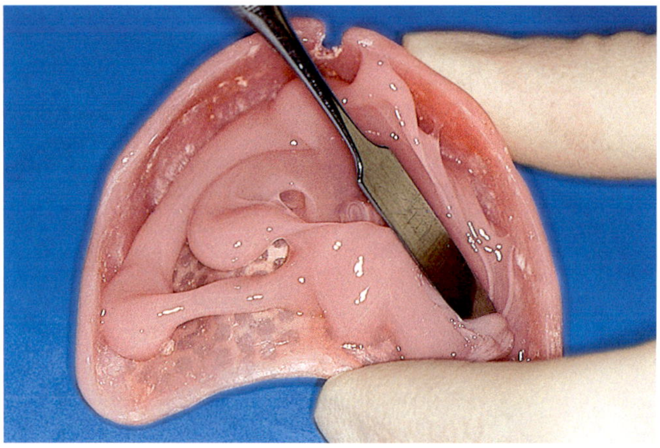

Fig 3-33o The material is spread evenly with a spatula.

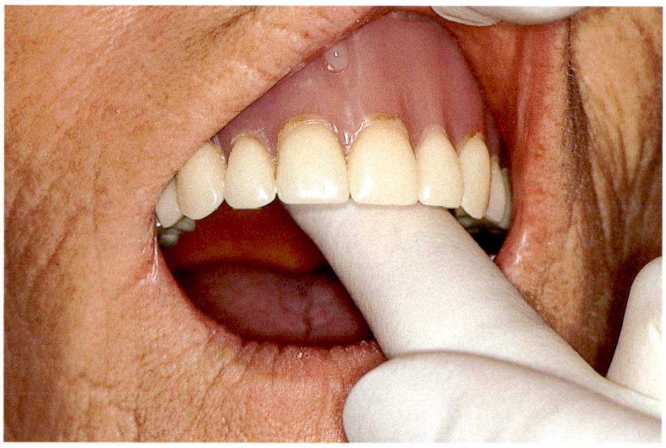

Fig 3-33p The denture is pressed centrally to the palate with increasing pressure.

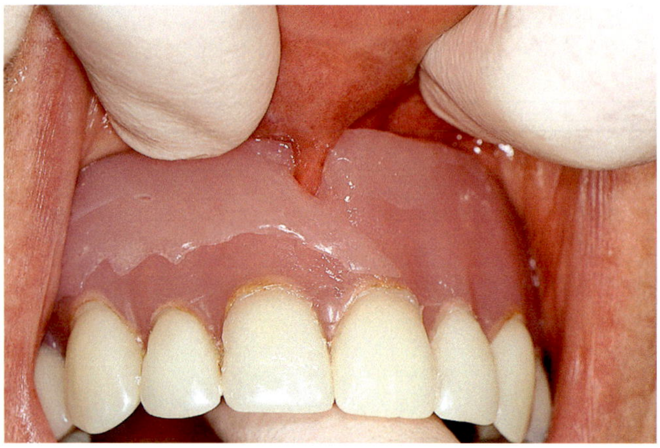

Fig 3-33q The functional impression is taken.

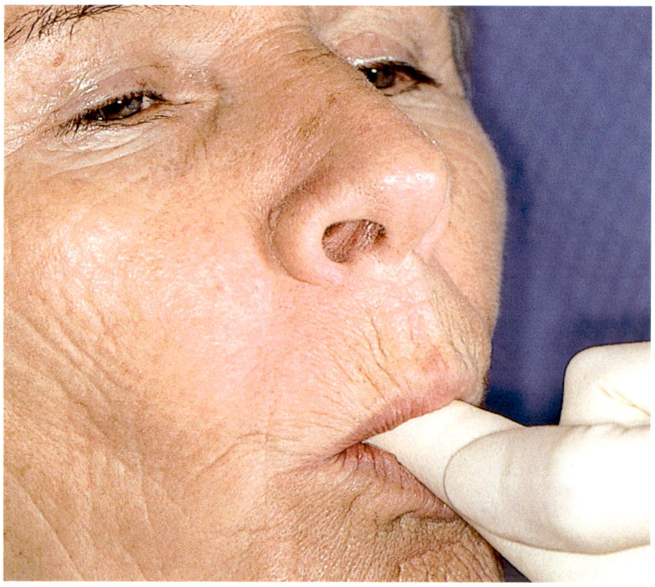

Fig 3-33r The impression is taken with the appropriate movements; here the patient is firmly sucking on a finger.

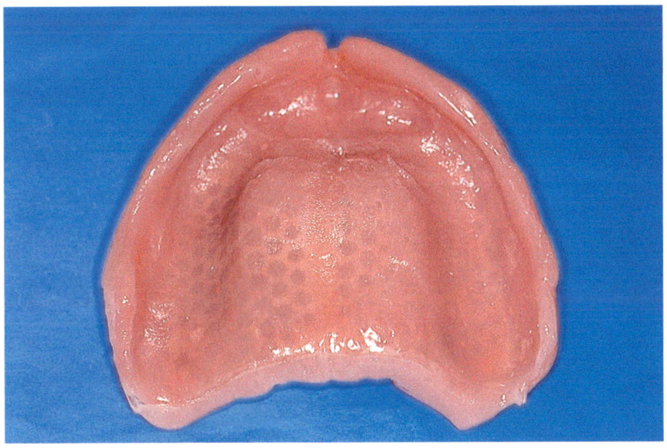

Fig 3-33s The functional impression is examined.

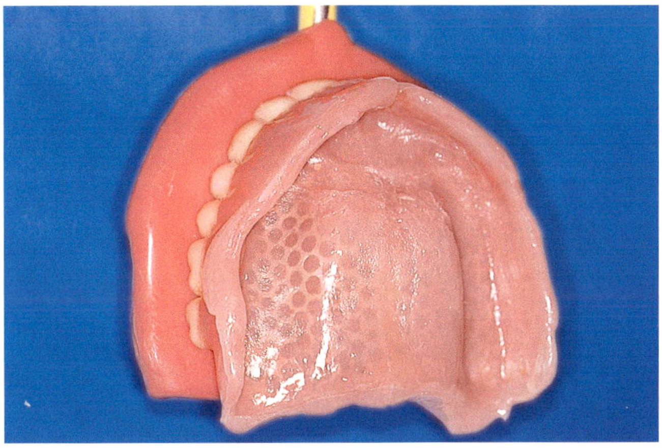

Fig 3-33t The bite fork is adjusted.

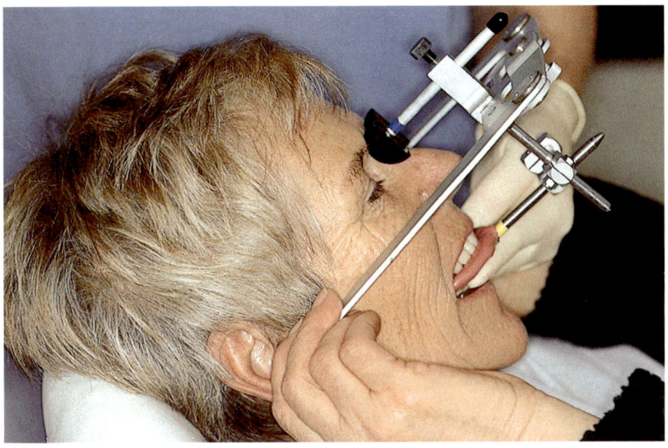

Fig 3-33u Registration is carried out with an arbitrary facebow system.

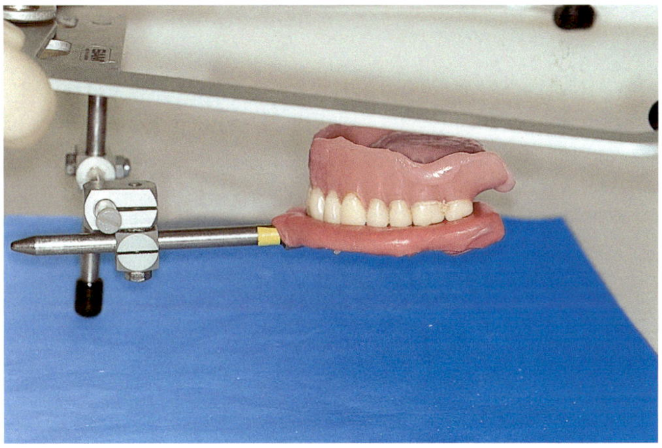

Fig 3-33v The denture in the correct position.

patient's mouth. It was not necessary to enlarge the margins that sealed the denture using impression material or other substances. The base was cleaned, and tray adhesive was applied (Fig 3-33l).

The functional impression was taken with Mollosil, a tooth-colored, long-term soft silicone liner (Figs 3-33m to 3-33r). All functional movements had to be made actively and passively (Figs 3-33s to 3-33p).

After 5 minutes the silicone was completely cured. The functionally reshaped denture was removed from the patient's mouth and checked, and any excess was removed (Fig 3-33s). Then the denture was reseated in the patient's mouth. A bite fork was covered with softened Beauty Pink Wax (Fig 3-33t); the denture was positioned in the middle, and the wax was allowed to cool. The ends of the Quick Mount facebow were inserted into the patient's ears, and the patient was asked to press it upward to meet the requirements of the Frankfort horizontal line as defined by Gutowski (Fig 3-33u).

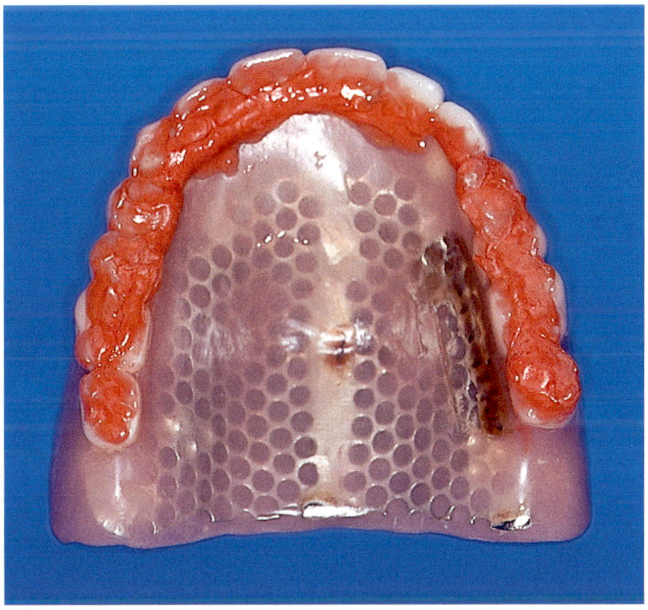

Fig 3-33w Denture with the bite registration.

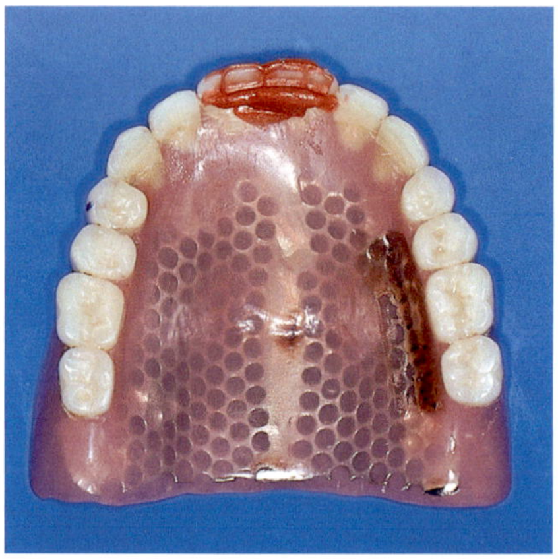

Fig 3-33x Protruded position and bite registration with the frontal jig.

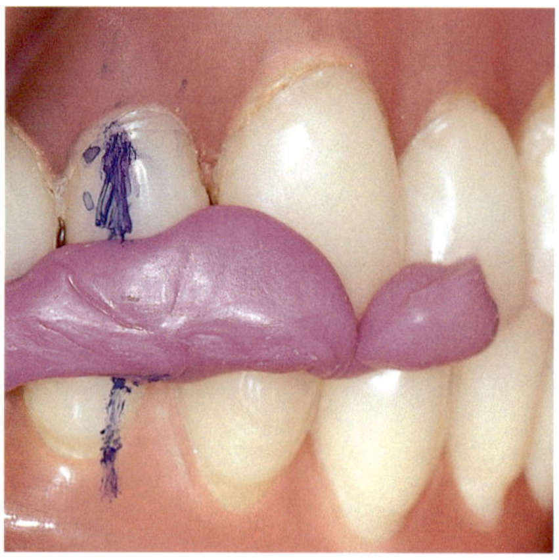

Fig 3-33y The protruded position is fixed with hard silicone.

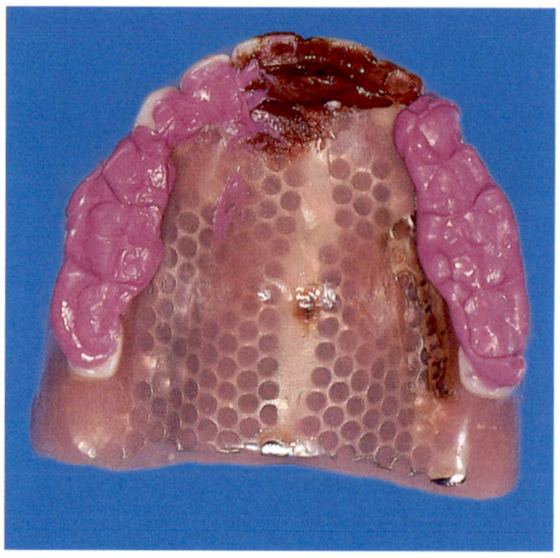

Fig 3-33z Denture with the protrusion registration.

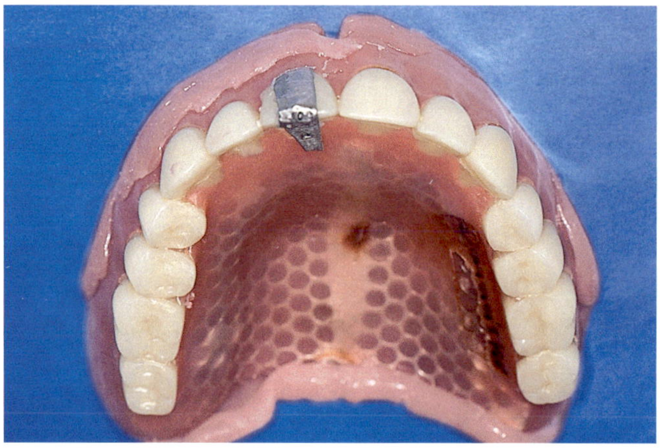

Fig 3-33aa The lead foil strip is bonded to the maxillary denture for functional analysis of the cephalogram.

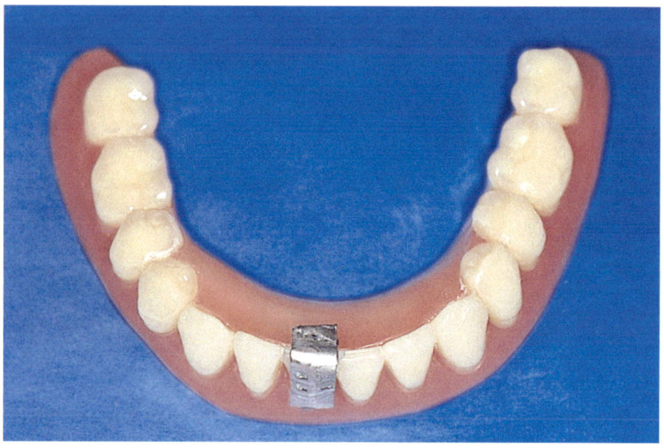

Fig 3-33bb A lead foil strip is bonded to the mandibular denture.

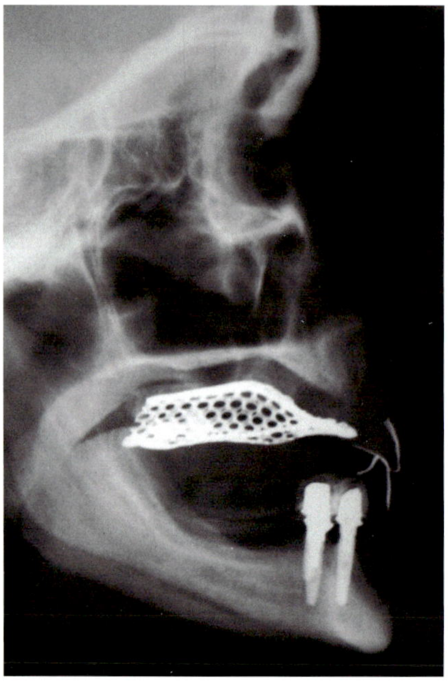

Fig 3-33cc Cephalogram.

The glabella was adapted, all screws were supported and tightened, and then the arbitrary registration was checked. If all positions are correct, the adjusted facebow can be removed (Fig 3-33v). An alginate impression of the mandibular denture was made and immediately filled with die stone.

Then the position of the mandible was determined with the registration of the centric occlusion. The habitual position of this patient was identical with the central position, so that it was possible to dispense with a registration of the central occlusion with a jig and special impression material (Gutowski). It was sufficient to register with Futar D hard silicone bite registration material (Fig 3-33w). The vertical dimension seemed to be correct according to the traditional measurement (normal occlusion = resting position –2 mm).

To adjust the inclination of the condylar path, a registration in a protruded position was required. The protruded position (protrusion 4 mm) for the mandible was

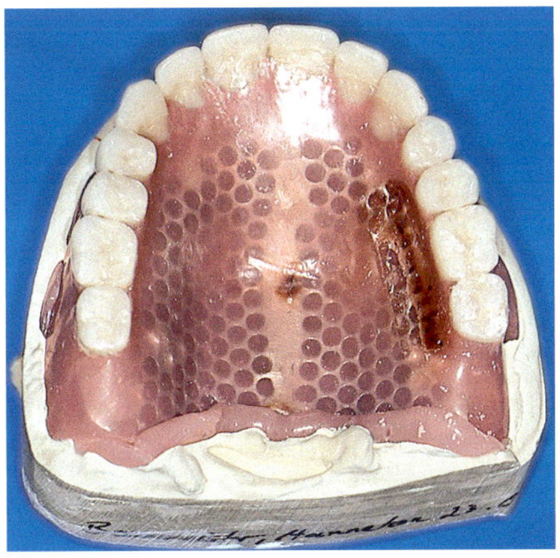

Fig 3-33dd Molded master cast.

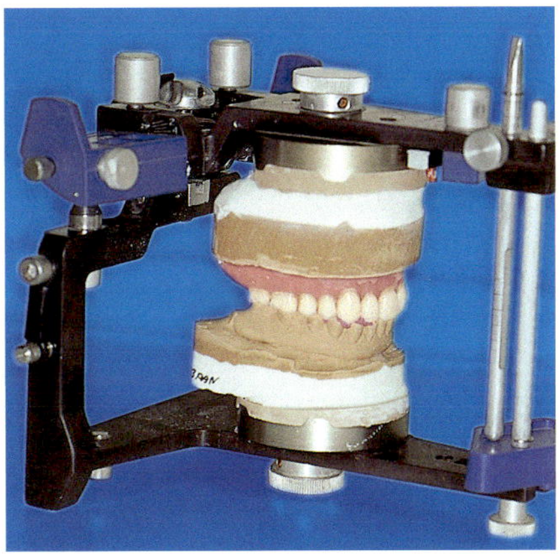

Fig 3-33ee Master cast mounted on the articulator.

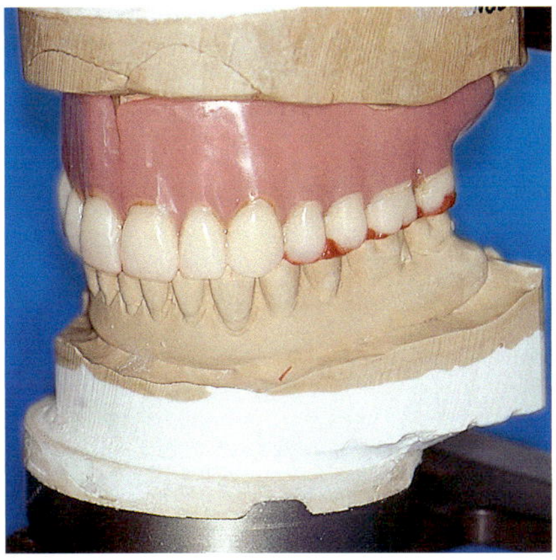

Fig 3-33ff Closeup view of the mounted cast.

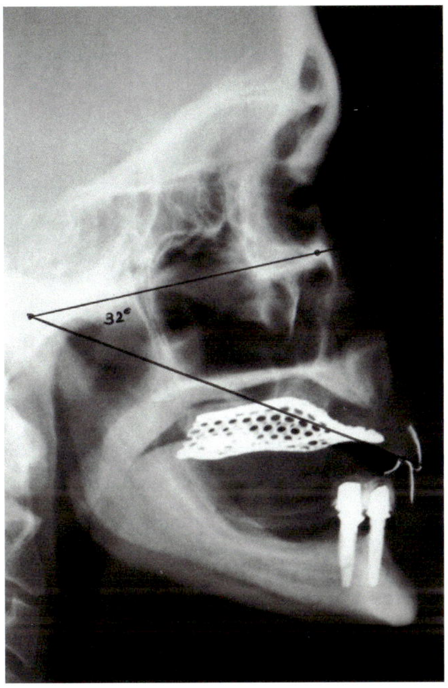

Fig 3-33gg *(left)* Functional analysis of the cephalogram.

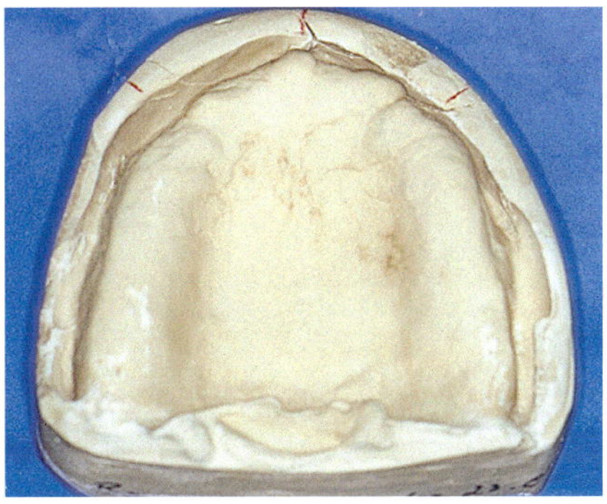

Fig 3-33hh *(top right)* Master cast.

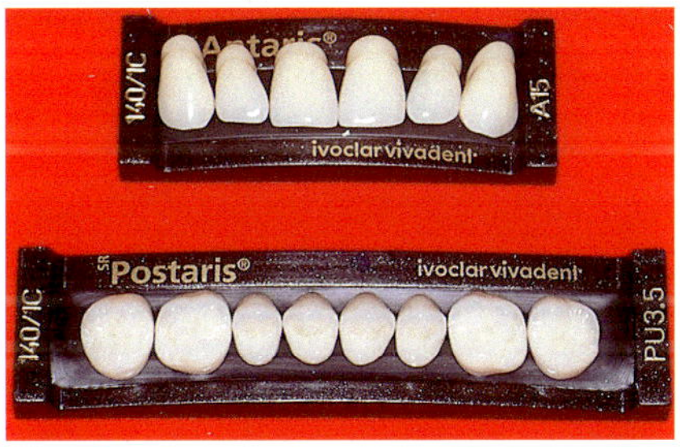

Fig 3-33ii *(bottom right)* Anterior and posterior teeth for the waxup.

determined with a jig of impression material. Then the position of the posterior teeth was registered with Futar D hard silicone (Figs 3-33x to 33z).

To allow functional analysis of the lateral cephalogram, the lead foil from an x-ray film for single-tooth radiographs was cut into strips and bonded to the maxillary right and the mandibular right central incisors (Figs 3-33aa and 3-33bb), and then a cephalogram was taken (Fig 3-33cc).

Laboratory work

The functional impression of the old maxillary denture was filled with die stone and removed after it was cured (Fig 3-33dd). Then the master cast was mounted to the articulator in correct relation to the skull with the help of the Quick Mount facebow, and the cast of the opposing jaw was positioned with the help of the centric registration (Figs 3-33ee and 3-33ff). The inclination of the condylar path was adjusted as usual on the articulator with the help of the protrusion registration (Fig 3-33gg).

Chairside work

After all the residual die stone was removed, the maxillary denture was seated back in the patient's mouth. Because the impression was taken with Mollosil, a tooth-colored liner, the patient was happy with the fit and color.

The tooth colors and shapes were jointly chosen by the patient, the dentist, and the dental laboratory techni-

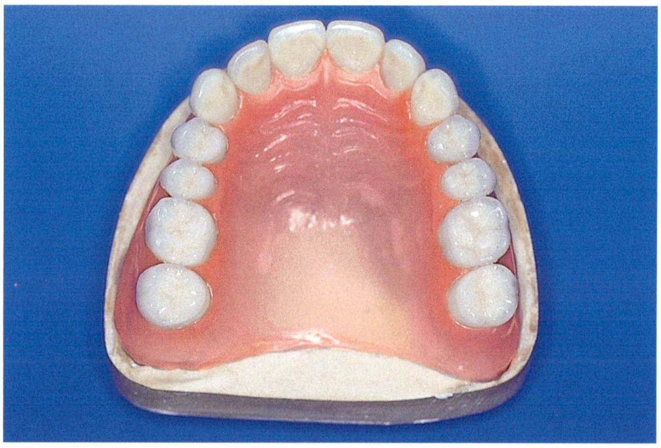

Fig 3-33jj Molded denture with the teeth fitted.

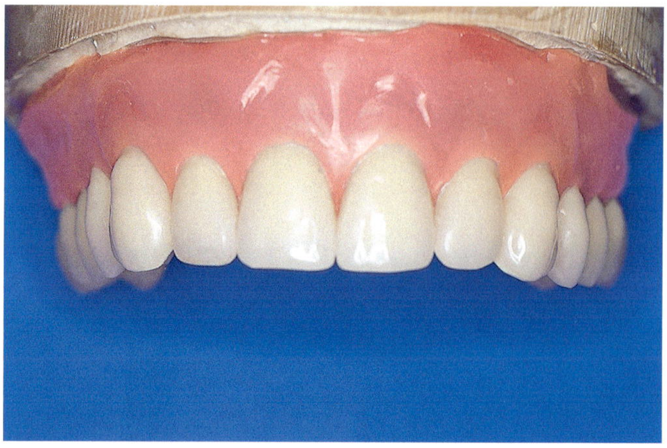

Fig 3-33kk Try-in of the waxed-up denture.

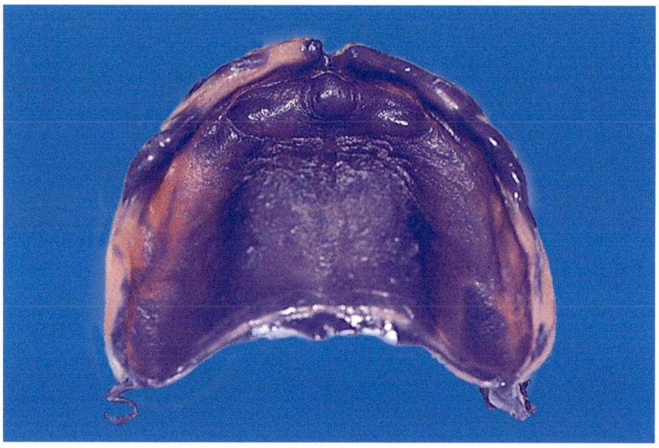

Fig 3-33ll Denture corrected with fine polyether impression material.

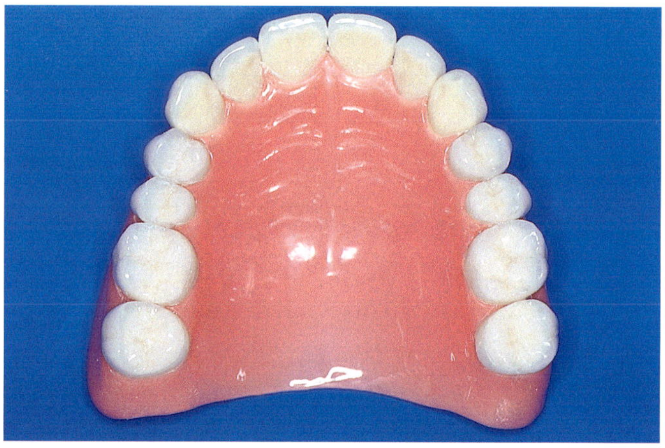

Fig 3-33mm Finished complete maxillary denture.

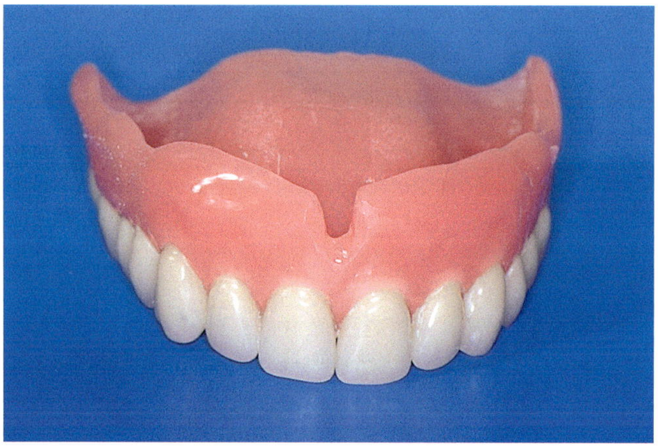

Fig 3-33nn Adaptation.

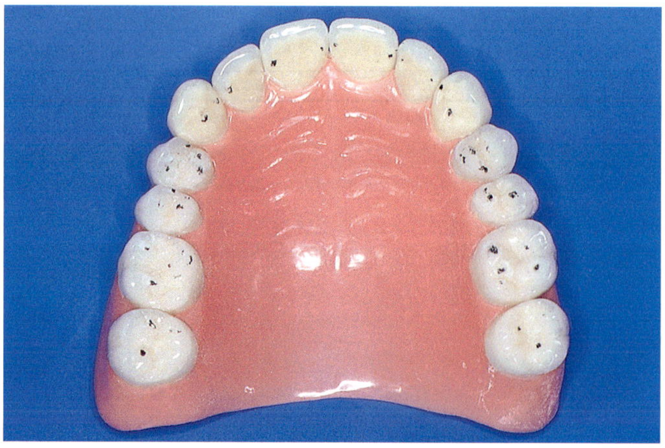

Fig 3-33oo The occlusion is checked.

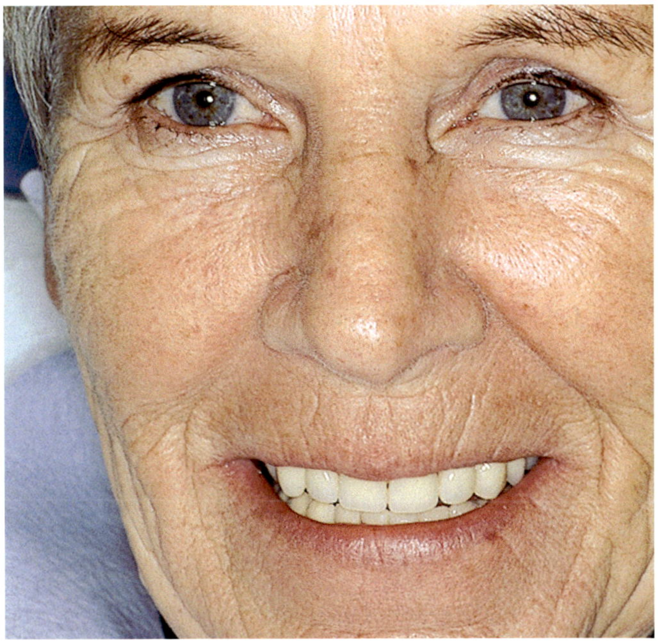

Fig 3-33pp The patient is happy with her new complete denture.

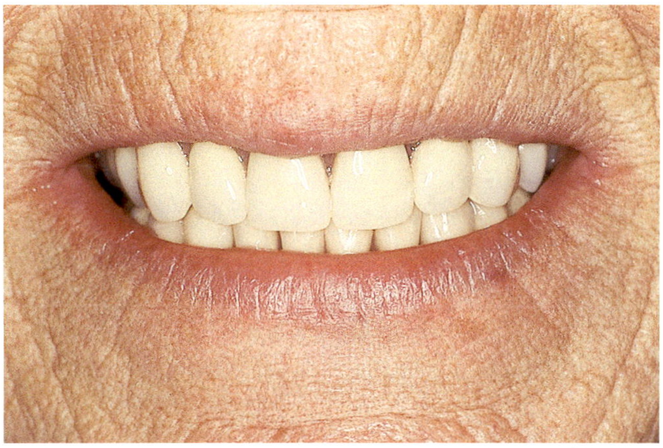

Fig 3-33qq Closeup view of the rejuvenated smile.

cian. Subsequently, a functional analysis of the cephalogram was performed (Fig 3-33hh), the information was forwarded to the dental technician, and the planned laboratory steps were reviewed with the dental technician.

The margins that were to later seal the denture to the gingiva were evaluated on the master cast, and any necessary adjustments to the cast were made by grinding or abrading. After the baseplate was made from light-curing tray material, the artificial teeth were waxed up. The author's principle of occlusion, which is also used for complete dentures, is anterior-canine guidance to allow for vertical chewing and the use of gnathologically sharp posterior teeth (Fig 3-33ii). Then the base was molded in pink wax.

Second day, in the morning

Chairside work

On the morning of the following day, the waxup with the teeth in their future positions was tried in (Fig 3-33jj). The positions were adjusted as necessary. The individual characterization of the teeth was discussed with the patient, and the teeth were ground accordingly. The color was characterized according to the patient's wishes (Fig 3-33kk). Last but not least, an impression of the denture base was made with fine polyether impression material (Permadyne blue; Fig 3-33ll).

Laboratory work

The wax denture was invested, filled, and polymerized. When it was cured, the investment was carefully removed from the cast, and the denture was finished and polished (Fig 3-33mm).

Second day, in the evening

In the evening, the finished complete maxillary denture (Fig 3-33nn) was tried in the patient's mouth. Any small adjustments were made immediately. The occlusion was checked with articulating paper and Shimstock foil to decide whether the denture should be remounted immediately or after the patient had worn the denture for a time. This decision can vary from patient to patient. Special attention must be paid to occlusion, because occlusion is what governs stability for chewing, and that can help to prevent atrophy of the alveolar ridges (Fig 3-33oo).

A complete maxillary denture was thus successfully fabricated and seated within 2 days (Figs 3-33pp and 3-33qq).

Conclusion

Through logical integration of the individual treatment steps, it is possible to make the fabrication of complete dentures considerably more expedient while maintaining a high standard of quality.

Materials

Mollosil plus, tooth-colored soft lining material (Detax)
Finishing burs with staggered teeth (Brasseler)
Beauty Pink Wax, extrahard, aged (available from dental wholesalers)
Quick Mount facebow (Whip Mix)
Bite compound material in syringes for central registrations (American Dental)
Brown impression compound for the frontal jig (Kerr Dental)
Futar D, hard bite registration silicone (Kettenbach)
Panadent articulator (Panadent)
Antaris anterior teeth/Postaris posterior teeth (Ivoclar Vivadent)
Permadyne light body polyether impression material (3M ESPE)
Hanel articulating paper (Coltène Whaledent)
Shimstock foil: emergency shock protecting blanket from a car first aid kit, cut into thin strips

Causes of Bruxism

Common problem: Is bruxism caused by emotional or occlusal issues?

Bruxism, temporomandibular joint (TMJ) disease, and any form of malpositioning between the mandible and maxilla are among the most difficult cases to deal with in everyday practice (Figs 3-34a to 3-34c). If a patient arrives at the office with a box full of bite guards, cursing 10 previous dentists, it is likely that, the day after tomorrow, he or she will be cursing you. What lies at the foundation of this problem?

Dentists receive little or no training in treating functional disorders of the masticatory system. This forces dentists to face a problem that they cannot truly solve. Should they refer the patient elsewhere? If so, where? How can dentists still analyze and treat patients with functional disorders successfully and in keeping with their ethical and medical responsibilities?

Proven solution: Analysis of the cause of bruxism using Lüscher Color Diagnostics

The statistical breakdown of patients who grind their teeth is depicted in Fig 3-35, which was created by Graber.[8] The 50% of patients whose bruxism is caused by occlusal factors can be helped quickly and easily through restoration of their teeth without further ado. Another 12% of patients have a TMJ disorder and have to be treated accordingly. In 30% of patients with bruxism, the cause is primarily psychogenic, and in 8% the cause of bruxism is purely psychogenic. These 38% are dentistry's greatest challenge.

If clinicians provide this group with purely functional treatment, it is bound to fail in most cases, because dentists are not trained in psychological assessment. How can practitioners clearly determine which of these patients fall into the 38% whose bruxism has psychogenic origins? The author's long-lasting experience is that unequivocal results can be achieved with the Lüscher color test, the psychological assessment tool developed by Max Lüscher.

"The preference for certain colors and shapes provides a sound assessment of a patient's current state of mind, thus allowing the dentist to unequivocally classify the

Figs 3-34a to 3-34c Severe bruxism has resulted in substantial vertical damage in a 55-year-old man.

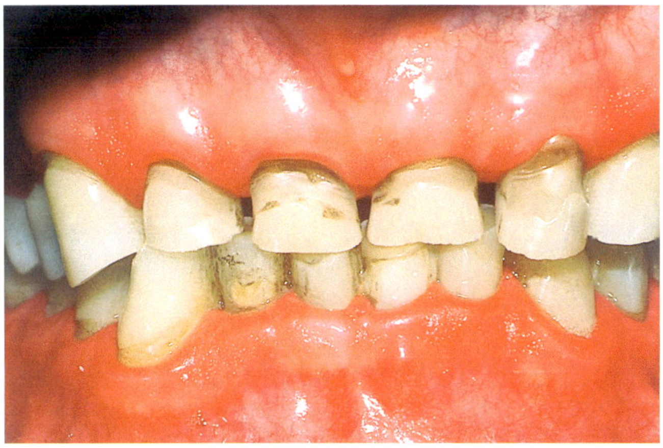

Fig 3-34a

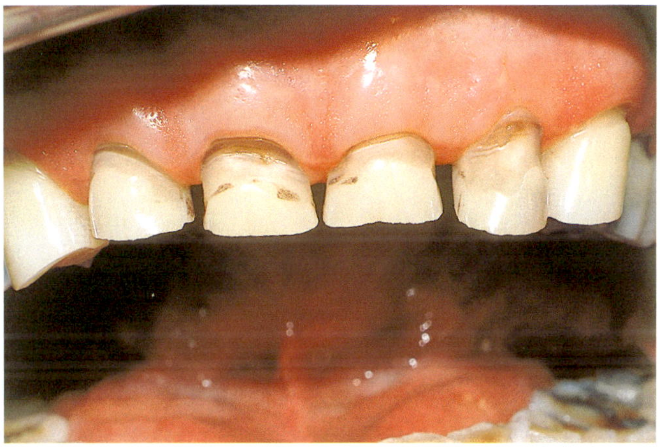

Fig 3-34b

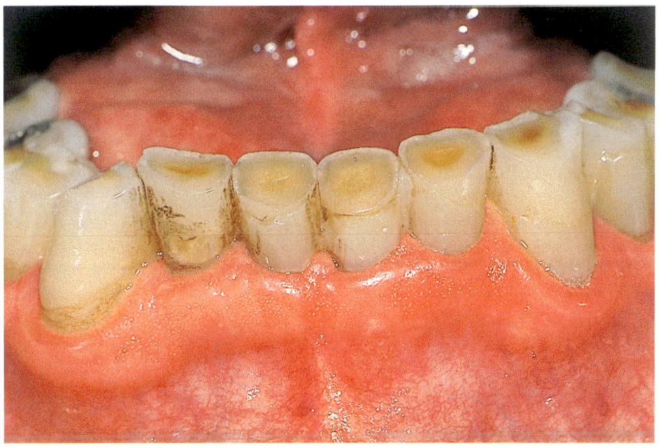

Fig 3-34c

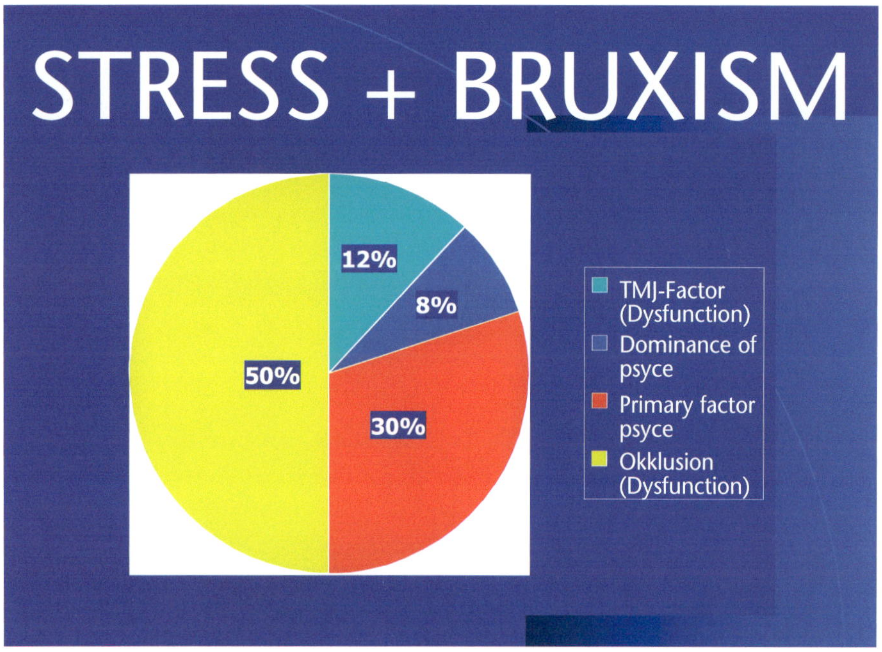

Fig 3-35 Role of stress in bruxism. (Courtesy of G. Graber, Basel, Switzerland.)

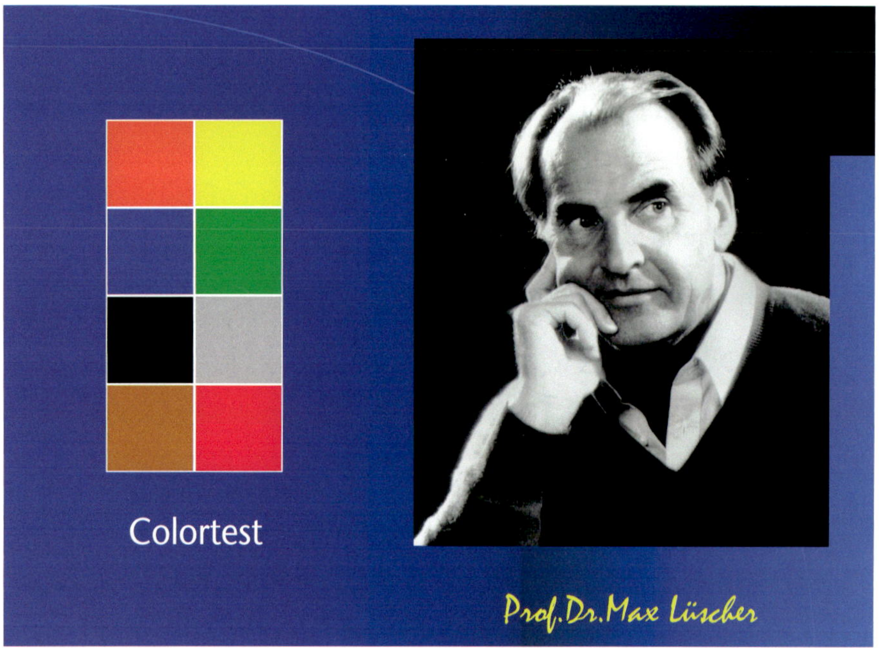

Fig 3-36 Lüscher color test.

causes of the bruxism. Lüscher has explained it in this way: Which of the colors shown in [Fig 3-36] is your favorite color? Red or yellow, blue or green or…? You will be surprised to see what you have revealed about your character by answering this question! The Lüscher test, with its 8 color cards, is offering more than 40,000 possible combinations. Its computer-based analysis provides you with a fast and exact analysis of your present emotional and physical condition and of the basic structure of your personality. The Lüscher test is based on color-psychology principles that have been confirmed by experiments. It is founded on the fact that liking or disliking a color is a subconscious but valid statement about a person's emotional and physical condition as such.

The nonverbal Lüscher Color Diagnostics System is an appropriate means acknowledged in the fields of psychology, psychiatry, and psychotherapy to quickly provide you with an impression of the emotional and psy-

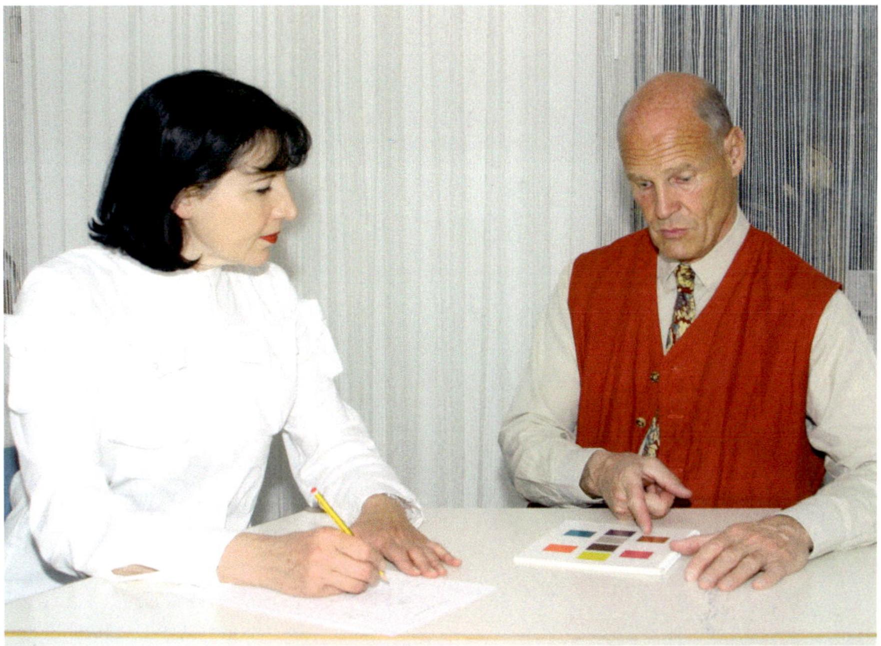

Fig 3-37a Performing the Lüscher color test.

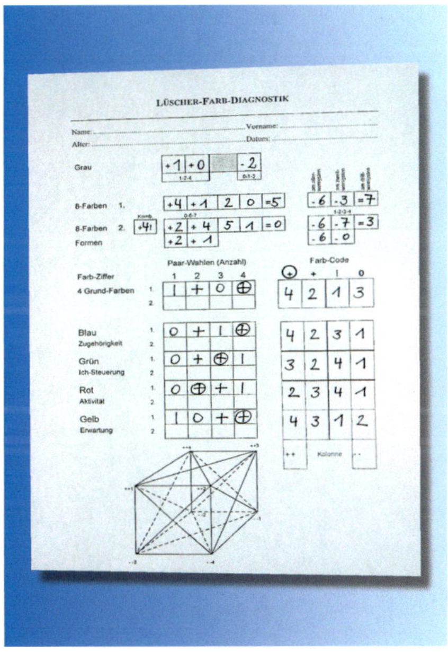

Lüscher-Farb-Diagnostik

Name: Vorname:
Alter: Datum:
Grau
8-Farben 1.
8-Farben 2.
Formen
Paar-Wahlen (Anzahl)
Farb-Code
Farb-Ziffer
4 Grund-Farben
Blau
Zugehörigkeit
Grün
Ich-Steuerung
Rot
Aktivität
Gelb
Erwartung
Kolonne

Fig 3-37b Assessment form.

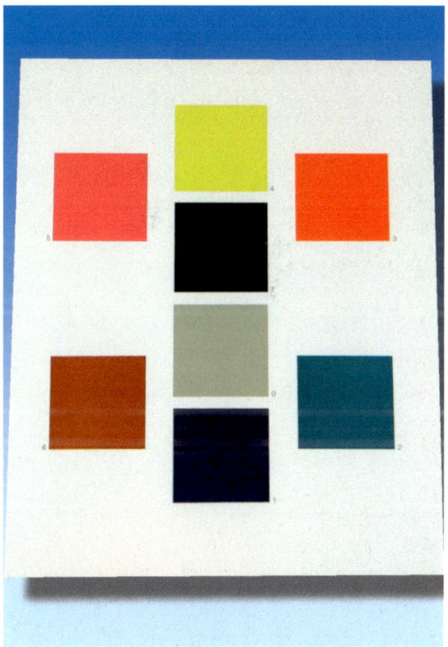

Fig 3-37c Basic colors.

chological state of the patient. The choice of color discloses any "subjective disturbances."

For example: Dark blue represents calm, quietness, relaxation, and regeneration. If the patient dislikes this color, then these states are unpleasant for the patient. Such people are restless, always in motion and incapable of relaxing; they may react with high blood pressure, sleep disorders, gastric disorders, and with bruxism, grinding, and other malfunctions of the jaws.

Since I presented my method to the scientific community at the international conference on psychology (Internationaler Kongress für Psychologie) in Lausanne in 1947, exhaustive research and large-scale surveys have confirmed the reliability of my testing method. For years, physicians, educators, psychologists, human resources managers, and advertising experts have been working successfully with the Lüscher Color Diagnostics System throughout the US and Europe in facilities such as doc-

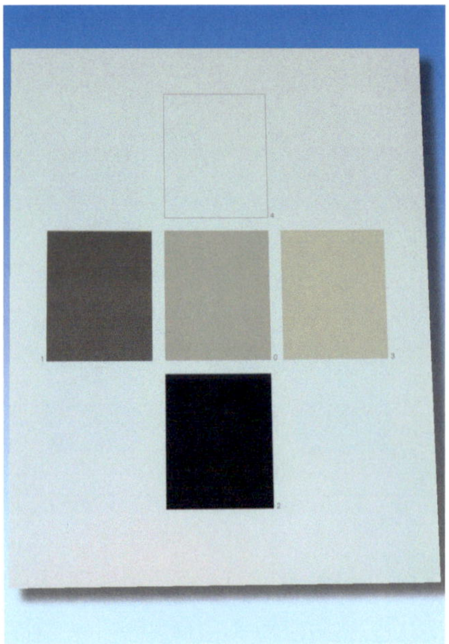

Fig 3-37d Grayscale sheets.

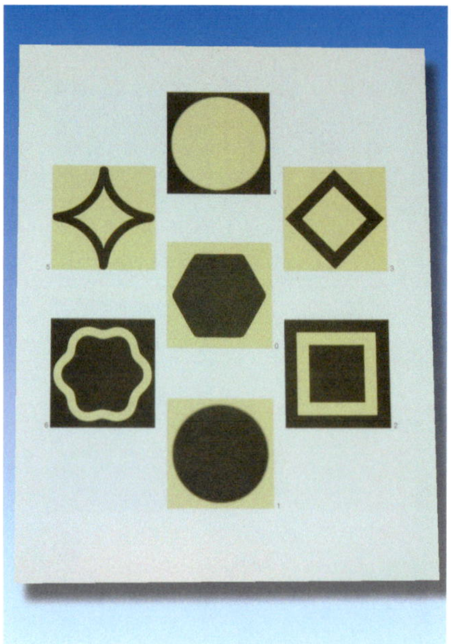

Fig 3-37e Shape sheets.

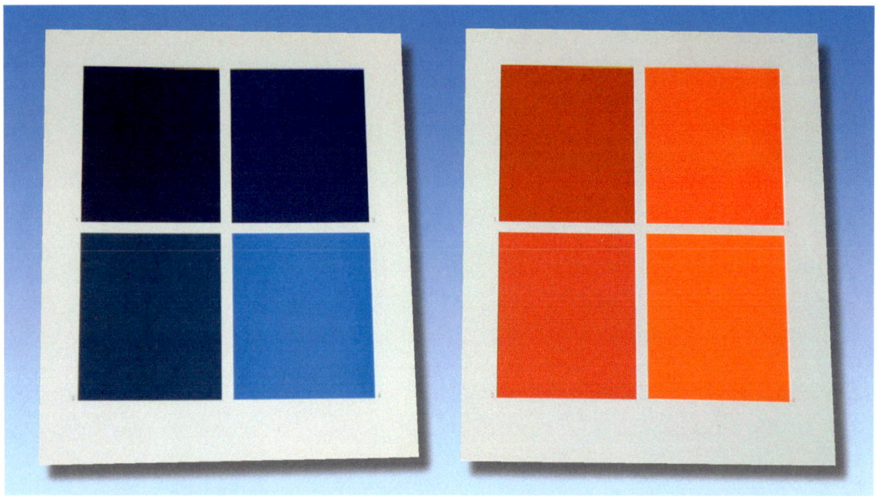

Fig 3-37f Two sheets of color combinations.

tor's offices, hospitals, schools, public authorities, and companies as well as in the fields of career counseling and product design."

Practical implementation of the Lüscher Color Diagnostics System

Before the test is actually used, it must be explained to patients very tactfully so that they are able to understand the whole purpose of the test. It is important to convey to the patients that they are not going to be made emotionally vulnerable in any way; the test is performed solely to establish the reasons for their bruxism. Any and all test results must be kept strictly confidential.

After the patient's consent is obtained, the test can be carried out by an appropriately trained assistant (Fig 3-37a). The following is required to perform the test: the Lüscher color test sheets, the assessment form (Fig 3-37b), a pencil, and an eraser. The person performing the test should work through the pages with the color test sheets one after another and write down the color, color combination or shape chosen with their respective numbers in the assessment form (Figs 3-37c to 3-37f). The test takes approximately 15 minutes and parts of it are reviewed again.

Thanks to the assessment software for the office computer (Fig 3-37g), the formerly time-consuming assessment procedure has now been streamlined so it takes no more than a couple of minutes: The values are entered

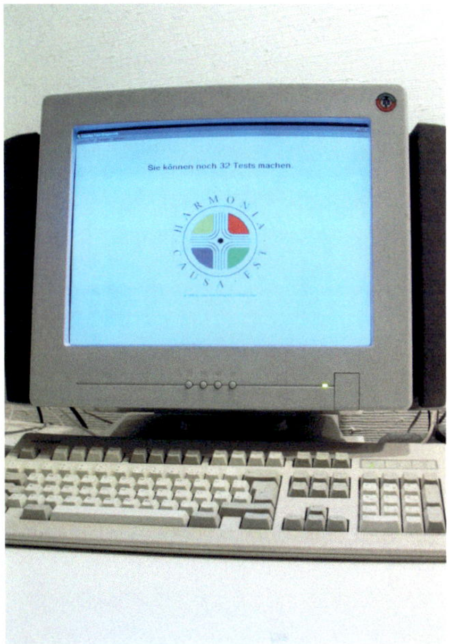

Fig 3-37g Assessment with the office computer.

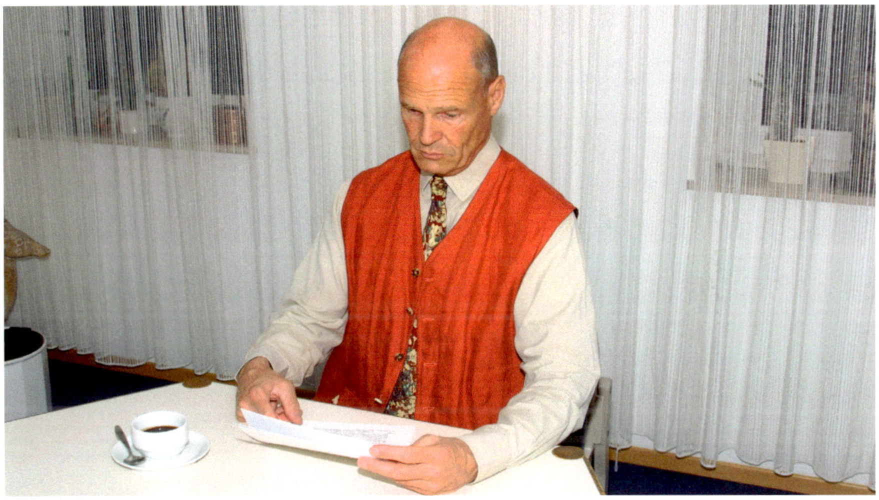

Fig 3-37h The patient reads his analysis print-out.

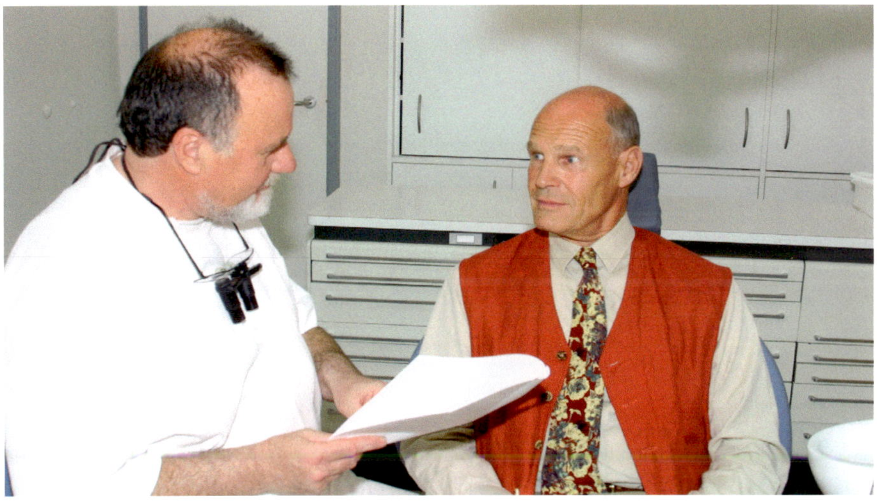

Fig 3-37i The results are discussed in a confidential conversation between patient and dentist.

and the test results are printed. The printout is about 10 letter pages. The author recommends handing it to the patient unread and having them study their analysis at leisure (Fig 3-37h). Afterward, the patient will want to talk about his or her condition in a confidential, one-on-one conversation (Fig 3-37i). For the dentist, the last page of the assessment (the summary) is the most relevant. The dentist should go through this page together with the patient to have a sound basis for the subsequent decision the clinician must make: Can the patient's bruxism can be helped directly with the methods available to a dentist, or is it necessary to initiate a different type of treatment or therapy?

The Lüscher Color Diagnostics System should be learned and practiced in a special training course. Information about the test can be obtained from the Lüscher Institute. Dentists may find that performing the test on themselves can lead to impressive results that may provide very valuable insights into their own personality.

Materials

Color test sheets, assessment forms, and assessment software (Lüscherdiagnostik), www.luscher.com

Fabrication of Centric Splints with Anterior Guidance

Common problem: Fabrication of splints with anterior guidance is very difficult

Bite guards and splints are an integral part of the pretreatment stage when it comes to treating functional disorders and conditions of the temporomandibular joint. The following forms of splints have proven useful: mouthguards, repositioning splints, and guidance splints.

The mouthguard serves as a means to relax the muscles involved in bruxism (clenching, grinding, and occlusal habits). This splint is an integral part of the initial treatment to relax the stomatognathic system to such a degree that it permits functional analysis, treatment, and restoration.

The repositioning splint is used when the functional unit of the disc and the condyloid process of the TMJ is disturbed. The splint is an attempt to achieve repositioning if dislocation occurs.

The guidance splint plays an important part in the more advanced stages of initial treatment, in which the stomatognathic system is already relaxed and the condyles are centrally positioned; this is the time to establish well-functioning anterior-canine guidance as a basis for successful rehabilitation. This is why anterior-canine guidance is established and ground into these types of splints.

Successful freehand creation of anterior-canine guidance and subsequent grinding is extremely difficult and very time consuming. Are there any other methods to do this more efficiently and expediently?

Proven solution: Establishment of anterior guidance with the Contour Curve Former

A new way of determining ideal anterior-canine guidance emerged when the Contour Curve Former (CCF) was developed in the 1980s. Anterior guidance was defined in the catenary model by Kubein-Meesenburg et al as follows: The anterior teeth of the mandible, which are correctly and harmoniously positioned in the dental arch, move in a vault formed by the anterior teeth of the maxilla that can be mathematically defined.

Research and practical experience led to a theoretical, biomechanically plausible model of anterior guidance, which in turn led to the excellent practical implementation of the CCF in establishing this anterior guidance for splints and permanent restorations.

Case report

The fabrication of a centric splint with anterior guidance (Figs 3-38a and 3-38b) will be demonstrated step by step through a patient case.

A 21-year-old woman was suffering from TMJ disease, migraine headaches, bruxism (clenching and grinding; the teeth were already abraded by 2 mm), and recurring bouts of insomnia (Figs 3-38c and 3-38d). Several mouthguards were unsuccessful; they even broke several times. The problem was a distance of 4 mm between the unguided centric condylar position (physiologic contact position) that the patient adopted herself and the habitual protruded position (intercuspal contact position) (Figs 3-38e and 3-38f). A guided centric registration revealed a long centric relation of 7 mm. Which centric position was suitable as an initial treatment?

The patient received a splint with centric plateau designed according to Shore[11] and wore it for 2 days. The plateau had been sandblasted to give it a matte surface; after the 2 days were over, shiny trace marks from the incisors were visible as a positioning guide. The regions of the anterior and posterior teeth were ground out to position the mandible in a defined centric position in relation to the maxilla (Fig 3-38g). This position was accepted by the patient and within 1 week led to significant improvement of her pain situation. In addition, her migraine headaches were treated successfully by hypnotherapy.

After 2 weeks, the patient was without pain and the centric splint, which had been successful so far, was to be rebuilt with the CCF so that it would provide anterior guidance. The appropriately contoured curve can be determined by *(1)* analyzing the palatal contour of the anterior teeth (Fig 3-38h); *(2)* analyzing the distal contour of the posterior teeth (the latter is determined by cutting a cast sagittally in a paramedian plane through the tips of the supporting cusps); or *(3)* arithmetically and geometrically analyzing the protrusion tracing of an axiographic evaluation.

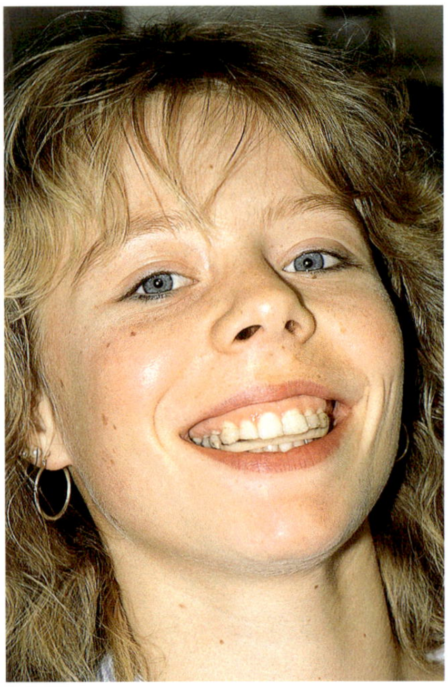

Fig 3-38a Patient with her centric guidance splint in place.

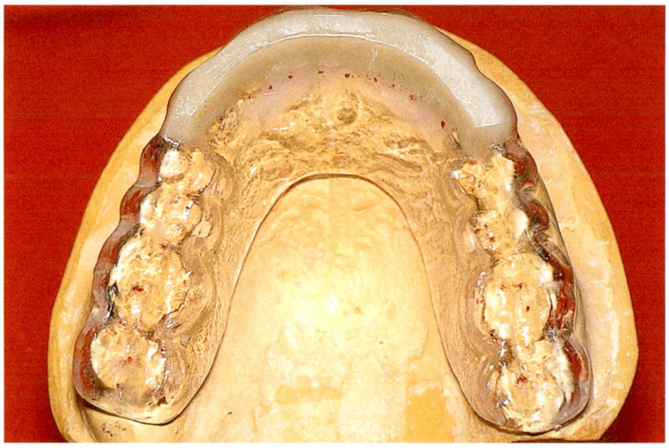

Fig 3-38b Centric guidance splint with anterior guidance.

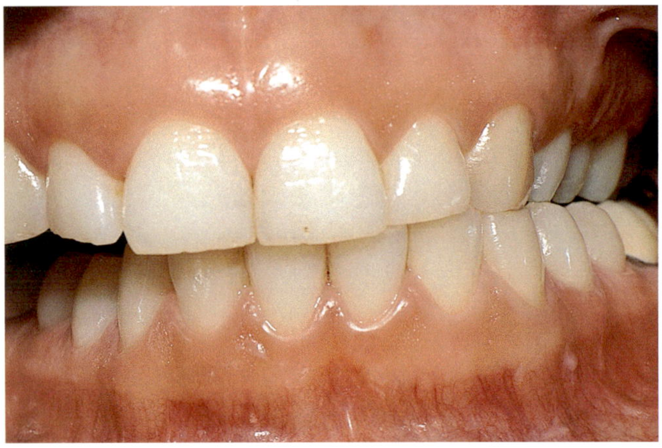

Fig 3-38c The patient exhibits eccentric bruxism.

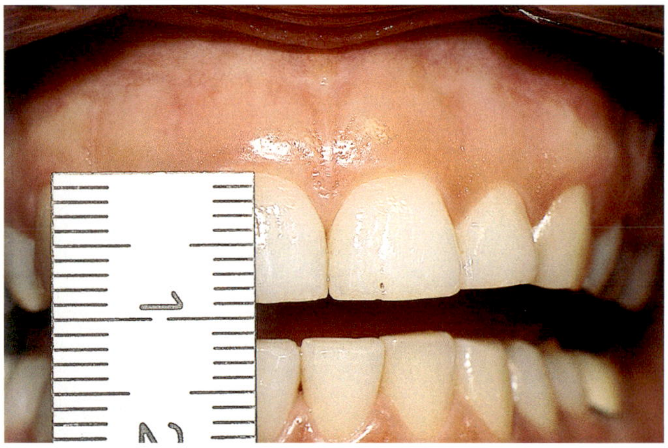

Fig 3-38d The teeth are already considerably worn down.

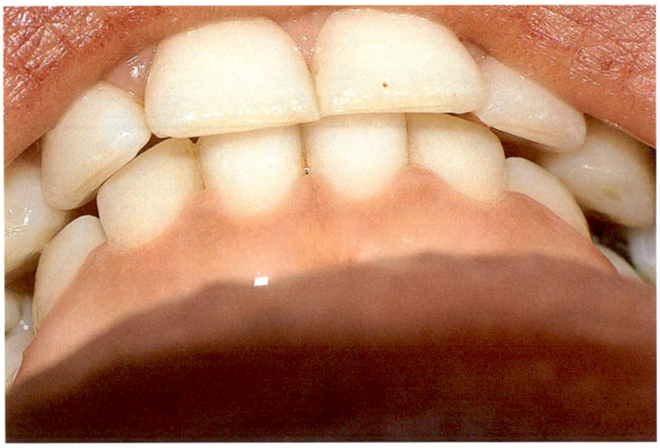

Fig 3-38e Habitual intercuspal contact position.

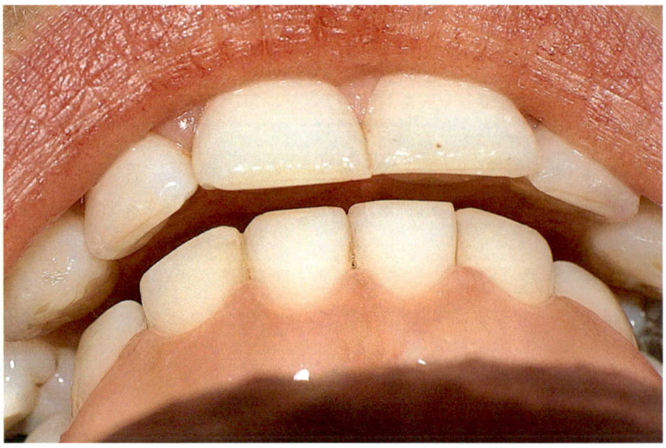

Fig 3-38f Centric position the patient has adopted herself (physiologic contact position).

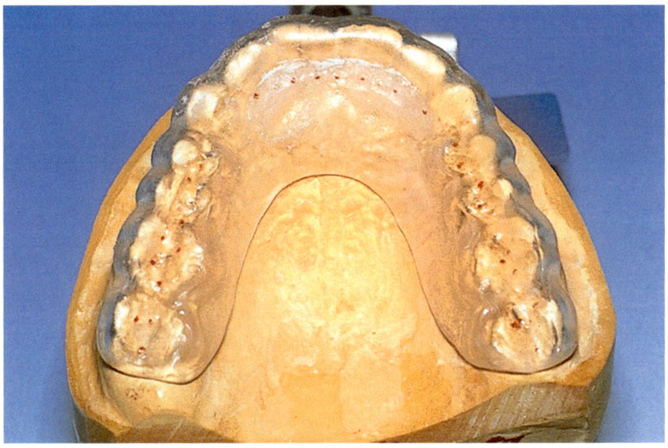

Fig 3-38g Centric splint with Shore plateau after selective grinding.

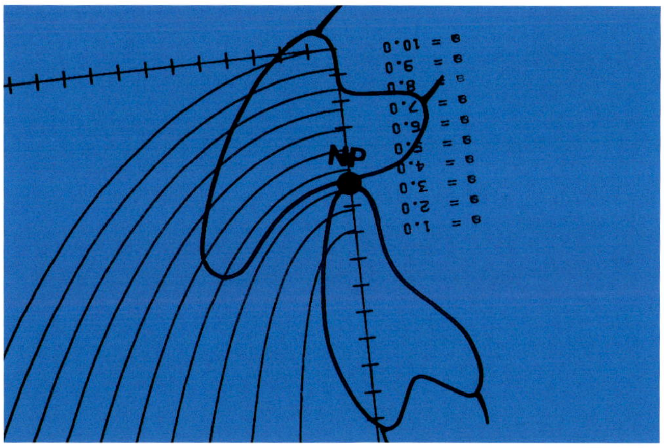

Fig 3-38h Analysis of the contour curve derived from the curve of the anterior teeth.

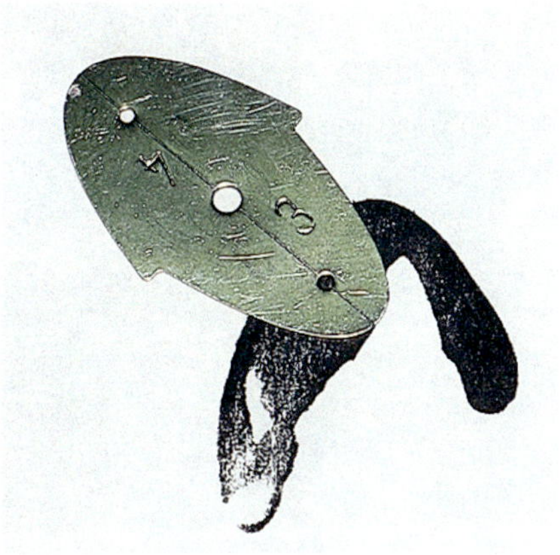

Fig 3-38i Analysis of the contour curve with the CCF disk on a stamped crosssection of the patient's anterior teeth.

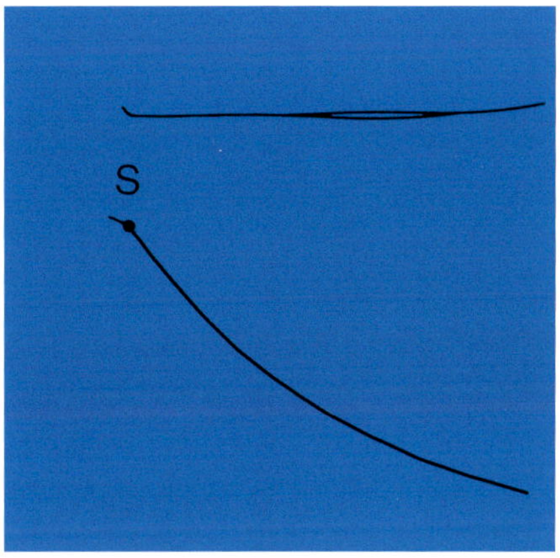

Fig 3-38j Patient's axiographic evaluation.

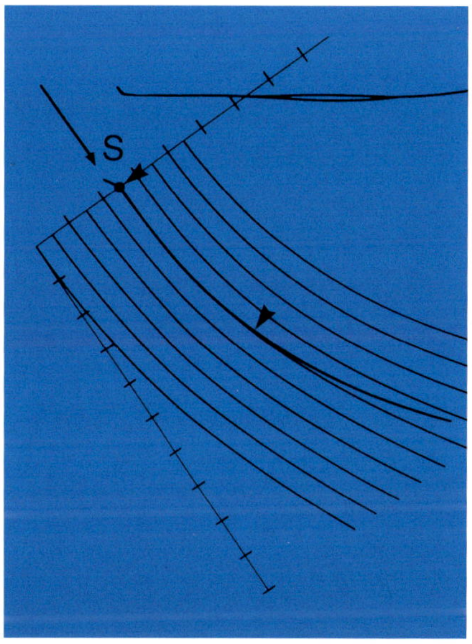

Fig 3-38k *(right)* Analysis of R_2 with the superimposed film and protrusion tracing.

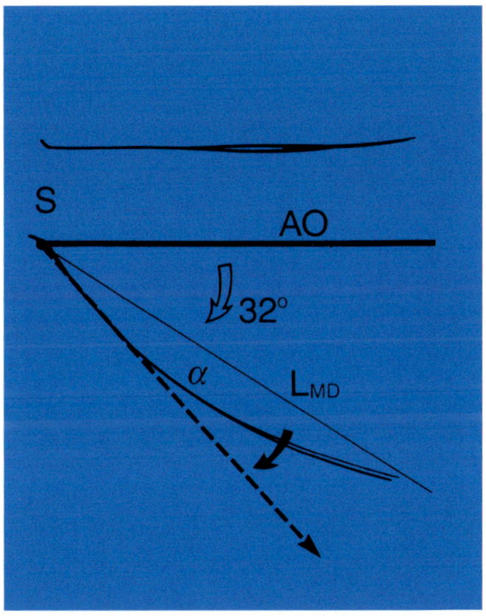

Fig 3-38l Determining the angle α.

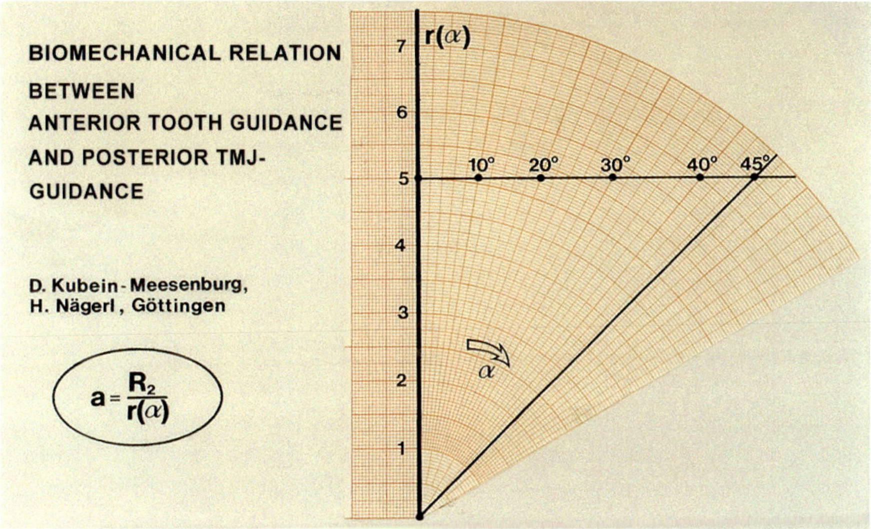

Fig 3-38m Calculation chart.

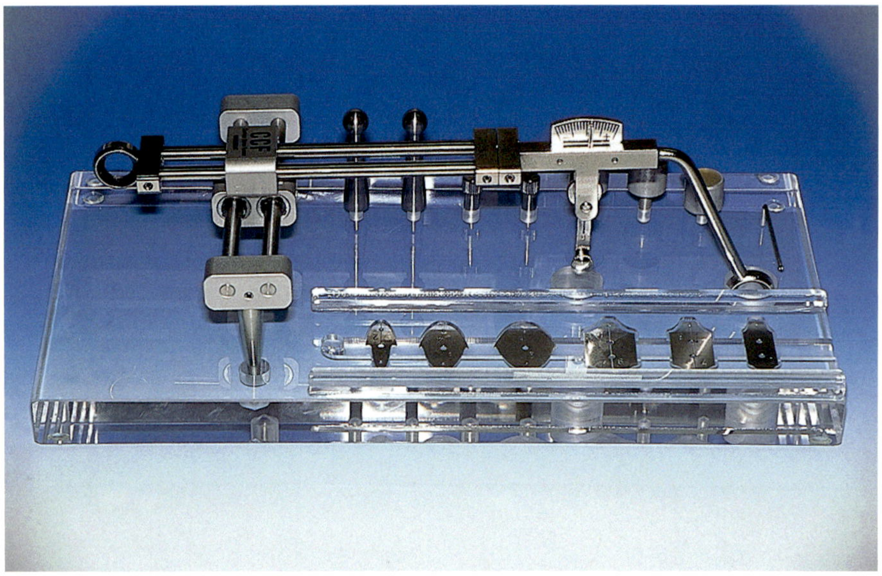

Fig 3-38n Contour Curve Former CCF (basic appliance).

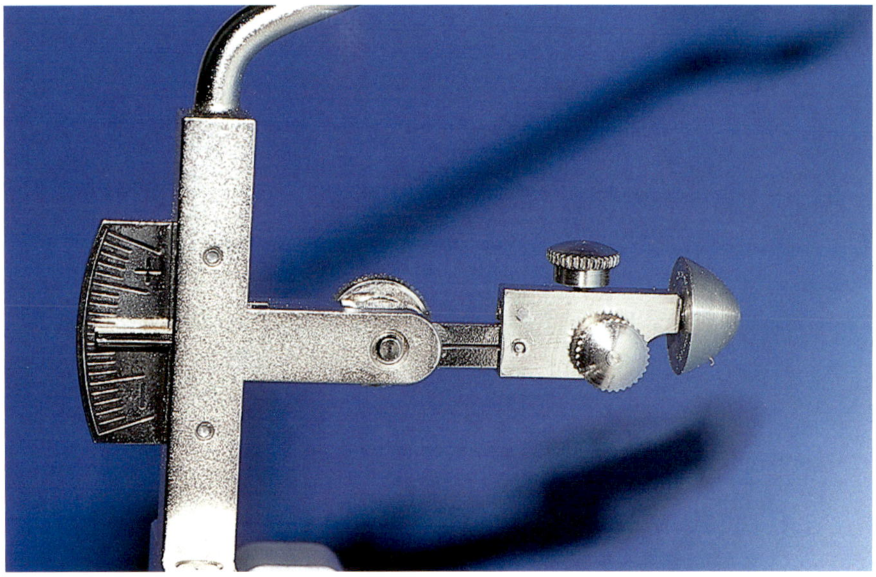

Fig 3-38o The appropriately sized tracing bud is mounted.

In this case, however, the posterior teeth were so flat as a result of bruxism that they did not lend themselves to analysis of the contour curve. The anterior teeth also were shortened considerably by bruxism so that the palatal curve, which could have been used for analysis, was also very short—too short, in fact, to allow clear determination of a contour curve (Fig 3-38i).

Furthermore the year-long experience with the CCF has shown that in patients with advanced bruxism, the axiographic tracings tend to be distorted, resulting in curves that are not consistent with the contour curves derived from the tooth shape. Therefore, it was decided to analyze the contour curve of the protrusion tracing from the patient's axiographic evaluation (Fig 3-38j).

The R_2 value of this protrusion tracing was determined by placing a clear foil over it; the value was 22 (Fig 3-38k). In addition, the angle between the coupling plane (coupling plane = auriculoinfraorbital plane – 32 degrees; see chapter 6) and the initial tangent to the curve was added to the axiography with the help of a protractor, with the hinge axis point as the angular point (Fig 3-38l). The a value (4) of the contour curve was taken from the chart (Fig 3-38m).

The CCF consists of a basic appliance (Fig 3-38n) that can be adapted to almost any articulating-condyle (ARCON)–type articulator. It is used for shaping the frontal vaults for crowns and fixed partial dentures. An additional set of buds was developed for shaping the anterior vaults of centric splints.

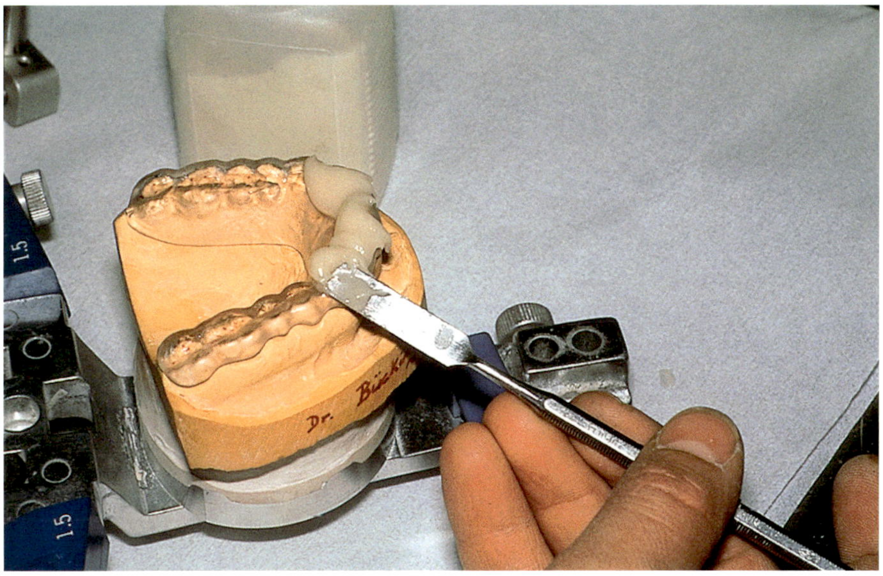

Fig 3-38p The cold-cure acrylic resin is applied.

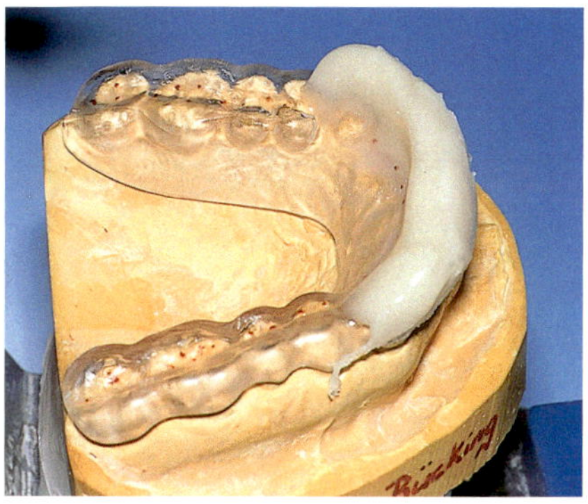

Fig 3-38q The plastic cold-cure acrylic resin is preshaped into a rim.

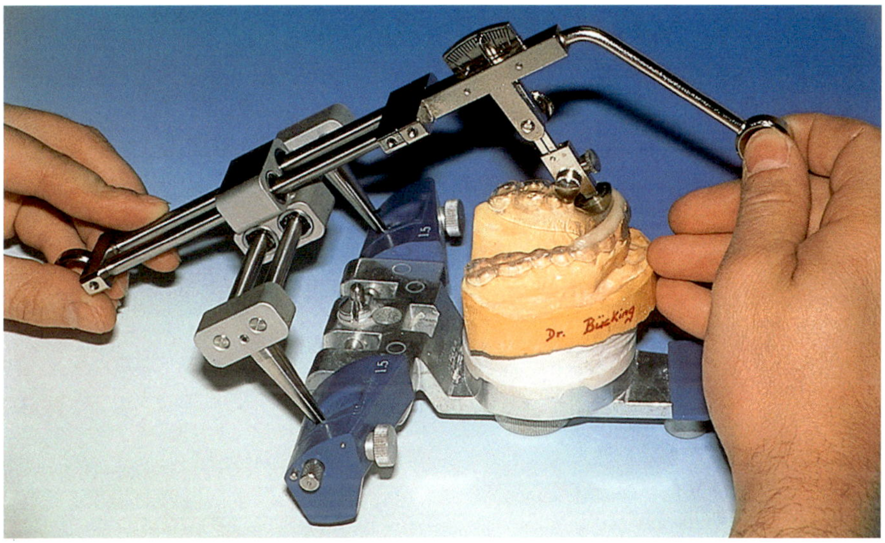

Fig 3-38r The CCF device is locked centrally in the articulator.

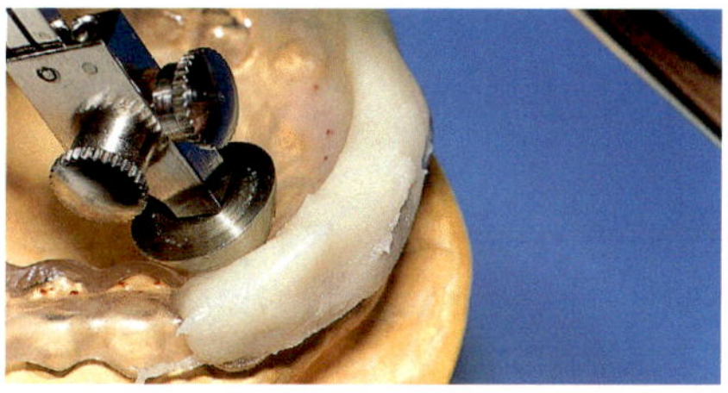

Fig 3-38s The anterior vault is shaped with the CCF (lateral view).

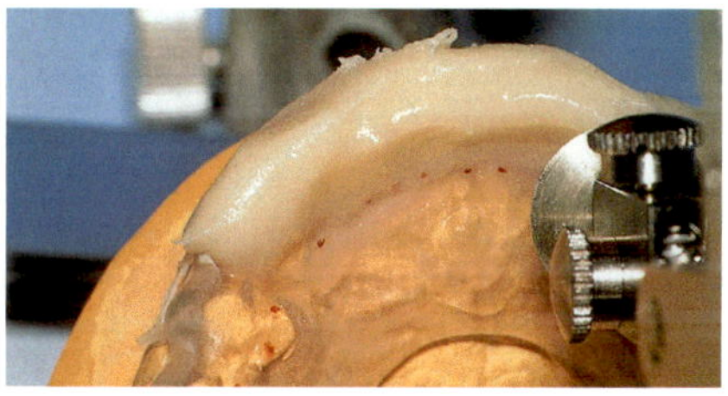

Fig 3-38t The anterior vault is shaped with the CCF (top view).

In the present case, the appropriate bud was selected and mounted onto the CCF device (Fig 3-38o) after it was determined that a = 4. The splint was selectively ground out again and remounted centrically into the articulator with the cast. The anterior region with the plateau was abraded and cleaned. A slow-curing butyl methacrylate (provisional crown and bridge resin) was mixed, applied to the anterior area as a flexible rim, and preshaped with thefingers (Figs 3-38p and 3-38q).

The CCF device was locked in the articulator in a central position. The tracing bud was moistened with monomer to ensure shaping of the anterior vault without its getting stuck (Figs 3-38r to 3-38t). The tip of the mounted bud was now led exactly along basal points that had been ground—the baseline—until a smooth and even vault was created to guide the teeth. After curing, it was trimmed to the correct height and carefully polished (Fig 3-38u).

At the try-in, the patient tested her new splint with anterior guidance by moving her jaw back and forth in all directions (Figs 3-38v to 38x), signaling her appreciation with a contented "mmmh." This is always the best compliment a dentist can get for successful treatment measures!

At the follow-up examinations, the patient was without pain and felt good. After a few months with regular follow-up visits, the plan is to begin the permanent prosthodontic restoration that will take place if the patient continues to be without pain.

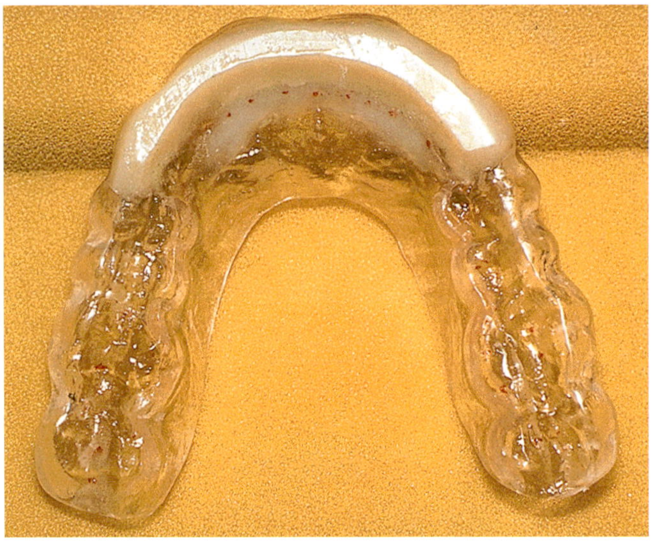

Fig 3-38u Finished centric splint with anterior vault.

Figs 3-38v to 3-38x The patient tests the splint in all functional dimensions: It allows harmonious, frictionless movements.

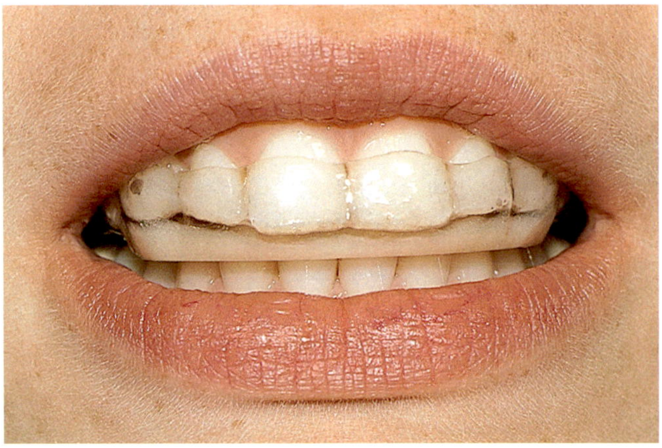

Fig 3-38v

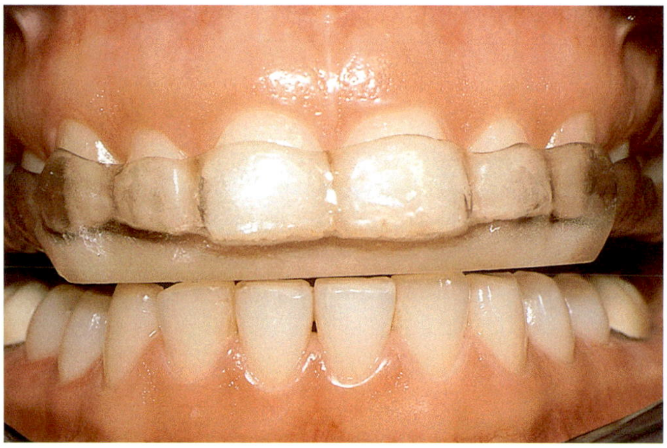

Fig 3-38w

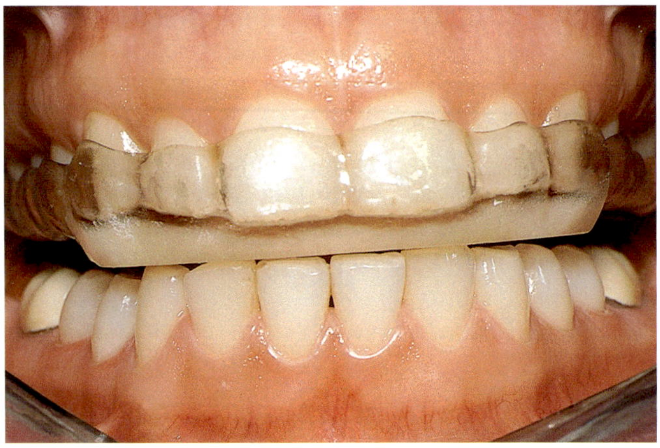

Fig 3-38x

Materials

Contour Curve Former (available directly from Dr Wolfram Bücking, Wangen, Germany)
Dentalon Plus prousional crown and fixed partial denture resin (Heraeus Kulzer); alternatively, Snap (Coltène Whaledent)
Hanel articulating paper (Coltène Whaledent)
Vacuum-forming foil (Erkodent)

Diagnostic Measures in Implant Prosthodontics

Common problem: Evaluation of the oral conditions for implant prosthodontics

The field of implant prosthodontics is essentially prosthetic dentistry with a surgical component. This means that dental implants are used to create abutments as anchors for the planned restorations. The procedure consists of the following individual steps:

1. Determination of the patient's wishes
2. Examination of the possible solutions with an implant-supported restoration
3. Prosthetic planning (setup, waxup) in conjunction with the dental laboratory technician
4. Evaluation of the implant bed (height, width, profile, and quality)
5. Fabrication of surgical templates consistent with the prosthodontic planning and diagnosis
6. Placement of implants with the help of a surgical template (with prior or concurrent augmentation, if necessary)
7. Allowance for healing time, depending on the diagnosis and the course of the surgical intervention
8. Exposure of the implants (mucogingival surgery)
9. Impression taking and occlusal registrations
10. Try-in of the denture framework
11. Assessment of the esthetics
12. Final restoration

The main focus of the two following subsections on planning implant procedures will be on evaluation of the implant bed. In this context, the following questions arise: How can the dentist obtain exact values for the height, width, profile, and quality of the bone bed? How exhaustive a diagnosis is needed for the various indications in implant prosthodontics? Is a computed tomogram (CT) really necessary for a single-tooth implant? Is a panoramic radiograph or a single-tooth radiograph sufficient to fulfill the aforementioned criteria? What kind of risk arises when the clinician does not have this information about the bone bed? How much more expensive does the implant procedure become when complex solutions from the dental laboratory are needed?

Proven solution: Acquisition of as much diagnostic information as necessary but no more than necessary

The expense of work and costs associated with different indications will be shown through some patient cases. The main focus is on the question as to how dentists can obtain all the information needed about the height, width, profile, and quality of the implant bed in different indications so that they can provide their patients with predictable implant-supported restorations.

Indication: Single-tooth implant for a maxillary incisor

A 17-year-old girl was missing her maxillary lateral incisors because of aplasia. The patient had been treated elsewhere with a cast framework removable denture that she was far from happy with. She wanted to have her spaces closed with a fixed denture (Figs 3-39a to 3-39d). In cases such as these, the following treatment options are available:

1. Orthodontic space closure by advancing the canines mesially. The author strongly advises against this treatment option, because it affects more than function and esthetics. The canines are half incisors and half posterior teeth, and their location is enormously important for the proprioceptive control of the stomatognathic system during chewing (Fig 3-39e).
2. Resin-bonded fixed partial denture. This is certainly an option, but it is esthetically problematic. Apart from that, resin-bonded fixed partial dentures also have a tendency to dislodge.
3. Cast framework denture. The patient was already wearing one and was dissatisfied with it.
4. Implant-supported ceramic crowns. This treatment option was the patient's dearest wish, which she had already inquired about.

The first step was to close the diastema between the central incisors to create a space for implantation of the lateral incisors. This was done with braces (Figs 3-39f to 3-

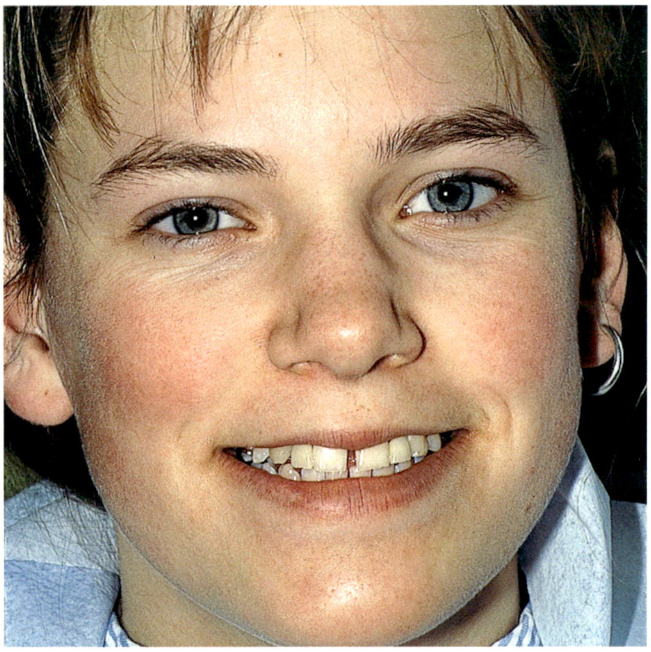

Fig 3-39a The 17-year-old patient is missing her maxillary lateral incisors.

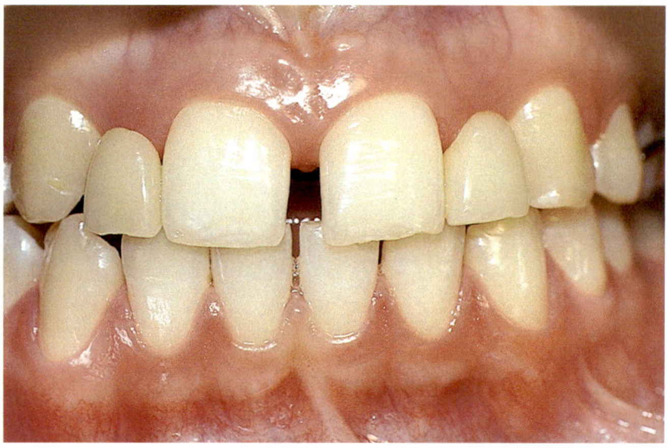

Fig 3-39b View of her mouth with partial denture in place.

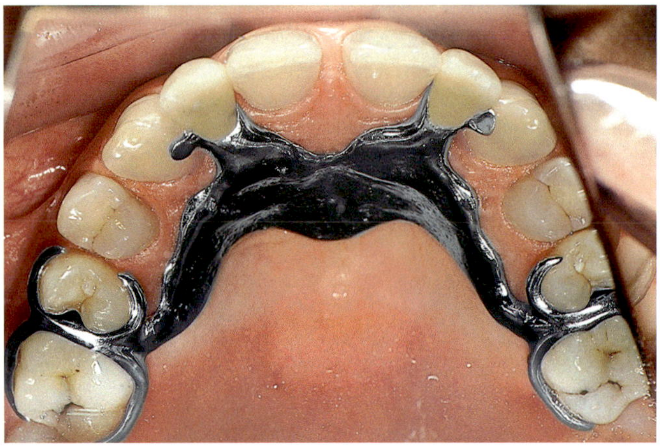

Fig 3-39c Occlusal view of the partial denture in the patient's mouth.

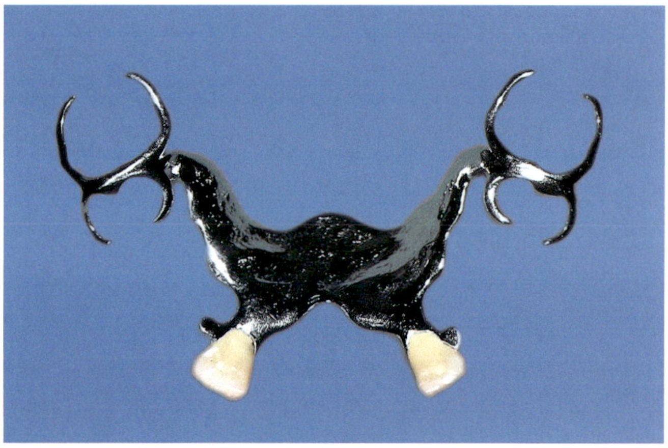

Fig 3-39d Cast-framework removable denture.

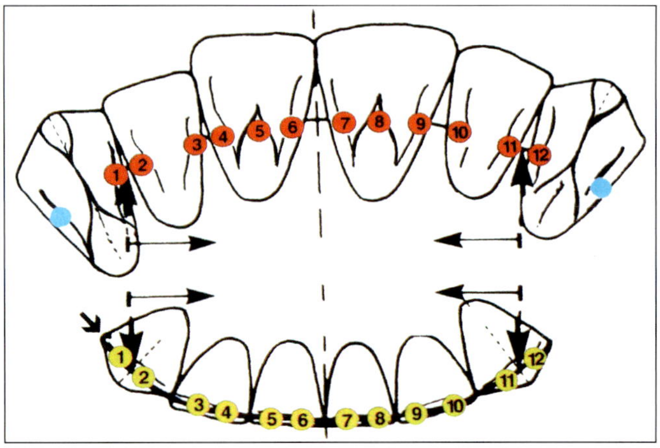

Fig 3-39e Ideal occlusion of the anterior teeth.

39i). The single-tooth radiographs in bisecting angle technique revealed the spaces that were opened (Figs 3-39j and 3-39k). The spaces should have been opened wider in the apical region, which would have been possible if retraction arch wires with loops had been used. The dentist should discuss this option with the patient's orthodontist.

When radiographs of anterior teeth are taken with the bisecting angle technique, it is essential not to adhere to the standard values issued by the manufacturer of the x-ray unit but to select the setting for when the tooth plane is parallel with the x-ray plane and parallel with the film plane. This permits both a protrusive plane and a retrusive plane to be rendered correctly in full size. The dental team must be instructed accordingly.

When this technique is used correctly, radiographs taken with the bisecting angle technique provide information about the height and the width of the implant bed in full size. How can the dentist acquire information about the profile? The measurement of the mucosal thickness is an appropriate means. Five readings must be taken: one centrally on the alveolar ridge, two vestibular points, and two oral points. Usually the values are determined, after administration of local anesthesia, by puncturing the mucosa with a sterile cannula or a sterile reamer with a silicone stopper. The stopper is pushed up the instrument and its position can be measured with a ruler (Figs 3-39l and 3-39m).

It is faster and more exact, however, to use a sharpened and sterilized periodontal probe with millimeter calibration for determining the mucosal thickness (Figs 3-39n to 3-39r). For this patient, the established values were marked on a cut cast, which was used to determine the implant position and diameter as well as to select the abutments (Figs 3-39s and 3-39t).

The position on the cast was marked in keeping with the guidelines for the "esthetic window" as defined by Gomez (see chapter 5). Once this position was determined and the bone bed was analyzed, a surgical template was created from a 2-mm steel jacket from a building supply store (Figs 3-39u to 3-39w). The bone quality that can be expected in the anterior region of the maxilla is class D3, which was confirmed at the time of the implant placement in this patient. The implants were placed, the wound was closed, and a diograph was made for verification (Figs 3-39x and 3-39y). After the implants were uncovered, the healing abutments were placed to shape the gingiva (Fig 3-39z). In this case, angled abutments and metal-ceramic crowns were used for the prosthetic restoration (Figs 3-39z and 3-39aa).

Figures 3-40a and 3-40b show a successful, esthetically optimum restoration 10 years after placement. As far as esthetics is concerned, much progress has been made in the last 10 years.

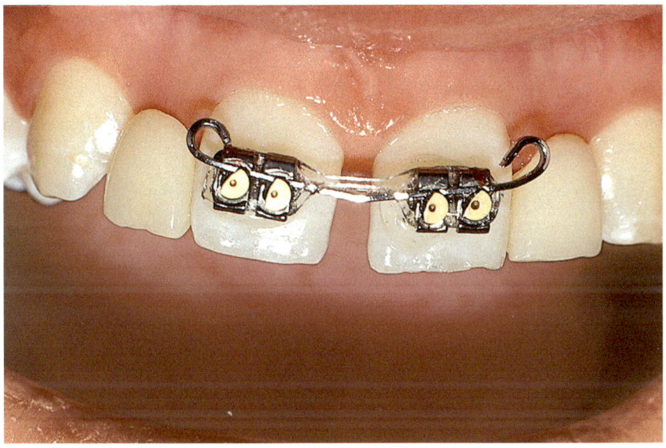

Fig 3-39f The diastema is closed with an orthodontic appliance.

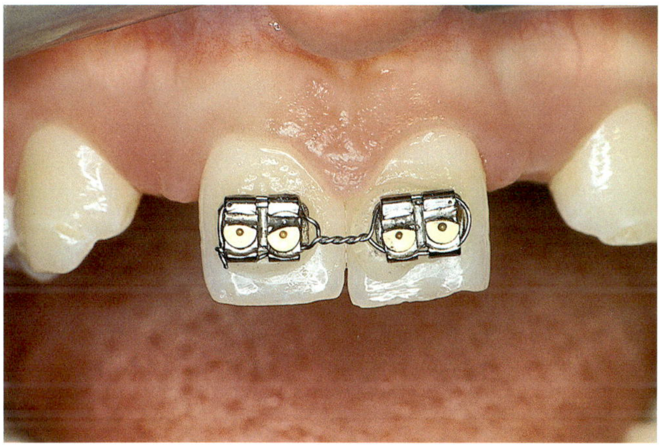

Fig 3-39g Closed space.

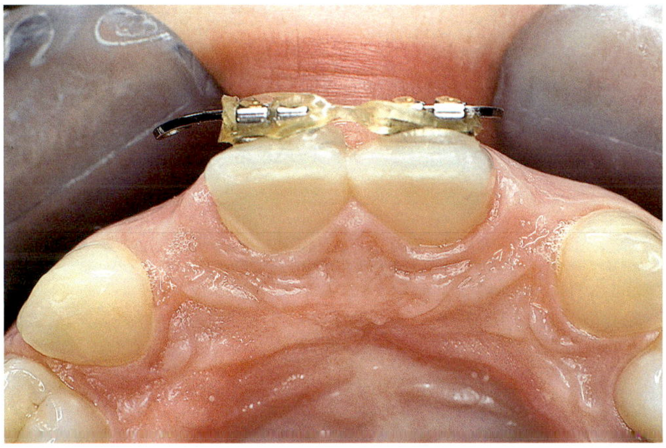

Fig 3-39h Palatal view of the spaces.

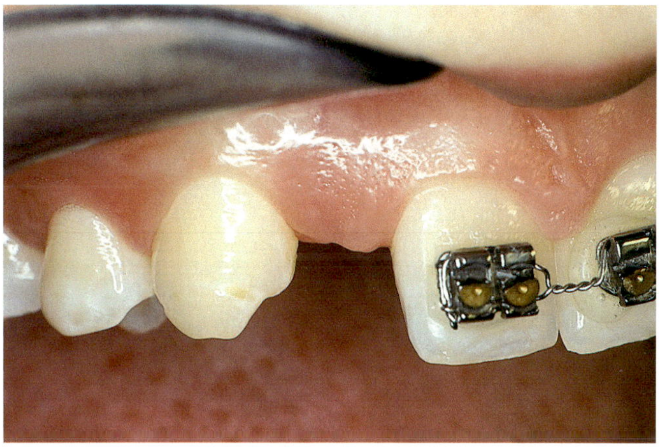

Fig 3-39i Frontal view of the spaces.

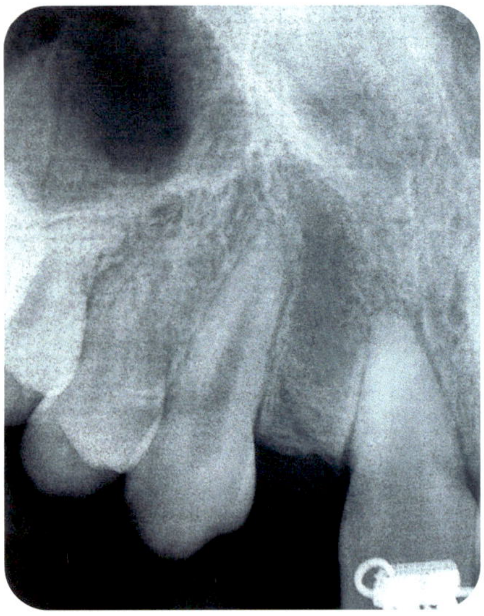

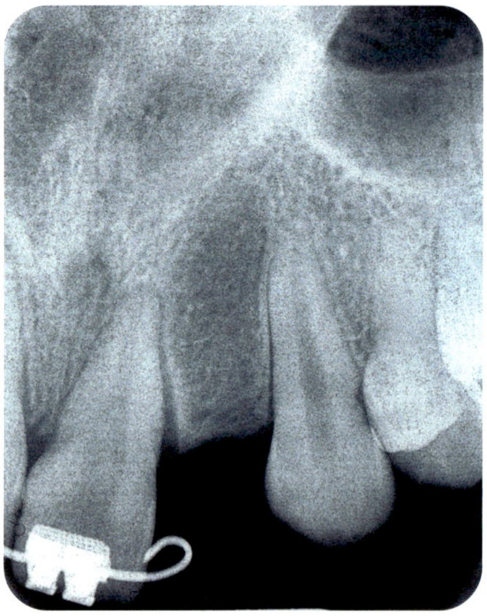

Fig 3-39j *(left)* Space at the position of the right lateral incisor.

Fig 3-39k *(right)* Space at the position of the left lateral incisor.

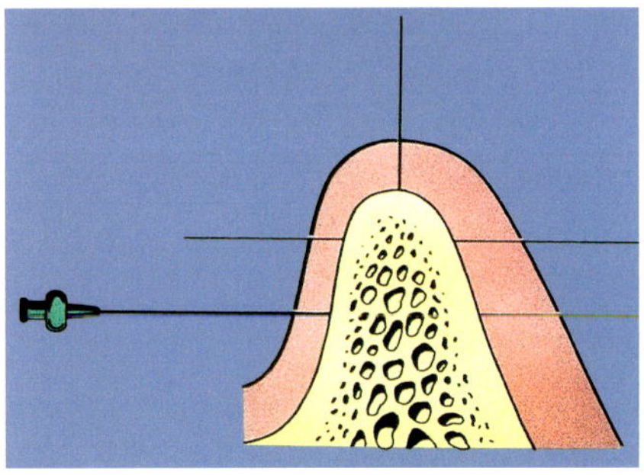

Fig 3-39l The mucosal thickness is measured.

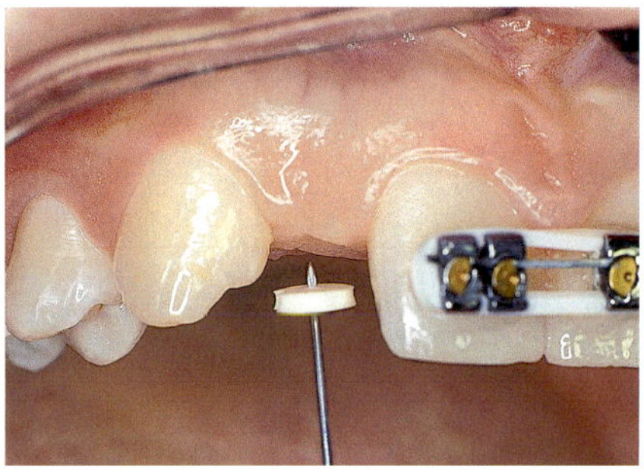

Fig 3-39m The mucosal thickness is measured with a sterile cannula and a silicone stopper.

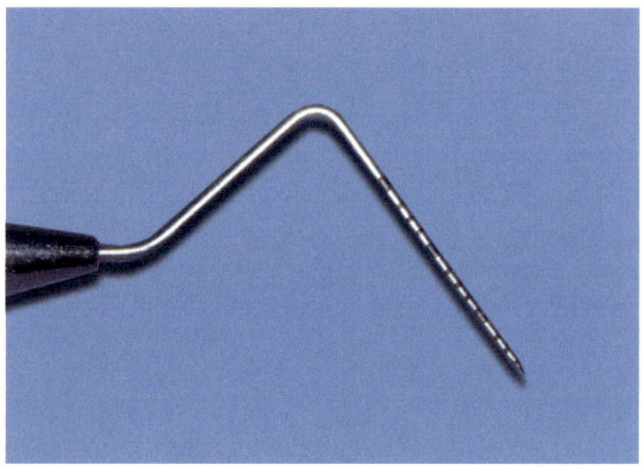

Fig 3-39n Sharpened periodontal probe with millimeter calibration.

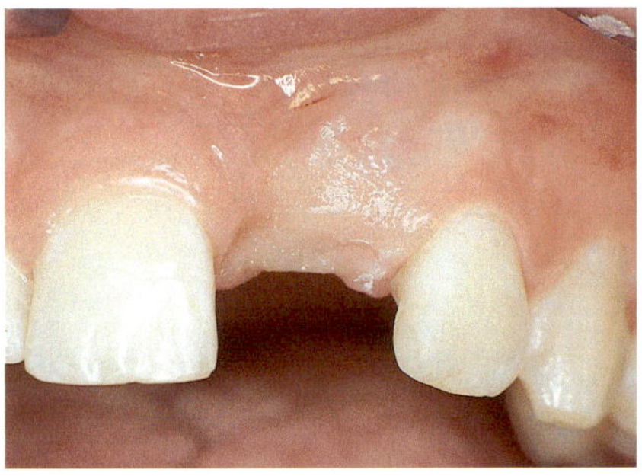

Fig 3-39o Mucosal thickness is measured at the position of the maxillary left central incisor after anesthesia was administered.

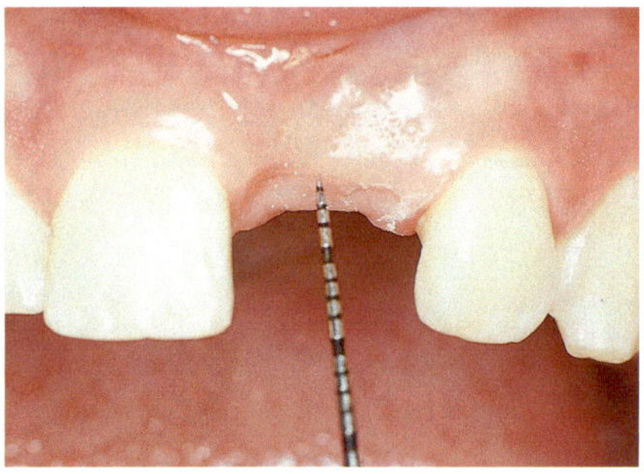

Fig 3-39p The mucosal thickness is measured with the sharpened periodontal probe (ridge measurement).

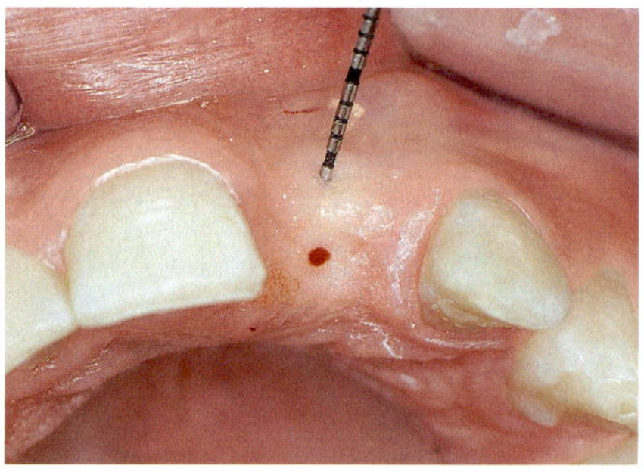

Fig 3-39q The buccal mucosal thickness is measured with the sharpened periodontal probe.

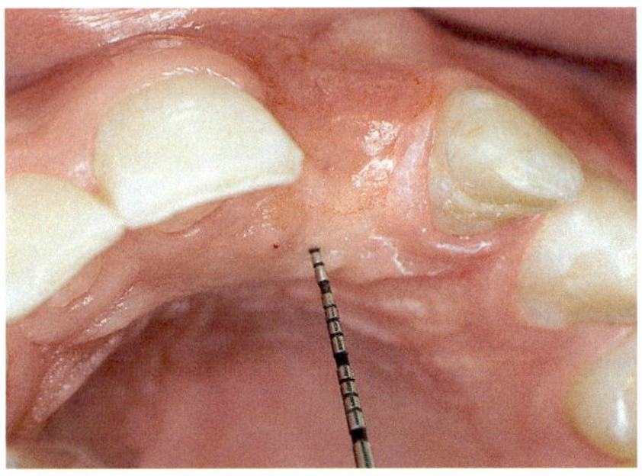

Fig 3-39r The palatal mucosal thickness is measured with the sharpened periodontal probe.

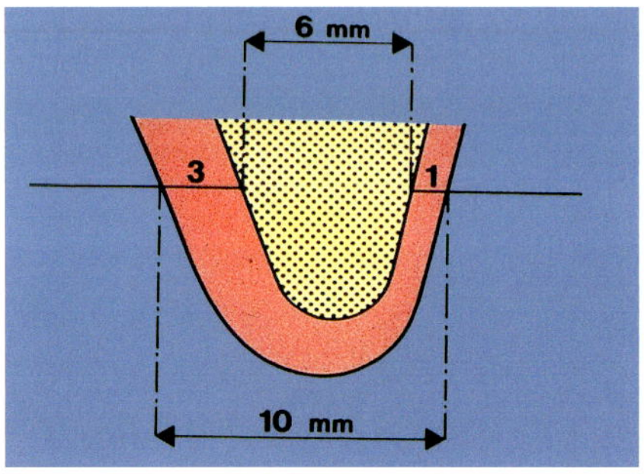

Fig 3-39s Diagram of the measurements taken for this patient.

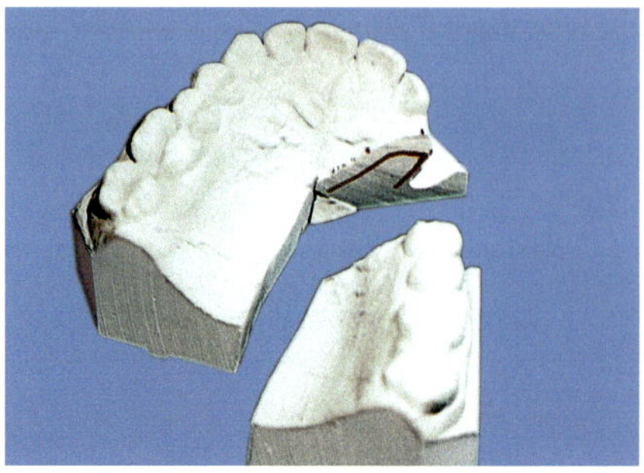

Fig 3-39t Measurements are transferred to the cut cast.

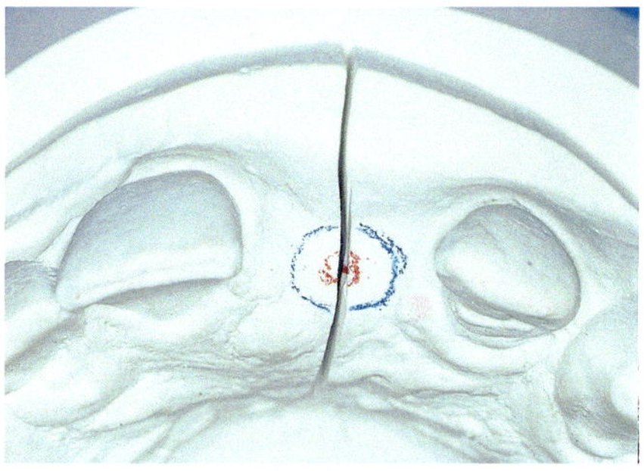

Fig 3-39u The implant position is marked on the cast.

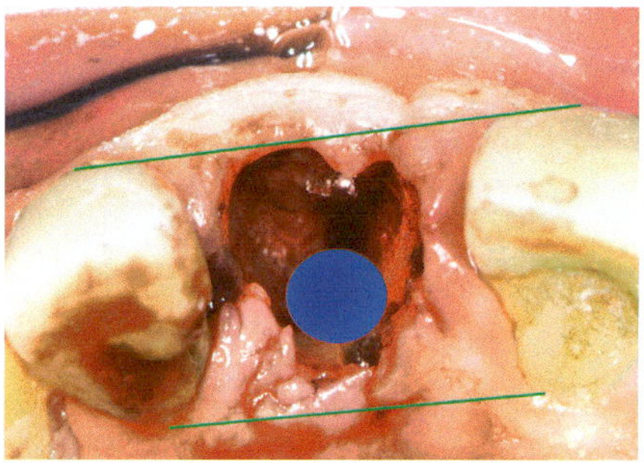

Fig 3-39v The esthetic window according to Gomez.

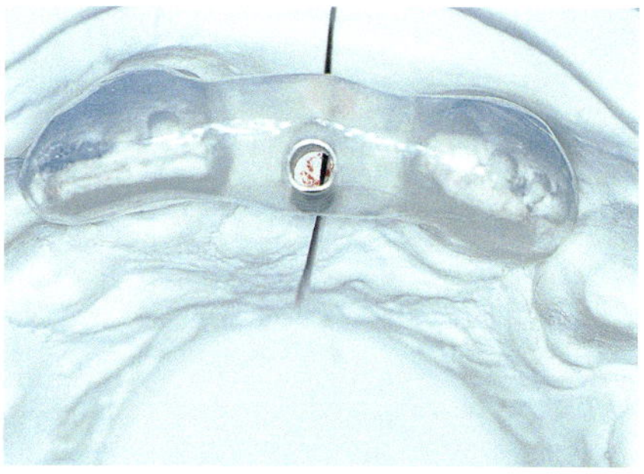

Fig 3-39w The surgical template is placed on the cast.

Fig 3-39x *(left)* Buccal radiograph of the implants in place.

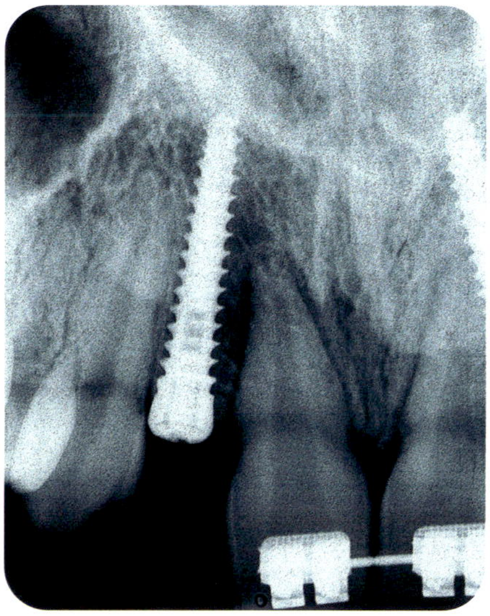

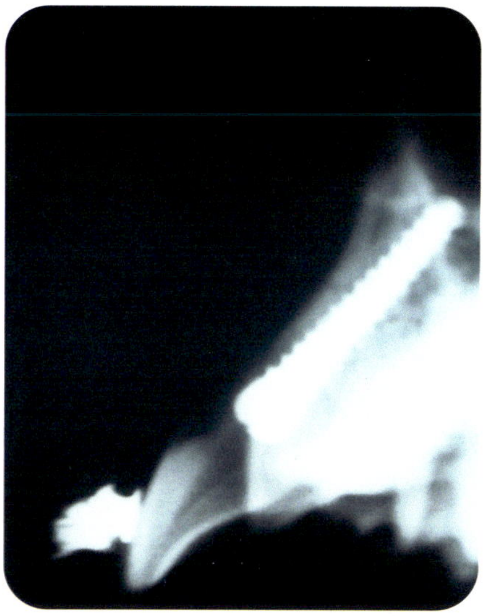

Fig 3-39y *(right)* CT of the implants in place.

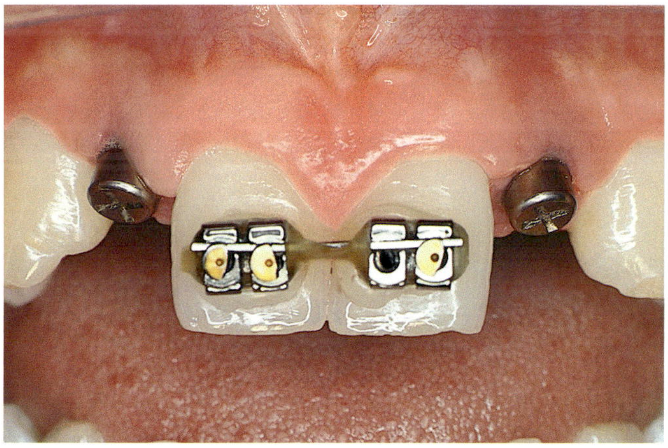

Fig 3-39z Implants after surgical exposure. The concept of the esthetic window was not known at the time of this surgery, which is why there are buccal recessions.

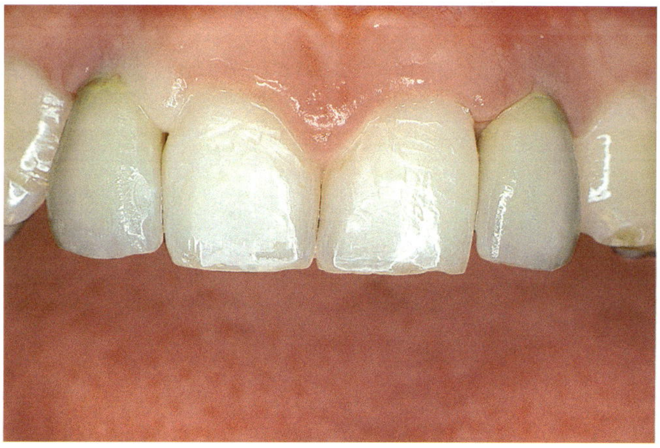

Fig 3-39aa Permanent restorations with metal-ceramic crowns.

Indication: Edentulous mandible

A 75-year-old patient was complaining about the lack of retention of his complete mandibular denture. If it were up to him, he would have the denture "hammered and soldered into place," as he put it (Figs 3-41a and 41b). How does the dentist establish the parameters required for height, width, profile, and quality of an edentulous mandible?

The height and width of the available bone can be determined with a panoramic radiograph (Fig 3-41c). The radiograph should be put in a transparent slipcover so that the dentist can mark the implant positions with felt-tip pens as a basis for the patient's informed consent (Fig

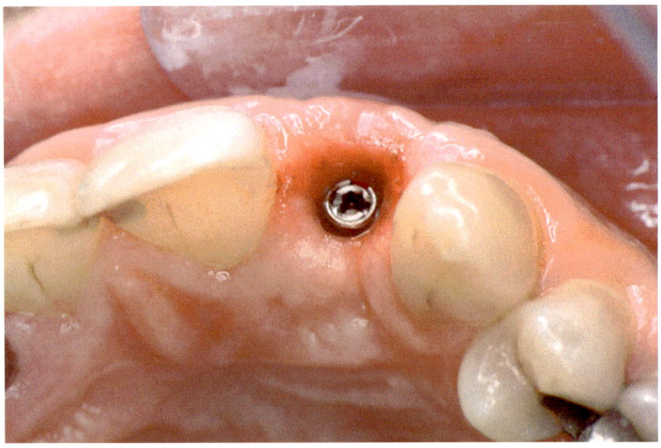

Fig 3-40a Anterior implant, positioned correctly.

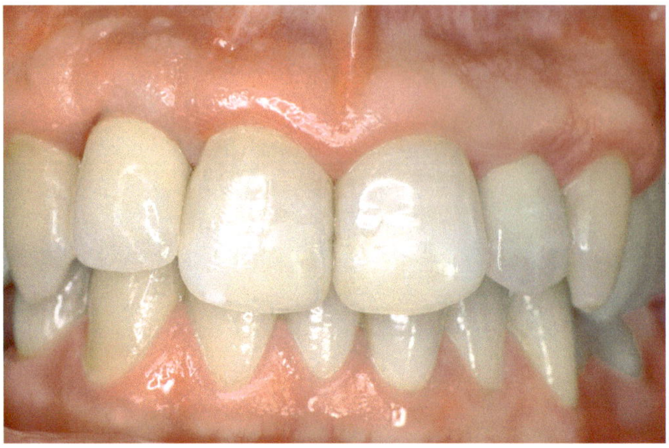

Fig 3-40b Good esthetics.

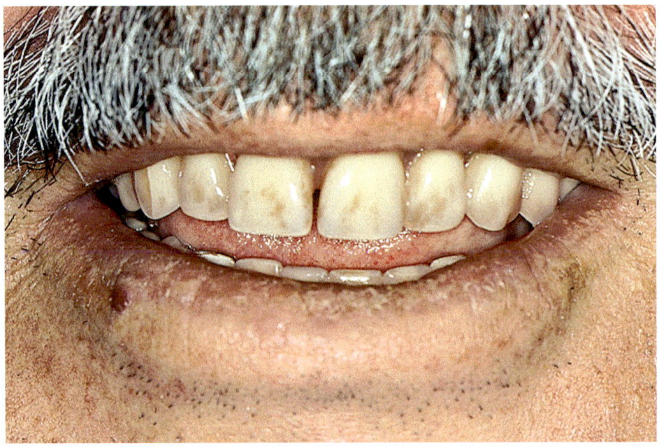

Fig 3-41a The 75-year-old patient is dissatisfied with his mandibular denture.

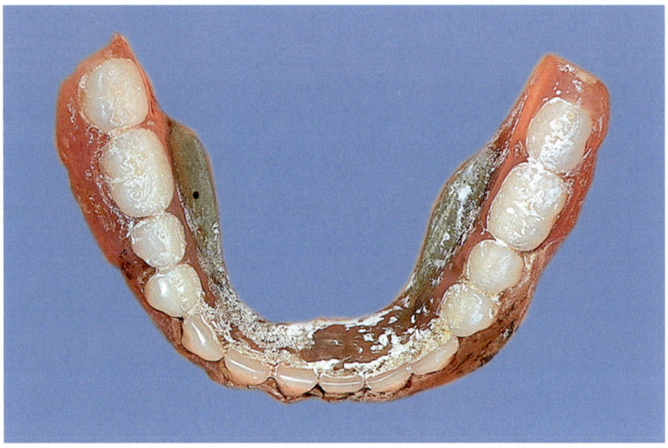

Fig 3-41b Poorly fitting complete mandibular denture.

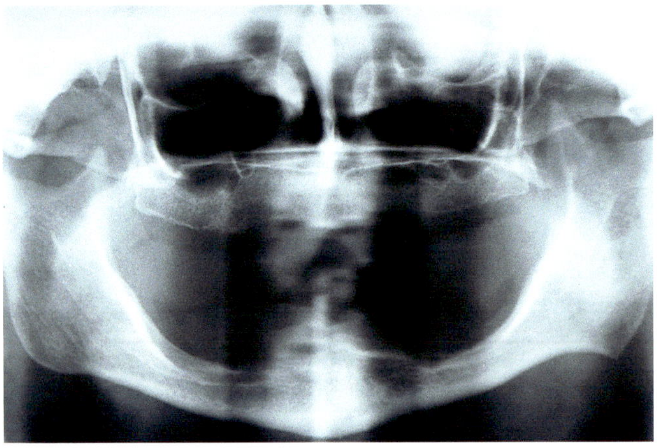

Fig 3-41c Panoramic radiograph of the patient.

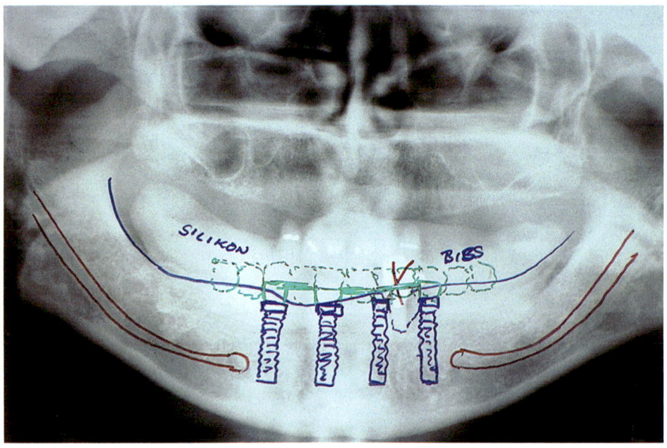

Fig 3-42 Implant positions are marked on a transparent file to obtain the informed consent of an edentulous patient.

3-42). Then the patient is provided with a cost estimate according to the dentist's usual price list. If the patient agrees to the planned restoration, the mandibular profile can be assessed (Figs 3-43 and 3-44).

The quickest method is to take a lateral cephalogram with lead foil strips (as described earlier in this chapter and in chapter 6). This tomography provides a midsagittal analysis of the bone bed in the mandible, thus allowing planning of the esthetic setup of the teeth and any

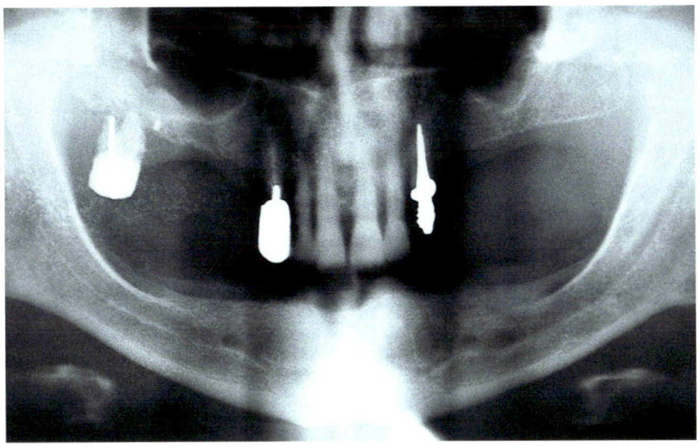

Fig 3-43 Panoramic radiograph of a patient with an edentulous mandible.

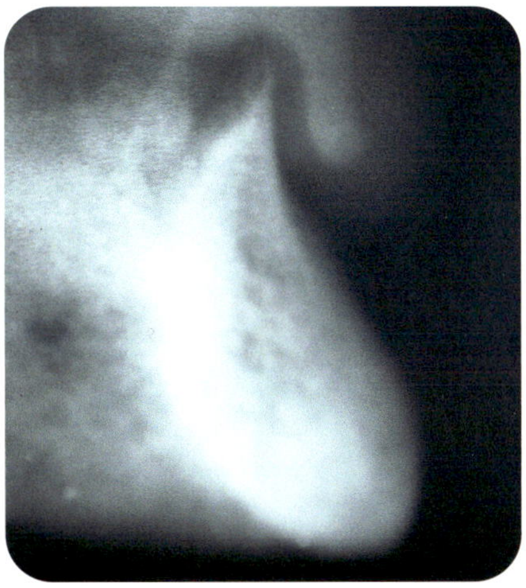

Fig 3-44 "Midsagittal tomography": detail from a lateral cephalogram.

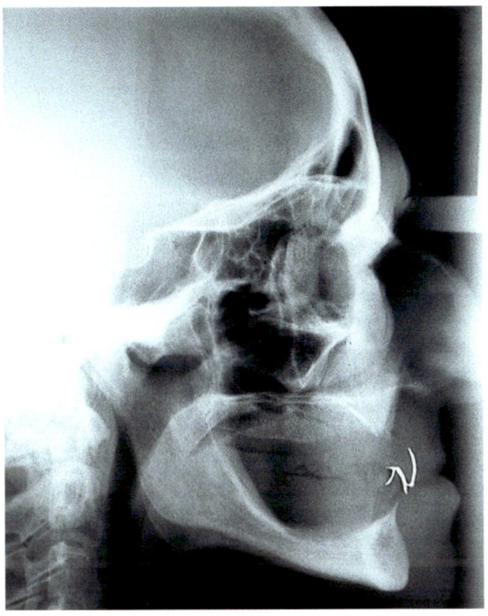

Fig 3-45a Lateral cephalogram with the anterior teeth marked with lead foil.

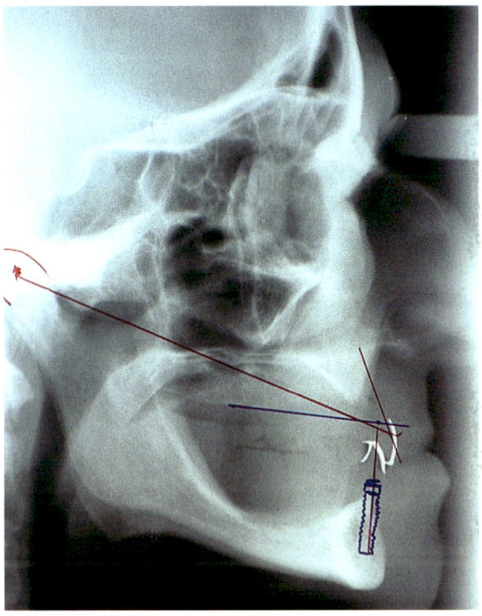

Fig 3-45b Functional analysis of the cephalogram.

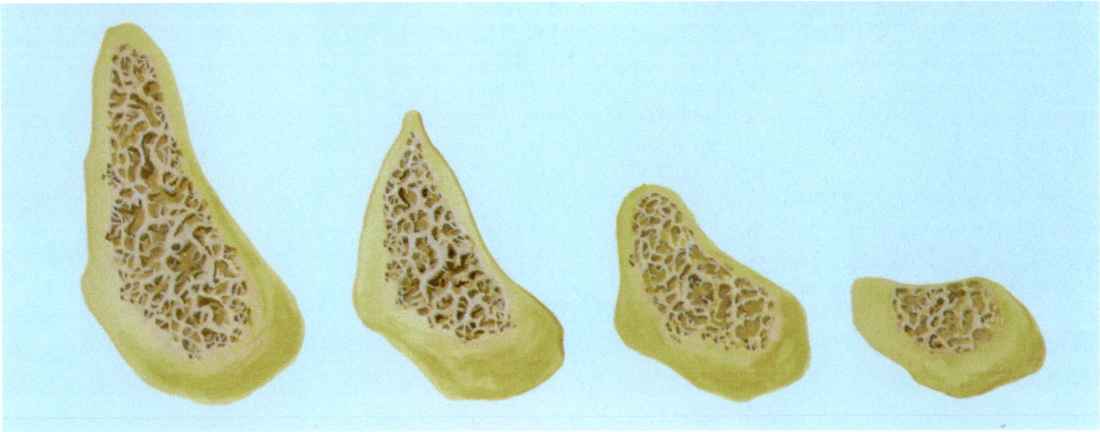

Fig 3-46 Cross sections of edentulous jaws.

implant positions required. It can also be used to measure vertically and perform a sagittal functional analysis (Figs 3-45a and 3-45b). This completes the analysis of the profile (Fig 3-46). The bone density to be expected in an edentulous jaw is class D1.

Indication: Posterior space in the mandible

In the posterior region of the mandible, the placement of implants is limited not only by the available bone but also by the path of the inferior alveolar nerve (Figs 3-47 and 3-

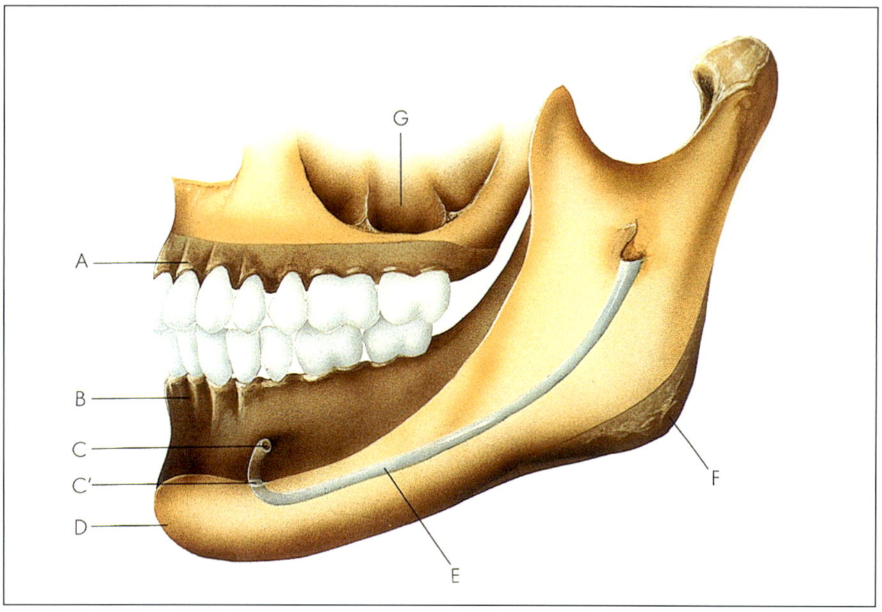

Fig 3-47 Path of the inferior alveolar nerve.

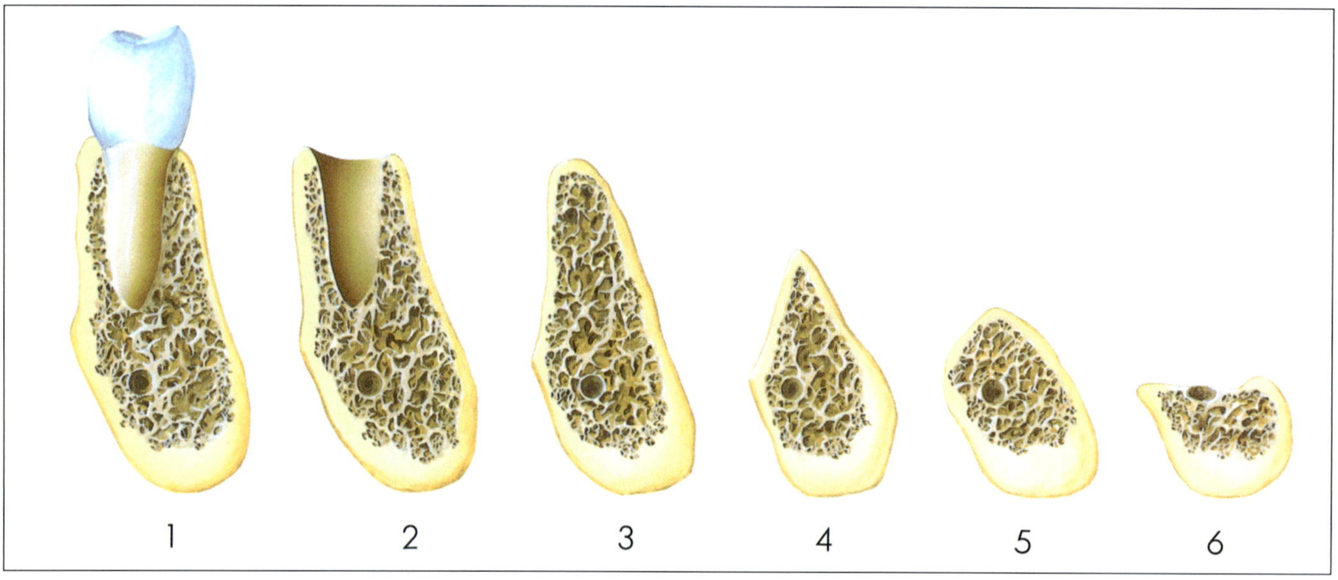

Fig 3-48 Atwood grades of resorption (1 to 6) in the posterior region of the mandible. (From Watzek. Reprinted with permission.)

48). Correct placement of the implants is difficult, especially if the mandible is already in an advanced state of resorption (Figs 3-49 and 3-50). In other words, the most important factor in planning implants in the posterior region of the mandible is to avoid damaging the inferior alveolar nerve (Fig 3-51). Taking the aforementioned into consideration, how can dentists obtain the necessary information about the available bone bed in the posterior region of the mandible with respect to height, width, profile, and quality?

A panoramic radiograph with measuring devices such as balls or pins is an absolute must (Fig 3-52). As the quality of panoramic x-ray units has increased enormously in the last couple of years, the distortion created by the rotation of the devices during exposure has been almost eliminated, thus allowing metric evaluation of panoramic radiographs. The manufacturers provide transparent templates with the lengths and diameters of implants (Figs 3-53a and 3-53b).

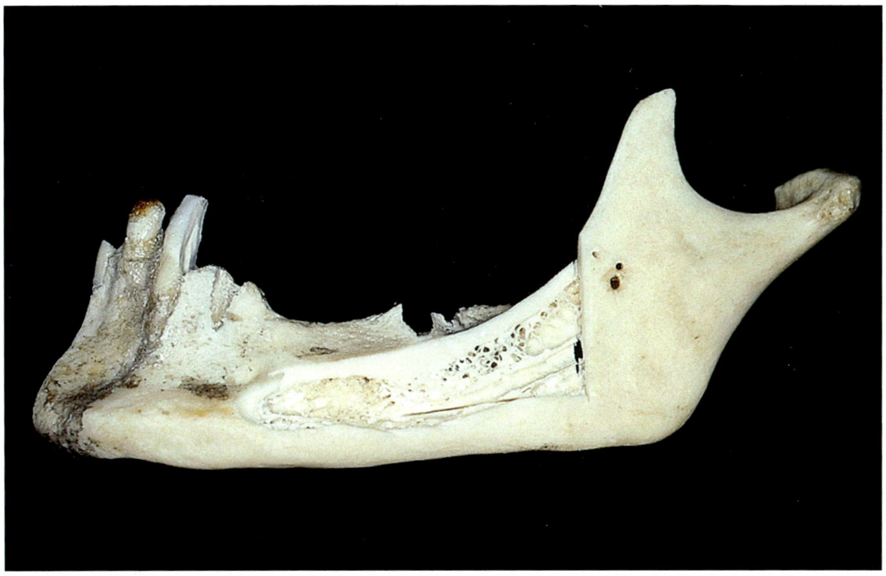

Fig 3-49 Severely resorbed mandible.

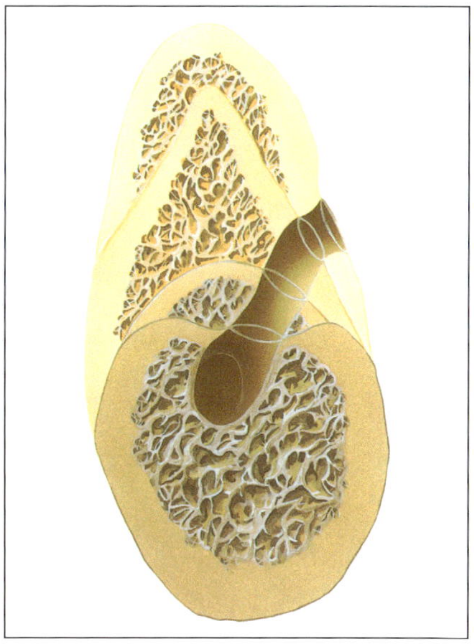

Fig 3-50 Progression of resorption at the mental foramen. (From Watzek. Reprinted with permission.)

In addition, a ruler was developed with both the full scale (1:1) and the scale of the panoramic radiograph (1:1.25) engraved in it (Fig 3-54). This lets the clinician take the last measurements (even during the surgical procedure) in a sterile environment.

On the panoramic radiograph, the mandibular canal and the mental foramen can usually be very clearly identified. The latter is always located underneath the buccal cusp of the second premolar in the mandible, straight down in a perpendicular line. Thus the height and width of the implant bed are defined. How can the dentist acquire the profile? The sharpened periodontal probe can be used (as described earlier) to measure the mucosal thickness of the edentulous part of the jaw. This method, however, is of limited use because the anatomic situation of the floor of the mouth and the vestibule do not permit a more extensive diagnosis (Figs 3-55 and 3-56).

With modern panoramic units it is now possible not only to take panoramic radiographs but also to create tomograms of the profile. These tomograms (Figs 3-57 and 3-58) usually have a magnification factor of 1:1.4 (Scanora 1:1.17). Their previously rather poor quality has improved considerably in the meantime and still continues to develop (Figs 3-59a and 3-59b).

It is essential to always have a clear idea about the anatomy of the mandible in all dimensions. It is vital for the dentist to have another close look at a prepared model of a skull in these cases. The inferior alveolar nerve enters lingually via the foramen in the ascending mandibular branch, diagonally follows the mandible

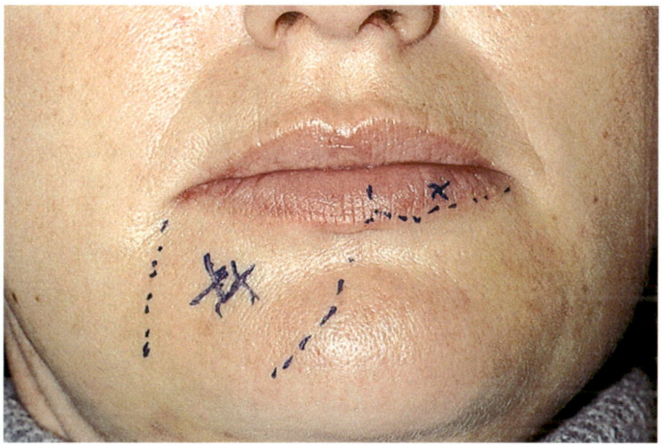

Fig 3-51 Paresthetic regions of the mandible after injury of the inferior alveolar nerve.

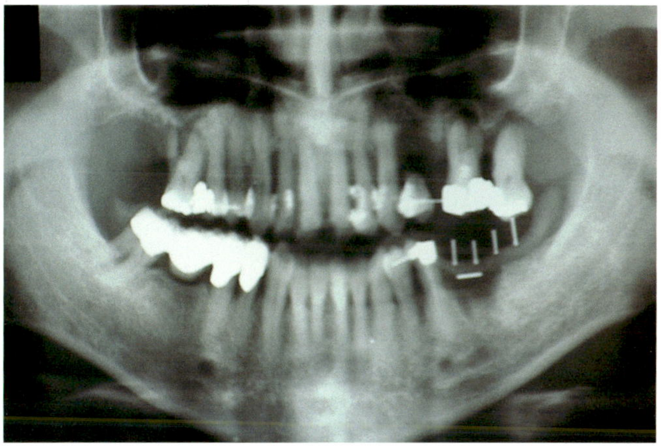

Fig 3-52 Panoramic radiograph with measuring pins.

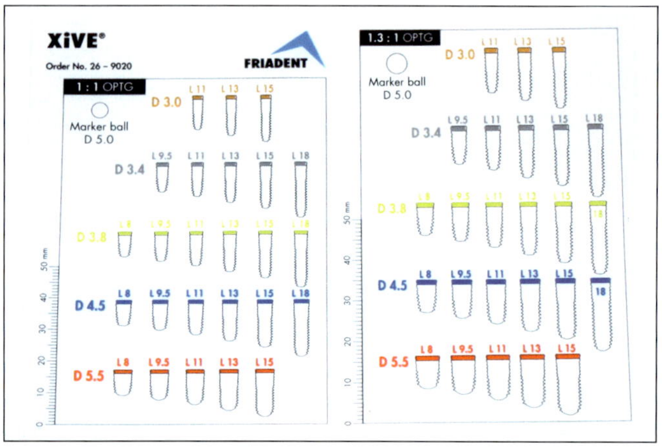

Fig 3-53a Transparent templates.

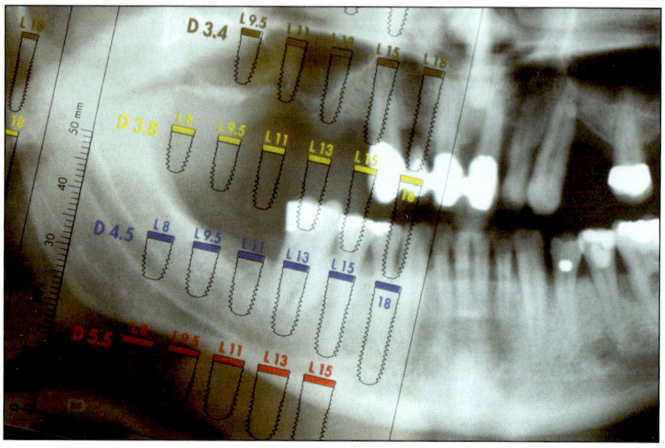

Fig 3-53b Transparent template on the panoramic radiograph.

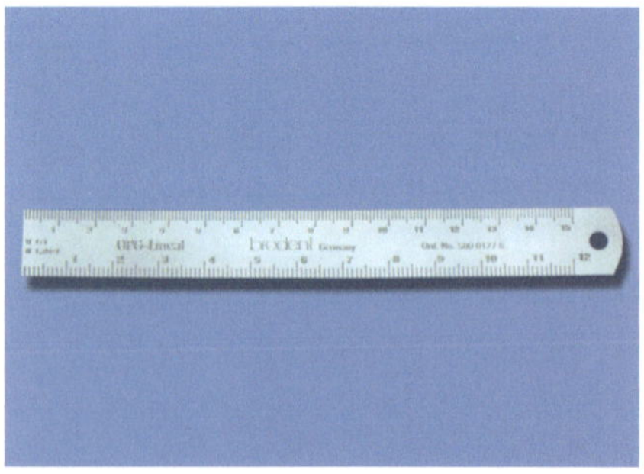

Fig 3-54 Ruler with scales of 1:1 and 1:1.25.

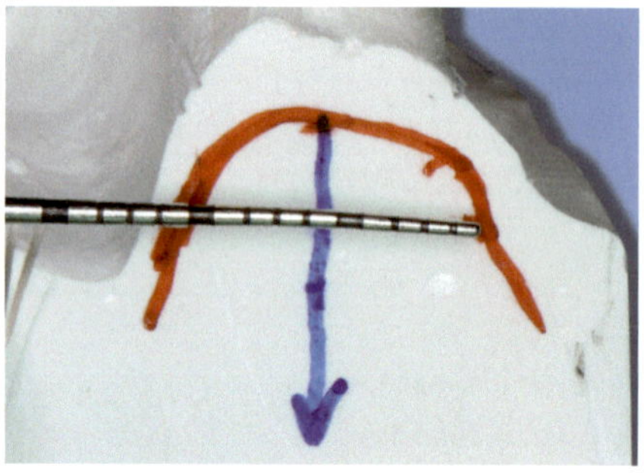

Fig 3-55 Mucosal thickness marked on the cast in the posterior region of the mandible.

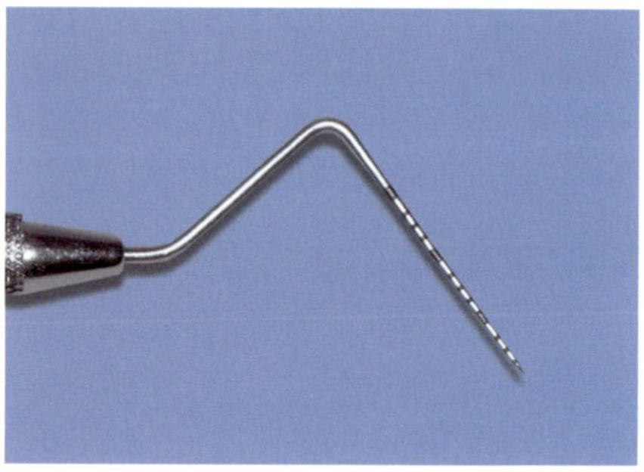

Fig 3-56 Sharpened periodontal probe.

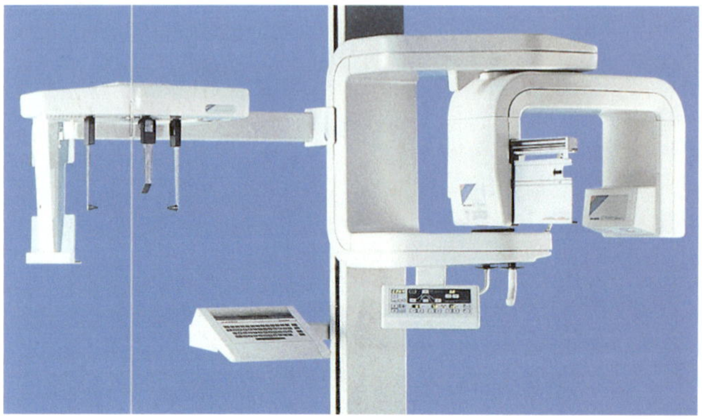

Fig 3-57a Modern panoramic x-ray unit.

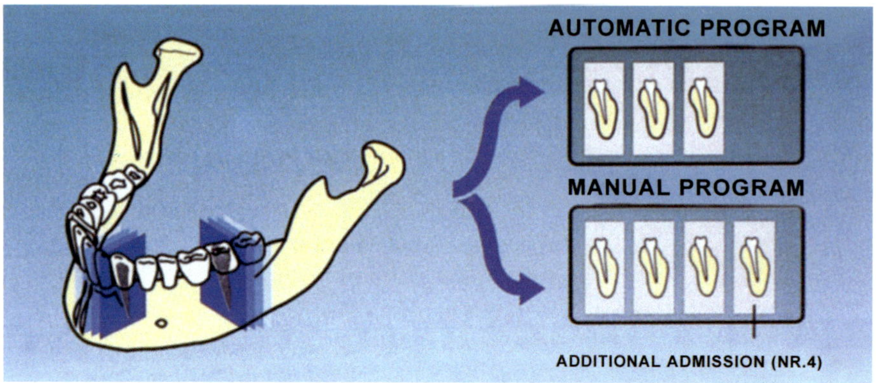

Fig 3-57b Transverse sections in the anterior and posterior region.

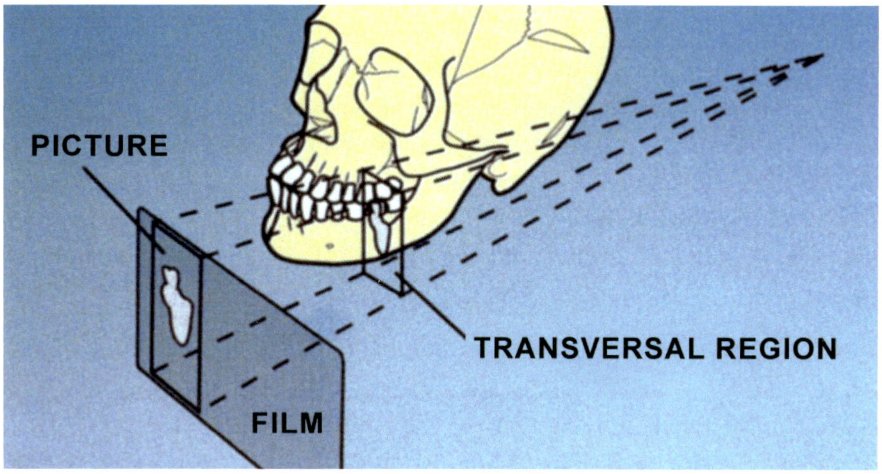

Fig 3-57c Tomography from the posterior region of the mandible.

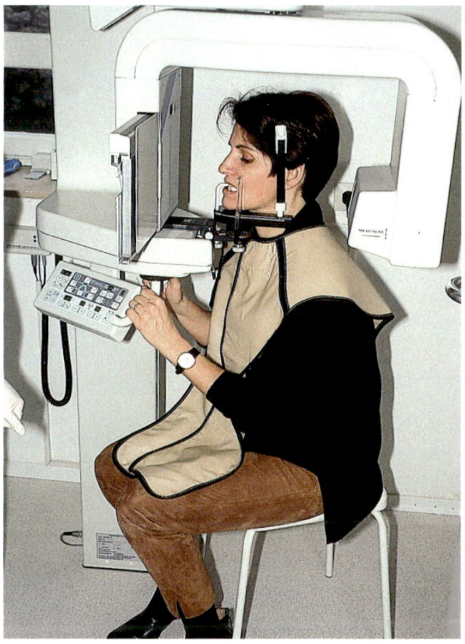

Fig 3-57d *(left)* Patient sitting in the unit during the x-ray.

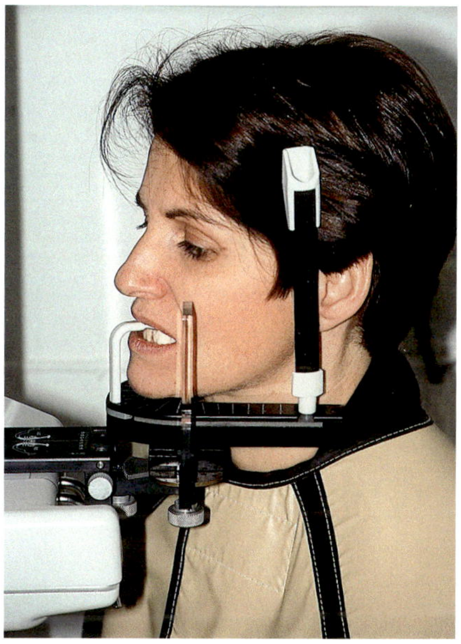

Fig 3-57e *(right)* Adjustment of the light visor.

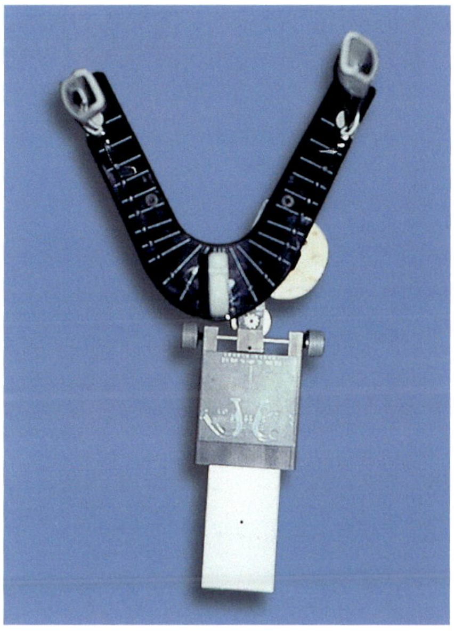

Fig 3-57f *(left)* Chin rest with scale for cross sections.

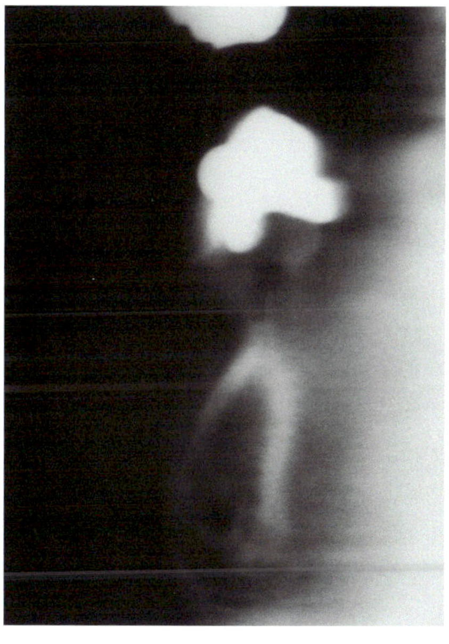

Fig 3-58a *(right)* Tomogram of the region of the mandibular right second premolar (mental foramen).

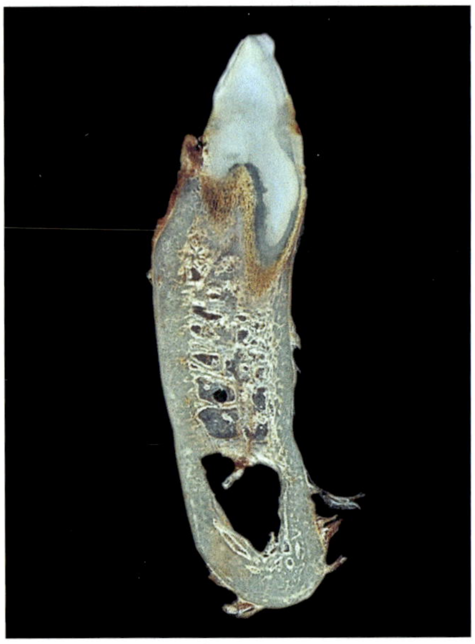

Fig 3-58b Anatomic crosssection of the same region. (From the archives of Dr Benner, Munich, Germany.)

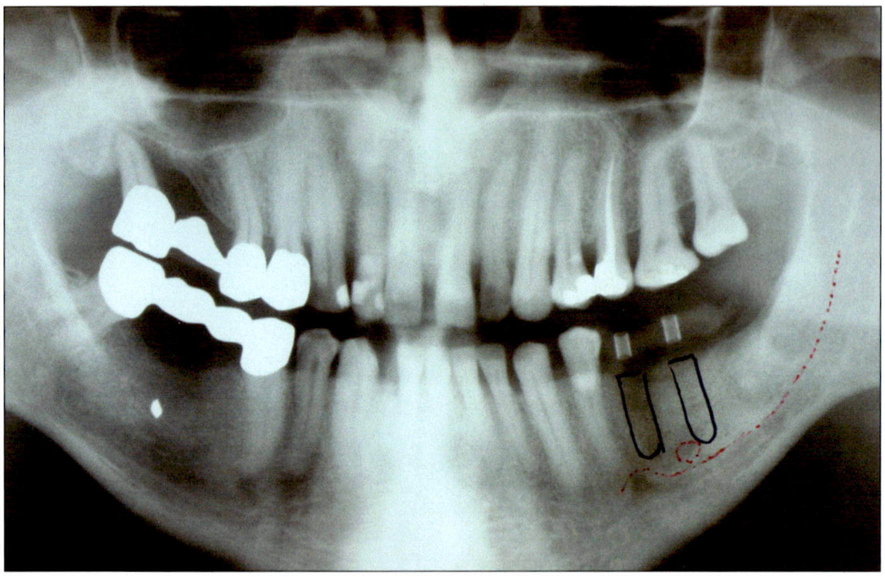

Fig 3-59a Panoramic radiograph with planned implants.

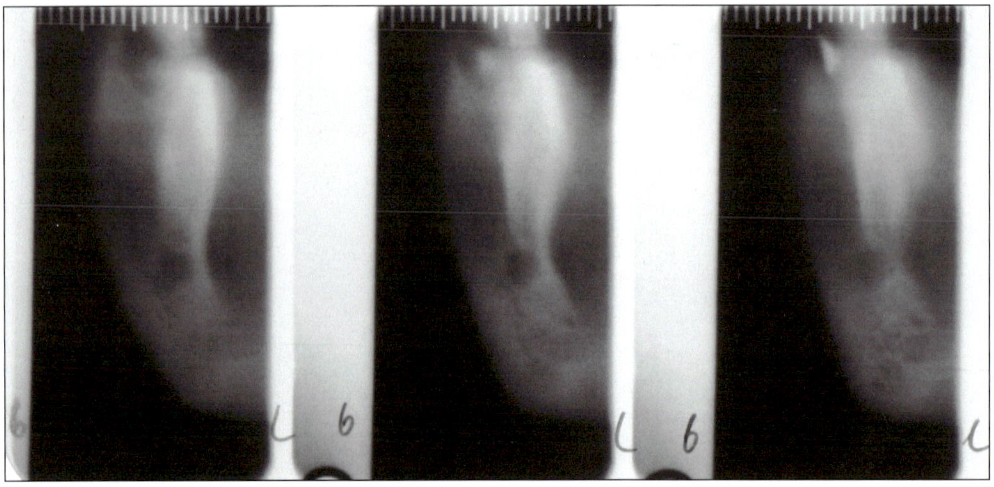

Fig 3-59b Tomography of the implant region. *(left)* Distal; *(center)* middle; *(right)* mesial.

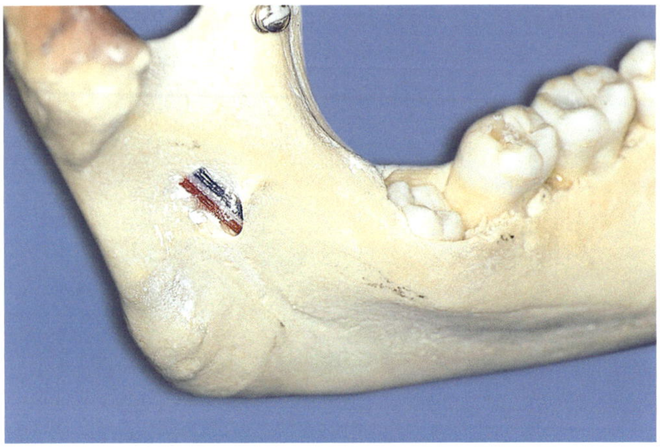

Fig 3-60 Mandibular foramen in the ascending branch.

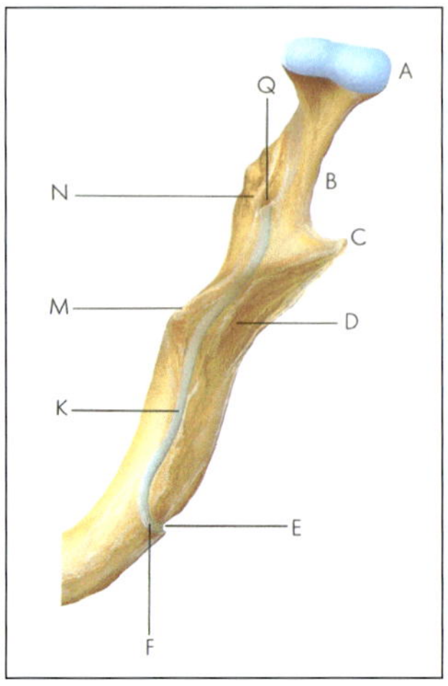

Fig 3-61 Diagonal path of the mandibular canal (inferior alveolar nerve). (From Watzek. Reprinted with permission.)

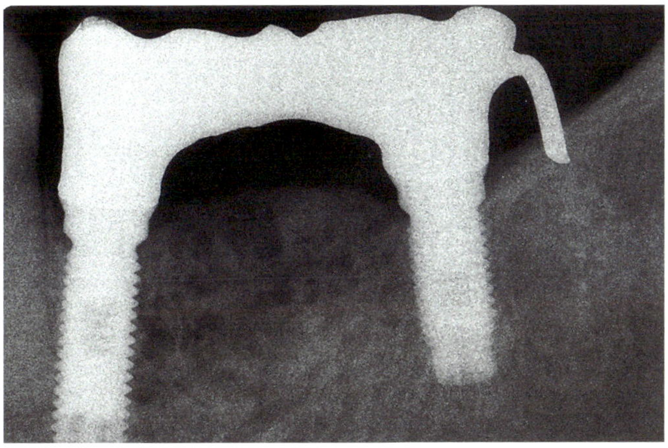

Fig 3-62a Implants in the region of the mandibular left first and second molars (framework try-in).

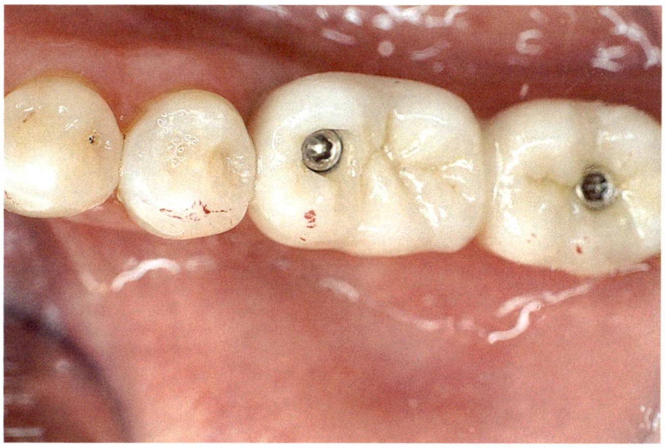

Fig 3-62b Implant-supported restorations in the molar region.

mesially, and leaves it at the mental foramen in the vestibule (Figs 3-60 and 3-61).

The bone quality to be expected here is D2, though hollow spaces must be reckoned with in elderly patients if they have been edentulous for a longer period. If in doubt, a CT should be obtained. Most patients, however, can be treated adequately with the diagnostic means suggested previously (Fig 3-62a and 3-62b). The following recommendations apply to the surgical procedure:

1. The surgeon should always use drills with a depth-limiting feature to prepare the implant channel.
2. Instead of nerve block anesthesia, infiltration anesthesia should be used in the surgical field, and the bone should be made more permeable with a substance containing hyaluronidase (Fig 3-63). In this way, the patient will only be able to feel the drilling when it has come within approximately 2 mm of the mandibular canal. This provides additional piece of mind to the surgeon.

Indication: Implants for the anterior and posterior regions of the maxilla

In edentulous segments of the maxilla, dentists very often find very unpleasant surprises. A seemingly compact maxilla often gives the impression of optimum conditions for insertion of an implant because of its thick and strong connective tissue (Fig 3-64a). Once the surgeon has reflected the flap, however, he or she may find razor-sharp alveolar ridges with irregular spots of resorption. In such a situation, implantation becomes extremely difficult (Fig 3-64b).

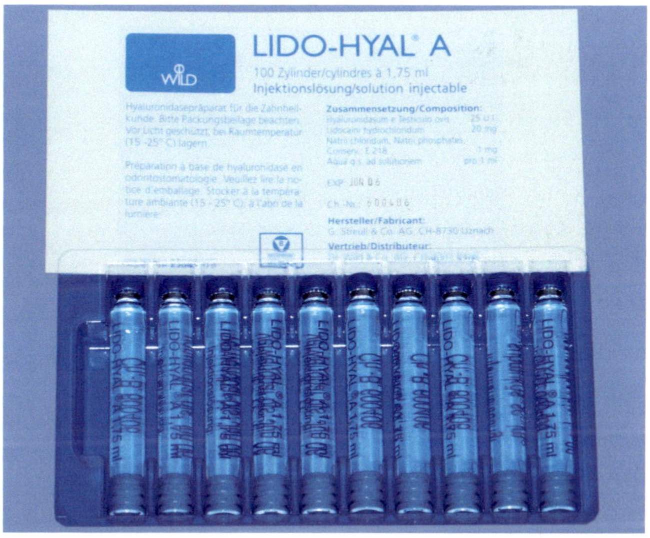

Fig 3-63 Lido-Hyal A, the hyaluronidase preparation to enhance permeability of the bone.

How can dentists acquire the relevant parameters for height, width, profile, and bone quality? Because resorption in the maxilla is irregular and often involves strongly collapsed areas, use of computed tomography is absolutely essential, because it is the only way to accurately plan an implantation. The dental industry offers various planning tools, including the Simplant software, which is currently very popular.

Radiologists with the appropriate equipment and training offer CTs at flat rates that follow previously determined criteria. The images are then sent via a Digital Imaging and Communications in Medicine (DICOM) interface to a processing center, and then they are sent back to the office, where they can be assessed with the appropriate software (Figs 3-65a to 3-65f). This proce-

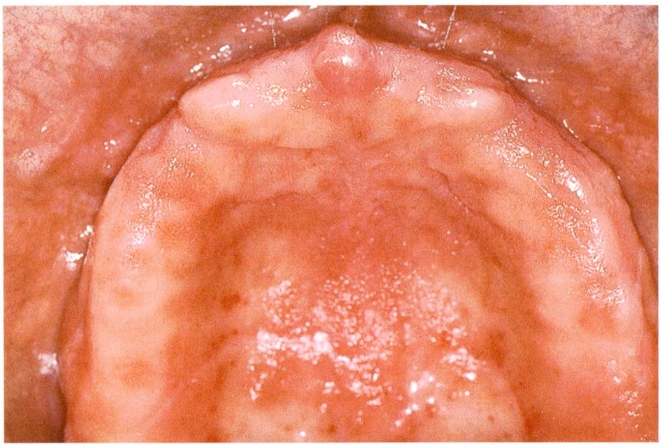

Fig 3-64a Edentulous maxilla with marked alveolar ridges.

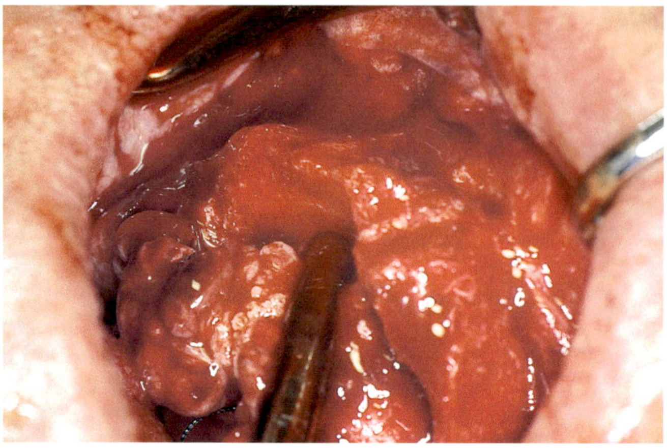

Fig 3-64b Edentulous maxilla after reflection. Resorbed alveolar ridges with sharp edges make implantation difficult.

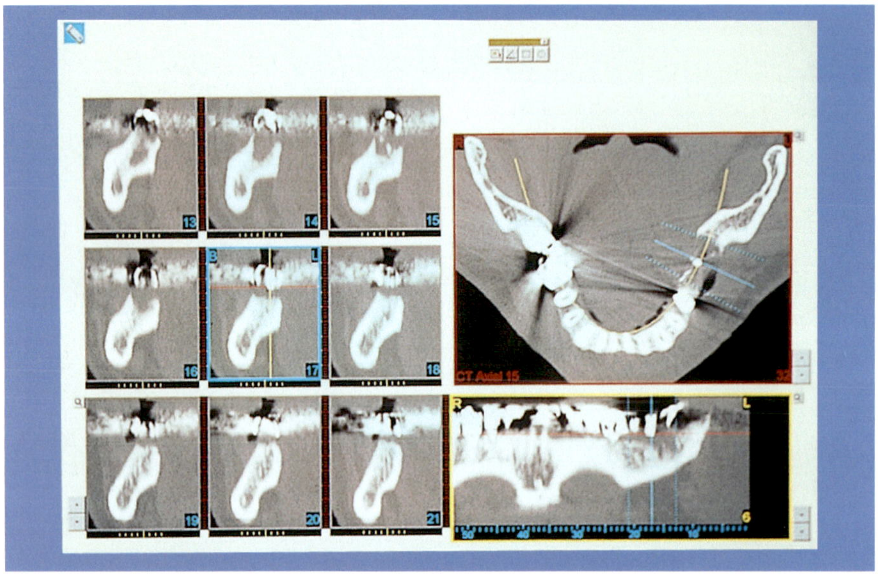

Fig 3-65a Simplant system: CT analysis in three dimensions.

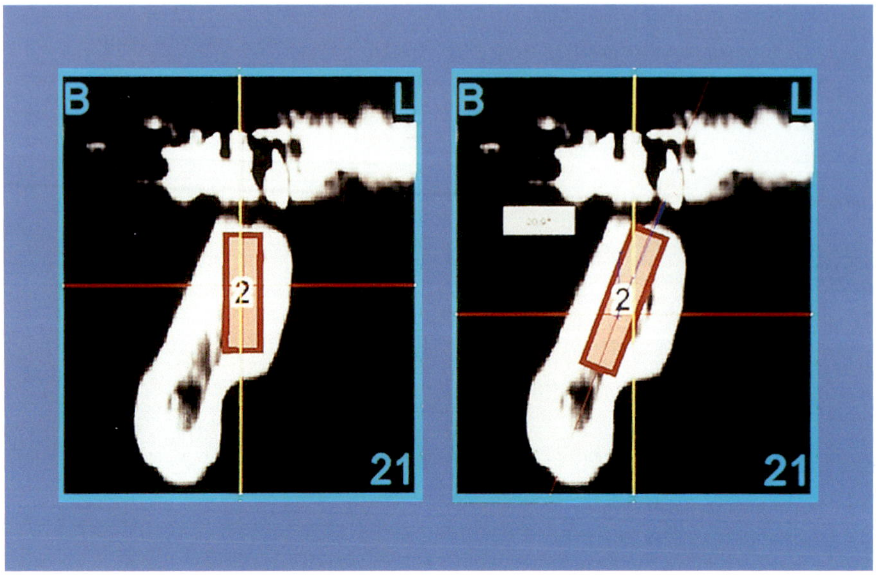

Fig 3-65b Determining the implant position at the office computer with the Simplant system. B = buccal; L = labial.

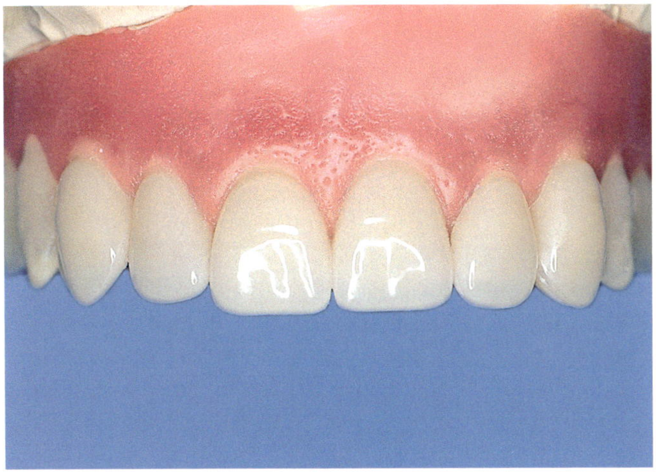

Fig 3-65c Esthetic prosthetic planning.

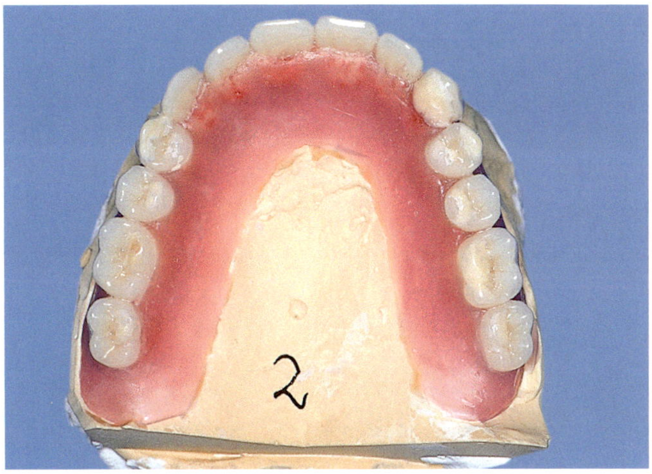

Fig 3-65d Functional prosthetic planning.

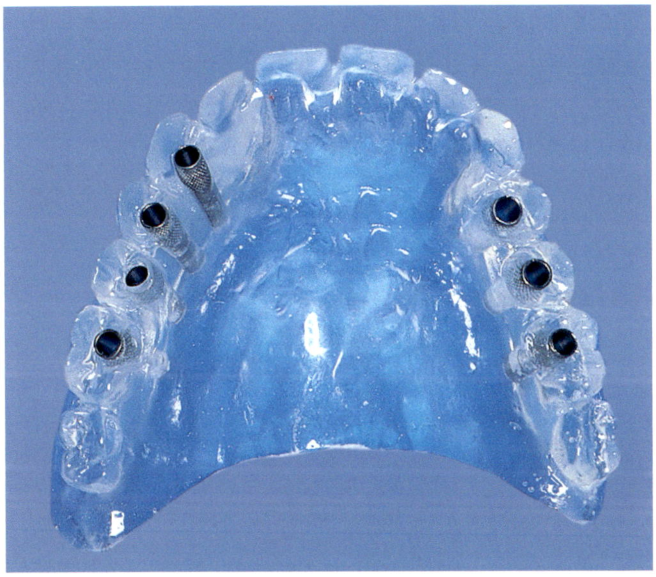

Fig 3-65e The implant position is determined with drilling guides in conjunction with prosthetic planning.

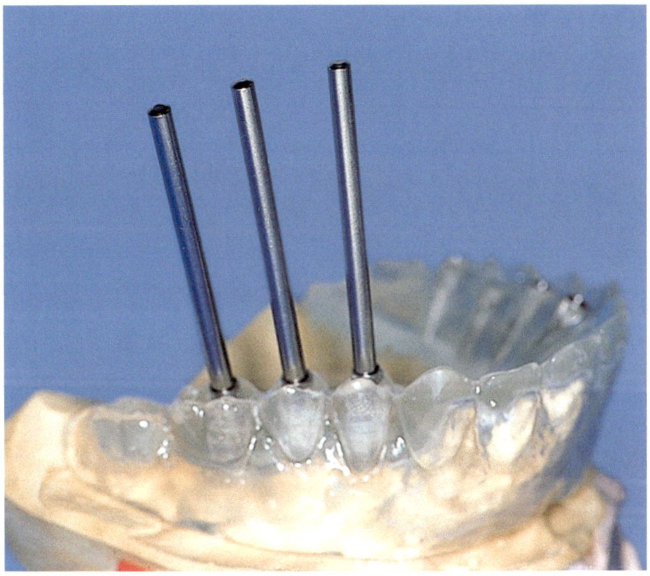

Fig 3-65f The drilling guides reveal the angulation of the implants.

dure is both expensive and time consuming, so it can be recommended only for dentists who frequently perform implant placement. For dentists who do not perform many implant placements, the author recommends asking a colleague who already has this system. The colleague can do the assessment and send the referring dentist a printout so that the implantation can be planned.

Today, a very vivid picture to help plan surgery can come from three-dimensional imaging of the surgical site. As these systems become more and more common, their prices will certainly drop, while the quality will undergo further improvement.

To summarize, more extensive implant procedures in the anterior and posterior regions of the maxilla should be planned in painstaking detail with CTs to eliminate the risk of unpleasant surprises during surgery. With CT technology, the dentist can predictably determine the height, width, profile and quality (density measurement according to Hounsfield) of the bone bed.

In the near future, a major step forward will take place with the new navigation systems, which are already being successfully tested. With any luck, they will soon be affordable for the average dentist's office (Fig 3-66a to 66c).

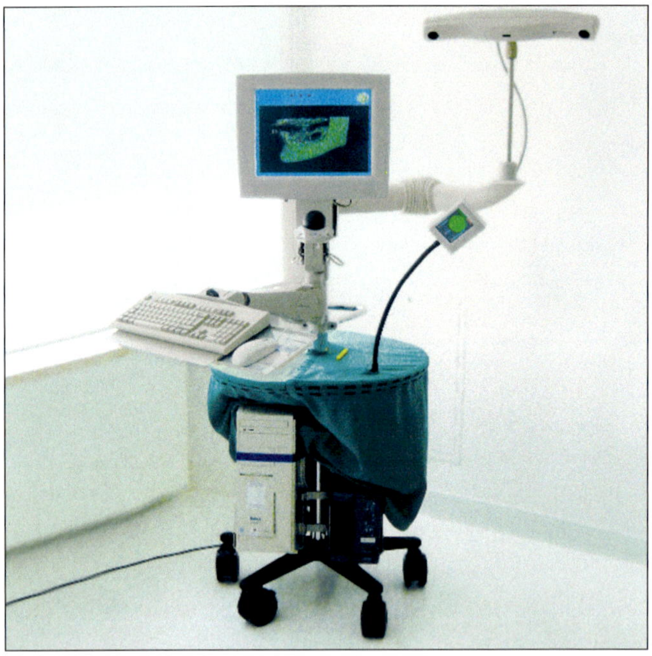

Fig 3-66a RoboDent navigation system. (From Kniha et al. Reprinted with permission.)

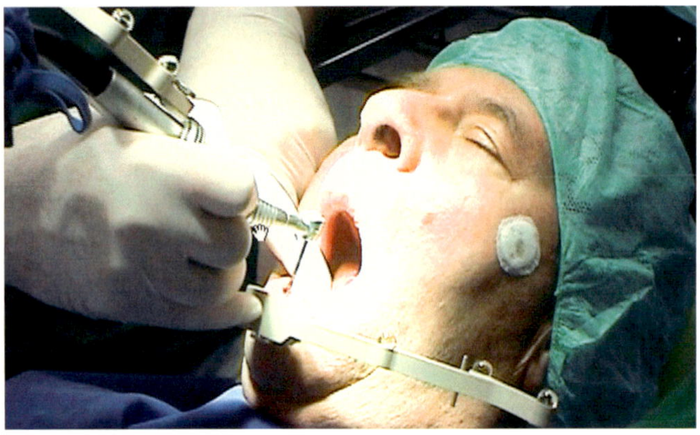

Fig 3-66b Implantation with the navigation system, shown on a three-dimensional model. (From Kniha et al. Reprinted with permission.)

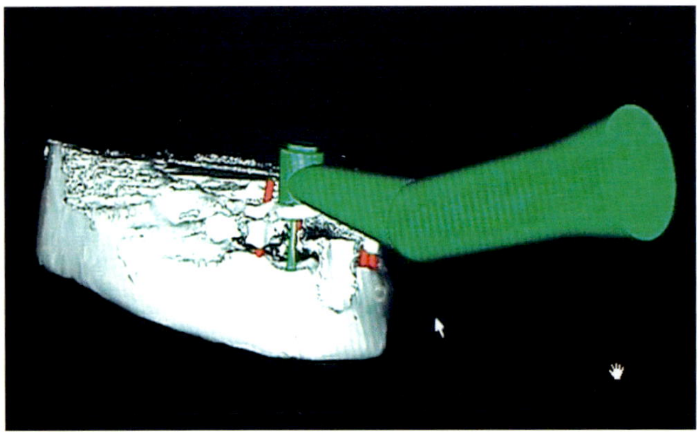

Fig 3-66c Implantation with the navigation system, shown on a patient. (From Kniha et al. Reprinted with permission.)

Materials

Brackets (Forestadent USA)
Single-tooth x-ray film (Eastman Kodak)
Panoramic x-ray film (Eastman Kodak)
Periodontal probe, sharpened (Hu-Friedy)
Implant systems used in this chapter: HATI (Thommen Medical); Brånemark (Nobel Biocare); Xive (Friadent)
High grade steel drilling jackets (building supply store)
Titanium surgical guides (Friadent; also available from other manufacturers)
Panoramic x-ray unit (Planmeca) with features for lateral cephalograms and tomography (www.trophy-digital.com)
Measuring instrument for panoramic radiographs (Bredent)
Scanora radiography system (Soredex)
Ultracain local anesthetic (Sanofi-Aventis)
Lido Hyal A hyaluronidase preparation (Wild)
Simplant computer tomography analysis (Materialise)
Navigation system (Robodent)
Anatomic model of the skull (available from medical supply stores)

4

Periodontics

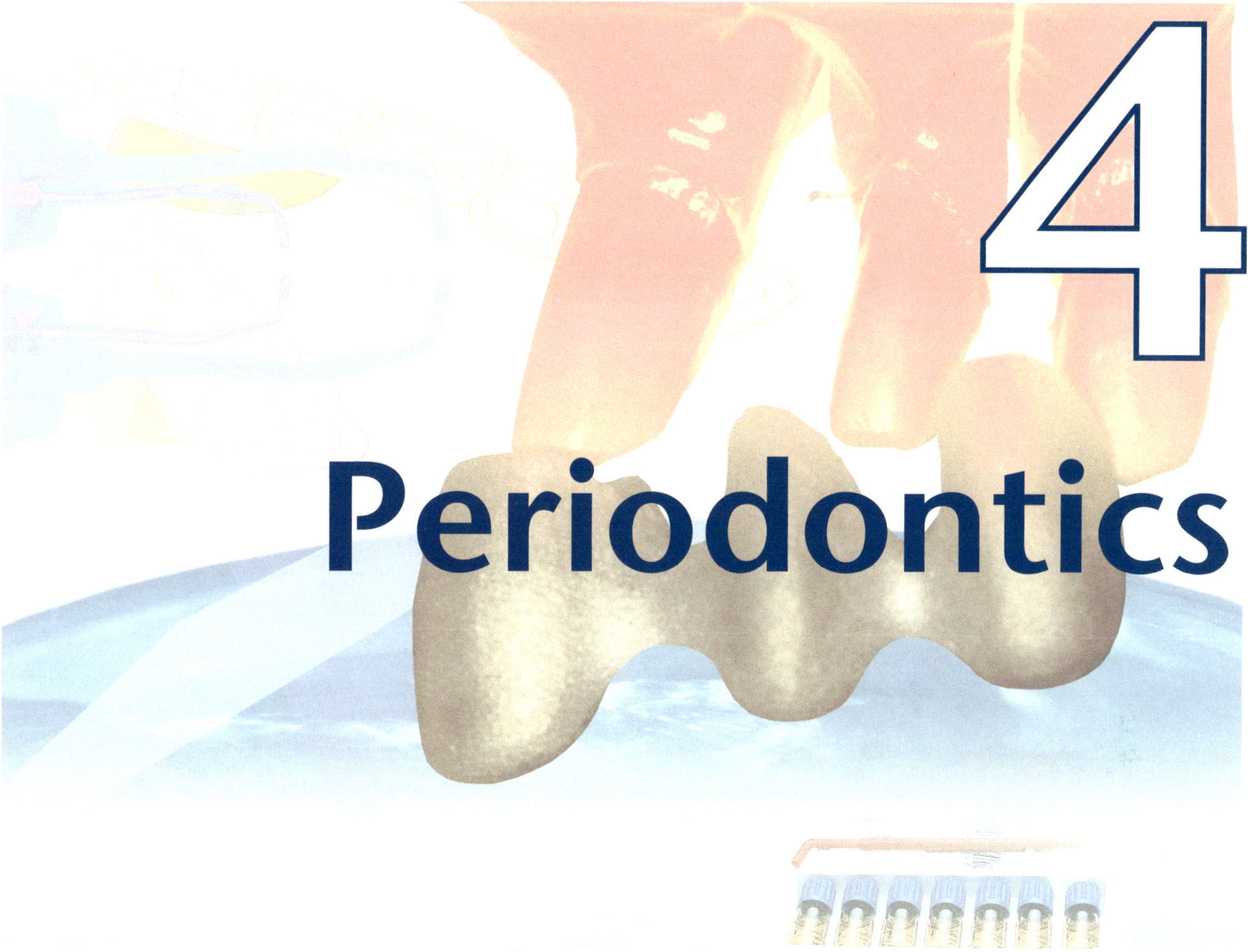

4

Interincisal Periodontal Splinting

Posterior Periodontal Splinting

Predictable Papillary Regeneration

Tooth Bed Versus Implant Site

Interincisal Periodontal Splinting

Common problem: Creation of functional and esthetic splints for mobile anterior teeth

Splinting periodontally involved teeth is an integral part of periodontal treatment today. If the resorption of the alveolar bone has already progressed to an advanced state, periodontal treatment has to begin with pretreatment measures (especially oral hygiene and a correlating decrease in inflammation) and splinting of the teeth with increased mobility (Figs 4-1a and 4-1b). Today it is known that simple improvement in oral hygiene and use of splinting can lead to success in treatment. There are two ways to create a splint:

1. Indirect splinting: Indirect splints are usually created by deep-drawing and are worn mainly at night. A disadvantage is that there is no guarantee that the mobile teeth will be splinted 24 hours a day.
2. Direct splinting: Direct splints are created with resin composite and adhesive bonding reinforced with wire, a metal or plastic net, or glass fibers. The advantage of this method is that the permanent splinting of mobile teeth leads to the desired treatment success.

During treatment, it is important to make sure that the planned fixed splint neither interferes with the patient's ability to perform oral hygiene nor negatively affects the patient with respect to pronunciation of words or creation of parafunctions. This goal can be achieved best with the help of an intradental splint with adhesive resin composite. This intradental and interincisal technique has proven very successful for splinting anterior teeth.

Proven solution: Fiber-reinforced resin composite splinting technique for mandibular anterior teeth

This technique can be used for anterior teeth with a mobility of degree 1 or higher and abraded incisal edges with exposed dentin.

First, the teeth are cleaned. A fine diamond is used to prepare 1- to 2-mm-deep grooves in the incisal edges of the teeth to be splinted (Figs 4-1c and 4-1d). Special care must be taken to avoid injury of the pulp. The height of the pulp chamber should be determined first on a radiograph.

The site that will receive the splint is etched, rinsed, and carefully dried (Figs 4-1e and 4-1f).

The silanized and bonded glass fiber bundle is removed from the blister pack, thinned out with a scalpel, and cut to the desired length. In general, these glass fibers are extremely hard to cut. If they are stretched first, they can be cut easily (Figs 4-1g to 4-1i). The trimmed glass fiber bundle should be kept out of the light as much as possible, because it will otherwise start to cure. It should be kept on a light-protected mixing slab (Figs 4-1j and 4-1k).

The advantage of the glass fibers used in this technique is that they form a firm chemical bond with the resin composite through silanization and bonding; thus, they can be polished very easily. In addition, no individual fibers are sticking out and poking the patient.

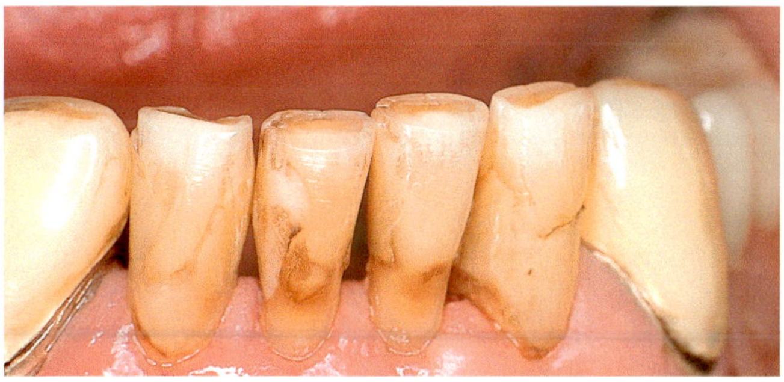

Fig 4-1a Mobile mandibular anterior teeth.

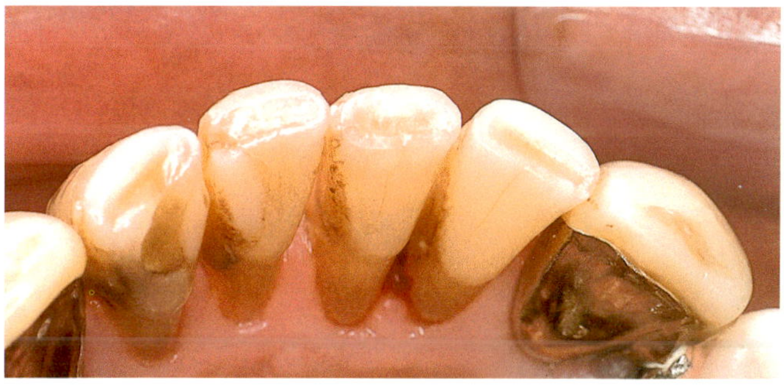

Fig 4-1b Incisal edges with exposed dentin.

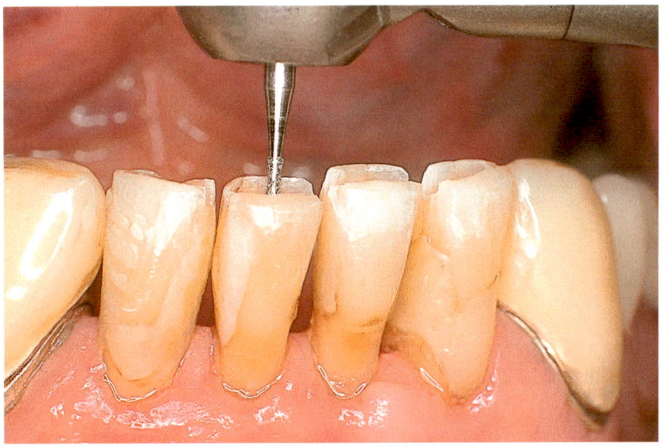
Fig 4-1c The incisal groove is prepared.

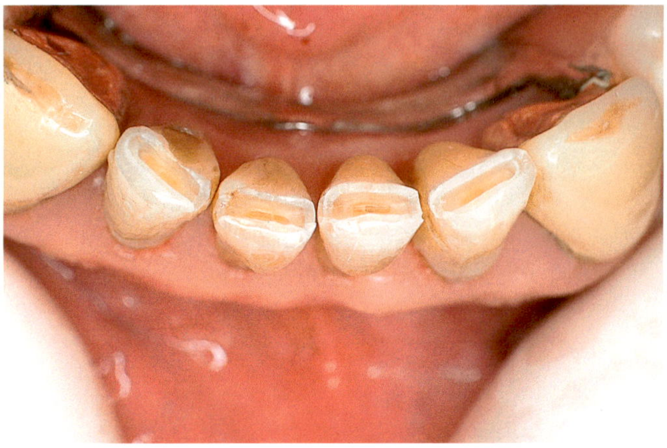
Fig 4-1d Incisal view of the preparation.

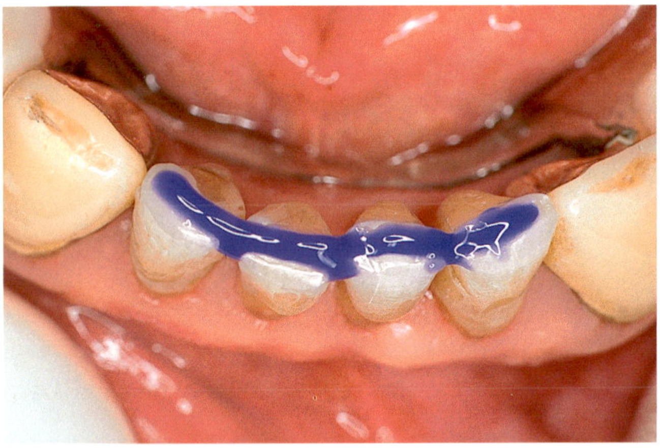
Fig 4-1e The cavity preparations for the splint are etched.

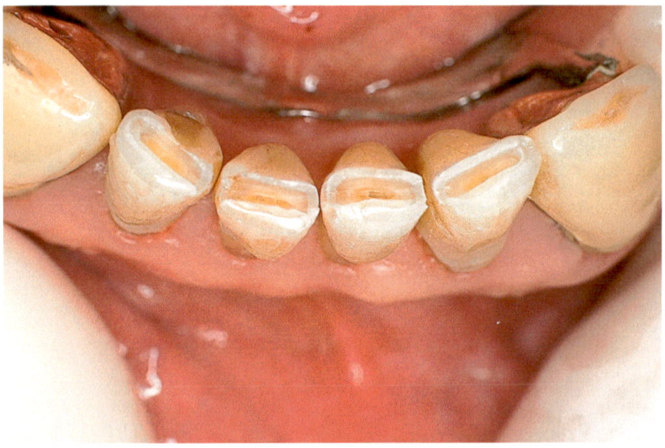
Fig 4-1f Appearance after rinsing and careful drying.

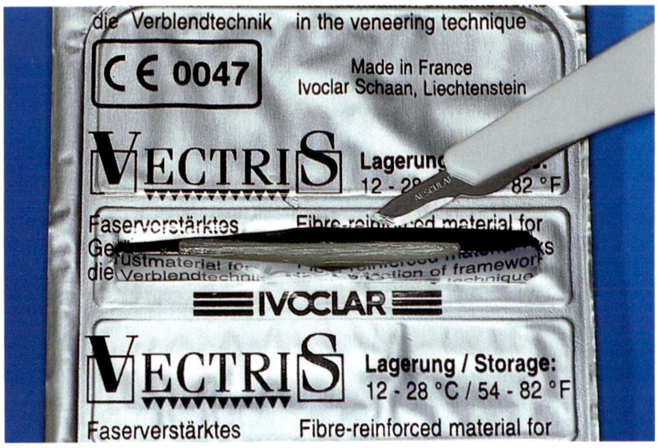

Fig 4-1g The blister pack with the glass fiber bundle is opened.

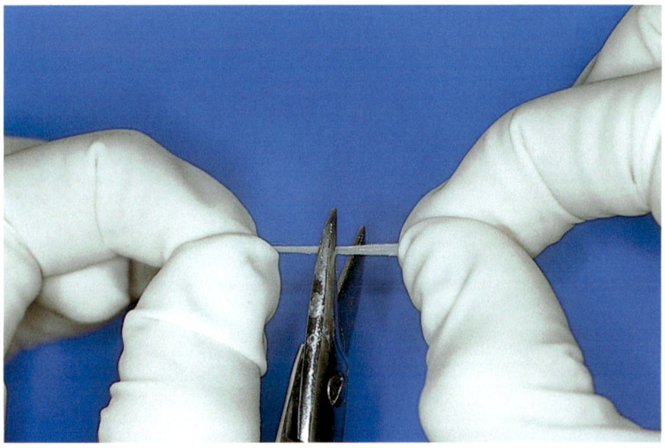
Fig 4-1h The thinned and stretched bundle is shortened with a pair of scissors.

Dentin adhesive is applied and cured (Fig 4-1l). The first layer of flowable resin composite is syringed into the groove (Fig 4-1m). The prepared glass fiber bundle is embedded in this still uncured layer of composite (Fig 4-1n). The incisal edge is shaped with a coat of resin composite and then light cured carefully (Figs 4-1o and 4-1p). Splinting is completed with a check of the occlusion and the appearance of the splint (Figs 4-1q and 4-1r).

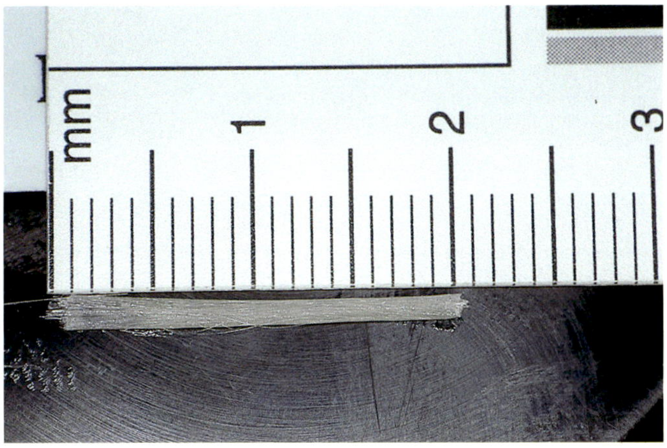

Fig 4-1i The length of the glass fibers is measured.

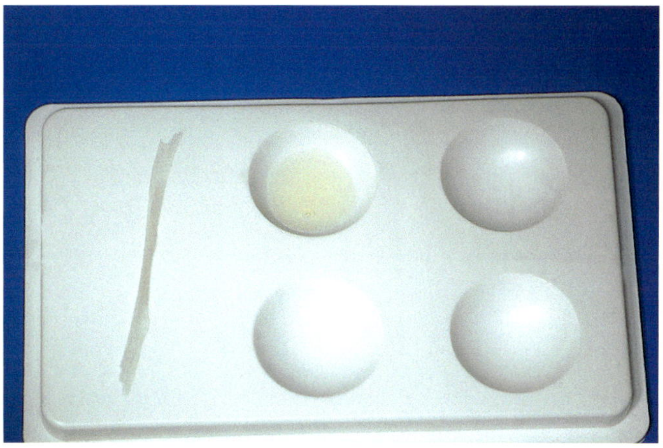

Fig 4-1j The fiber bundle is kept on a mixing slab.

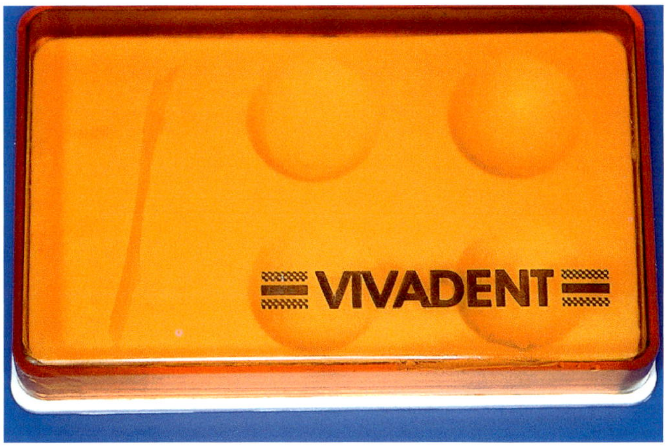

Fig 4-1k The fiber bundle is protected from light with a cover.

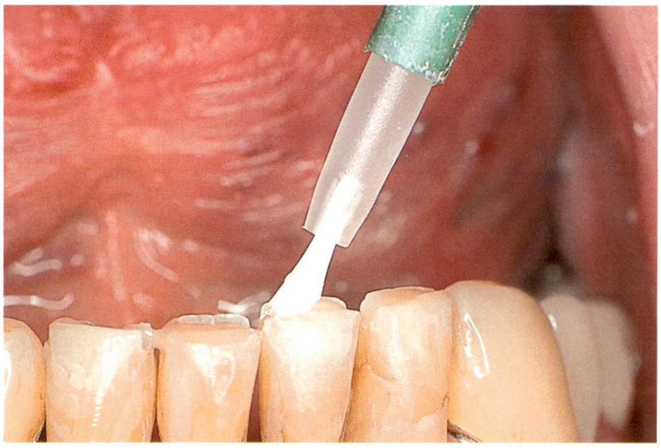

Fig 4-1l The dentin adhesive is applied.

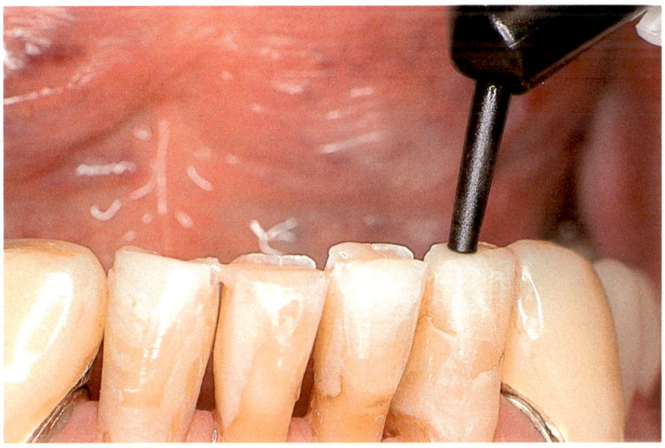

Fig 4-1m The first layer of the flowable resin composite is syringed into the groove.

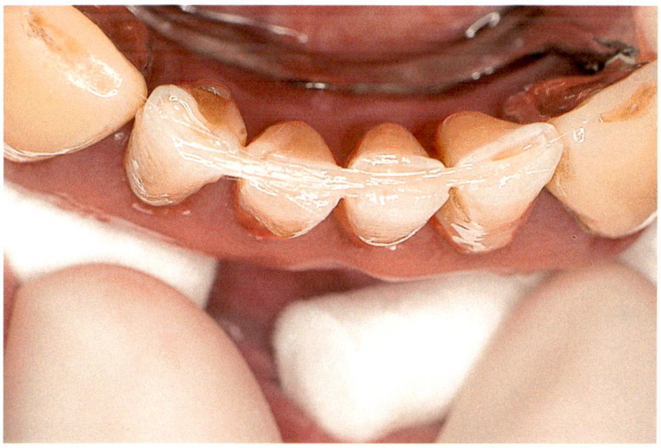

Fig 4-1n The fiber bundle is placed in the groove.

Covering the exposed incisal dentin also prevents the discoloration of the teeth from progressing. If the teeth are already severely discolored, bleaching can be considered (Fig 4-1s).

For further discussion of the principles of dental splinting, readers are referred to the relevant literature in periodontology textbooks and professional journals. For further details about the technique using fiber-rein-

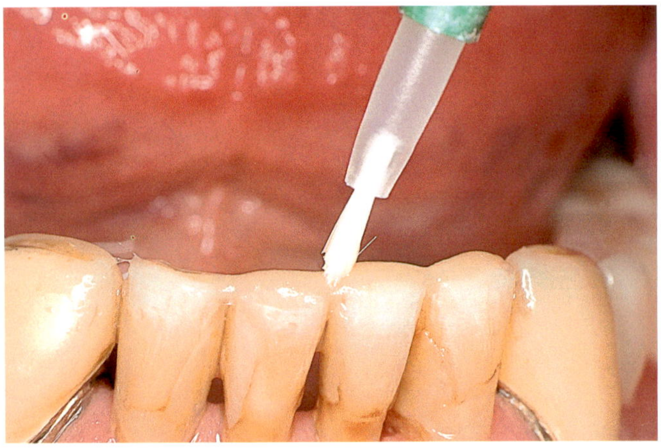

Fig 4-1o The covering layer is contoured.

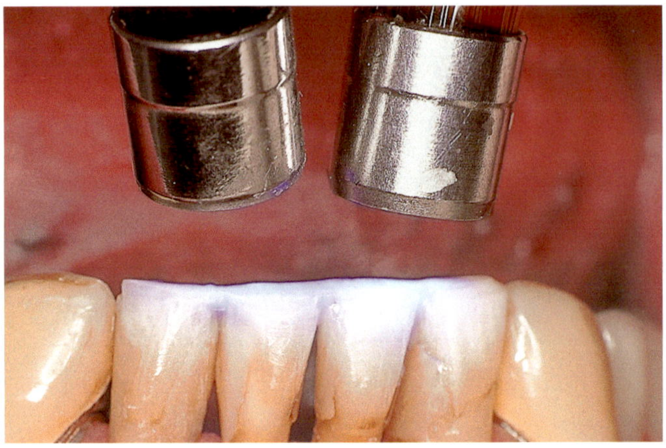

Fig 4-1p The restoration is carefully light cured with two light sources.

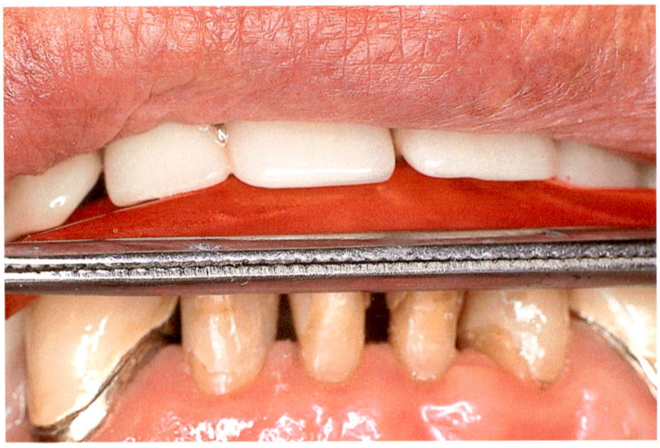

Fig 4-1q The occlusion is assessed.

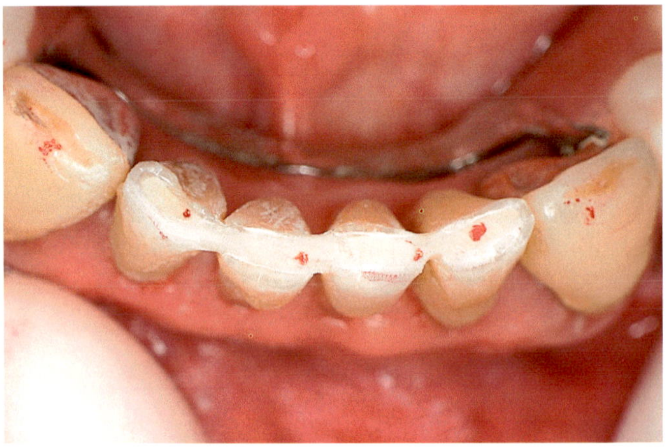

Fig 4-1r The occlusal stops are indicated in red.

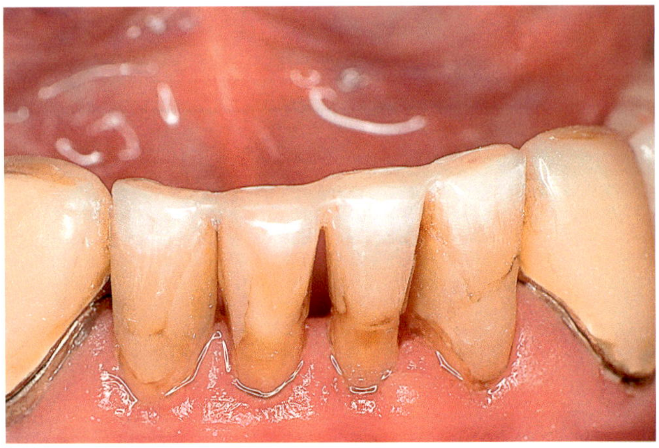

Fig 4-1s Final appearance of the anterior teeth with the interincisal splint.

forced resin composite materials, described in this section, readers are referred to the author's previously published book,[1] which also describes other techniques for periodontal splinting.

Materials

Ultra-Etch (Ultradent)
Excite dentin bonding agent (Ivoclar Vivadent)
Tetric Flow resin composite (Ivoclar Vivadent)
Everstick glass fiber system (Stickteck)

Posterior Periodontal Splinting

Common problem: Creation of functional and esthetic splints for mobile posterior teeth

Splinting of teeth with increased mobility plays an important role in the systematic treatment of periodontal disease. Especially in advanced cases of periodontitis, a basic rule is to splint first and treat later; otherwise, the periodontium of a mobile tooth cannot heal completely.

At one time, fibers and wires were the only means of creating intradental splints; they were fixed inside or on the teeth with adhesives. However, these fibers and wires did not bond to the resin composite (that is, did not form a chemical bond), which resulted in frequent breakage of these splints.

Because the glass fibers used in the procedure described in this section are already silanized and coated with a bonding agent, they offer new possibilities for periodontal splinting. The splints are stable, durable, easily accessible for oral hygiene, and esthetically inconspicuous. They therefore meet the basic requirements of periodontal splints.

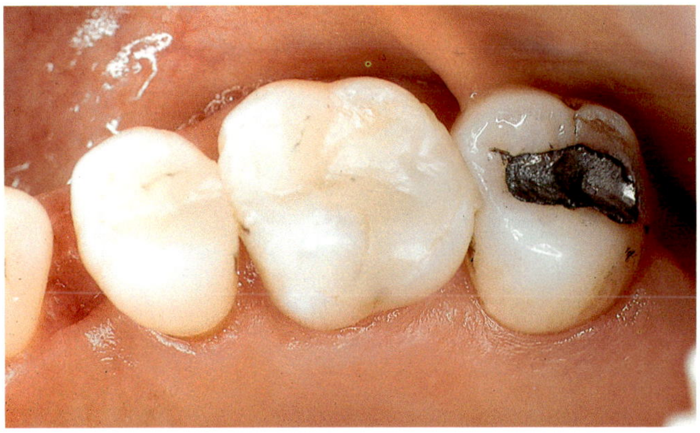

Fig 4-2a The periodontally compromised teeth are to be splinted.

Proven solution: Internal adhesive splinting of posterior teeth

Internal periodontal splinting, also referred to as *A-splinting*, comprises the following steps. First, occlusal grooves are ground into the interproximal areas of the posterior teeth to be splinted (Figs 4-2a and 4-2b). The length of the grooves is measured with a periodontal probe (Fig 4-2c) and the glass fibers are cut to the required length (Figs 4-2d and 4-2e). The glass fiber bundles must be protected from light once they have been cut, because polymerization is initiated with every exposure to light, including the operating light, sunlight, and the curing light (see Fig 4-1k).

The grooves are etched with phosphoric acid for 30 seconds, rinsed for 15 seconds, and dried carefully (Fig 4-2f). Wedjets are coated with petroleum jelly and inserted into the interproximal spaces to preserve their shape (Fig 4-2g). If there is exposed dentin, a dentin adhesive is applied.

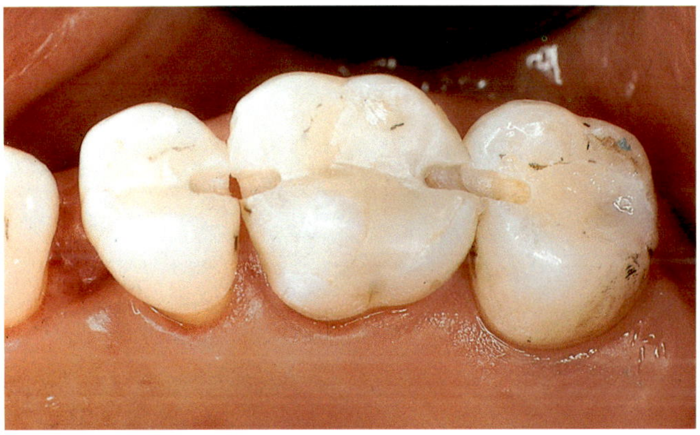

Fig 4-2b Occlusal grooves are ground into the proximal areas to receive the splint.

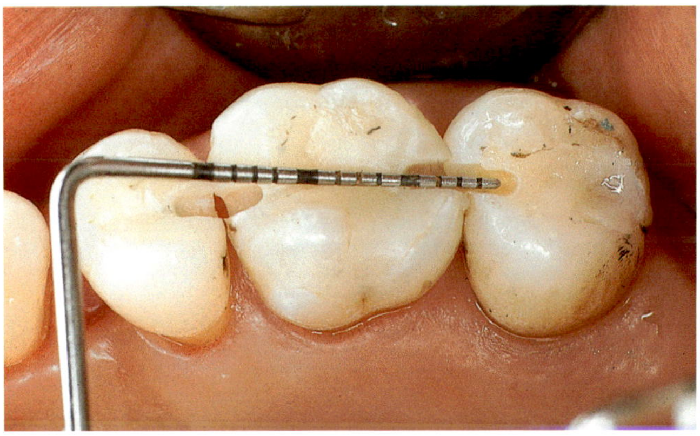

Fig 4-2c The required lengths of the fibers are measured with a periodontal probe.

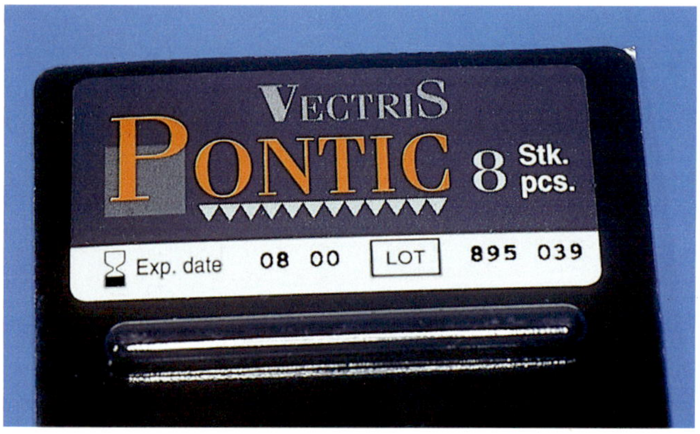

Fig 4-2d Glass fibers in their blister pack.

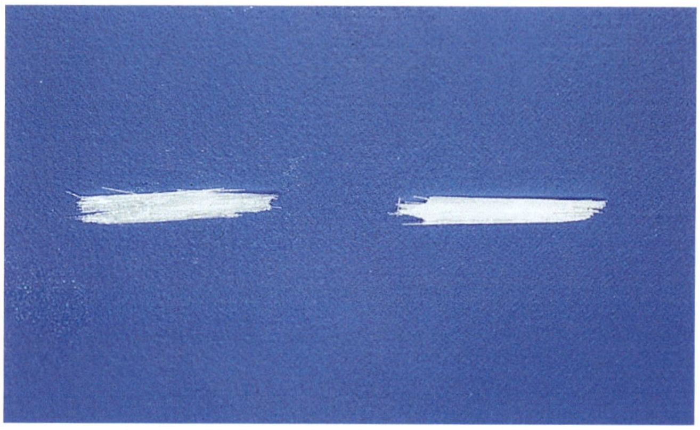

Fig 4-2e The cut glass fibers are ready for use.

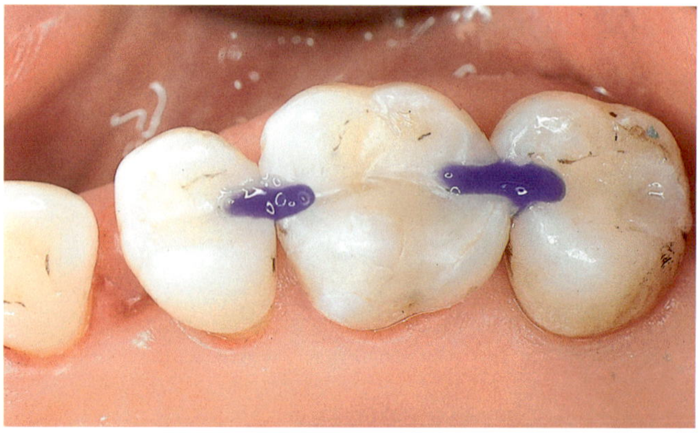

Fig 4-2f The retention cavities are etched with phosphoric acid for 30 seconds.

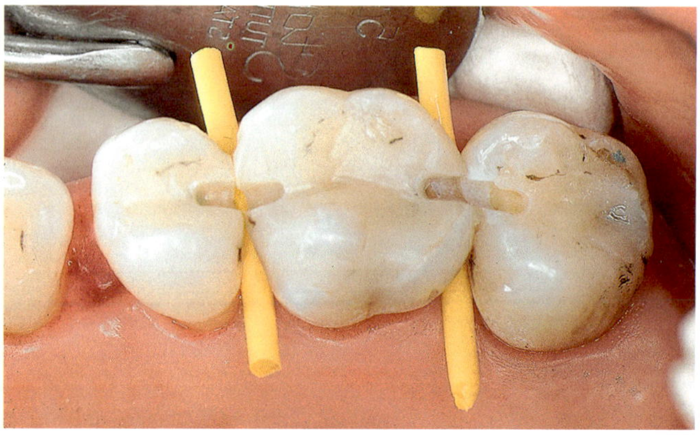

Fig 4-2g Wedjets are inserted to preserve the shape of the embrasure spaces.

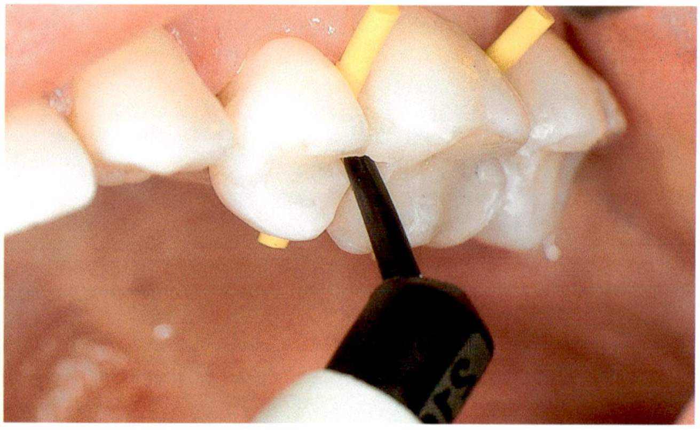

Fig 4-2h A base layer of flowable resin composite is applied, and interim curing is performed.

A base layer of flowable resin composite is applied, and interim curing is performed (Fig 4-2h). The prepared glass fiber bundles are laid in the etched cavities and positioned with a disposable brush (Fig 4-2i). The fibers are covered with a second layer of flowable resin composite and the etched cavities are completely filled (Fig 4-2j). The covering layer is contoured with the disposable brush (Fig 4-2k).

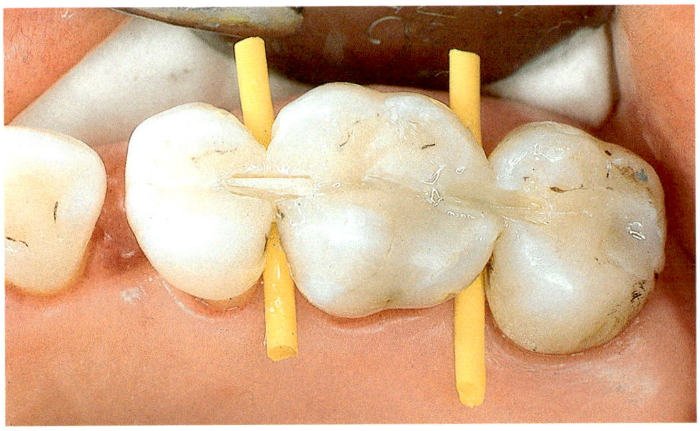

Fig 4-2i The fiber bundles are placed lengthwise in the cavities and subsequently adapted.

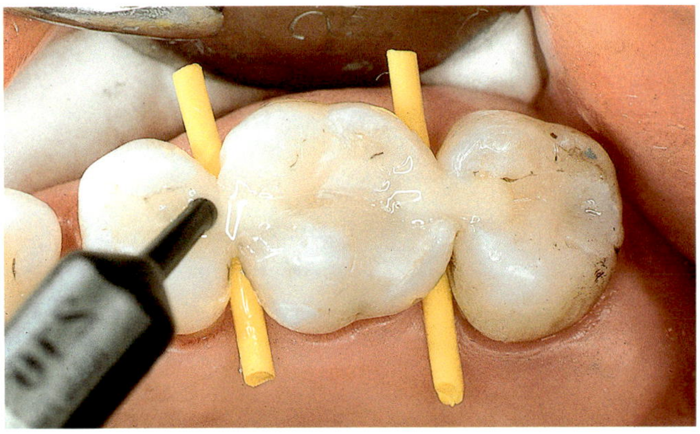

Fig 4-2j The fiber bundles are covered with resin composite.

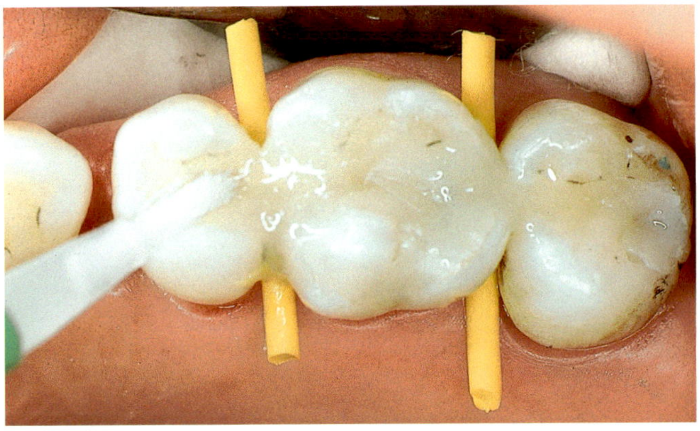

Fig 4-2k The covering layer is contoured with the disposable brush.

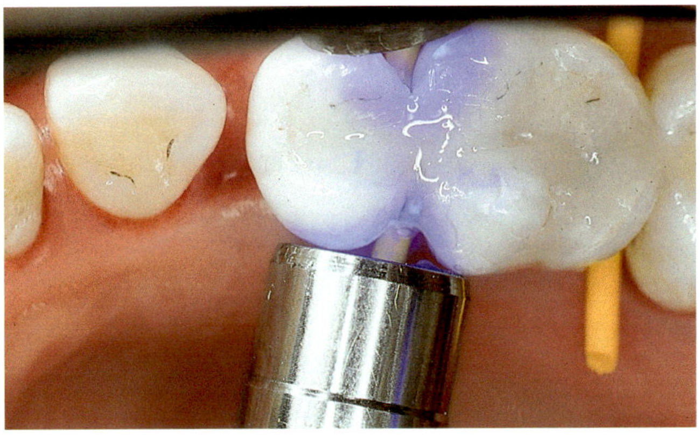

Fig 4-2l Careful final curing is carried out with two light sources.

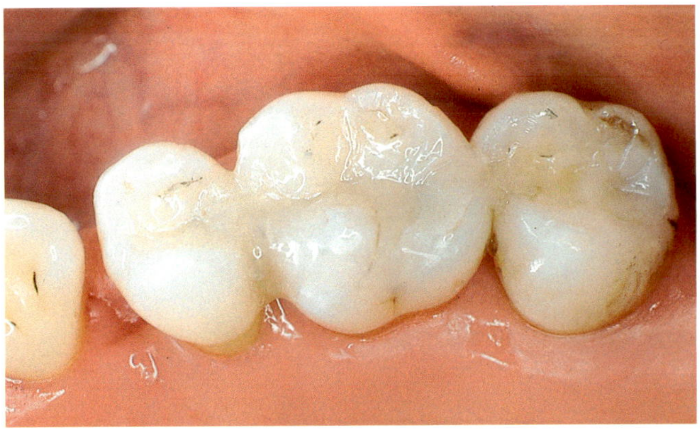

Fig 4-2m Finished splint.

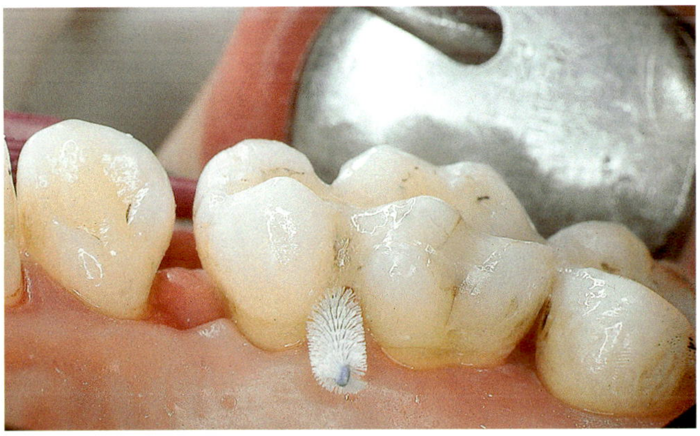

Fig 4-2n The embrasure spaces are examined to ensure that they can be cleaned with an interdental brush.

The splint is carefully cured with two curing lights from opposite sides; this process should begin laterally through the enamel (Fig 4-2l). The splint is finished and, if necessary, polished. The occlusion is checked, and the patient is shown how to clean the embrasure spaces. The patient should practice the use of an interdental brush in front of the dental team (Figs 4-2m and 4-2n).

If this splint breaks, which can at times occur with mobile teeth, it can easily be repaired with resin composite and glass fibers.

Materials

Tetric Flow (Ivoclar Vivadent)
Everstick glass fiber system (Sticktech)
Wedjets from a dispenser (Hygenic, Coltène Whaledent)

Predictable Papillary Regeneration

Common problem: Loss of the interdental papillae and appearance of "black triangles"

The loss of the interdental papillae, especially in the anterior region of the maxilla, is a serious esthetic problem. This is a source of great psychological distress for patients whose smiles reveal extensive gingiva.

The World Health Organization defines health as physical and mental well-being. Dentists therefore should make every possible effort to provide patients with an improved appearance through restorations of both the teeth (through fixed partial dentures, veneers, and resin composite restorations) and the gingiva (through appropriate soft tissue management). In other words, the aim is to reestablish the physical and emotional well being of patients through an esthetic optimization of both the tooth and the gingival portion of the restoration.

Is it really possible to reconstruct the missing interdental papillae in a predictable way? Can patients be relieved from the unattractive "black triangles" that plague them? The condition is widespread and is even referred to as *black triangle disease* (Figs 4-3a and 4-3b).

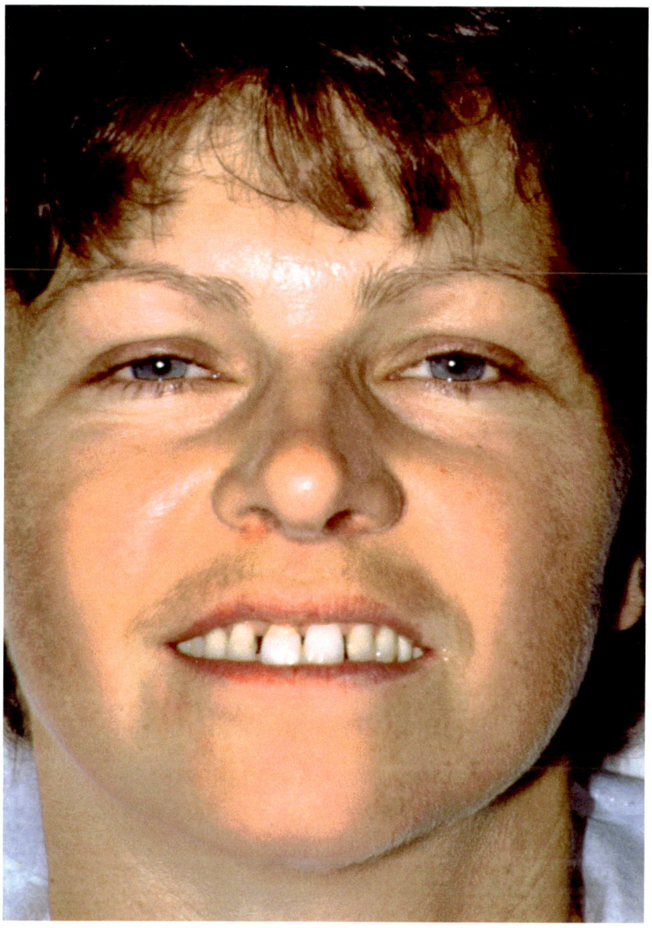

Fig 4-3a The unhappy patient shows a forced smile. Black triangles are visible interdentally.

Proven solution: Bone sounding–Measurement of the interdental biologic width

In 1961, Gargiulo et al[2] published their research about the biologic width and the relationships among the sulcus, the epithelial attachment, the connective tissue attachment, and the alveolar bone (Fig 4-3c). Further research revealed that a shortfall in the respective minimal distances inevitably leads to gingivitis and periodontitis, even when oral hygiene is optimal (Fig 4-3d). Furthermore, research by Tarnow et al[3] found precisely defined relationships between the interproximal contact points of the teeth and the alveolar bone (Fig 4-3e).

In the past, clinicians used to pay attention to the interproximal contacts only as far as esthetics and the prevention of food impaction were concerned, and anterior teeth were reconstructed accordingly (Figs 4-3f and 4-

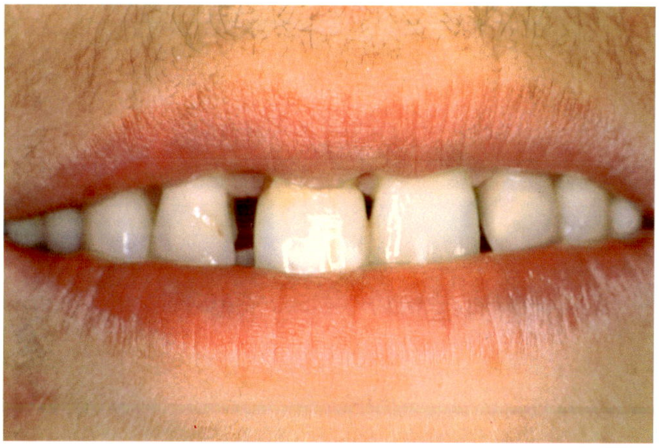

Fig 4-3b Patient's lip line.

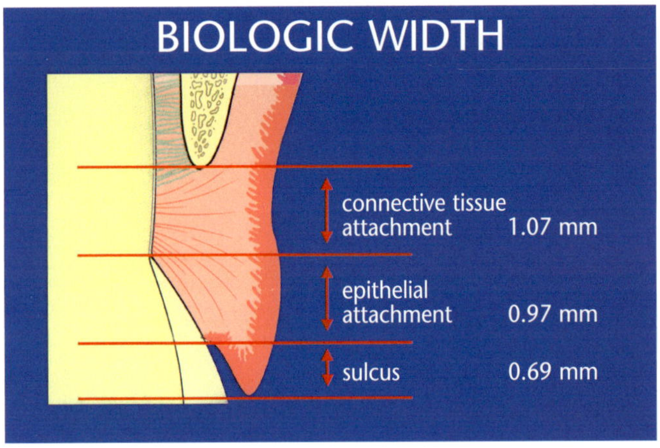

Fig 4-3c Biologic width. (From Gargiulo et al.[2] Reprinted with permission.)

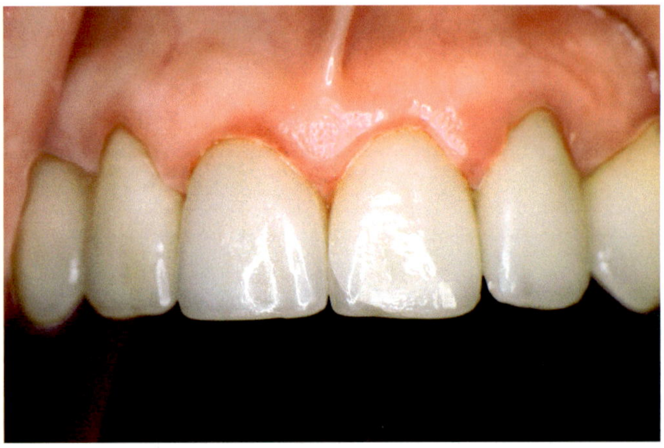

Fig 4-3d The biologic width was ignored. Chronic gingivitis ensued, despite excellent oral hygiene.

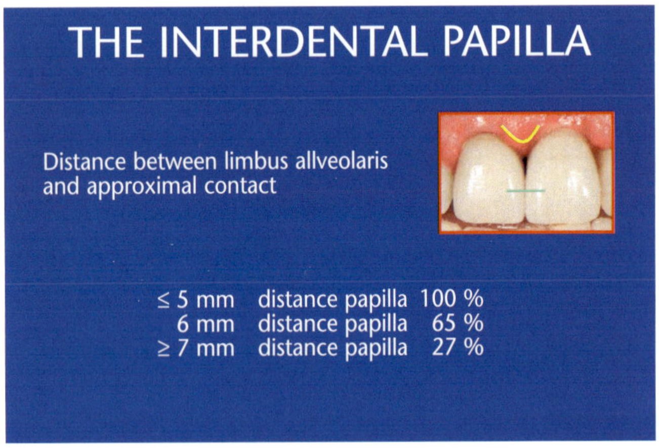

Fig 4-3e Relationships of the papilla, the contact point, and the alveolar bone, according to Tarnow et al.[3]

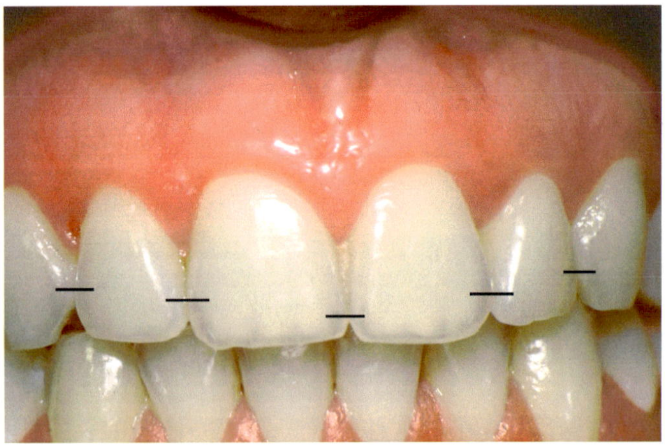

Fig 4-3f The interproximal contact points of the maxillary anterior teeth are rising symmetrically and esthetically.

3g). The distances between the contact point and the alveolar bone, as defined by Tarnow et al,[3] led to the creation of a contact area: The upper end of the contact area is defined by esthetic criteria, whereas the lower end is defined by the distance to the alveolar bone (Fig 4-3h).

How can this periodontal standard be respected when restorations are designed? How can the distances to the alveolar bone be determined? Kois[5] did just that in a publication about the dentogingival complex, which encompasses all tissues involved. He introduced the concept of "sounding to the osseous crest" to restorative dentistry.

With this concept, after local anesthesia is administered to the patient, the dentist sounds with a millimeter-calibrated probe until the upper ridge of the alveolar bone is reached (Figs 4-3i and 4-3j). The measured values are entered on a form (Fig 4-3k). These values now serve as a basis for the reconstruction, no matter who performs the procedures and how. The restoration may involve a dentist using an indirect technique with resin composite, an orthodontist who strips and lateralizes the teeth, or a dental technician who works with veneers or crowns (Figs 4-3l and 4-3m).

When these relationships within the dentogingival complex are clearly defined, they provide the key to predictable, successful regeneration of the interdental papillae (Fig 4-3n).

The aforementioned criteria were followed for the patient presented in this section, and a good result is achieved (Fig 4-3o).

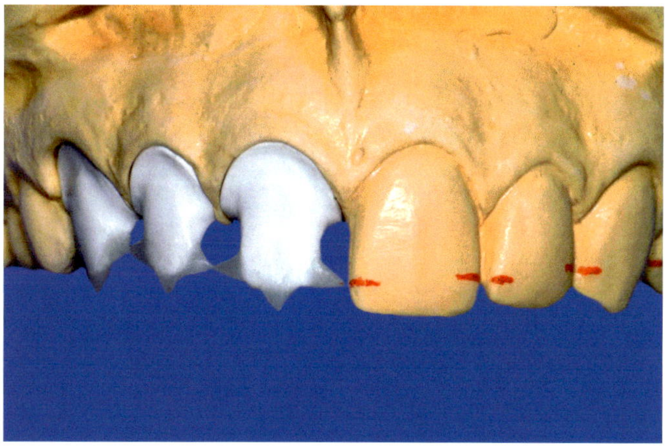

Fig 4-3g Concept for waxing up the maxillary anterior teeth, as defined by Kubein-Meesenberg et al.[4] The contact points are defined with proximal cones.

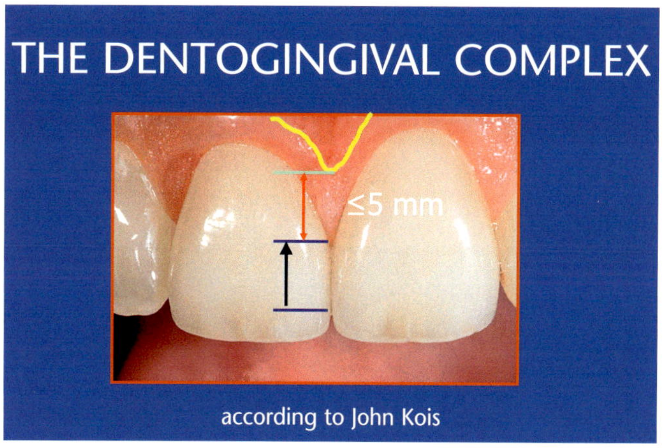

Fig 4-3h Relationships between interproximal contact points and the alveolar bone, as presented by Tarnow et al.[3]

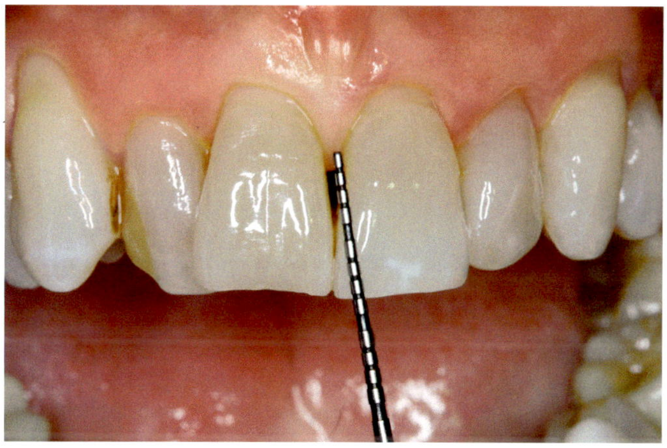

Fig 4-3i The papilla and the contact area are measured toward the incisal edge.

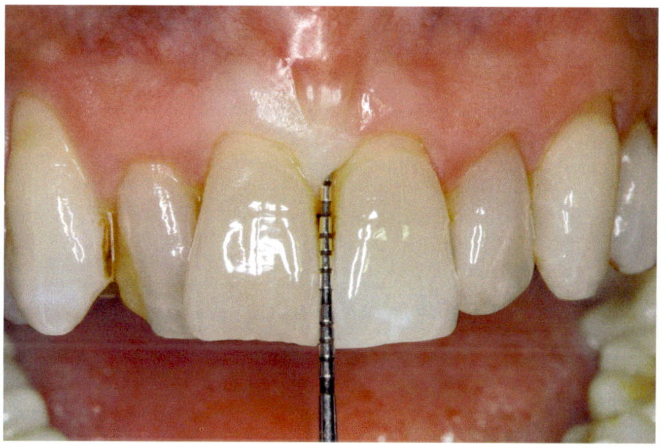

Fig 4-3j Sounding to the osseous crest.

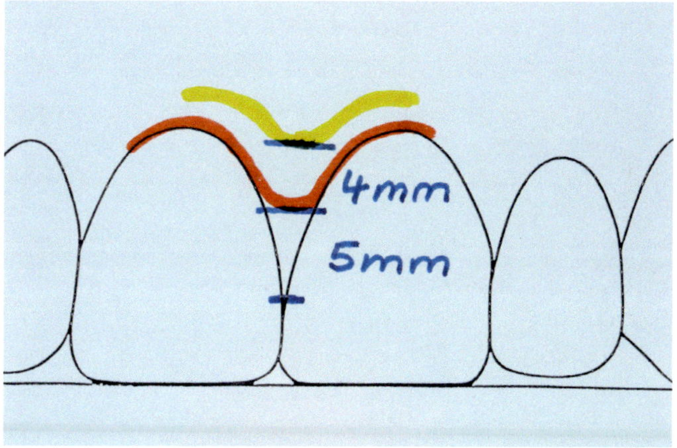

Fig 4-3k The values are entered on a form.

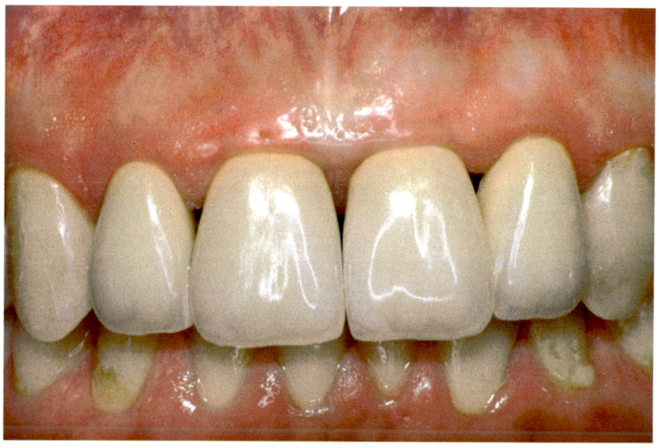

Fig 4-3l The maxillary anterior teeth of this patient have been restored. After 1 week, black triangles are still visible.

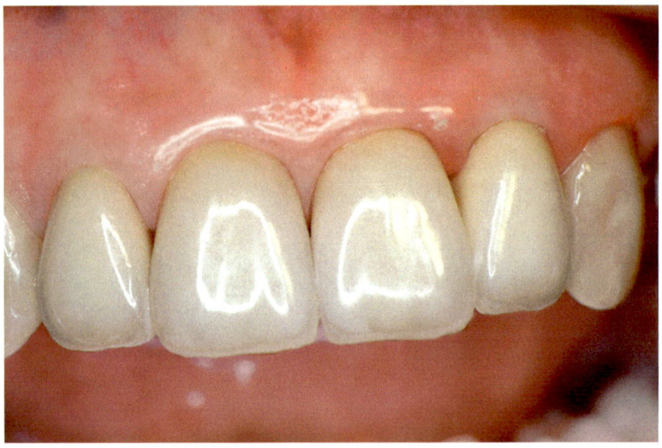

Fig 4-3m Three months later, the interdental papillae are regenerating. It is safe to assume that regeneration eventually will be complete.

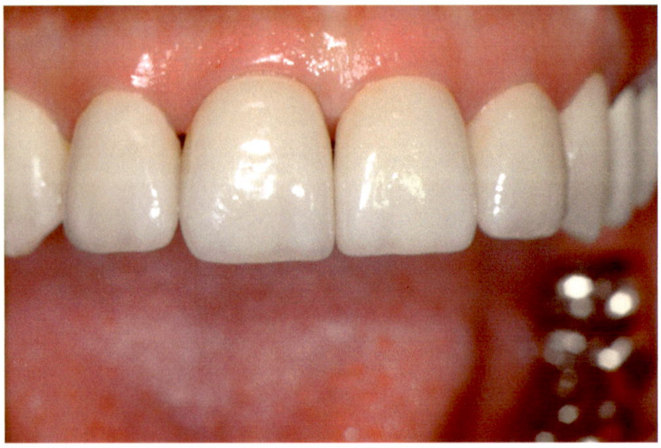

Fig 4-3n Closeup view of the restored maxillary anterior teeth: The papillae have regenerated almost completely.

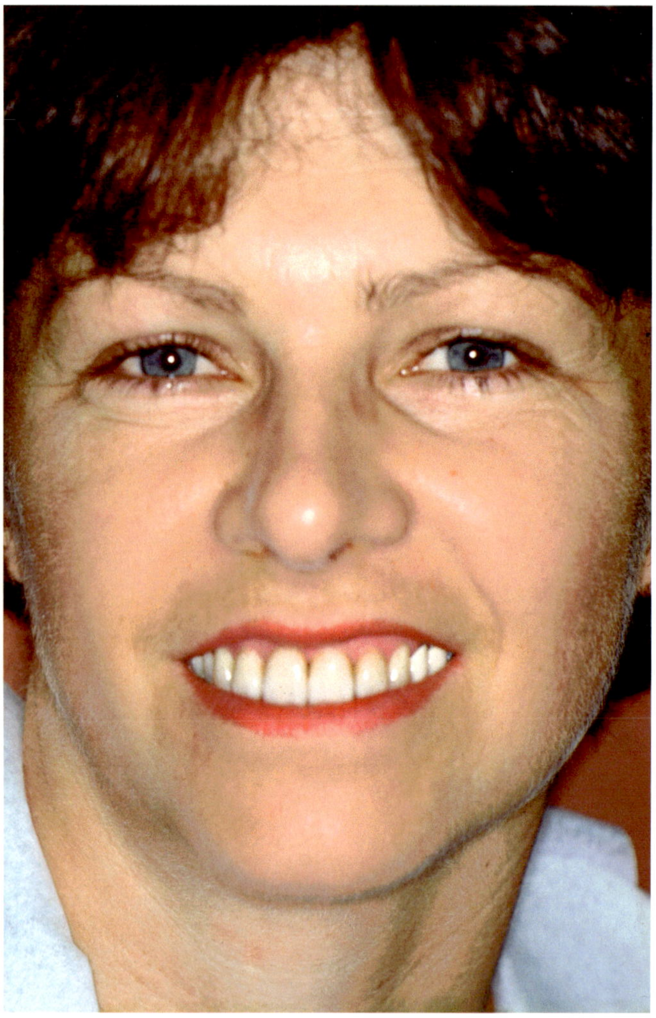

Fig 4-3o The patient displays a happy smile after the restoration.

Materials

Periodontal probe with millimeter calibration (Hu-Friedy)
Form: The biologic width (produced by the author's office; to be published)

Tooth Bed Versus Implant Site

Common problem: How long can the dentist fight to preserve the periodontium without losing too much valuable bone for implantation?

A systematic periodontal treatment was successfully completed in a 45-year-old woman 10 years ago. She was a heavy smoker. Her oral hygiene was good, and she regularly used an electric toothbrush, Superfloss, and interdental brushes. Despite all the efforts on her part and on the part of the dental team, a continuous resorption of the alveolar bone was diagnosed at the regular examination. The author tried to make it clear to the patient that her teeth would have to be extracted early enough to maintain a sufficient amount of bone available for an implantation. However, the patient wanted to keep her teeth by all means.

Soon, however, the teeth had to be extracted anyway, but by then the alveolar bone was severely atrophied (Fig 4-4a). The teeth of the mandibular third quadrant had already been replaced with an implant-supported restoration, which seemed to be stable, despite the use of very short implants with long crowns. Suddenly the periodontal degeneration accelerated enormously, leading to the loss of all of her maxillary dentition (Fig 4-4b). Moreover, the patient also suffered psychologically, because she was unable to wear a complete denture because of an extremely strong gag reflex which could be triggered simply by touching the palate. Thus, the situation in the patient's maxilla was almost hopeless.

The residual height of the alveolar bone in the anterior region from canine to canine was 10 to 12 mm. Four implants (length: 10 mm; diameter: 3.75 mm) placed in the regions of the right and left canines and central incisors failed. After they had been exposed and temporarily loaded on the healing abutments, the implants became loose and had to be explanted. The small amount of bone available (bone quality: D3 to D4) had not withstood the occlusal forces.

Bone augmentation by the oral surgeon was the last resort. However, the patient was unwilling to accept this treatment plan, and she left the office in complete frustration with the remark: "You are the most incompetent dentist I have ever met!"

How can dentists avoid such a situation? What mistakes were made? What other diagnostic options are available in the earlier stages of treatment? How can dentists achieve predictable treatment success in such extremely difficult cases?

Proven solution: Clear diagnosis is the key to successful treatment

A few years ago, the paradigm shifted in periodontology: Scientific research clearly showed that periodontal destruction not only is caused by bacterial agents, but also is determined by genetic predisposition. The results of further research showed that heavy smoking accelerat-

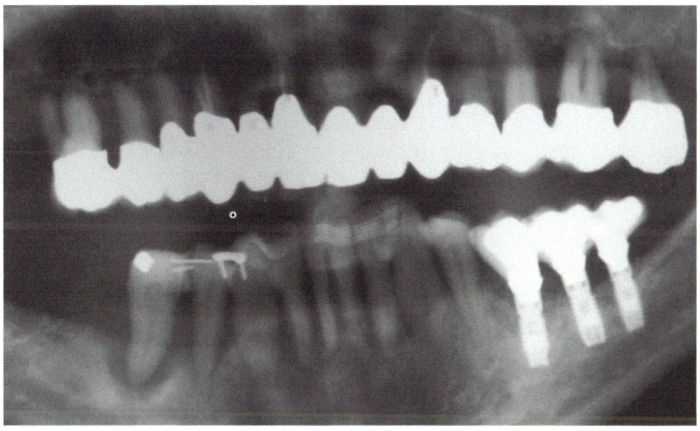

Fig 4-4a The rapid progress of bone resorption is visible on the panoramic radiograph.

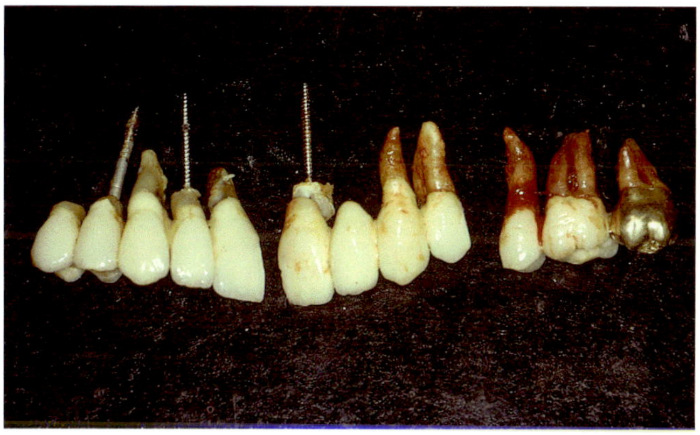

Fig 4-4b Complete loss of the dentition in the maxilla.

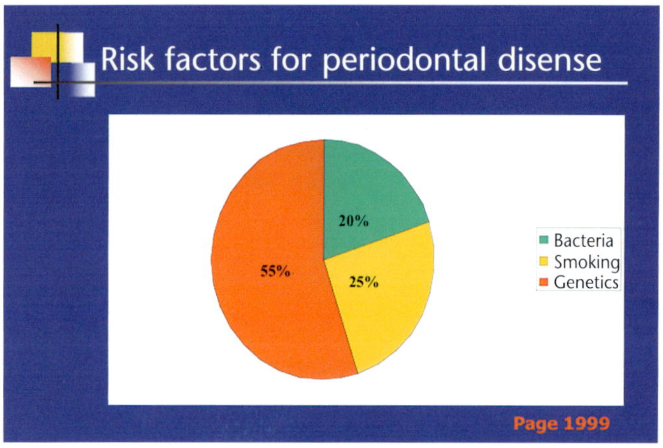

Fig 4-5 Causes of progressive periodontal resorption.

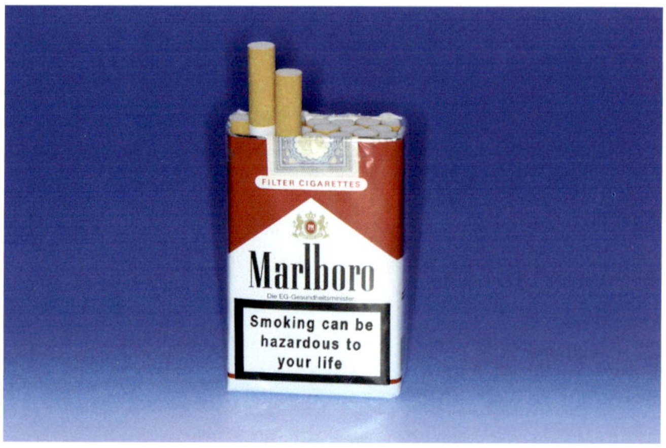

Fig 4-6 Smoking can kill—both the patient and the periodontium!.

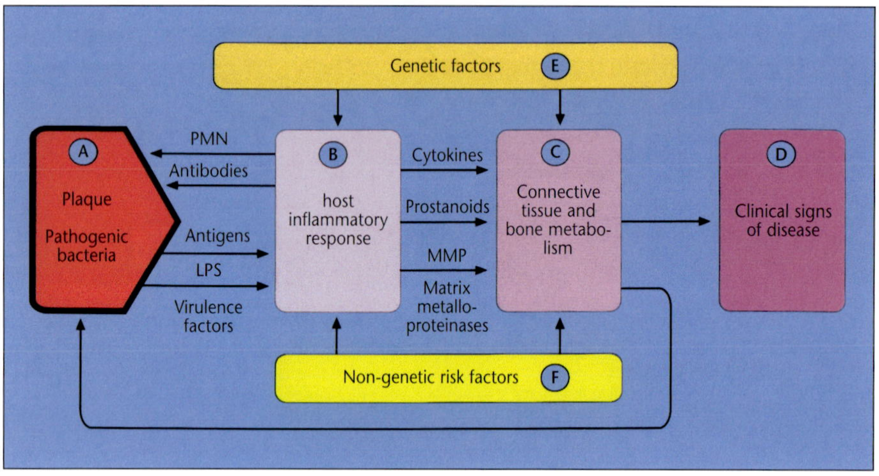

Fig 4-7 Pathogenesis of periodontitis in humans, as defined by Page and Kornman.

ed periodontal resorption (Fig 4-5). Thus, smoking by patients is one of the most critical issues a dentist faces in daily practice, both in periodontology as well as implantology (Fig 4-6).

Researchers have identified the individual resorptive processes in the tissues involved (Figs 4-7 and 4-8). As a consequence of these findings, in the author's private practice, the sequence of diagnostic procedures changed to the following protocol:

1. Complete diagnostic assessment, including clinical evaluation, gingival status, papillary bleeding index, and complete-mouth radiograph series
2. Professional dental hygiene and instructions for oral hygiene over the course of several appointments
3. Bacterial testing of the periodontia that are still compromised by inflammation (Fig 4-9)
4. Patient education, emphasizing the role of smoking as an accelerator of periodontal disease and strongly encouraging the patient to quit smoking (Fig 4-10)
5. Genetic assessment of the interleukin-1 genotype (Fig 4-11)
6. Reevaluation of the dental and periodontal state in a thorough discussion with the patient based on all the available data

This discussion with the patient aims at reviewing the treatment plan together with the patient and reaching a consensus based on the available information. It does not make sense to treat patients as if they were unable to make decisions themselves; instead, the dentist should clearly explain the diagnosis and make clear-cut treatment suggestions. This empowers them. The dentist should also talk and reach an agreement with patients about alternatives in case of failure.

In the words of Dr Myron Nevins: "You have to make decisions! You have to make your dentistry predictable!" This phrase has been ringing in the author's ears since attending Dr Nevin's courses in Swampscott, Massachusetts. He kept preaching the same idea: "In Germany, you like to try things out a lot. But a doctor who is just trying things out is not good for much. Compromises lead to incalculable risks. Our patients want a clear-cut treatment and a prognosis for success for at least 10 years—so let's give it to them!"

Therefore in the author's practice, the treatment strategy was rearranged as follows:

1. Make clear decisions: Which teeth can be preserved in the long term? Which have to be extracted as soon as possible?
2. Augment immediately after the extraction to preserve bone (with antibiotic prophylaxis).
3. Have the patient quit smoking (wait for 6 months).
4. Implant where necessary and where possible. Talk with the patient about the possible loss of implants and how to proceed with any repeat implantations.
5. Allow longer periods for healing.

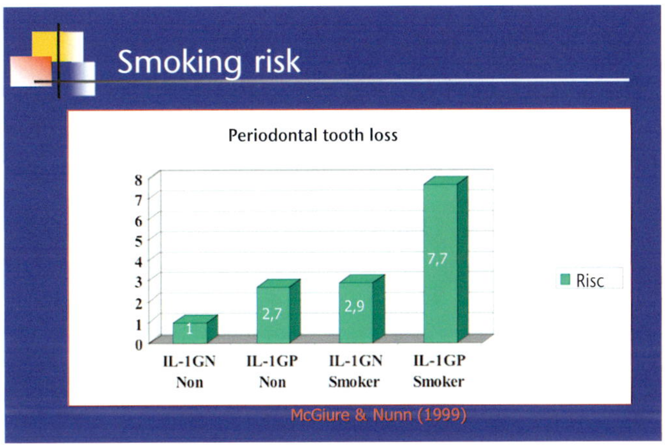

Fig 4-8 Risk factors for the loss of periodontally compromised teeth. (Data from McGuire and Nunn.)

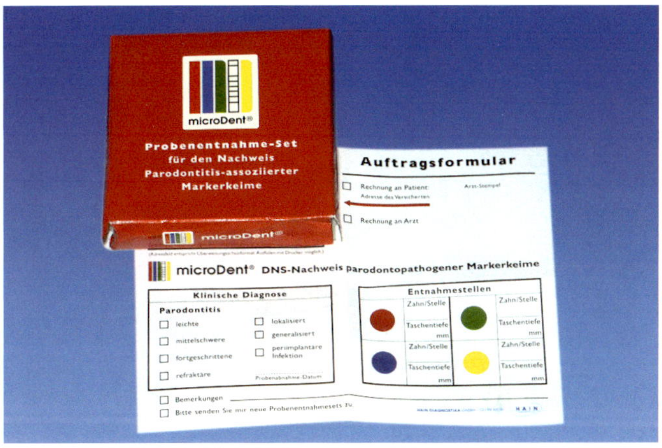

Fig 4-9 MicroDent bacteria test kit.

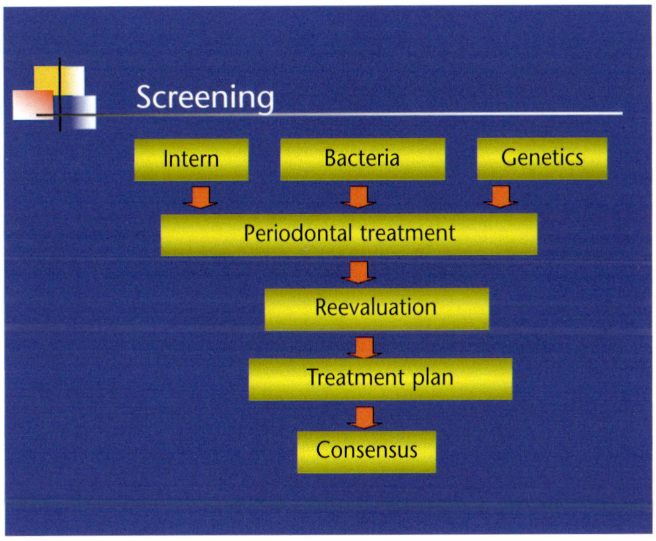

Fig 4-10 Smoking is an accelerating factor in periodontal disease.

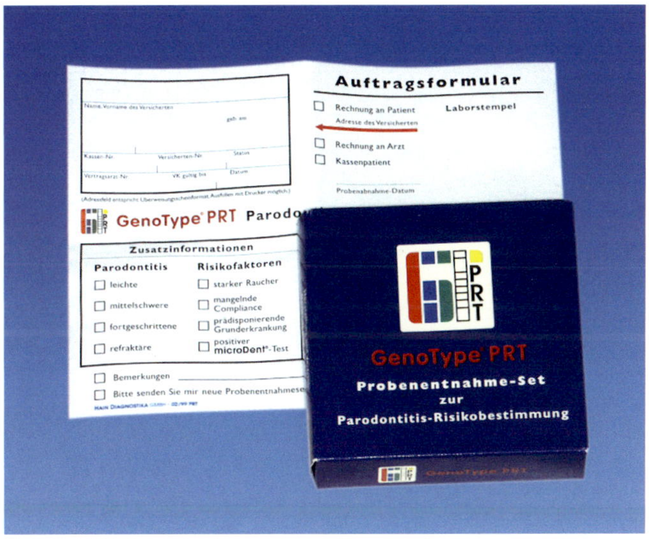

Fig 4-11 GenoType PRT genetic test kit.

6. After healing, measure the implants with the Periotest device.
7. Place provisional restorations.
8. Reevaluate the oral conditions.
9. Place permanent restorations.
10. Follow up.

The author cannot claim not to have had any failures since this protocol was instituted, but failures have markedly decreased in number. Dentists also must learn to say no in cases when patients do not want to follow treatment suggestions and the dentists cannot bear the risk of treating them according to their wishes. Dentists should not be tempted by patients to treat them by indulging in high-risk experiments. Both dentists and patients almost always regret it.

Materials

MicroDent bacteria test (Hain Lifescience); bacteria test kits can also be obtained from other manufacturers
GenoType PRT and PST genetic tests (Hain Lifescience); genetic test kits can also be obtained from other manufacturers
Periotest device (Medizintechnik Gulden)

5

Implant Dentistry

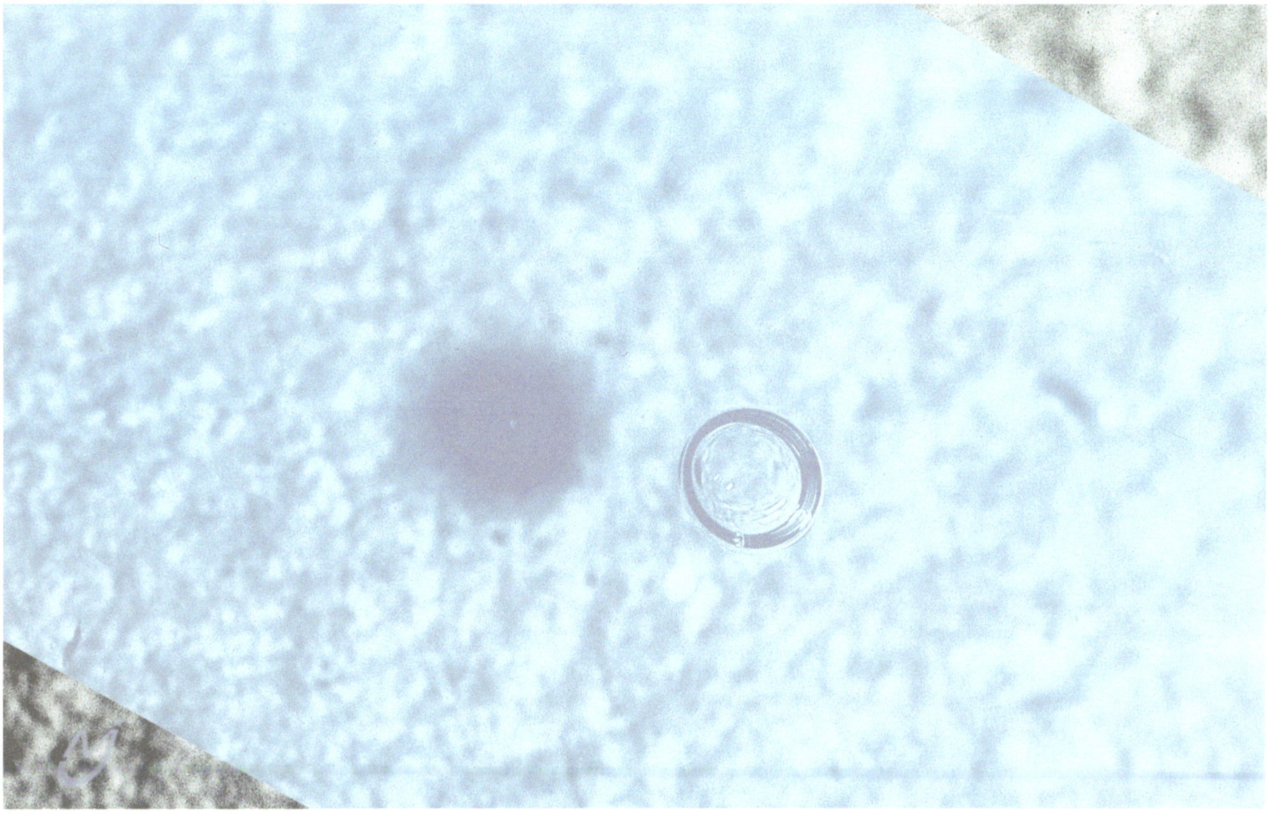

5

Congenitally Missing Maxillary Lateral Incisors

Improvement of the Implant Site Using the Osteotome Technique

Implant Prosthodontics: Tightening of Screws

Immediate Implant Placement

Selection of an Implant System

Congenitally Missing Maxillary Lateral Incisors

Common problem: When and how to treat the spaces

The absence of maxillary lateral incisors is a treatment challenge for every dentist, orthodontist, and dental technician (Fig 5-1a). Statistically, this anomaly seems to be growing more and more frequent. Two different treatment concepts are still debated: closing the spaces by moving the canines into the position of the lateral incisors or opening the spaces to allow prosthetic restoration. In this context the following questions arise:

1. At what age can it be recognized that teeth are congenitally missing?
2. Are there any orthodontic pretreatments?
3. When should the actual orthodontic treatment commence?
4. Does it really make sense from an esthetic and functional point of view to move the canines mesially to act as lateral incisors?
5. After the spaces have been opened, when and how can they be closed with restorations?
6. At what age can the spaces be closed with crowns on single-tooth implants?

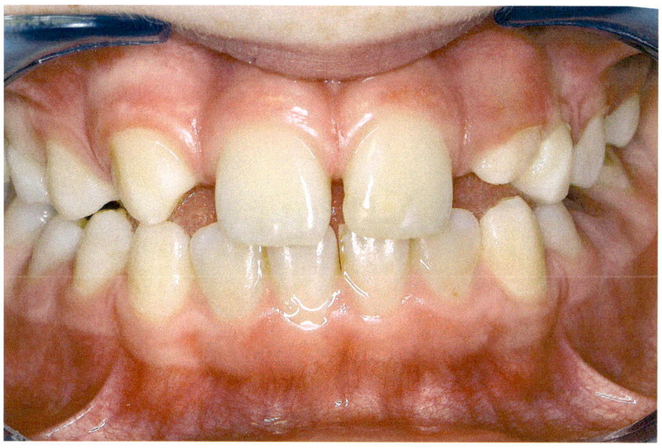

Fig 5-1a Patient with congenitally missing lateral incisors. (Courtesy of A. Breunig, Memmingen, Germany.)

Treatment concept 1

The first treatment option is to close the space by moving the canines into the position of the lateral incisors (Fig 5-1b). The treatment result is unattractive and thus not satisfactory, because, with its shape and color, the canine looks very much out of place at the position of the lateral incisor. It is certainly possible to achieve a good result with adhesive resin composite or ceramics that can be further improved by bleaching, if necessary. This treatment concept, however, does not respect the principle of minimally invasive treatment in modern dentistry. Most of the time, the functional result is a narrowing of the dental arch in the maxilla and thus a reduced overbite or even an edge-to-edge bite. The desired anterior-canine guidance therefore cannot be achieved satisfactorily. The first premolar can only take over lateral guidance in part. Most of the time, the reduced or nonexistent overbite results in abrasion or recessions. Therefore, long-term success cannot be attained with this treatment concept.

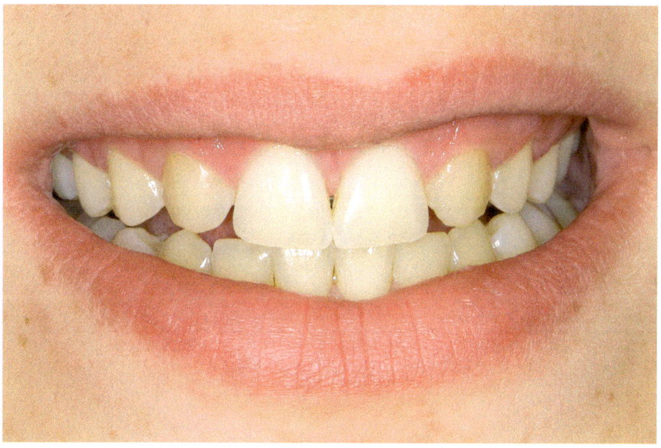

Fig 5-1b Canines moved into the position of the lateral incisors. (Courtesy of A. Breunig, Memmingen, Germany.)

Treatment concept 2

The second option, ie, opening the spaces or keeping them open orthodontically and subsequently providing a prosthetic solution, leads to an attractive and functional long-term result. For reasons of both esthetics and function, the maxillary canines belong in their natural posi-

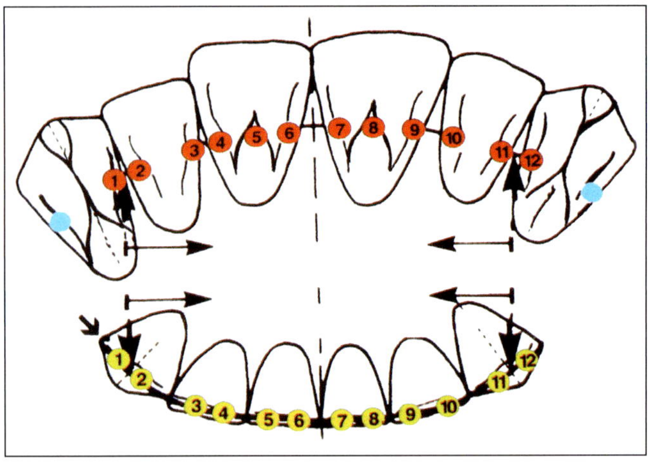

Fig 5-2 Occlusal contacts of the anterior teeth in a normal occlusion. The occlusal vault is shown from the mesial side of the maxillary right canine to the mesial side of the maxillary left canine. The distal halves of the canines belong to the posterior segment

tion. Only there can they fulfill their function as a means of lateral and protrusive guidance. Only half of the maxillary canine is an anterior tooth—the distal half of the tooth belongs to the posterior segment (Fig 5-2).

Proven solution: Opening the spaces for a prosthetic restoration

The procedure is demonstrated step by step through a case report. Both maxillary lateral incisors were congenitally missing in a 13-year-old patient. The spaces had been opened orthodontically and were to be restored with two single crowns on implants (Figs 5-3a to 5-3e).

The desired implant-supported single-tooth restoration is contraindicated at this age, however, because there

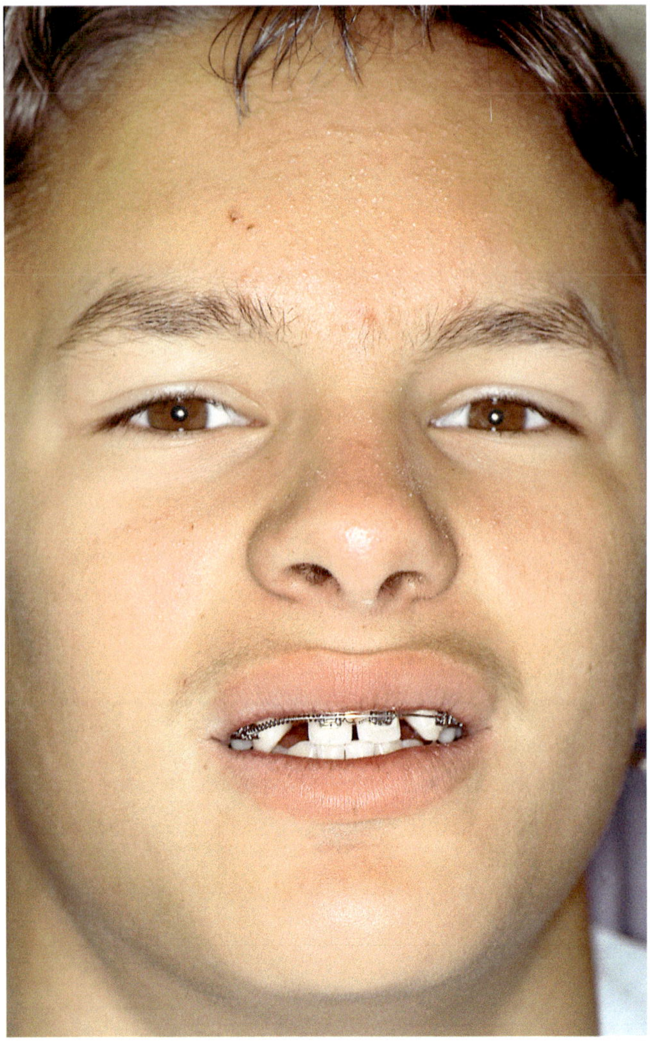

Fig 5-3a Thirteen-year-old patient with congenitally missing maxillary lateral incisors.

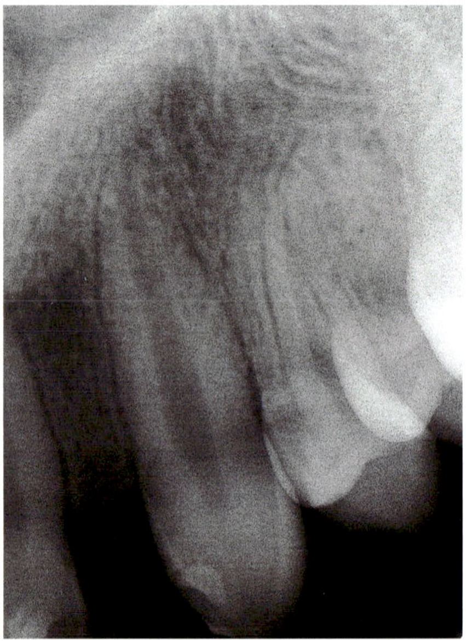

Fig 5-3b Radiograph of the lateral incisor area.

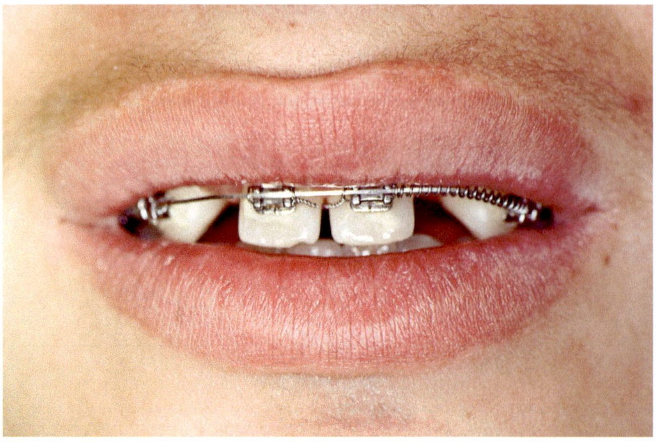

Fig 5-3c Patient's lip line.

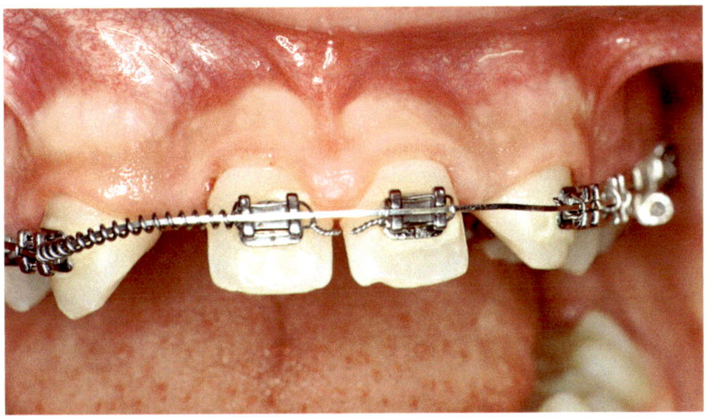

Fig 5-3d Appearance after the spaces have been opened orthodontically.

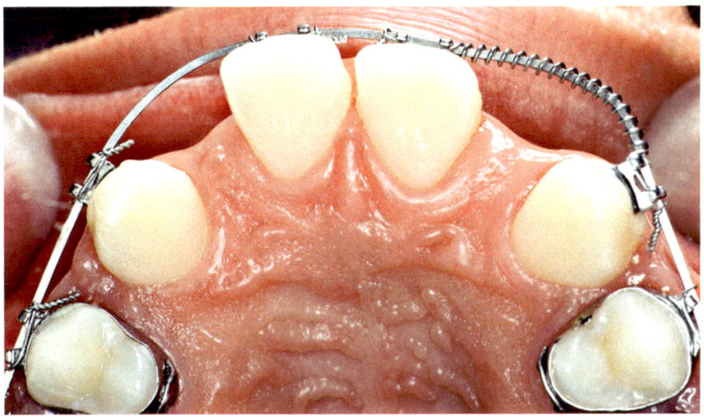

Fig 5-3e Opened spaces (palatal view).

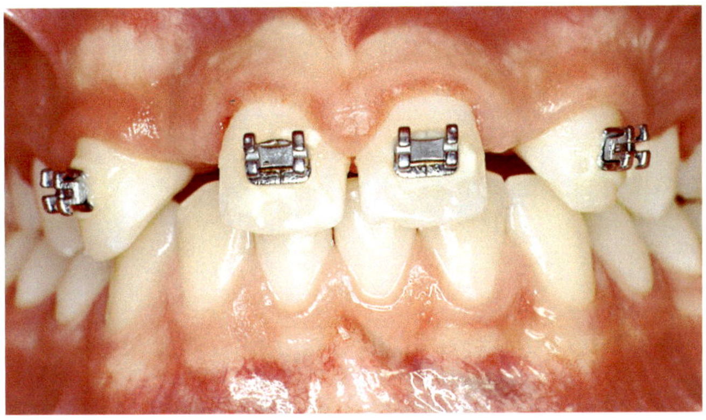

Fig 5-3f The retraction arch wire is removed.

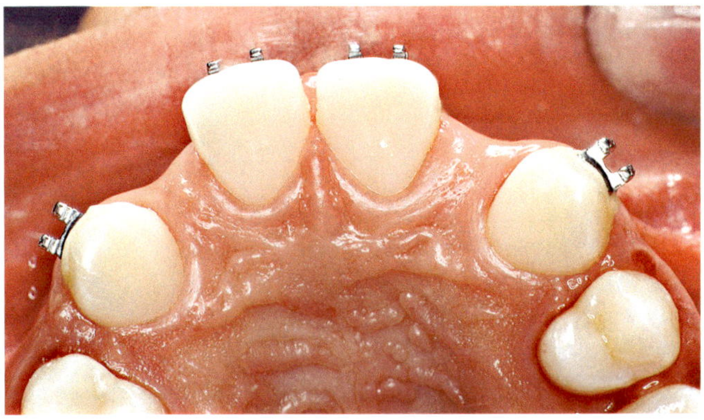

Fig 5-3g Small guide grooves are prepared on the abutment teeth.

is the risk that the alveolar ridge will keep growing with the teeth while the implant-supported crown will remain in its position. This would be a disastrous result, both esthetically and functionally, and it would not be possible to correct later. Most of the literature specifies an age of 17 or 18 years as the earliest appropriate age for an implantation.

Because this patient was not old enough yet, the spaces were restored bilaterally with an interim prosthesis consisting of a resin-bonded fixed partial denture made of Targis/Vectris. The Targis/Vectris system is a glass fiber resin composite system that is suitable for this kind of interim restoration. When the patient reached the age of 18 years, the spaces were to be permanently closed with two implant-supported single crowns. The patient and his parents were informed in detail and agreed to the procedure.

The retraction arch wire was removed (Fig 5-3f), and small guide grooves were prepared in the palatal surfaces of the canines and central incisors (Fig 5-3g). Before the impression was taken, the brackets were blocked out with wax (Fig 5-3h). The impression was taken with polyether and filled with die stone to create the master cast (Figs 5-3i and 5-3j). The retraction arch wire was reseated for continued retention (Fig 5-3k).

A framework was made from Vectris fibers in the laboratory. Only the interwoven Vectris frame fibers could be utilized, because there was not enough space to use the Vectris pontic fibers (Fig 5-3l). The glass fiber frameworks were laminated with Targis and finished (Figs 5-3m to 5-3o).

The retraction arch wire was removed for the adhesive cementation and rubber dam was placed (Figs 5-3p and 5-3q). The tooth surfaces to which the fixed partial dentures were going to be bonded were etched with phosphoric acid for 30 seconds (Fig 5-3r), rinsed, and dried. A marked etching pattern was visible (Fig 5-3s). For adhesive cementation, a dual-cure luting resin composite of medium viscosity was applied and completely polymerized carefully from all sides (Fig 5-3t).

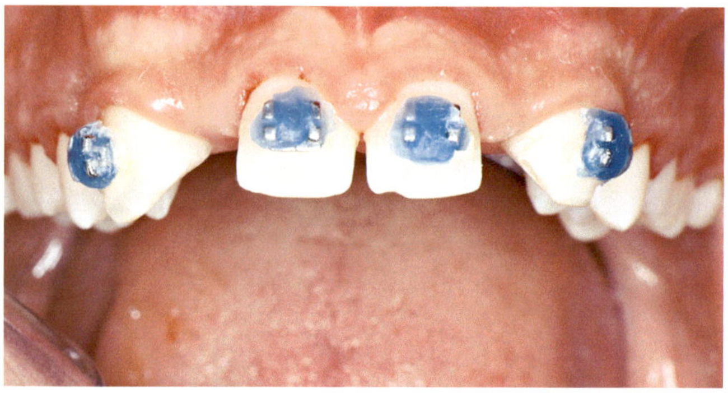

Fig 5-3h The bonded brackets are blocked out with wax.

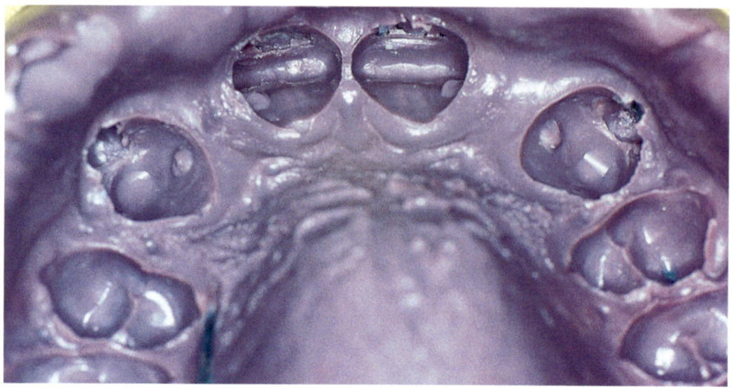

Fig 5-3i Impression.

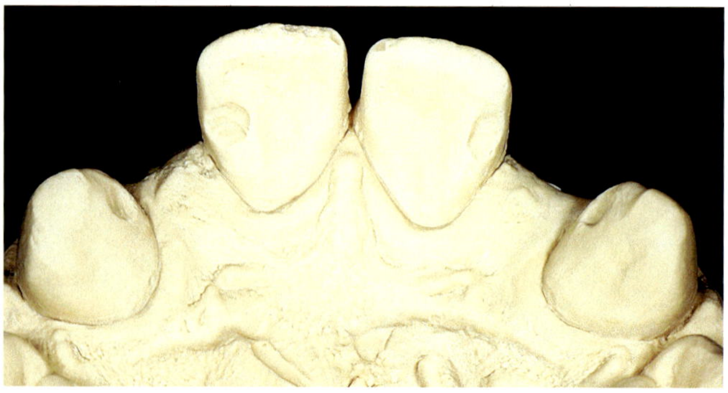

Fig 5-3j Master cast.

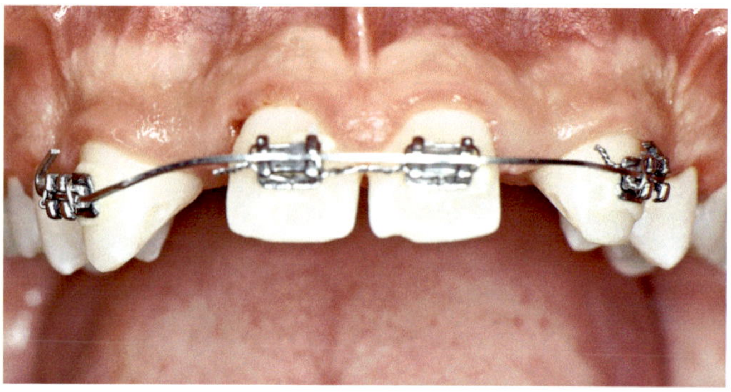

Fig 5-3k The retraction arch wire is reseated to retain the position of the abutment teeth.

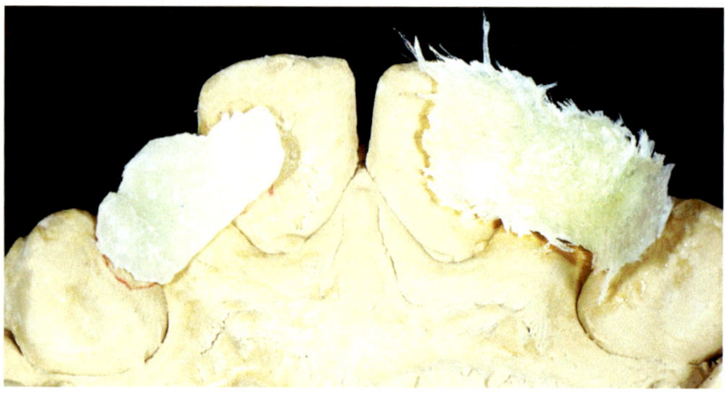

Fig 5-3l Framework construction with Vectris frame glass fiber mats.

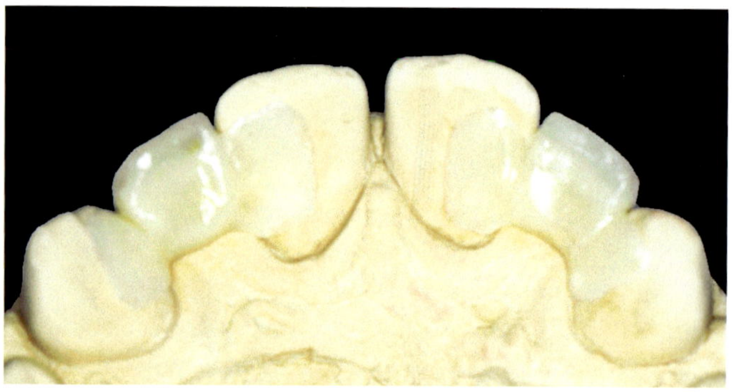

Fig 5-3m Palatal view of the finished fixed partial dentures.

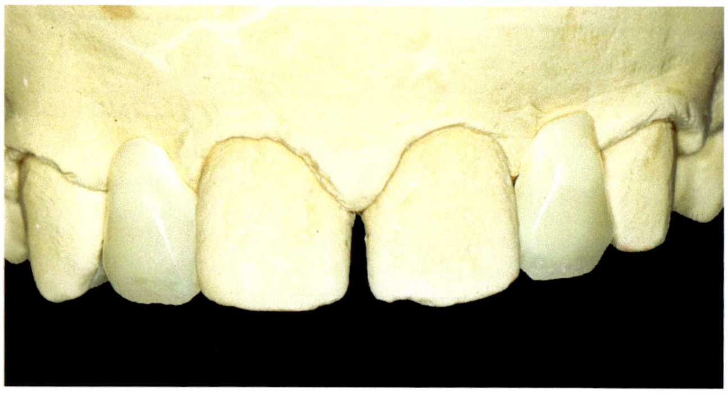

Fig 5-3n Labial view of the finished fixed partial dentures.

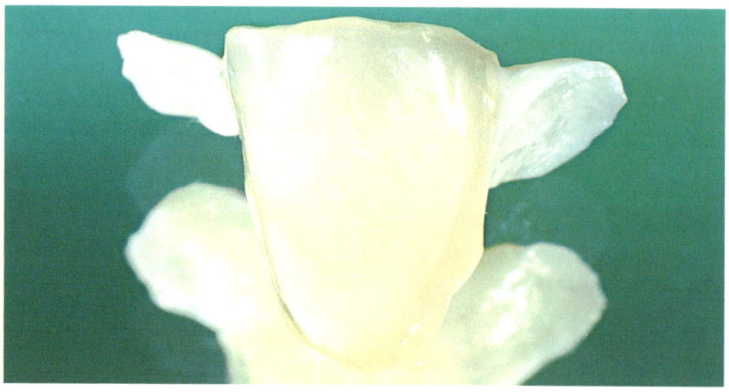

Fig 5-3o The resin-bonded fixed partial dentures are ready to be cemented.

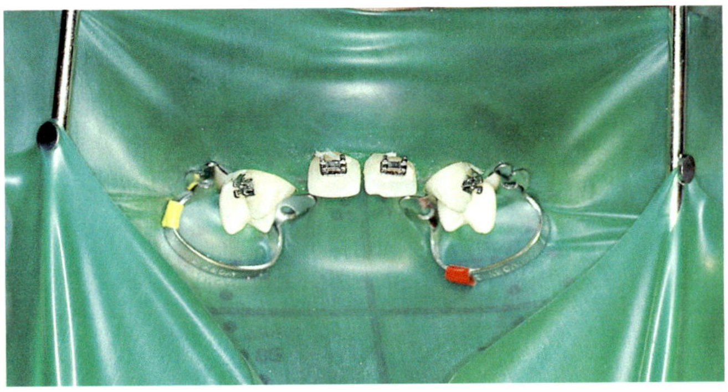

Fig 5-3p Rubber dam and frame.

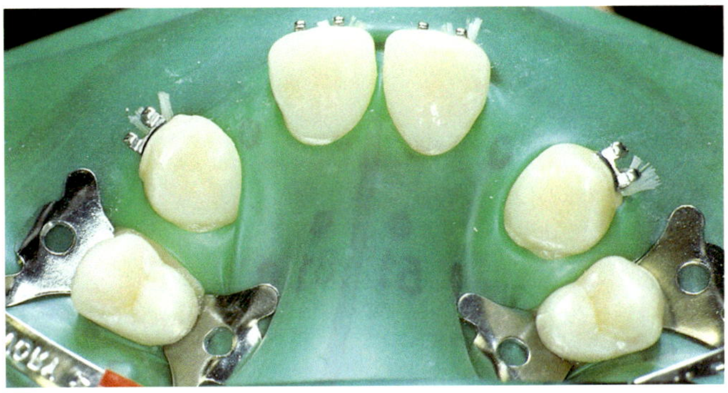

Fig 5-3q Rubber dam is held in place with clamps and ligatures.

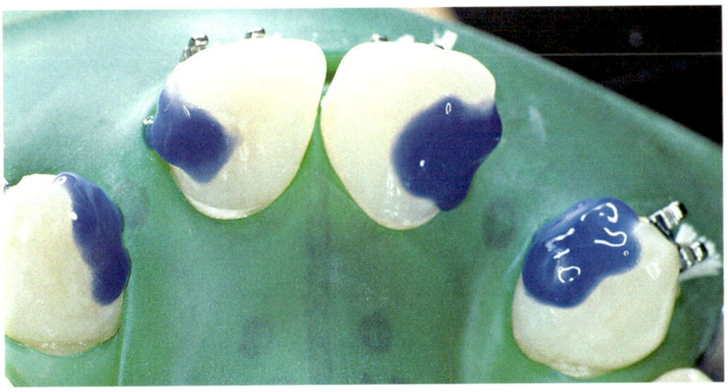

Fig 5-3r Etching of the bonding surface with phosphoric acid for 30 seconds.

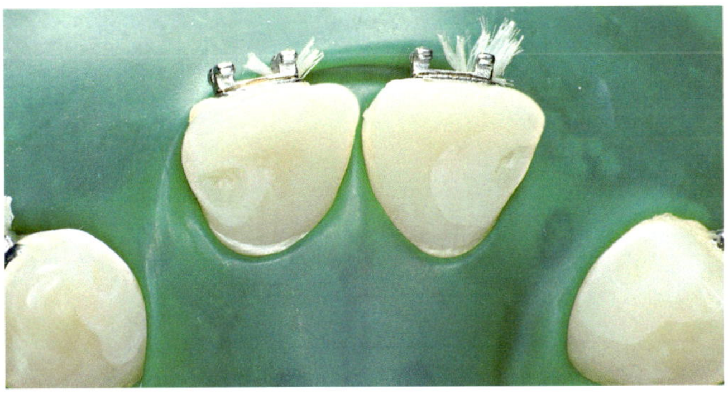

Fig 5-3s The etching pattern is checked.

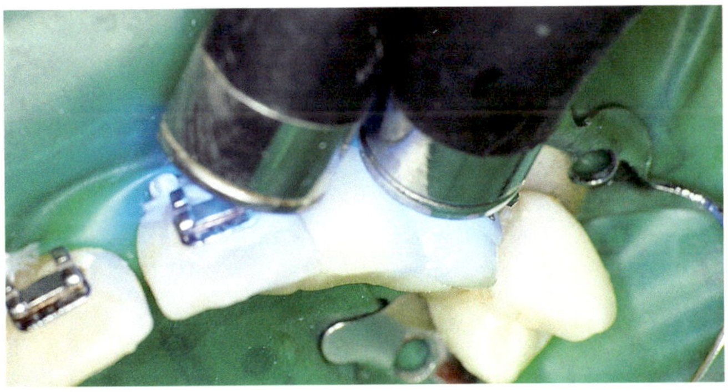

Fig 5-3t The fixed partial dentures are adhesively bonded with careful polymerization.

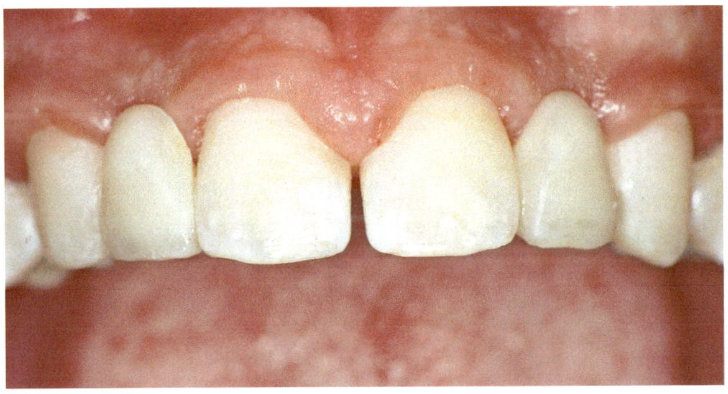

Fig 5-3u The finished fixed partial dentures are in place.

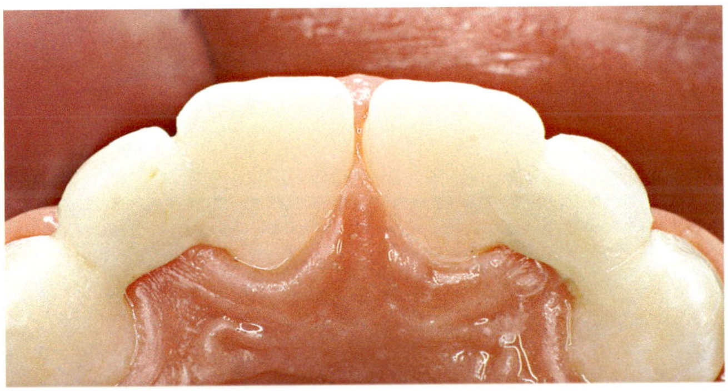

Fig 5-3v Palatal view of the finished fixed partial dentures in place.

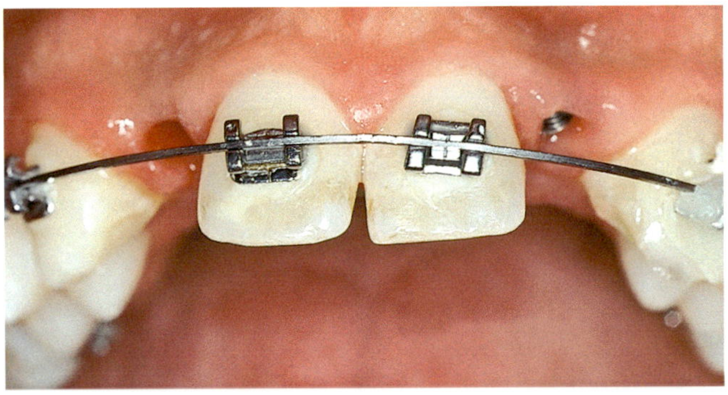

Fig 5-3w New brackets have been placed to further open the spaces after implant insertion.

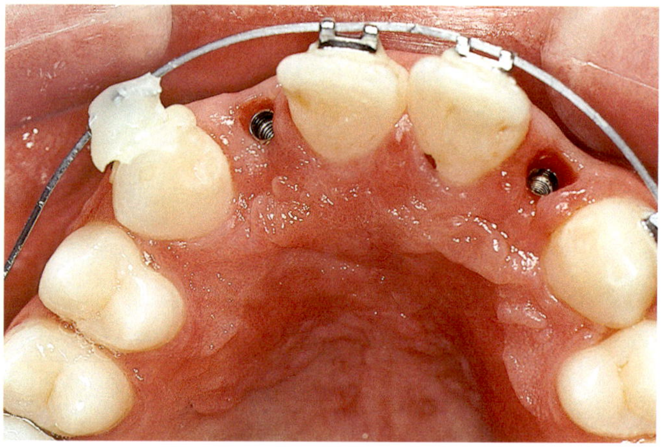

Fig 5-3x Palatal view of new brackets.

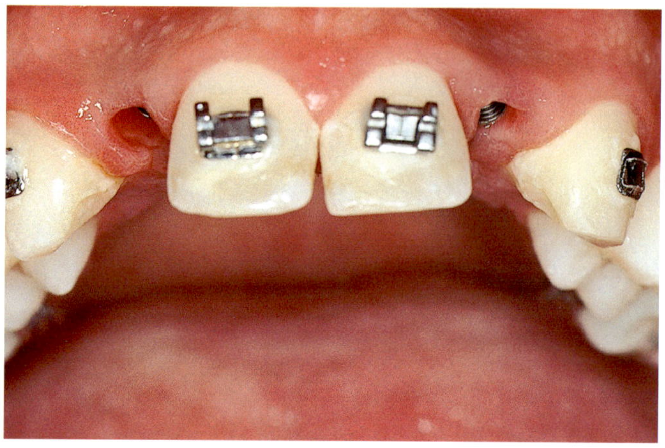

Fig 5-3y The retraction arch wire is removed prior to removal of the brackets.

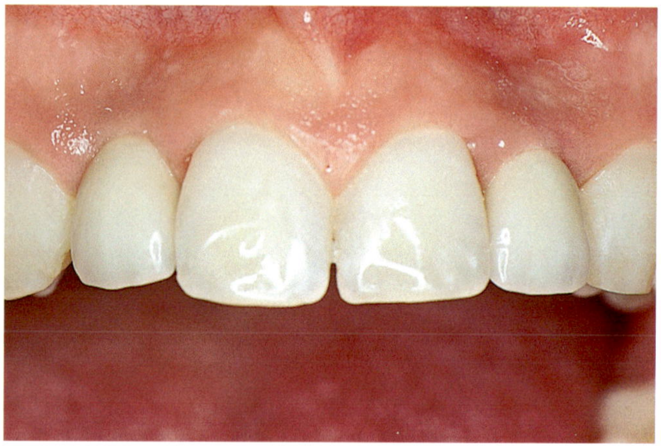

Fig 5-3z Implant-supported all-ceramic crowns.

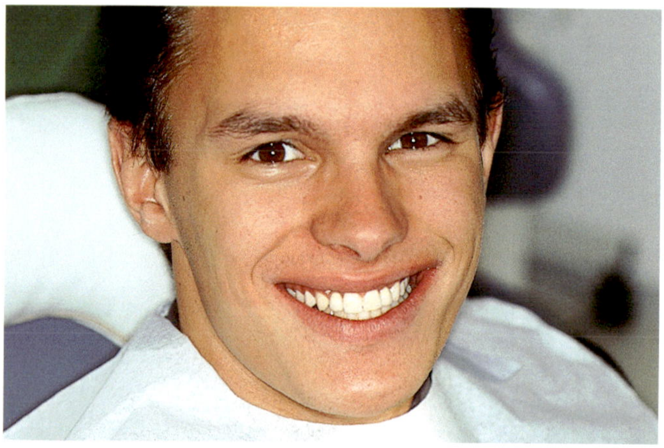

Fig 5-3aa Beaming patient.

The patient was sent home after the restoration was carefully checked and fluoride was applied to the teeth. A good interim result was achieved (Fig 5-3u and 5-3v).

Like most resin-bonded fixed partial dentures, these fixed partial dentures had to be recemented occasionally over the following years. Both fixed partial dentures were constantly at risk because the patient played a lot of sports. When the patient was aged 17 years, brackets were placed once again for a short period of time to further open the spaces for the planned implantation in the region of the lateral incisors (Figs 5-3w to 5-3y).

When the patient was 18 years old, the implants were inserted. After a healing period of 3 months, the permanent restorations were successfully placed (Fig 5-3z). Figure 5-3aa shows the final treatment result: A happy, smiling young banker.

Materials

Targis/Vectris system (Ivoclar Vivadent)
Impregum (3M ESPE)
Variolink Ultra luting cement (Ivoclar Vivadent)
Micro Miniplant implants, 3.25 mm in diameter and 15 mm long (3i Implant Innovations)

Improvement of the Implant Site Using the Osteotome Technique

Common problem: Inadequate implant site

In the course of the diagnosis for a planned implantation, dentists frequently encounter patients with porous bone (Fig 5-4) and/or too little bone substance both horizontally and vertically (Fig 5-5).

Lekholm and Zarb created a system for classifying bone quality in implant dentistry (Fig 5-6), and their classification is a safe guideline to judge the quality of the bony site. On radiographs and computed tomograms, the bone quality can be determined with the help of histograms using the Hounsfield scale. However, even a cursory inspection of the radiographic images will indicate the bone quality that is likely to be expected. Judy and Misch summarized the properties of the different categories of bone (Figs 5-7a to 5-7d).

Wolff's law reveals that unloaded bone degenerates; under a physiologic load, bone formation occurs until a stable equilibrium is reached; bone that is overloaded also degenerates. With teeth and implants alike, forces are transmitted within the bone and therefore contribute to the conservation and reinforcement of the bone. A load distributed over a larger area leads to external bone resorption at the loaded surface, as with complete dentures (Fig 5-8). The absence of a load, on the other hand, leads to a reduction in bone quality, ie, to the resorption of internal supporting structures (Fig 5-9). In conclusion, an intraosseous physiologic load preserves bone volume and quality.

One great challenge in implant dentistry today is bone type D4, which is encountered mainly in the maxilla, especially in the distal region. If the implant site is prepared only with drills and mills, so much of the little bone available is usually lost that neither primary stability nor sufficient osseointegration is ensured (bone-implant interface 25%). What opportunities does the dentist have to optimize the designated bony bed with respect to quality and quantity in the extremely problematic class D4 bone (see Figs 5-7a to 5-7d)?

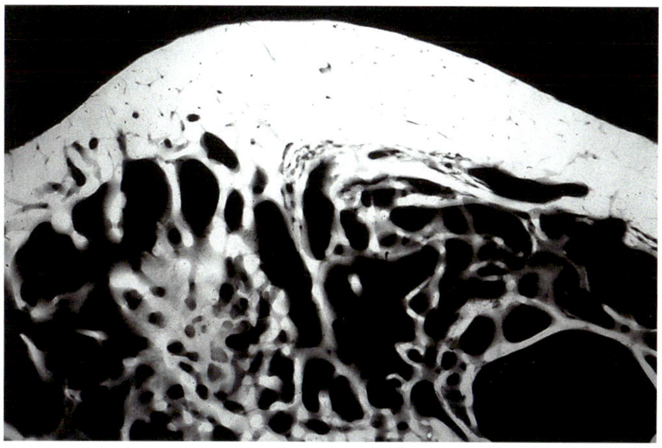

Fig 5-4 Porous bone, class D4. (Courtesy of Prof Klaus-Ulrich Benner, Munich Anatomical Institute.)

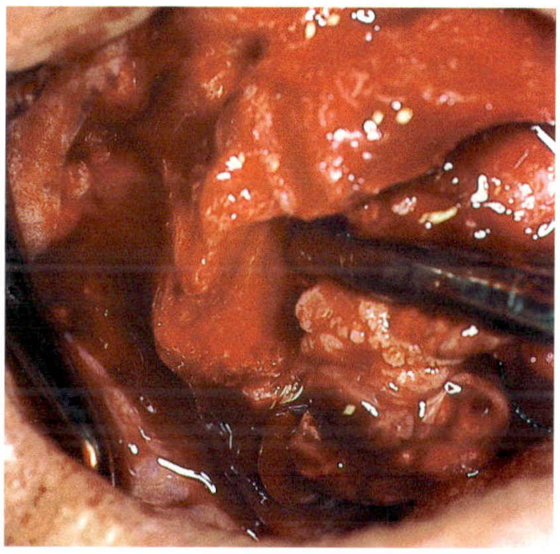

Fig 5-5 Thin alveolar ridge in the maxilla after surgical exposure.

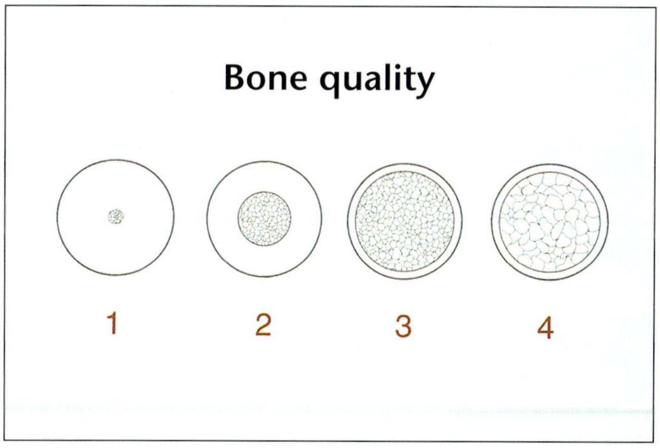

Fig 5-6 Classification of bone quality, as defined by Lekholm and Zarb.

Features of bone quality	
D1 dense cortical bone, little cancellous bone	Anterior mandible, atrophied, edentulous
Advantages:	**Disadvantages:**
Primary stability BIC 90 % Shorter implants	Poorer blood supply (prolonged healing) Reduced bone height for osteotomy preparation Risk of overheating

Fig 5-7a Features of bone quality D1, as defined by Judy and Misch. BIC = bone-to-implant contact.

Features of bone quality	
D2 dense cortical bone, dense cancellous bone	Anterior and posterior mandible, palatal region of the maxilla
Advantages:	
Primary stability BIC 75 % Bone healing Simple preparation technique	

Fig 5-7b Features of bone quality D2, as defined by Judy and Misch. BIC = bone-to-implant contact.

Features of bone quality	
D3 thin cortical bone, close-meshed cancellous bone	Posterior maxilla
Advantages:	**Disadvantages:**
Blood supply	Osteotomy preparation Bicortical anchorage BIC 50 %, more implants required, splinted superstructures

Fig 5-7c Features of bone quality D3, as defined by Judy and Misch. BIC = bone-to-implant contact.

Features of bone quality	
D4 thin cortical bone, wide-meshed cancellous bone	Anterior and posterior maxilla
	Disadvantages:
	Primary stability BIC 25 % Monocortical anchorage Internal sinus floor elevation Osteotome technique

Fig 5-7d Features of bone quality D4, as defined by Judy and Misch. BIC = bone-to-implant contact.

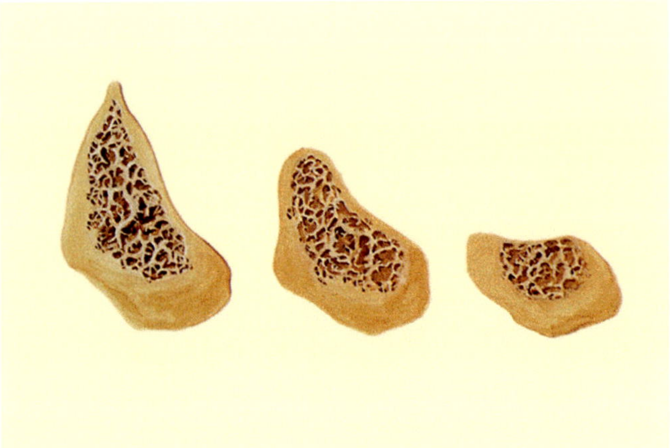

Fig 5-8 Atrophied alveolar crest in the mandible.

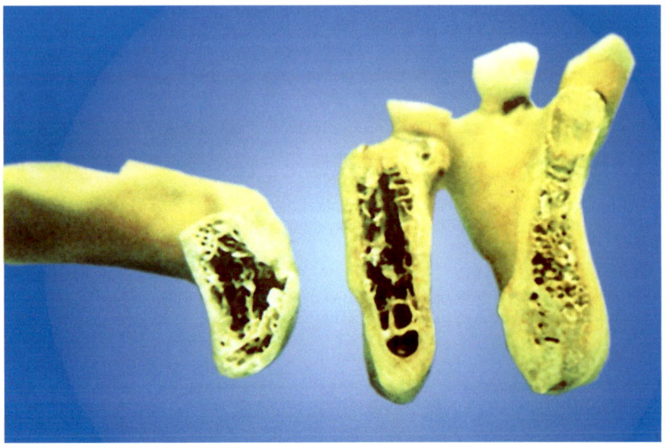

Fig 5-9 Internally atrophied bone showing hollow spaces.

Proven solution: Osteotome technique

In the early 1990s, Robert B. Summers developed a technique known as the *osteotome technique*. It involves using hollow chisels of a conical shape, or osteotomes, to cut, condense, and spread the bone. A set of osteotomes contains five standardized sizes with depth demarcations (Figs 5-10 to 5-12).

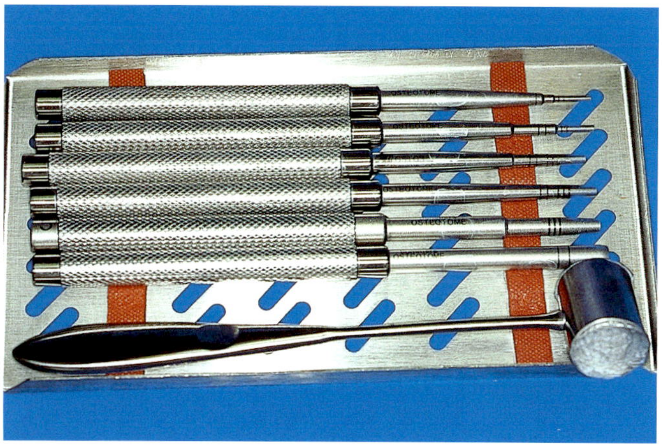

Fig 5-10 Osteotome tray with hammer.

Indications

Bone compaction

During preparation, the bone is not removed but condensed, both vertically and horizontally (Fig 5-13).

Internal augmentation

Hollow spaces in the bone can be internally augmented with autologous bone or a bone replacement material to reinforce the implant site and to increase the contact area with the implant (Fig 5-14).

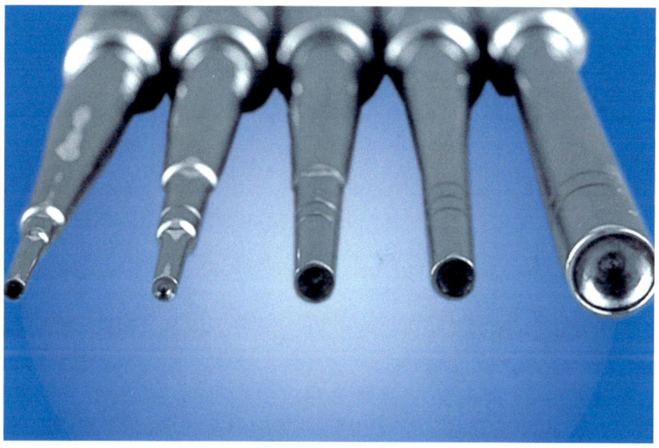

Fig 5-11 Osteotome kit with five standardized osteotomes.

Bone spreading

Bone spreading can only be performed with thin and flexible compact bone (bone types D3 and D4, resorption classes A, B, and C in the maxilla; Fig 5-15). The bone's response to spreading has to be observed closely to prevent the bone from breaking off unintentionally (Fig 5-16). The method of choice for dealing with strong compact bone is bone splitting.

Indirect vertical sinus floor elevation with implant insertion

This procedure is indicated if the floor of the sinus is at least 5 mm thick. Furthermore, the patient should be able to open the mouth far enough to allow the use of osteotomes. The clinician can also work with offset osteotomes, although these are more difficult to handle, if he or she has to "feel" the way through the bone (Figs 5-17 and 5-18).

Future site development (indirect vertical sinus floor elevation as a preparatory measure for future implantation)

The floor of the sinus is scored with a large-diameter trephine mill, 6.5 mm or larger (Fig 5-19a), and malleted with the no. 5 osteotome (Fig 5-19b). The nasal mucosa is carefully prepared away from the bone with a fine sinus instrument from the tray for open sinus floor elevations (Fig 5-20). The elevated area is then filled with grafting material and covered with a resorbable membrane (Fig 5-

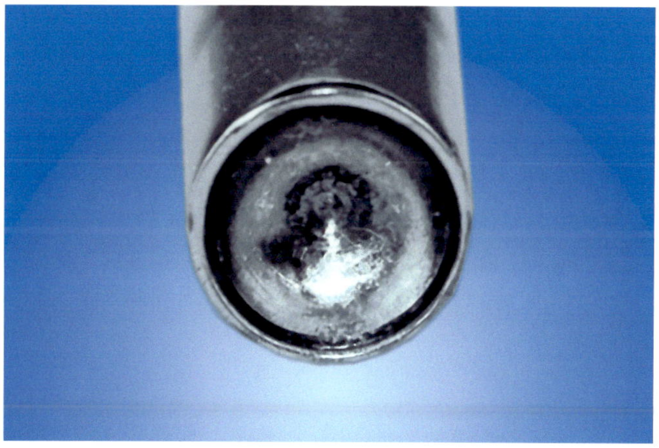

Fig 5-12 Cutting surface of the hollow chisel.

Improvement of the Implant Site Using the Osteotome Technique

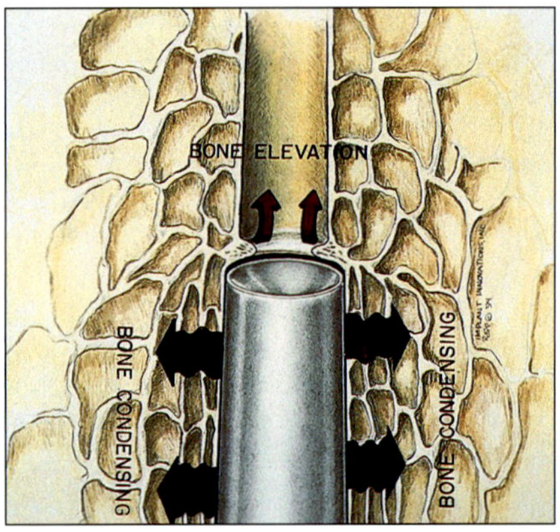

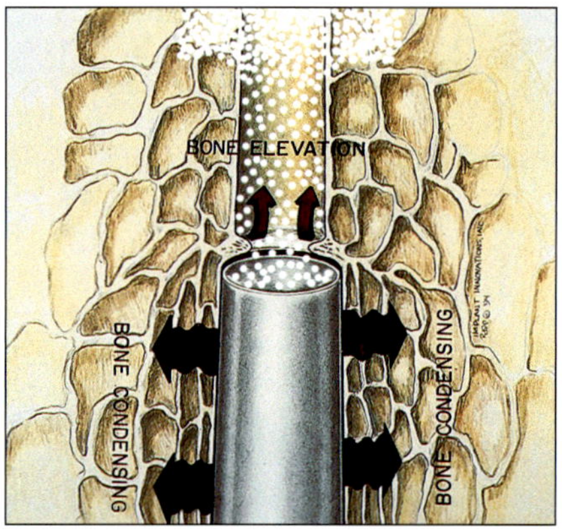

Fig 5-13 *(left)* Working principle of osteotomes: preparation and condensation. (Courtesy of Dr Richard Lazzara, 3i Implant Innovations).

Fig 5-14 *(right)* Internal augmentation. (Courtesy of Dr Richard Lazzara, 3i Implant Innovations.)

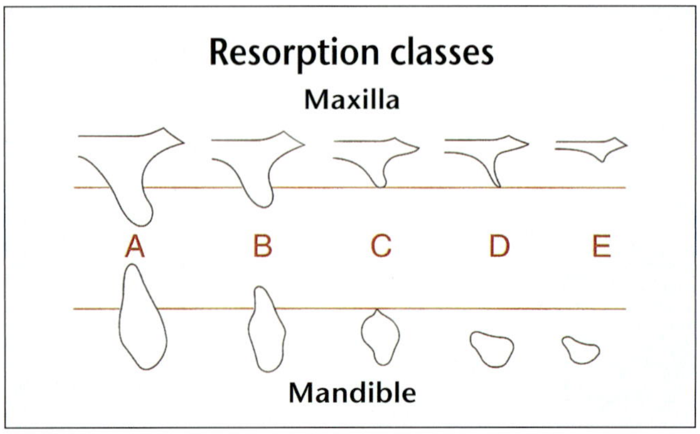

Fig 5-15 Resorption classes according to Lekholm and Zarb.[1]

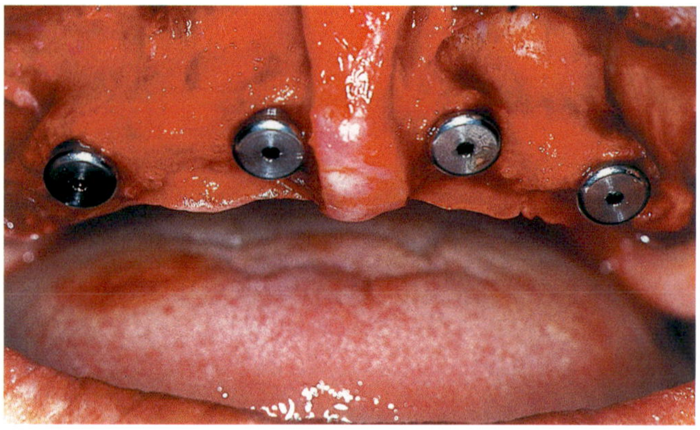

Fig 5-16 Implant placement after preparation with osteotomes.

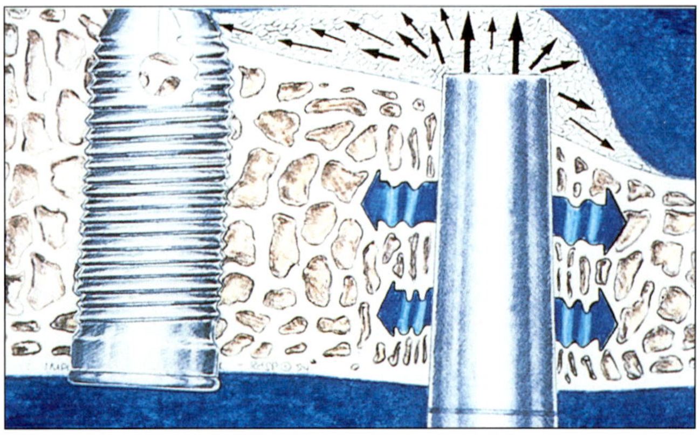

Fig 5-17a Indirect vertical sinus lift. (Courtesy of Dr Richard Lazzara, 3i Implant Innovations.)

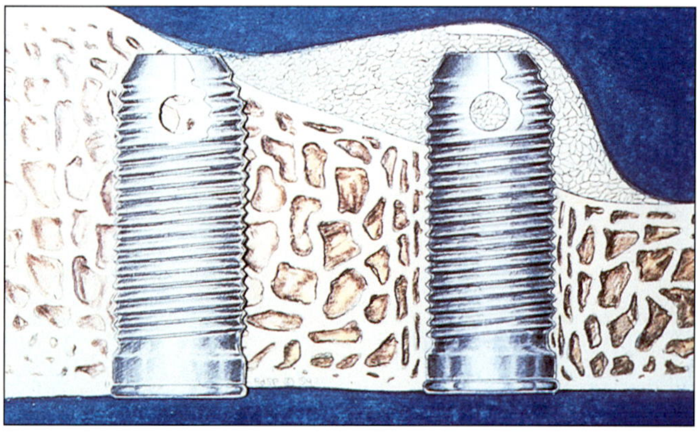

Fig 5-17b Indirect vertical sinus lift after implant placement. (Courtesy of Dr Richard Lazzara, 3i Implant Innovations.)

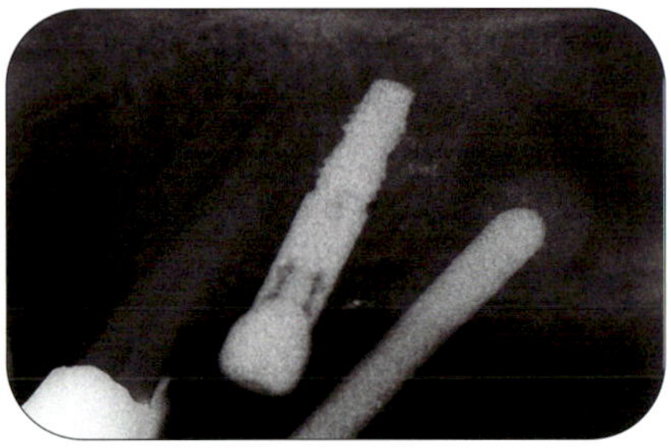

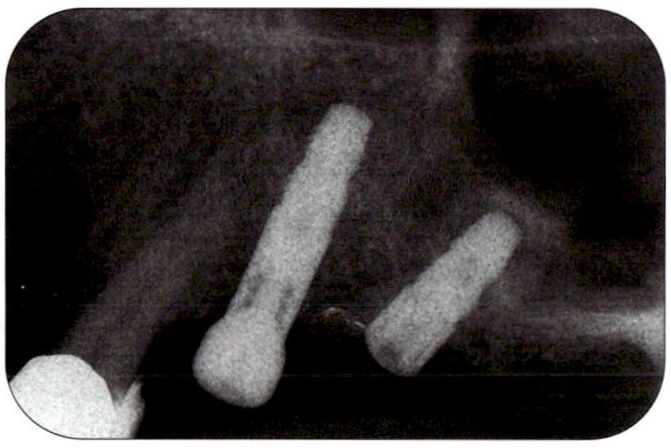

Fig 5-18a *(left)* Indirect sinus lift in a patient. Radiograph for calibration with a measuring pin.

Fig 5-18b *(right)* Indirect sinus lift after implant placement.

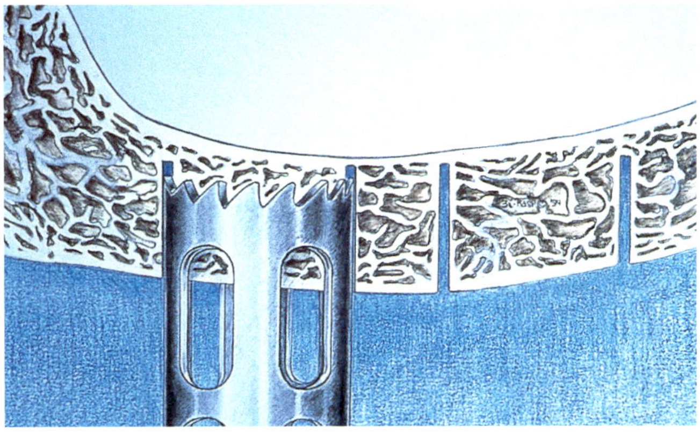

Fig 5-19a "Trephination" of the sinus floor. (Courtesy of Dr Richard Lazzara, 3i Implant Innovations.)

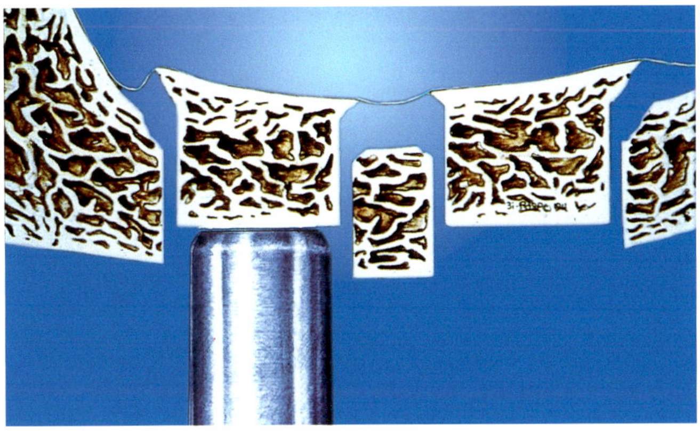

Fig 5-19b Malleting the trephined pieces of bone upward. (Courtesy of Dr Richard Lazzara, 3i Implant Innovations.)

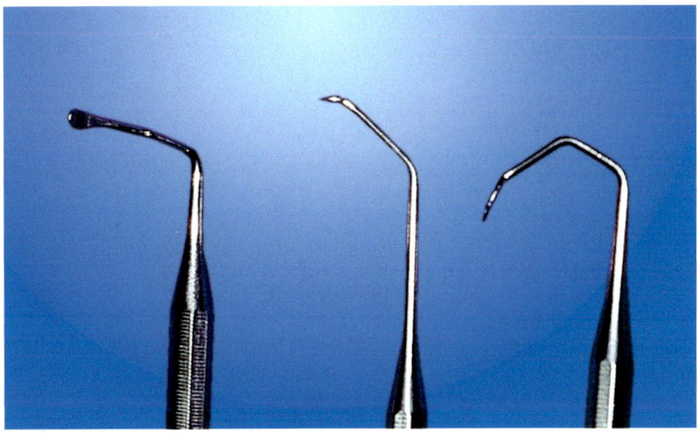

Fig 5-20 Sinus instruments from a sinus lift tray.

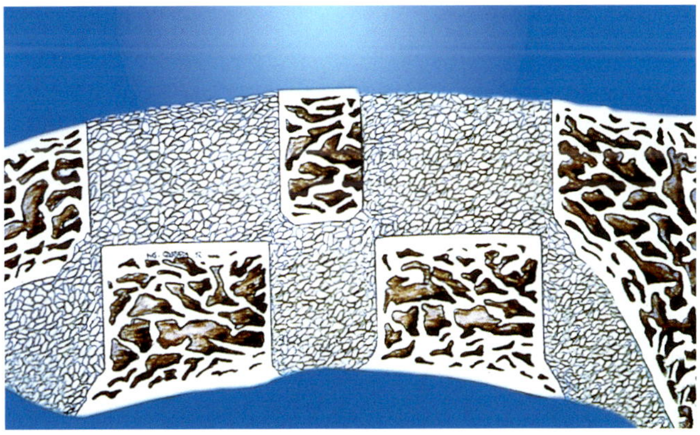

Fig 5-21 Vertical sinus floor elevation as preparation for a future implantation.

21). After a healing time of 4 to 6 months, the implants can be placed.

Figure 5-22 can serve as a guide to identify the individual indications based on their differential diagnosis.

Technique

It is critical to adhere to the individual steps for an indirect vertical sinus floor elevation slavishly, or the procedure will not be successful.

Single-tooth radiographs (full scale), a panoramic radiograph (scale 1:1.25 or other, depending on the dentist's x-ray unit), and a tomogram (scale depending on the x-ray unit) are taken to evaluate the available bone. Whenever possible, the images should be taken with metal balls of 5 mm diameter placed in the patient's mouth to enable the dentist to confirm the scale of the images.

The patient is informed about the procedure, especially the bone malleting, which may cause headaches in the days

Osteotome sinus floor elevation				
< 3 mm	3 mm	5 mm	7 mm	9 mm
sinus lift	sinus lift	sinus lift	sinus lift	sinus lift
Without implant	With implant	With implant	With implant	With implant
		Osteotome sinus lift	Osteotome sinus lift	Implant sinus lift
Future site	Future site			Osteotome sinus lift

Fig 5-22 Indications for open and closed sinus floor elevations.

following the procedure. If the dental assistant holds the patient's head with both hands, this can help to dampen the subjective sensation of "hammering". After anesthesia is administered to the patient, the flap is reflected and fixed buccally with a fixation suture.

The implant position is marked with a bud bur according to the surgical template. The pilot hole is prepared with a 2-mm twist drill to working length, just underneath the sinus floor. This step must be carried out very carefully because the floor of the sinus must not be perforated. A single-tooth radiograph with a calibrated depth gauge is taken and reviewed.

After the depth has been measured, the site is prepared with the no. 1 osteotome to working length. Preparation is continued with the no. 2 osteotome up to working length. The site is also prepared to working length using the no. 3 osteotome, and the floor of the sinus is worked free very carefully. The surgeon should pay attention to the sound when malleting; it gets duller when the bone starts to break. A cold dental mirror can be used to check if perforation has occurred; if this is the case, the mirror will steam up immediately and blood bubbles will emerge from the cavity.

The grafting material is inserted into the cavity with an amalgam carrier and condensed with a plugger. This step is repeated as many times as necessary. About 1 mm of membrane elevation of the nasal mucosa can be expected for each round of filling and condensing. A single-tooth radiograph can be taken, if necessary, to confirm the amount of elevation.

When the floor of the sinus is sufficiently elevated, grafting material is inserted one more time and condensed with the final osteotome (no. 3, 4, or 5, depending on the implant diameter).

The implant is removed from its sterile packing and placed in the prepared site. If a press-fit implant is used, it is carefully tapped to the desired depth. If a screw-type implant is used, the implant is screwed in carefully to avoid perforating the nasal mucosa. The implant is the last osteotome.

The wound is closed with an ordinary suture (eg, Gore-Tex CV-5). Finally, the implant position is confirmed on a panoramic or single-tooth radiograph. Figure 5-23 shows a fiber-optic image of the interior of the maxillary sinus after implantation and sinus lift with osteotomes.

Management of perforations

If the nasal mucosa has been perforated and augmentation material has escaped into the sinus, the implantation procedure must be stopped and tried again after 3 months. As an alternative, the surgeon can immediately create a lateral window, prepare the mucosa of the maxillary sinus, and switch to an open sinus lifting technique. The perforation site is then covered with a collagen membrane.

The patient must be informed about all surgical procedures and their consequences. In the following days, the patient may experience a slight nosebleed, and the graft material may flow out through the nose.

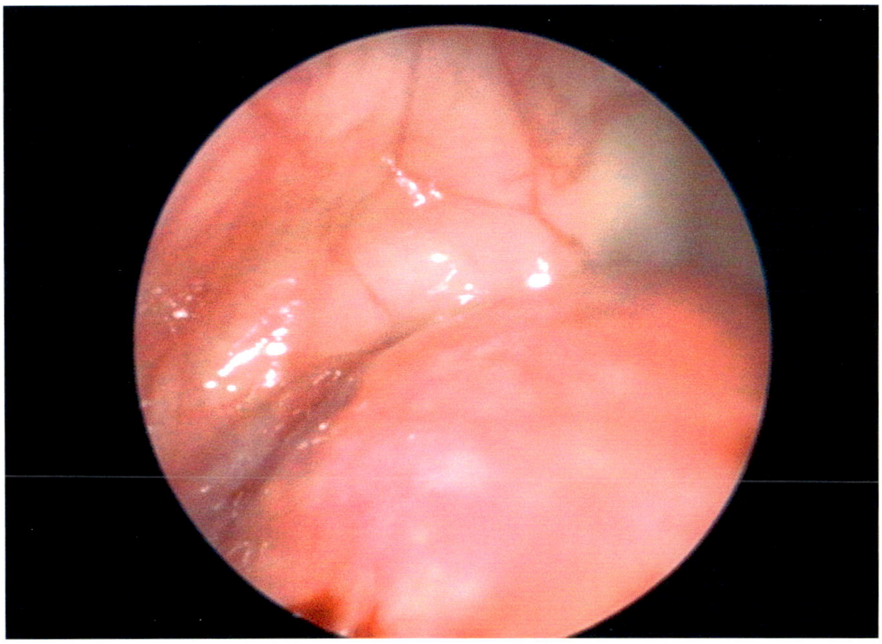

Fig 5-23 Fiber-optic image of the maxillary sinus after osteotome sinus lift and implantation. (Courtesy of Prof W. Engelke, Göttingen University.)

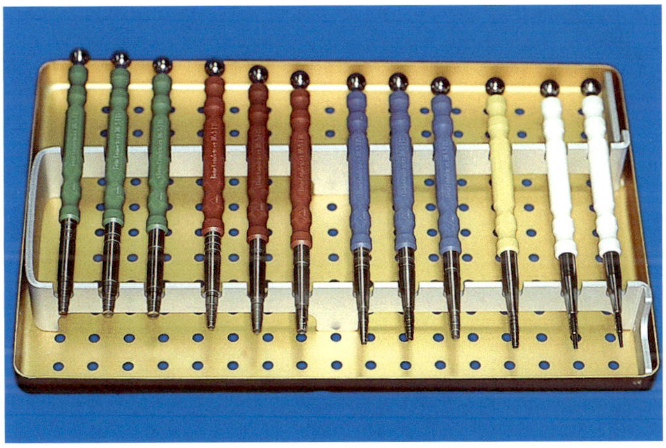

Fig 5-24 Bone condensers for the Frialit 2 system.

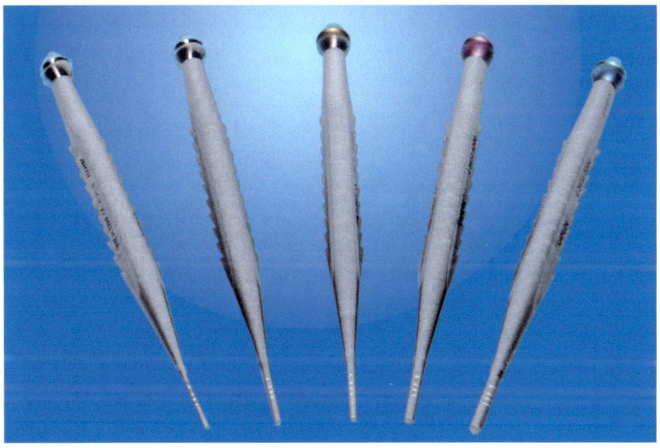

Fig 5-25 Osteotomes for the Camlog system.

Implant-specific osteotomes

The Summers osteotomes shown are suitable for all cylindrical implants with diameters from 3 to 5 mm. The manufacturers offer special osteotomes for other implant shapes. For example, bone condensers are available for the Frialit 2 system (Fig 5-24) and osteotomes for the Camlog system (Fig 5-25).

Conclusion

If an implantation is planned in type D3 or D4 bone, ie, in the maxilla, osteotomes should always be kept ready. It is almost always possible to achieve a significant improvement of the implant site with their help. To avoid failures, the clinician should practice the osteotome technique in training courses, on models, and on animals.

Materials

Summers osteotomes (3i Implant Innovations)
Osteotomes for the Camlog system (Camlog)
Bone condensers for the Frialit 2 system (Friadent)
Sinus floor elevation tray with trephine mills as designed by Kirsch and Ackermann (Friadent)
Bio-Oss augmentation material to be used with autologous bone (Geistlich)
Bio-Gide collagen membrane (Geistlich)
Frios System for pin fixation, if necessary (Friadent)
Gore-Tex CV-5 suture (Gore)

Implant Prosthodontics: Tightening of Screws

Common problem: Loosening or breakage of screws

When Brånemark developed his implant system with a hexagonal head (height 1.75 mm) in the 1970s, his idea was that the hexagonal head should provide only a moderate degree of retention and that the abutment should be fixed with the screw (Fig 5-26). The screw was meant to break, without damaging the implant, if overloaded (Fig 5-27). This was a predetermined breaking point between the implant and the abutment. Moreover, the abutment screws were slotted screws that could only be screwed in with a comparably weak force (maximum of 20 Ncm).

Koch et al wanted overloads to be absorbed by an intramobile element in the IMZ system. Up until the 1990s, they also used slotted screws, which allowed only a small amount of torque to be applied (20 Ncm) (Fig 5-28). Moreover, through the plastic intramobile element, the screw and the abutment were subjected to tensile stress, which frequently led to loosening of the screw. The screws rarely broke; in most cases, if anything broke, it was the intramobile element, which broke because of fatigue (Fig 5-29).

With the Frialit 2 system, which had a hexagonal socket (Fig 5-30), the screws rarely loosened or broke. The system utilized Allen screws that could be tightened somewhat better (25 Ncm).

The problem was the frictional lock between the implant and the abutment: How much centric and eccentric force does an implant endure? When does it break?

In the course of the 1990s, it became clear that implants that are successfully osseointegrated can absorb a lot more force without breaking than was believed. In particular, research involving finite element analysis has contributed greatly to knowledge and understanding of load leveling and force transmission (Figs 5-31a and 5-31b). It was determined that the important factor is not the length of the implant but its diameter in the contact area with the abutment. This load-bearing area should be equivalent to the diameter of the tooth at the level of the gingiva and thus lead to an ideal distribution of pressure on the implant with different masticatory forces (Fig 5-32a). This idea can be expressed as $P = F/A$, ie, the pressure equals the force divided by the unit of area. The larger the area, the more force can be absorbed.

Correspondingly, in most implant systems, it has now become commonplace to allow a choice of appropriate diameter for the tooth to be replaced (3.25 to 6.5 mm) (Fig 5-32b). Implant lengths of 10 to 13 mm are considered successful; longer implants are unnecessary, and shorter ones can be risky.

The question of whether the systems with an internal or an external hexagon were better was clearly decided in favor of the internal hexagon. Most manufacturers of implants with external hexagons now also offer internal hexagons, and the new implant systems exclusively have internal ones (Fig 5-33).

Given this knowledge and experience, how can the clinician prevent screws from coming loose or breaking?

Proven solution: Tightening of the screws with a defined torque

The solution is actually very much reminiscent of automobile technology. When new tires or wheels are put on a car, the garage has to tighten the wheel nuts with a defined torque (80 Nm), with the help of a torque wrench, and must check them again after a few miles. If there is an accident because the wheel nuts were inadequately tightened, in some countries the garage may be fully liable. Dentists should act accordingly in implant prosthodontics.

Cemented versus screw-retained crowns

Because the internal systems have proven so reliable that few screws loosen, in most cases the implant superstructure is now cemented instead of screw retained. Temporary cements, such as zinc oxide–eugenol cements, have proven inadequate for this application, because they can loosen very suddenly and tend to leak. The material of choice is Durelon, a carboxylate cement (Fig 5-34). It provides a tight seal and has sufficient adhesive force, and the crowns cemented with it can be removed. To ensure this, however, the crowns must be brushed with only a thin layer of cement and only in the lower part.

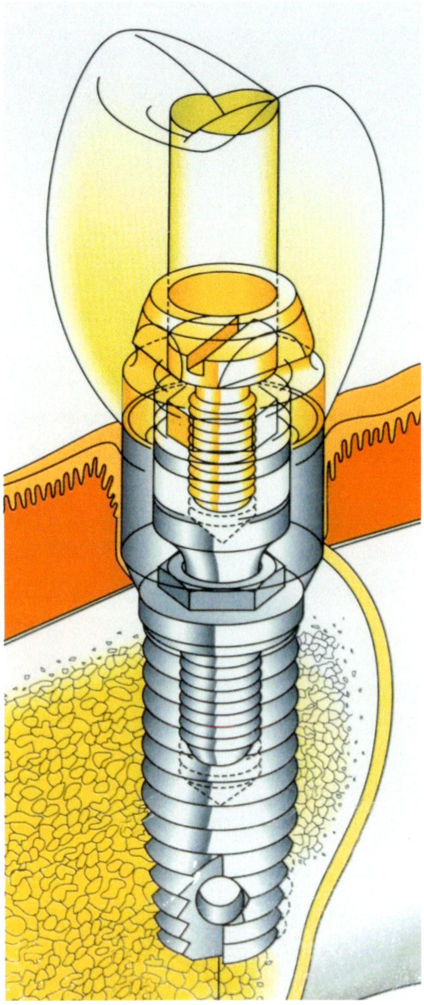

Fig 5-26 Brånemark implant with mesostructure and crown.

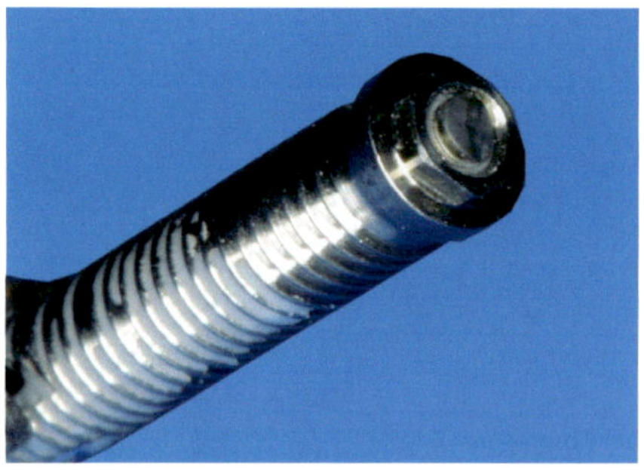

Fig 5-27 Broken screw of a external hexagonal implant. The implant had been supporting a molar crown and had to be explanted.

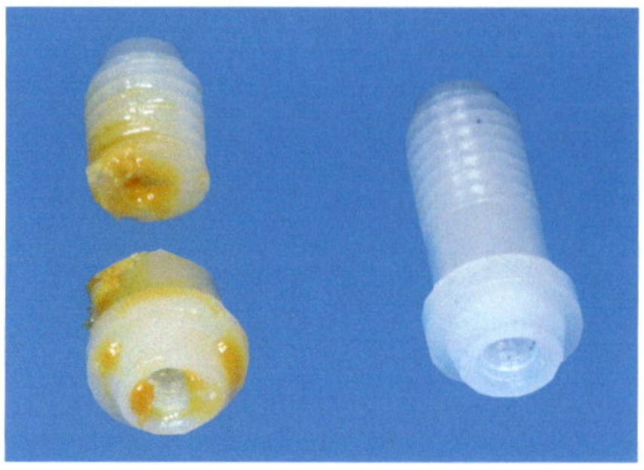

Fig 5-29 Broken intramobile element.

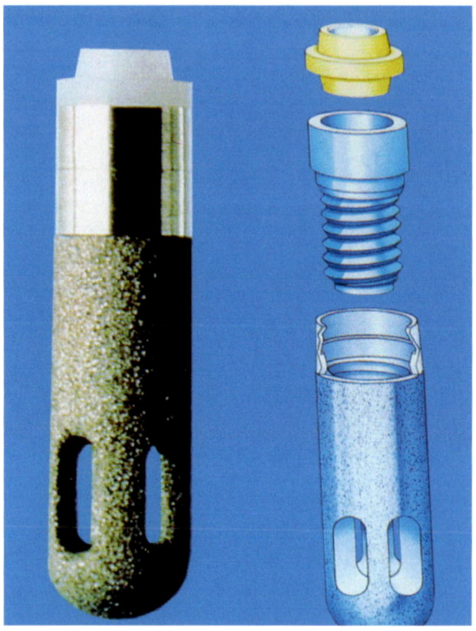

Fig 5-28 An intramobile element and its successor, the intramobile connector, which was developed because frequently the intramobile elements broke, provided inadequate hygiene, or came loose (see Fig 5-29).

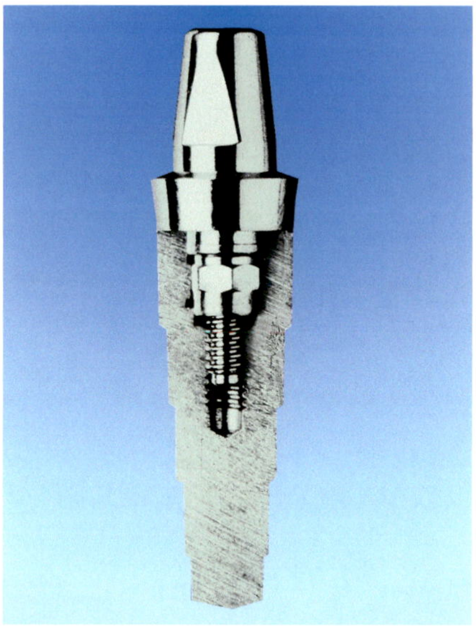

Fig 5-30 Implant with internal hexagonal socket.

Horizontal screws have not proven very useful. They are very difficult to screw into position inside the patient's mouth. Usually they are small slotted screws and their slots are ruined very quickly. Moreover, there is a higher risk that the patient will swallow or aspirate these screws.

Even cemented superstructures still have a vertical screw connection of the abutment. Therefore, the question arises as to what kind of screw and tool should be used, at what amount of torque, to prevent the screws from loosening or to minimize the occurrence of loose screws.

Table 5-1 Screws and their respective maximum torques

Type of screw	Maximum torque (Ncm)
Slotted	20
Phillips	30
Allen	60
Square socket	70

Selection of screws

Selection of screws is very easy if the list of different types of screws and their maximum torque in Table 5-1 is used as a guide. Slotted screws provide no adhesion to the screwdriver, while Phillips screws provide only some adhesion. It is therefore advisable to use screws with a hexagonal or square socket. Screws with a square socket, however, are more difficult to feel and unscrew inside their deep shaft. Because forces of up to 70 Ncm within the

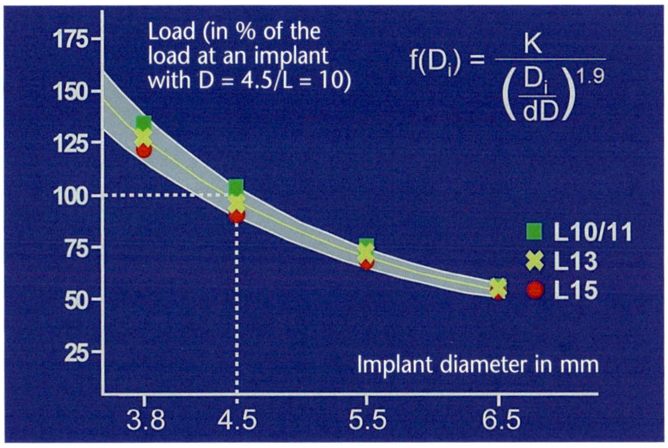

Fig 5-31a Influence of the implant diameter on the load to the bone. From Vizethum et al.

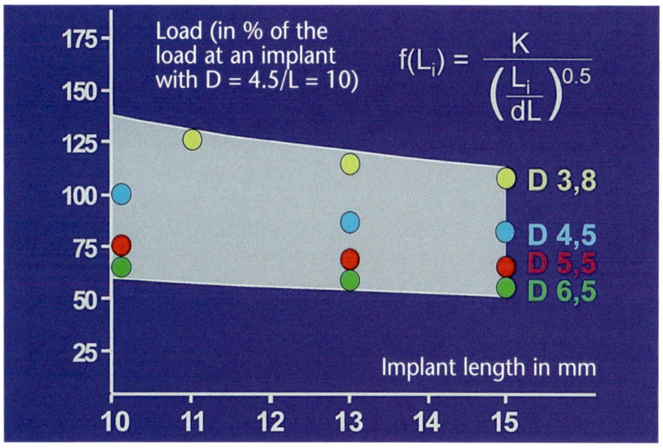

Fig 5-31b Influence of the implant length on the load to the bone. From Vizethum et al.

Fig 5-32a *(left)* Frialit 2: load-bearing area for the crown.

Fig 5-32b *(top right)* Implant diameter (D) analogous to the tooth diameter.

Fig 5-33 *(bottom right)* Camlog tube-in-tube system.

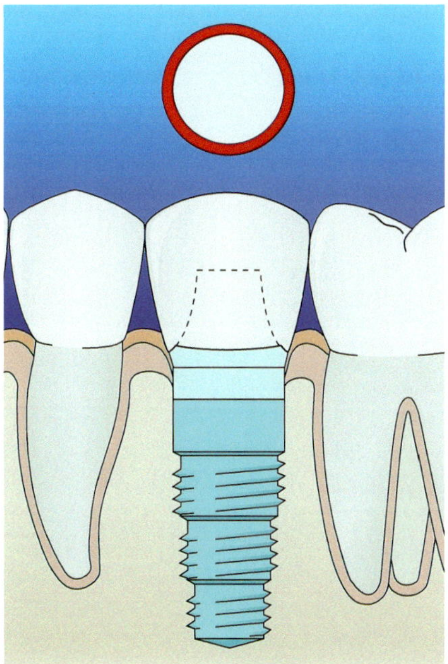

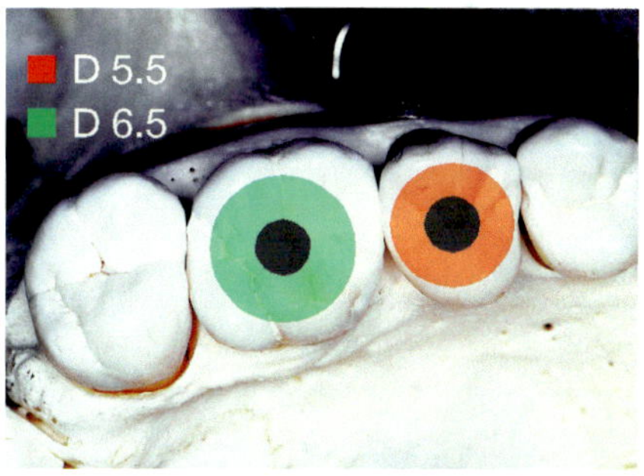

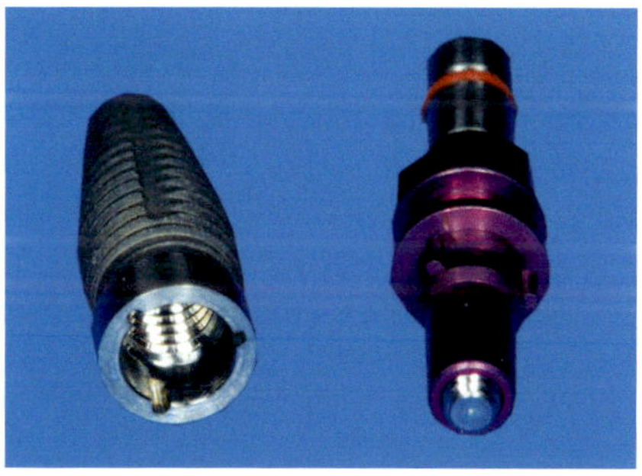

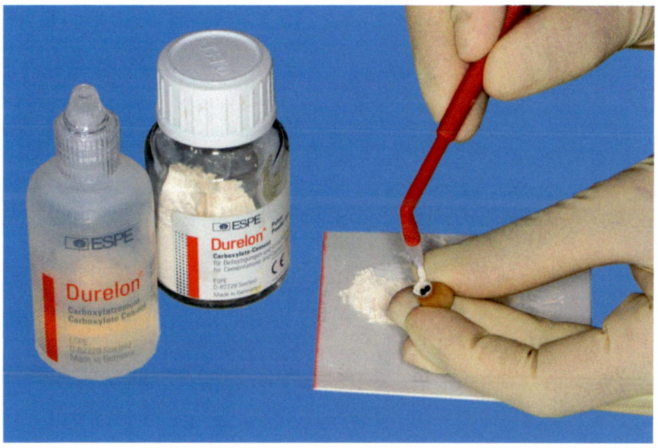

Fig 5-34 The crown is brushed with Durelon.

patient's mouth are not only unnecessary but also rather dangerous, the hexagonal socket screw is certainly the best choice (Fig 5-35). In the engineering world, screws known as *TORX screws* are utilized which allow a torque of more than 100 Ncm (Fig 5-36). In implant dentistry, this type of screw is only used with the ITI Bonefit implants.

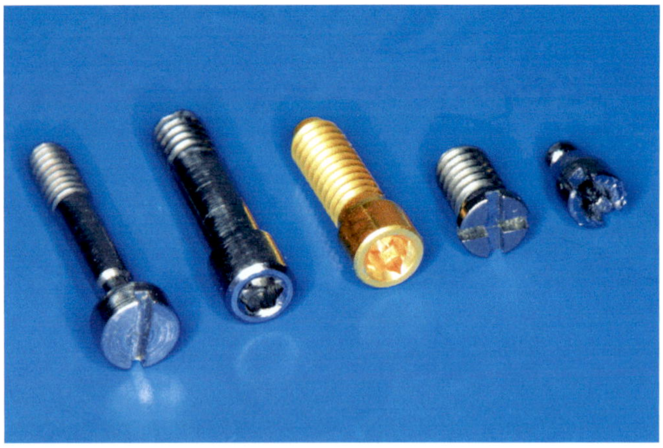

Fig 5-35 Different types of screws: *(left to right)* slotted screw, Allen screw, square socket screw, Phillips screw, horizontal screw (combined slotted and Allen screw).

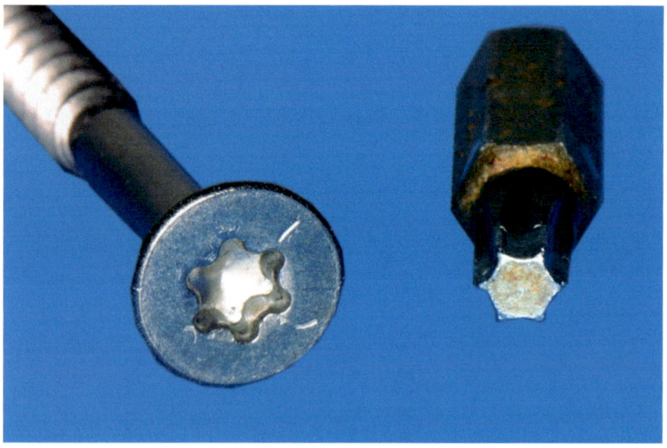

Fig 5-36 TORX screw with driver bit (building supply store).

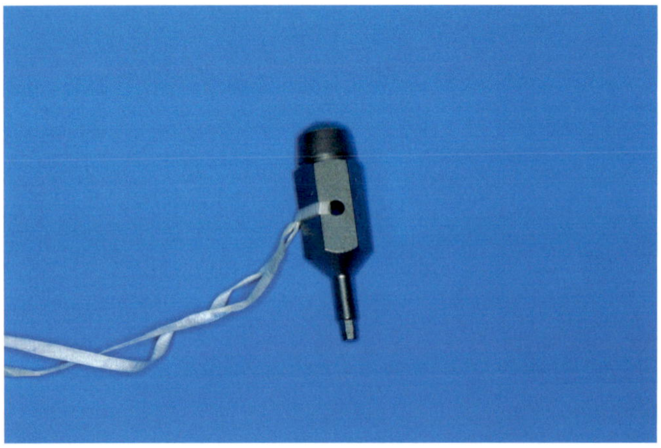

Fig 5-37a Manual screwdriver secured with dental floss.

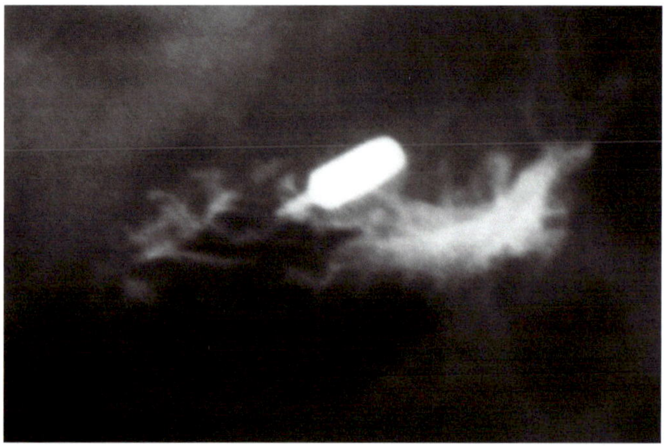

Fig 5-37b Manual screwdriver bit in the stomach of a patient. The bit was swallowed because it had not been secured.

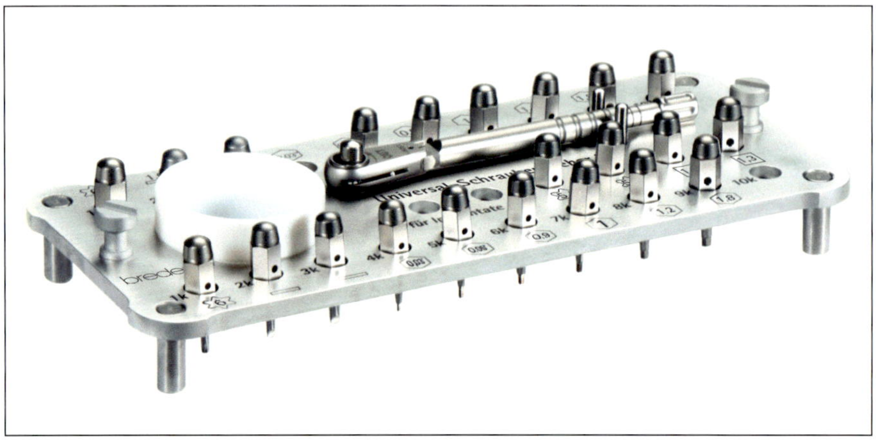

Fig 5-38 Ratchet with Bredent screwdriver bits.

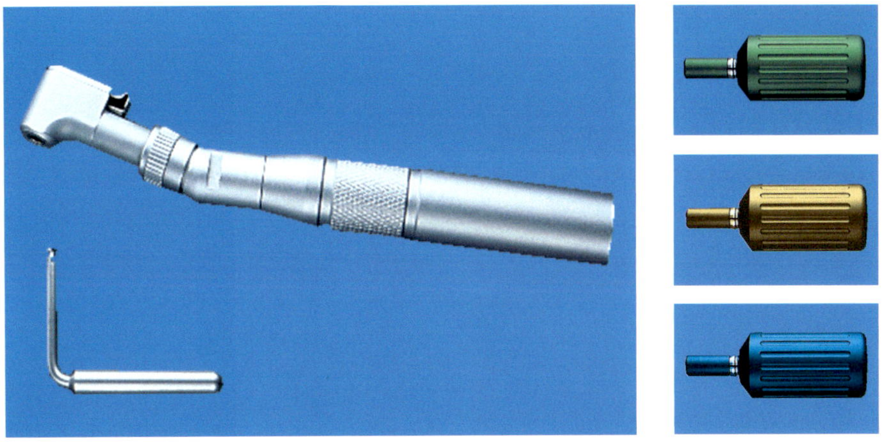

Fig 5-39a *(left)* Offset screwdriver (3i Implant Innovations).
Fig 5-39b *(top right)* Adapter for 10 N/cm torque.
Fig 5-39c *(center right)* Adapter for 20 N/cm torque.
Fig 5-39d *(bottom right)* Adapter for 30 N/cm torque.

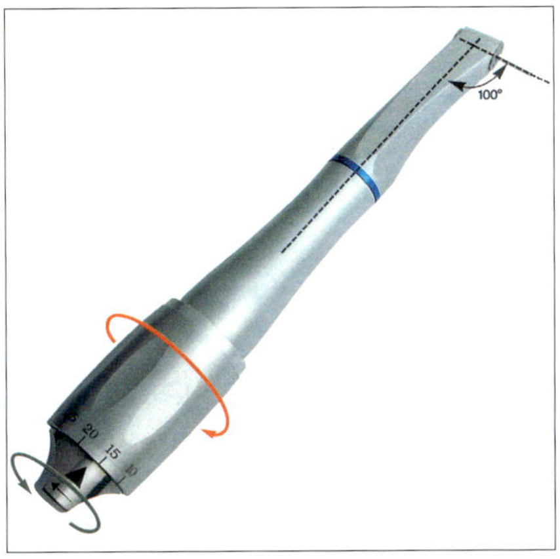

Fig 5-40 *(left)* Offset screwdriver with adjustable torque (American Dental).

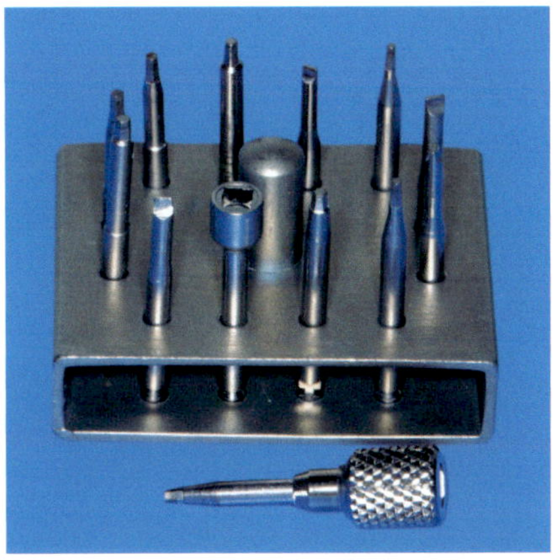

Fig 5-41 *(right)* Bücking kit for use with power tools for dentistry or with offset screwdrivers; a handle for manual use is shown in front.

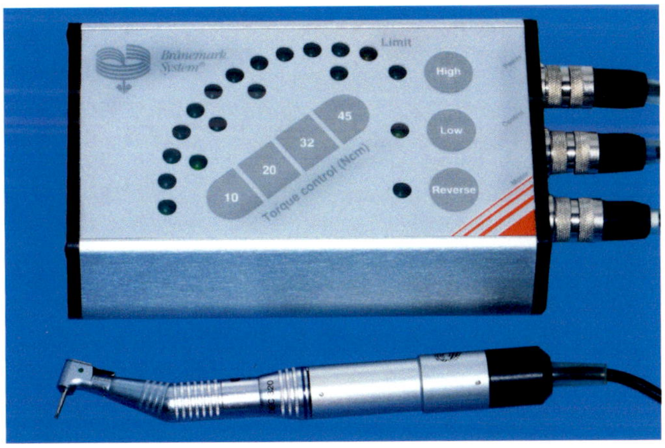

Fig 5-42 Brånemark Torque Controller.

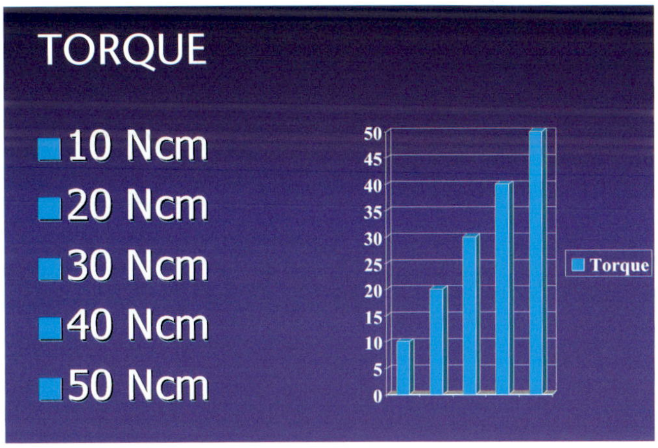

Fig 5-43 Torques used in dentistry.

Selection of tools

A clinician who places many implant-supported restorations and use these kinds of screws every day will find that the manual screwdrivers are very difficult and unwieldy to handle, especially in the posterior region of the mouth. Moreover, these screwdrivers should always be secured with dental floss to prevent the patient from swallowing or even aspirating the tool (Figs 5-37a and 5-37b). Because the dental floss tends to wind itself around the screwdriver and the screw and makes tightening the screws very difficult, many dentists dispense with this

Torque (N/cm)	Application
10	– Healing caps – Healing abutments – Impression posts – Horizontal retainer screws
20	– Two-stage implants – Removable abutments
30	– One-stage implants with healing abutments – Abutments for cemented superstructures
40	– One-stage implants with provisionally fixed restorations out of occlusion
50	– Immediately loaded implants with bar-retained superstructure, placed intraforaminally in the mandible

Tabelle 5-2 Recommended torgue values.

safety measure and risk swallowing or aspiration of the instrument by their patients and thus very serious legal consequences. Manual screwdrivers should be used only in the anterior region, where they can be secured at the floor of the mouth with an opened surgical sponge or with a gauze pad.

In the posterior region of the mouth, it is better to use ratchets (Fig 5-38) or offset screwdrivers (Figs 5-39 to 5-41) that are turned manually. There are simple tools without torque control and more elaborate ones with adjustable torque. They can be used with any screwdrivers that can be connected to a handpiece. To permanently screw in the vertical screws, the author recommends use of an implantation unit (Fig 5-42) with defined torques of 10 to 50 Ncm. Figure 5-43 depicts the torques used in dentistry.

The appropriate values for torque for different parts are shown in Table 5-2. These torque values should be used with caution, because the quality of the available bone must be considered. An osseointegrated implant in the maxilla may start to rotate when 30 Ncm of torque is applied to it. Currently there is also some discussion about whether torques of more than 20 Ncm for the insertion of screw-type implants cause pressure necrosis of the bone at the bone-implant interface. The screws should therefore be turned back one-quarter turn after they are screwed in, to avoid pressure on the bone.

The special characteristic of titanium known as the *self-lubricating effect* can cause the implant and abutment to be welded together as in a cold welding process; in this case, the abutment cannot be loosened again. Therefore, well-dosed torques between 10 and 30 Ncm should be used.

Units with torque control can be obtained from various manufacturers.

Materials

Set of long screwdrivers for slotted, Phillips, and Allen screws, for use on models and not inside the mouth (available at building supply stores)

Short and long screwdrivers for manual use (As the number of patients with implants is increasing and patients become increasingly mobile, it is useful to have the appropriate screwdrivers for the most common implant systems at hand. Many screwdrivers can be used for several systems. The author keeps screwdrivers available to work with the following systems: Brånemark [Nobel Biocare], Frialit 2 [Friadent], Paragon, Steri-Oss, Camlog [Camlog], Hati [Thommen], Osseotite [3i Implant Innovations], ITI Bonefit [Straumann], and IMZ [Friadent].)

Set of screwdriver bits with ratchet (Bredent)

Offset screwdrivers (3i Implant Innovations, Nobel Biocare, and American Dental)

Set of screwdriver bits for offset screwdrivers for all established systems (Bredent)

Implantation unit with torque control (Available from W&H, Nouvag, Nobel Biocare, XO Care, KaVo, and Braun Aesculap. This is only a selection of the torque controlled units; many other very good units are available for dental use.)

Durelon carboxylate cement, film thickness 10 µm (3M ESPE)

Immediate Implant Placement

Common problem: High risk and difficult placement of immediately loaded implants

In the course of many implantology conferences, there are presentations in which carefully selected case reports are shown to demonstrate the immediate placement of implants and abutments and even immediate loading of implants. These procedures are described as the routine and daily work of an implant dentist, as if to say, "Oh, you're not doing this yet?" After the conference, the humble, normal implant dentist returns to the office, tries the procedures shown at the conference, and is faced with enormous problems and any number of treatment failures. To some degree, this phenomenon is certainly due to speakers who want to distinguish themselves, but to a greater degree it is because the time constraints of such presentations prevent the speakers from adequately discussing the criteria for implementing the procedure. It is indeed possible to place implants successfully right after tooth extraction, but first the following questions must be answered:

1. Is the extraction socket free of inflammation, or does it instead show a chronic or even acute inflammation?
2. Are the bone walls around the socket strong enough?
3. Is there enough bone for an implantation beyond the apex to ensure primary stability of the immediately placed implant?
4. What kind of bone quality is present?
5. How can the height, width, and profile of the available bone be analyzed?
6. Which implant length and diameter are required?
7. How great are the distances to the adjacent teeth?
8. How deep does the implant need to be placed? How deep can it be placed?
9. How can the tooth be extracted without damaging the socket?
10. What kind of provisional restoration is suitable?

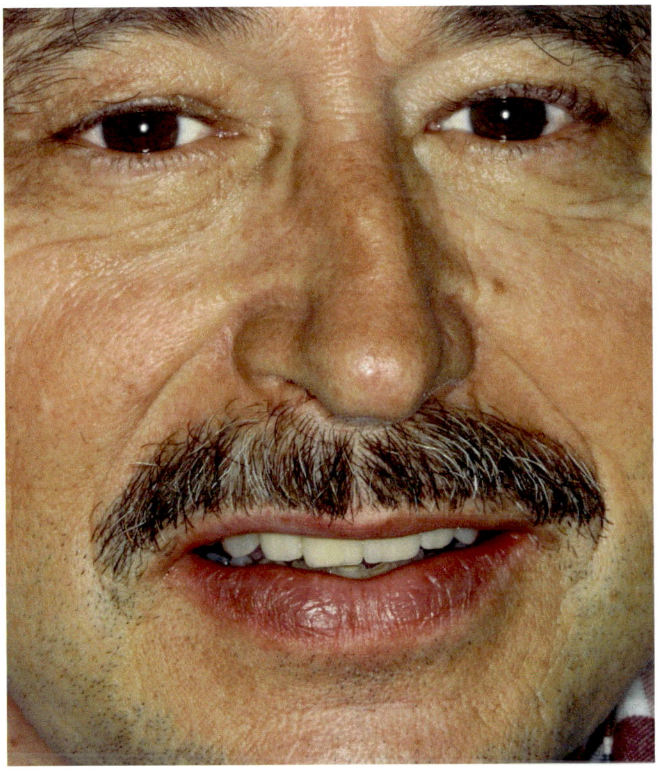

Fig 5-44a The 58-year-old patient has a central incisor that must be extracted.

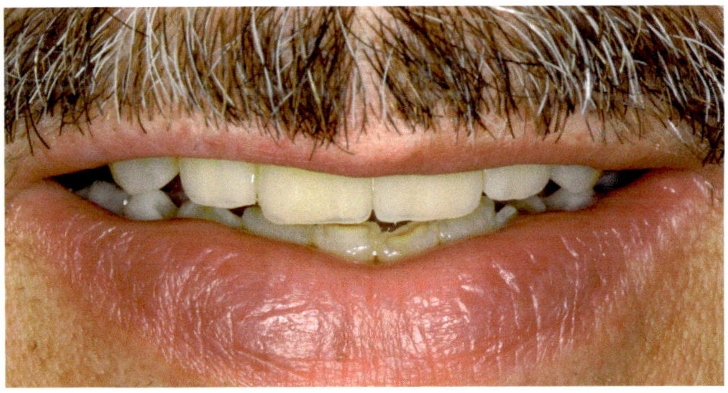

Fig 5-44b Patient's lip line.

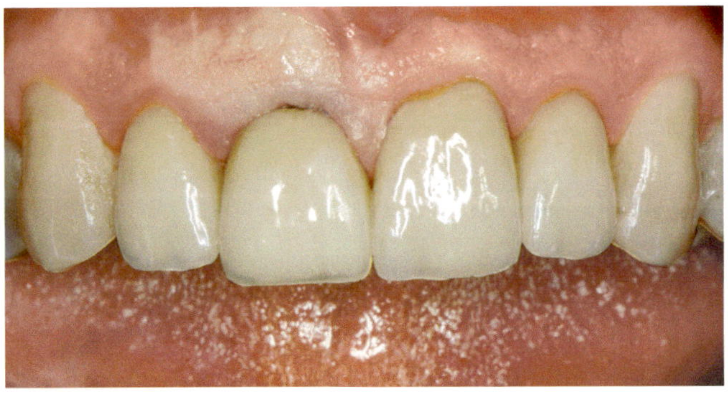

Fig 5-44c Maxillary anterior area.

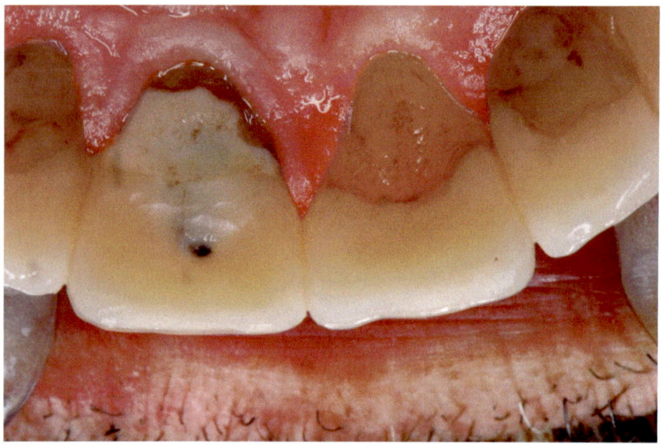

Fig 5-44d Palatal view of the maxillary anterior teeth.

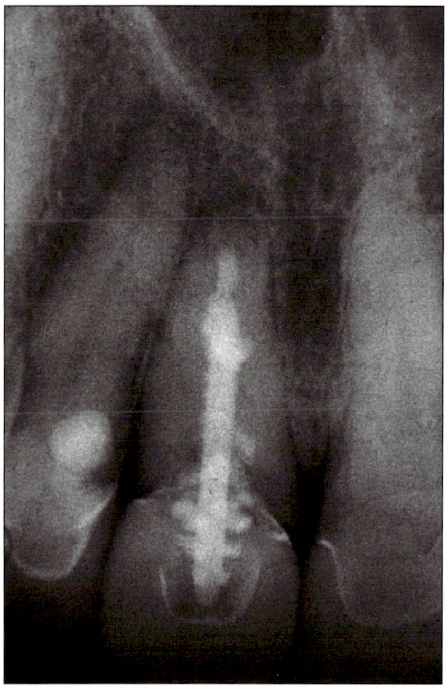

Fig 5-44e Single-tooth radiograph of the affected area.

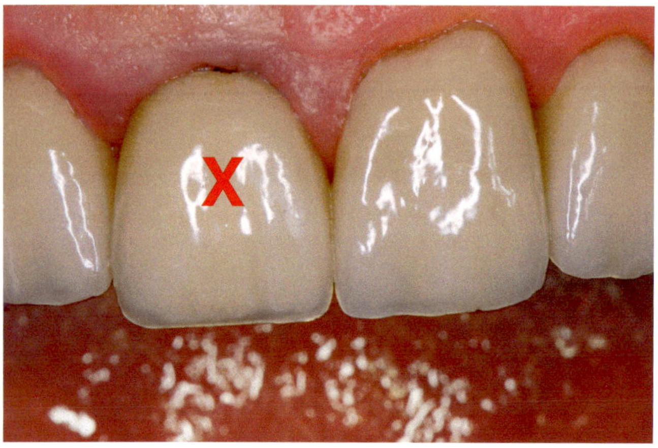

Fig 5-44f The maxillary right central incisor is to be extracted.

Proven solution: Careful planning, gentle extraction, and exact implantation

The following case report will show how an immediate implantation can be a success if it is planned and conducted carefully.

An all-ceramic crown was placed on the maxillary right central incisor in a 58-year-old patient several years previously. The tooth required endodontic treatment because of pulpitis, which had probably been caused by a blow during sports activities. The tooth was restored with a direct core buildup. This restoration worked well for a year, until the apex became very sensitive to pressure. The apex had changed for the worse to such an extent that an apicoectomy had to be performed.

After a few months, in which the patient had temporarily taken antibiotics, the tenderness in the apical region returned. This was the typical course of a tooth that had been "treated to death." A revision apicoectomy promised little success. As a result, after having been informed in detail, the patient decided to have the tooth extracted and an implant placed immediately (Figs 5-44a to 5-44f).

To remove the clinical crown, an extraction forceps for anterior teeth was wrapped with first-aid tape to prevent damage to the crown. The post crown was removed with a rotational movement (Fig 5-44g). To allow extraction of the root, the periodontal fibers were severed with the help of a periotome like the one designed by Schulte (Figs 5-44h to 5-44j). To prevent the alveolus from being damaged, under no circumstances should the tooth be luxated when it is removed.

To protect the alveolus, the remaining root was cut into quarters with the help of a bone bur used in a high-speed handpiece with water cooling (Figs 5-44k to 5-44m). The individual parts of the root were removed with diamond-coated tweezers and checked for completeness (Figs 5-44n and 44o). After the extraction, the socket was inspected carefully (Fig 5-44p).

In this case, the labial portion of the bone was reduced but completely intact on bone sounding. Incision with a scalpel, especially vertically on the labial side, should be avoided by all means.

The position for the guide drill was determined following the principle of the "esthetic window": 1.5 mm away from the cervical tangent on the labial side, at a position that was flush with the cervical tangent on the palatal side (Fig 5-44q). An implant with a diameter of 4.5 mm was used to enable a distance of 1.5 mm to the adjacent teeth (Fig 5-44r).

The pilot hole was prepared with a 2.0-mm drill (Fig 5-44s) and broadened with the next drill to 3.2 mm (Fig

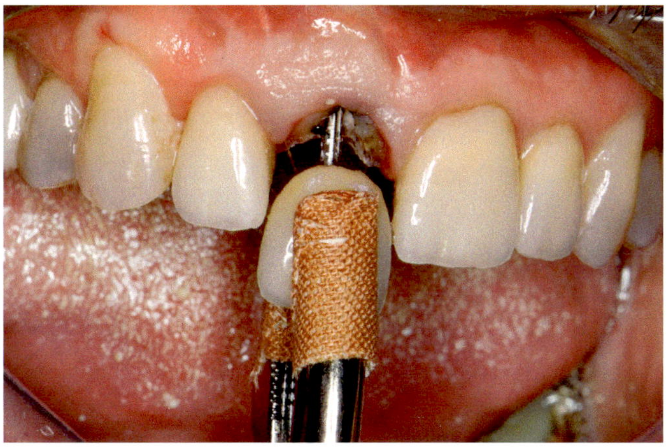

Fig 5-44g The post crown is removed with the wrapped extraction forceps.

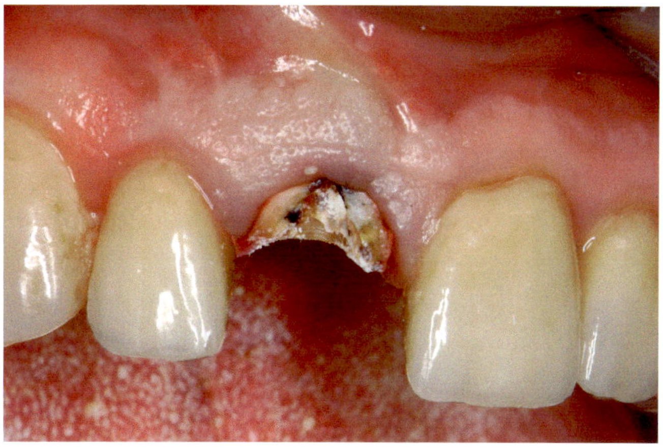

Fig 5-44h Remnant of the root.

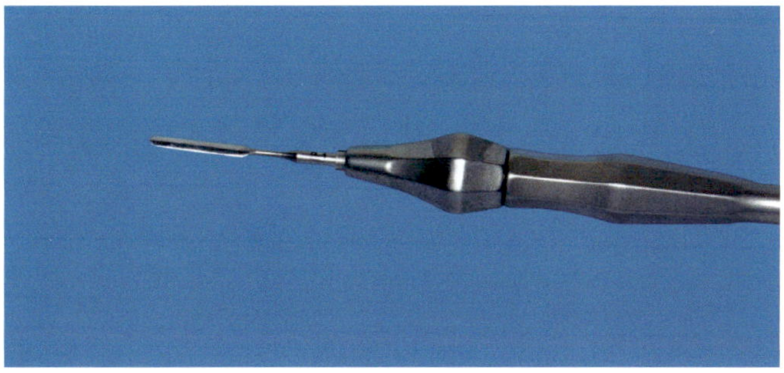

Fig 5-44i Periotome designed by Schulte.

Fig 5-44j *(right)* The circular fibers are carefully dissected with a periotome.

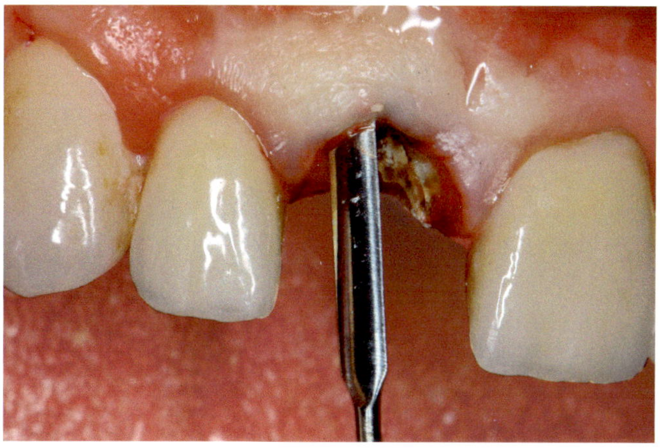

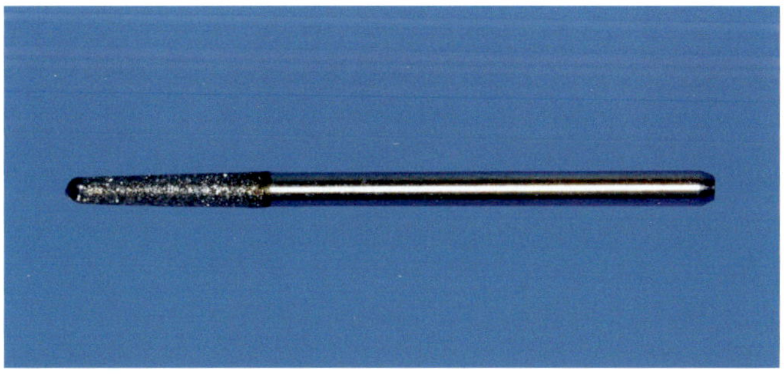

Fig 5-44k Extra-long bone bur.

Fig 5-44l *(right)* The root is cut into four parts with the extra-long bone bur.

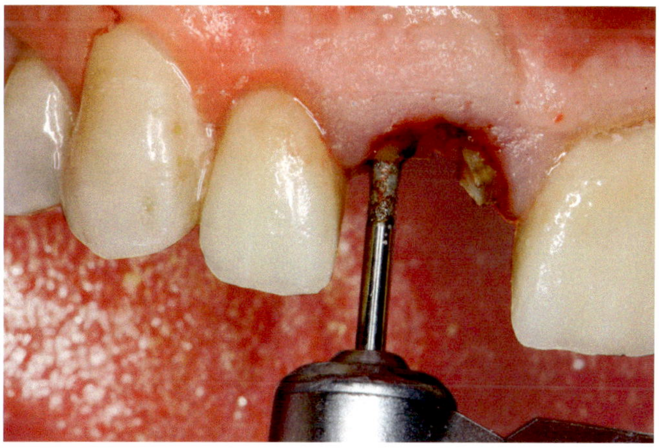

5-44t). To ensure sufficient primary stability, a 4.5-mm drill from the Xive system was used to prepare to a defined depth of 15.0 mm up to the floor of the nose (Figs 5-44u and 5-44v). The Xive implant was removed from its sterile packaging, taken from its glass vial with the handpiece, and gently inserted with slow speed using a torque of 30 Ncm (Fig 5-44w to 5-44bb). The implant position (height, distance, and depth) was checked (Figs 5-44cc to 5-44ee).

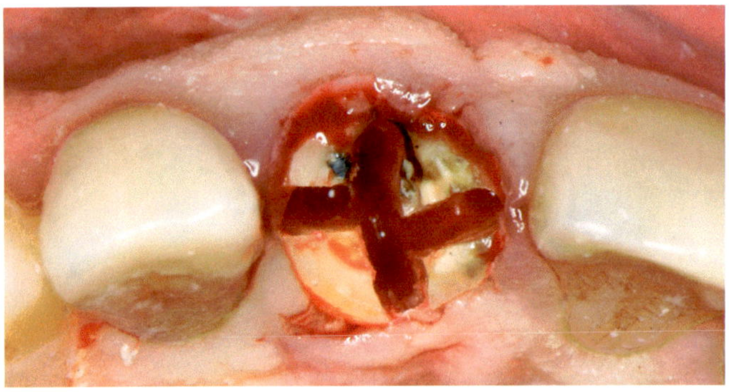

Fig 5-44m The root has been cut into quarters.

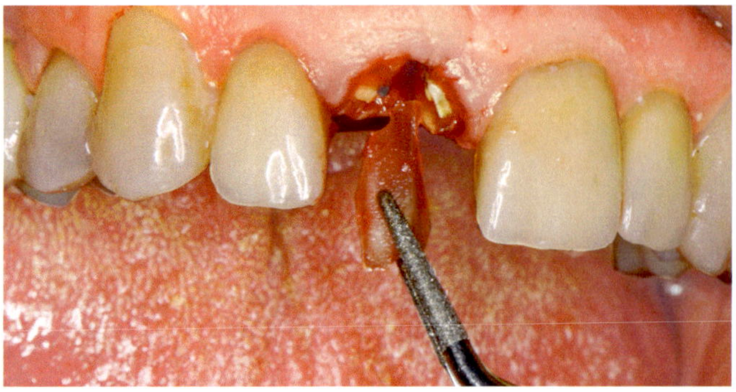

Fig 5-44n The root remnants are extracted with diamond-coated tweezers.

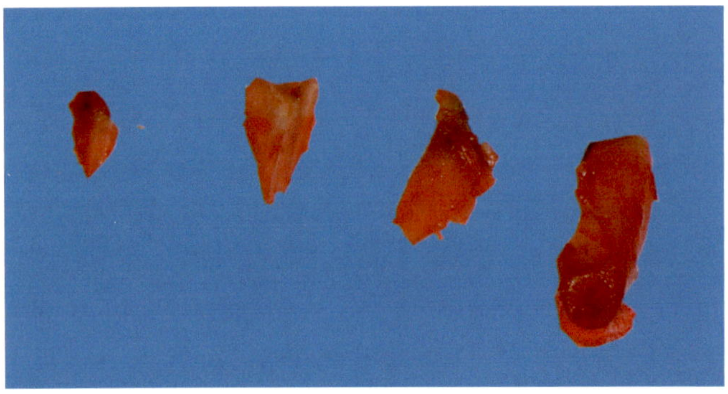

Fig 5-44o The extracted parts of the root are examined to ensure that they are complete.

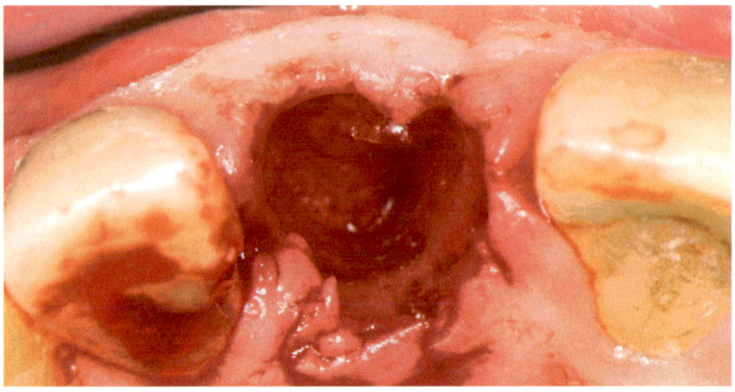

Fig 5-44p The empty socket is inspected.

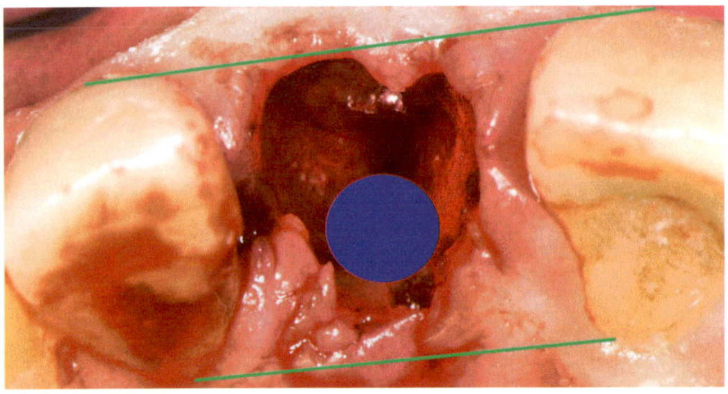

Fig 5-44q The exact location for the pilot hole is planned.

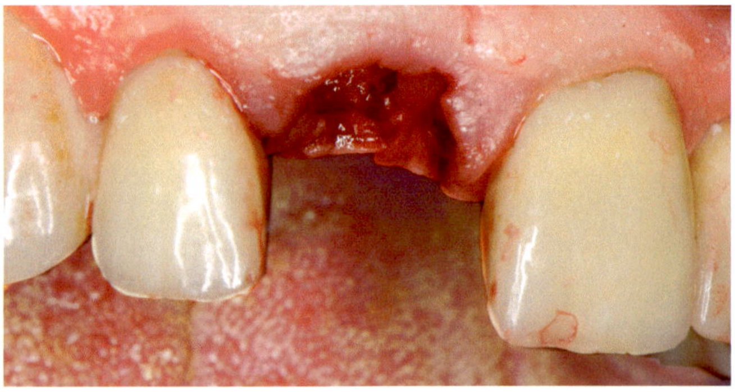

Fig 5-44r The implant diameter is chosen so that the distances to the adjacent teeth are correct.

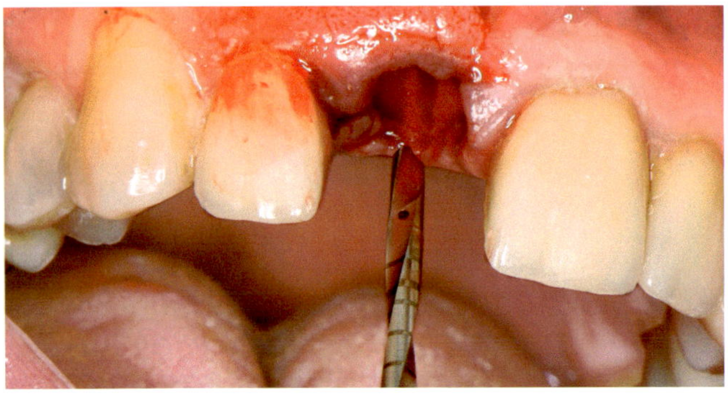

Fig 5-44s The 2-mm pilot hole is drilled.

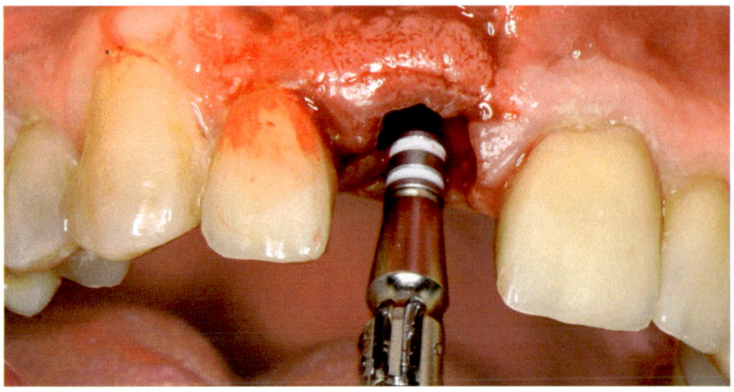

Fig 5-44t The pilot hole is enlarged to 3.2 mm.

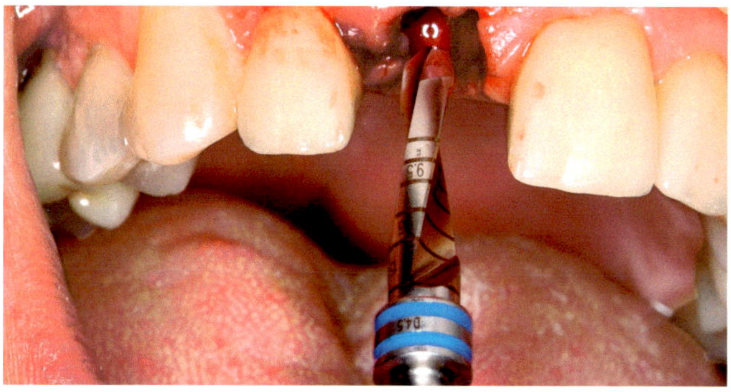

Fig 5-44u The hole is enlarged to 4.5 mm, the largest diameter.

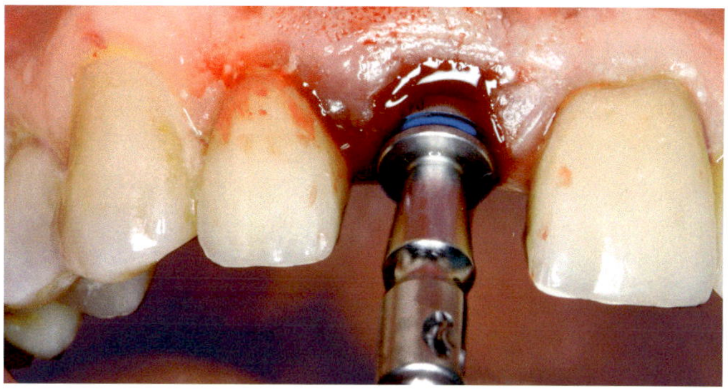

Fig 5-44v Drilling is continued to 15.0 mm depth, up to the floor of the nose.

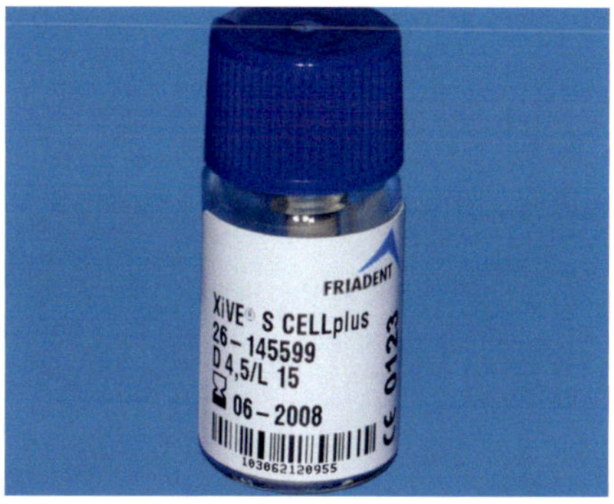

Fig 5-44w Xive implant in its sterile pack.

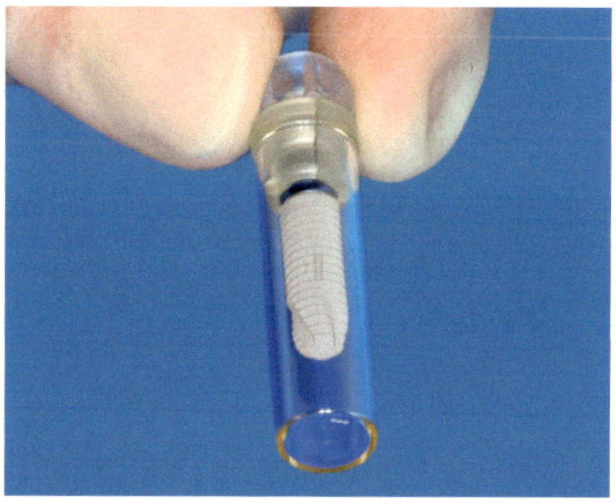

Fig 5-44x The vial containing the implant is removed.

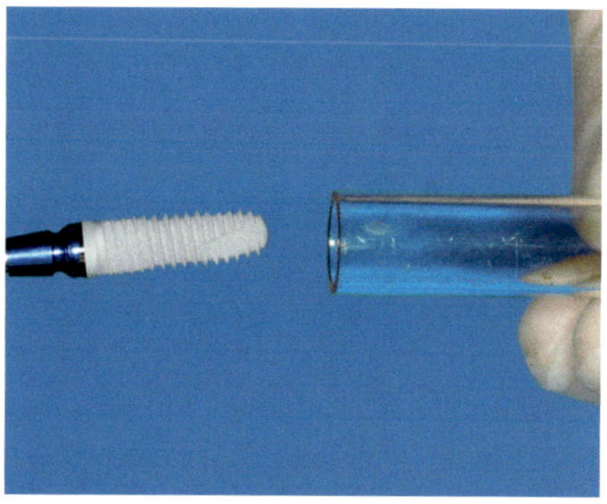

Fig 5-44y The implant is picked up with the handpiece.

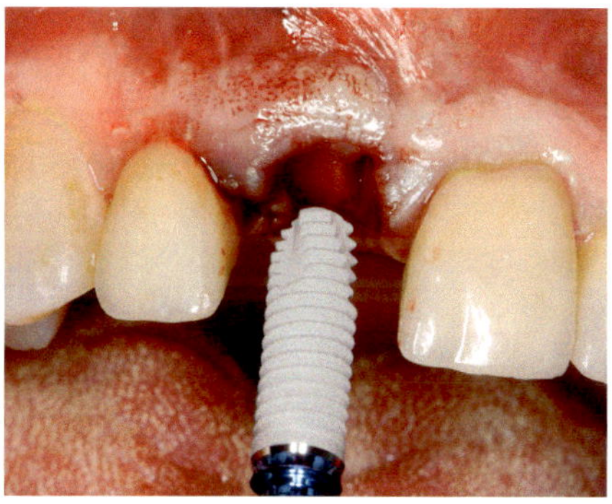

Fig 5-44z The implant is gently placed in the socket.

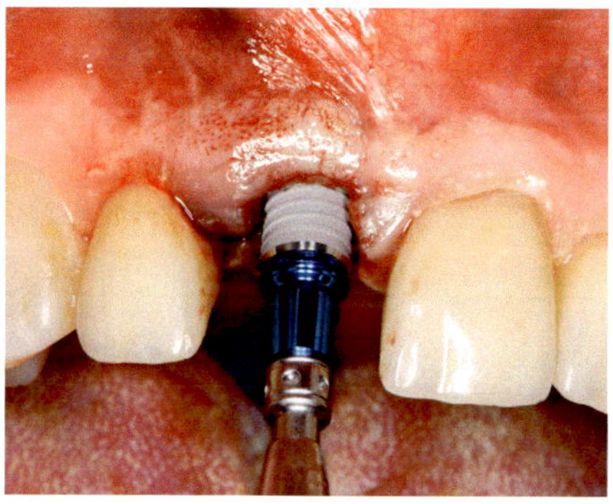

Fig 5-44aa The implant is inserted carefully and slowly.

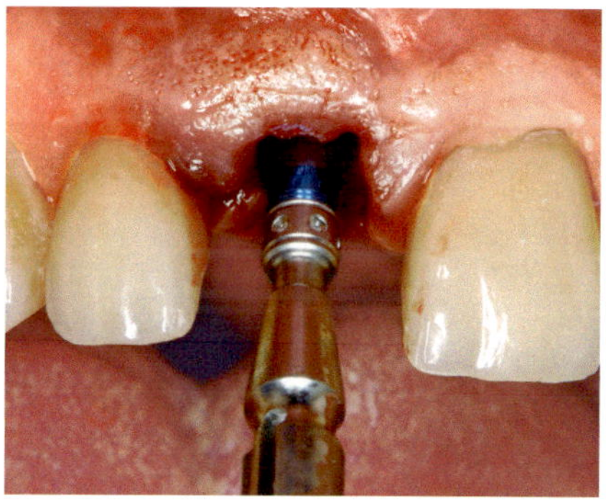

Fig 5-44bb The implant is tightened carefully.

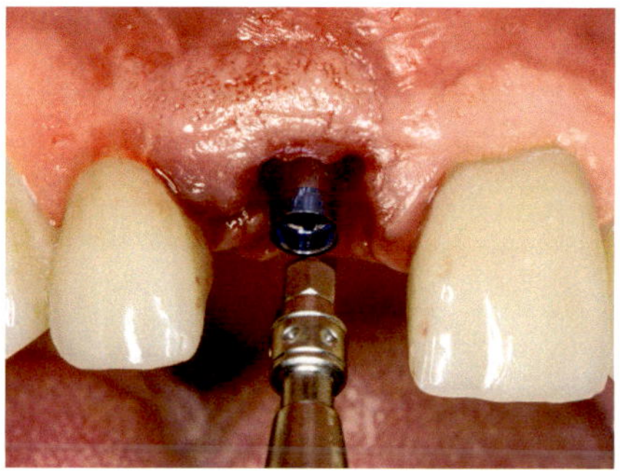

Fig 5-44cc The placement of the implant is complete.

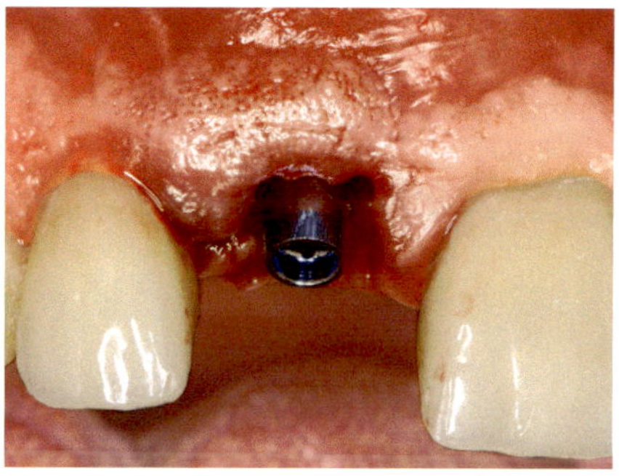

Fig 5-44dd Labial view of the fully inserted implant.

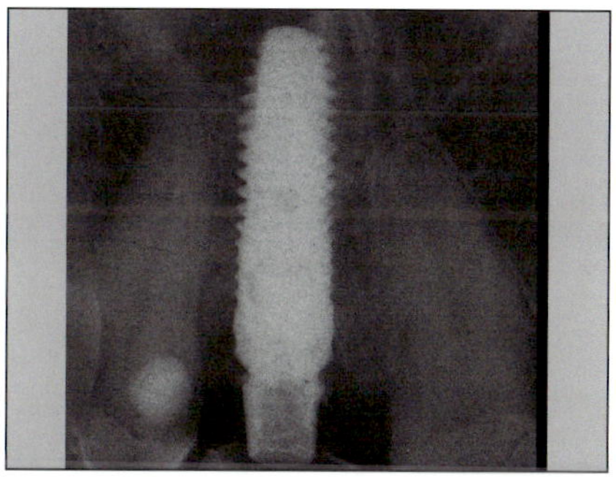

Fig 5-44ee Radiographic view of the implant.

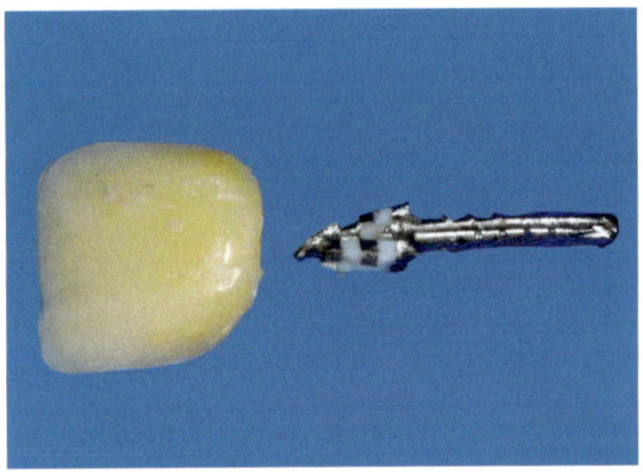

Fig 5-44ff After removal of the pin, the natural tooth crown is reworked to serve as a provisional restoration.

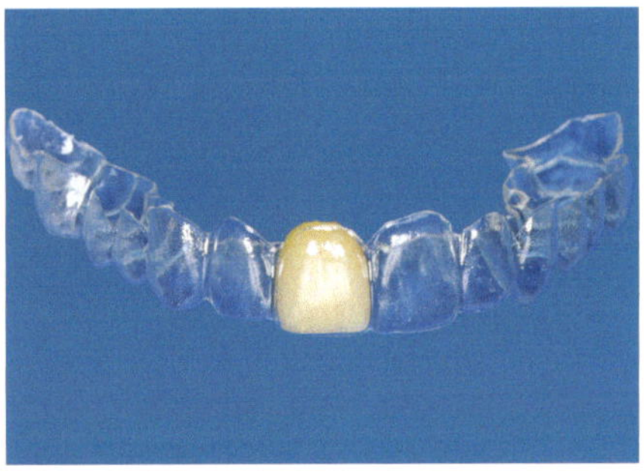

Fig 5-44gg The crown is placed in the vacuform template.

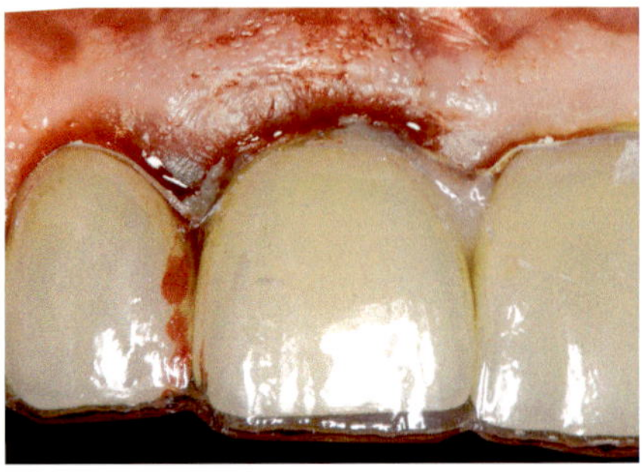

Fig 5-44hh The crown is covered with acrylic resin and placed in the splint.

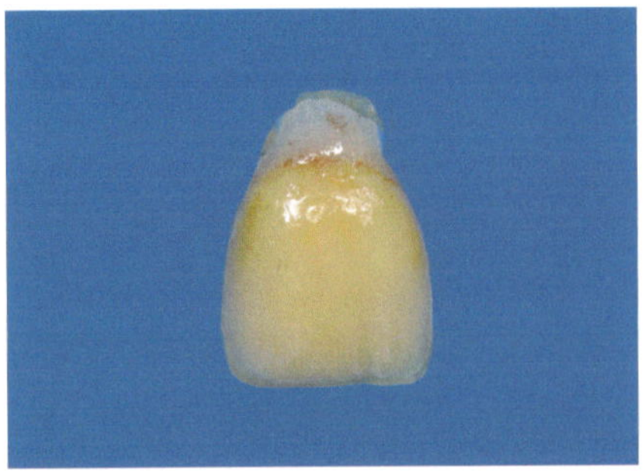

Fig 5-44ii The crown is finished with a subgingival elongation.

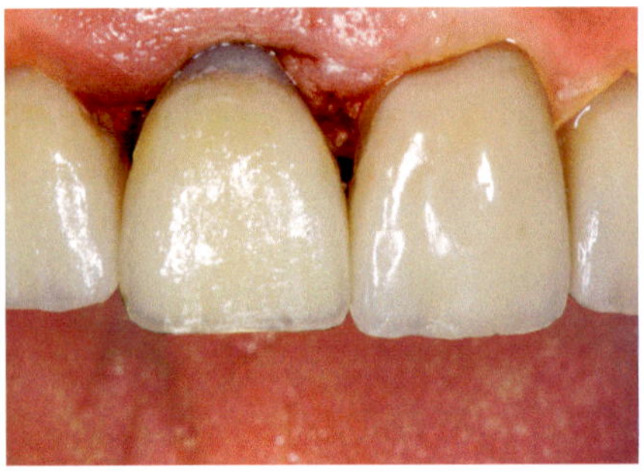

Fig 5-44jj The crown is cemented with temporary cement.

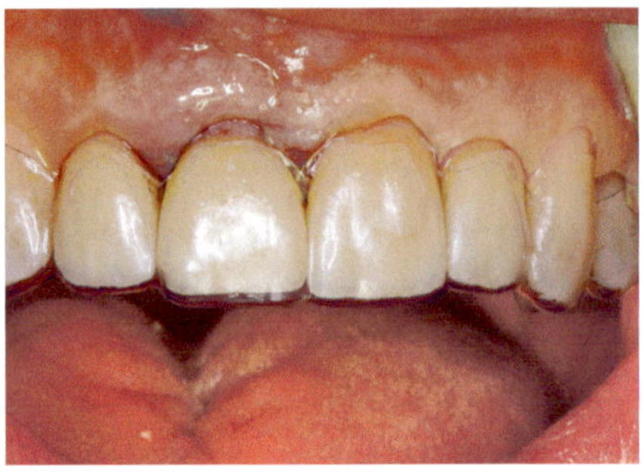

Fig 5-44kk A bite guard is used to protect the immediately placed implant.

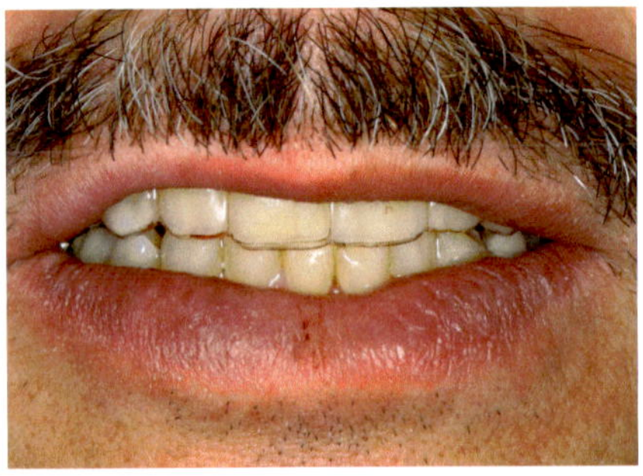

Fig 5-44ll The bite guard is barely noticeable in the labial view.

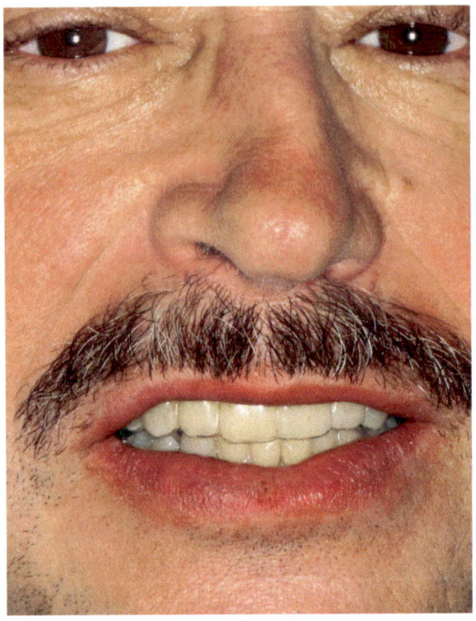

Fig 5-44mm The patient is somewhat tired but very pleased.

Because the patient depended on a complete dentition for professional reasons, the existing crown was used as a provisional restoration; the pin was removed and the interior of the crown was prepared. The crown was refashioned with the help of a vacuform template and slow-curing acrylic resin (Figs 5-44ff to 44ii). Once the crown was finished, it was cemented to the abutment with temporary cement (Fig 5-44jj). In the Xive system, the abutment is premounted. The bite guard placed to protect the immediately placed implant was not at all esthetically conspicuous (Figs 5-44kk and 44ll).

To avoid any form of overload, the patient was instructed to eat only soft foods, to avoid any loading of the implant, and to wear the bite guard 24 hours a day. In the end, the patient left the office in a somewhat exhausted state but was very pleased (Fig 5-44mm).

Countless articles have been published on the subject of immediate implant placement and loading, which cannot all be cited here. For further reading, the author recommends *The International Journal of Oral & Maxillofacial Implants* and extensive research on the Internet.

Materials

Periotome as designed by Prof Schulte (Friadent)
Extra-long bone bur with a carbide head and a diamond body with friction grip (Bredent)
Xive implant system (Friadent)

Selection of an Implant System

Common problem: Selection of the appropriate implant system

An implant system should be selected carefully, because it is not only a major investment for a dentist's office but also one with far-reaching consequences. Which criteria can help dental professionals in choosing the right implant system?

Proven solution: Consideration of all the characteristics required of a modern implant system

Recommendations

The dentist should choose a well-established implant system that has been on the market at least 10 years, so that it is past its testing stage and "growing pains." There should also be sufficient evidence to suggest that the implant system will remain on the market for another 10 years at least. It would be absolutely ruinous if an explantation were necessary only because the parts are not manufactured anymore or the implant system has ceased to exist.

The implant system should be bought only from a company whose representative can always be contacted and who will always be ready to answer any questions. The company should be able to deliver all parts within 24 hours.

The investment and the amortization to be expected should be calculated carefully, and the price-performance ratio should be examined.

The dentist should buy an implant system that a nearby colleague is also using. This allows colleagues to help each other with parts and advice. The dentist definitely needs a specialist (an oral surgeon or an oral and maxillofacial surgeon) who knows the chosen system, who can help in emergencies, and who will take the cases that are too difficult to be handled by a nonspecialist.

Necessary characteristics of a modern implant system

In the course of a career as an implant dentist from 1974 to the present, the author has used 10 different implant systems that can be judged without bias. Based on this and numerous discussions with experienced colleagues, the following checklist was developed.

Root shape

It has taken nature thousands of years to successfully develop the shape of the tooth. It is hardly ever possible to improve on nature; despite widespread assumptions to the contrary, nature knows no redundancy—the final shape is simply perfect.

With that in mind, it has taken available implant systems rather long to adopt the root form demonstrated by nature. Subperiosteal implants do not transfer the masticatory forces to the bone and were therefore problematic to use. Needle implants did not correspond to the root proportions. Blade implants did not offer three-dimensional stability. Cylindrical implants, especially those with a larger diameter, did not allow for sufficient blood supply to the cervical region of the implant, which resulted in bone resorption. Therefore the root shape (whether conical, rounded in the apical region and cylindrical in the mucosal region, or graduated as with the stepped cylindrical implants) is the only shape that should be chosen for an implant system (Figs 5-45 to 5-47).

Material

The competition between ceramics and titanium in the development of implants has been clearly settled in favor of titanium implants, because their mechanical properties are much better, especially with respect to breaking strength. Titanium is considered bioinert and bone-friendly because of the layer of titanium oxide that forms on it immediately after its processing (Fig 5-48). To date, no implant rejections resulting from allergic reactions have been reported in the scientific community worldwide. This fact also takes millions of hip joint endoprostheses into account, which is a good point to mention to skeptical patients who set a high value on natural materials.

Zirconium implants are currently attracting a great deal of interest. They seem to be an interesting metal-free alternative, although zirconium, too, is a metal and zirconium implants are made of zirconium oxide. With respect to healing, in the author's opinion this is more likely to be a step backward and leaves many questions unanswered. However, it will be interesting to see how these implants perform in the long run (Fig 5-49).

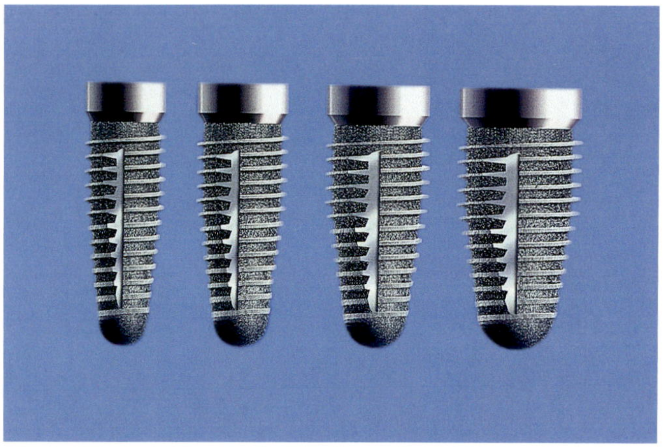

Fig 5-45 Camlog root-shaped implant (Camlog).

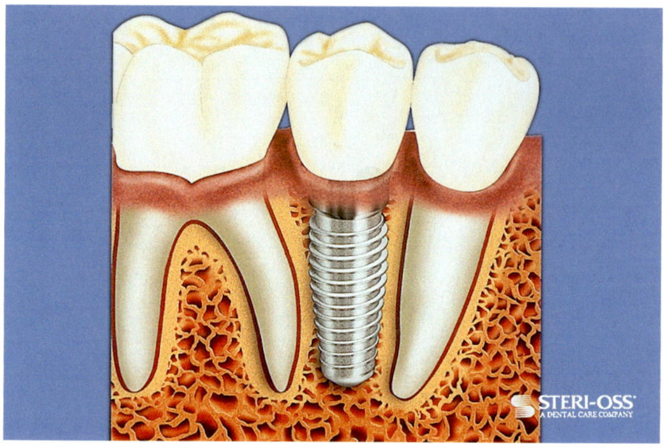

Fig 5-46 Steri-Oss root-shaped implant.

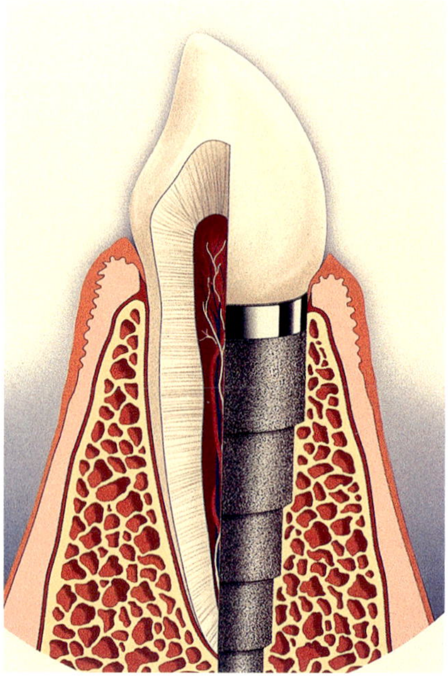

Fig 5-47 Frialit 2 stepped cylindrical implant (Friadent).

Rough surface

A rough surface is now standard for almost all dental implants, because it offers better mechanical retention and osseointegration. The implant should have a surface roughness between 2 and 20 µm (Fig 5-50). This is achieved by sandblasting and/or acid etching of the endosseous surface. The concept of coatings has been largely abandoned. Hydroxyapatite surfaces are known to heal more quickly but a bacterial infection on their surface can lead to rapid bone resorption around the implant. Titanium plasma spray–coated surfaces allegedly cause liver damage, but to the author's knowledge there are no scientific findings to confirm this assertion. Nowadays, smooth surfaces that have only been processed mechanically (such as the ones originally designed by Brånemark and intended solely for edentulous mandibles) are rarely used anymore. Thus, sandblasted and/or etched surfaces have become widely accepted for most implant systems.

Implant materials:

+ Commercially pure titanium, grades 1 to 4, typically contains 99.6 to 99.75% Ti; examples: Bonefit, Brånemark, IMZ, *3i*

+ Titanium alloys Ti/6A/4V 90% titanium, 6% aluminum, 4% vanadium; example: Corvent.

Fig 5-48 Titanium as an implant material.

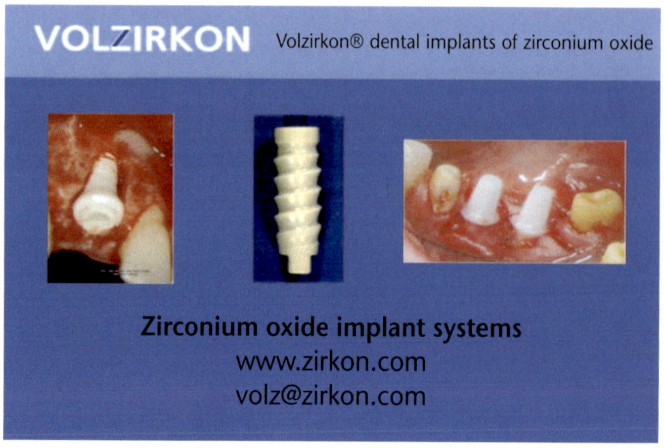

Fig 5-49 Zirconium implant.

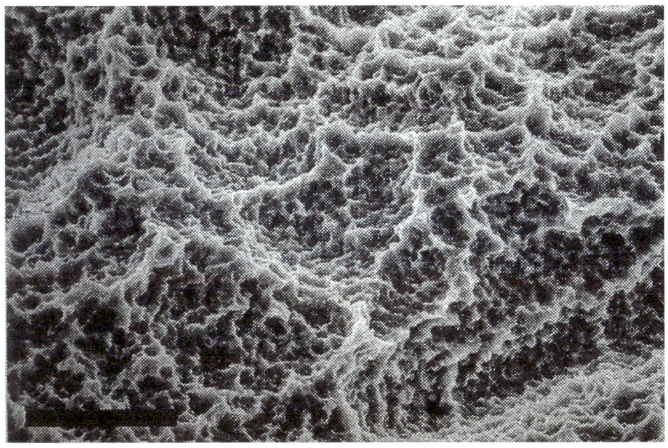

Fig 5-50 Implant surface (surface roughness of 2 to 20 µm).

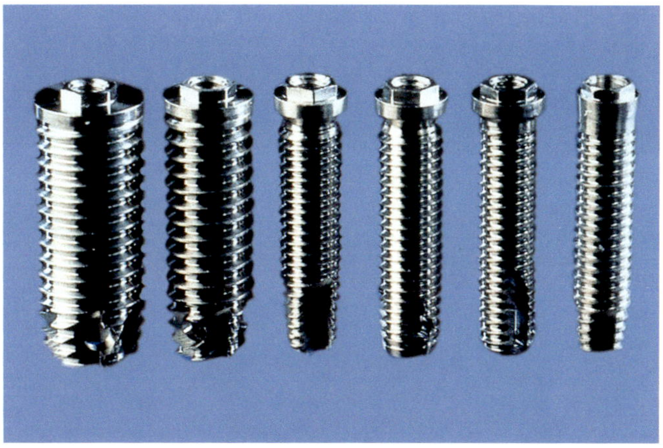

Fig 5-51 Brånemark implant with external hex (Nobel Biocare).

Internal fixation system

The classic hexagonal head introduced by Brånemark has outgrown its usefulness. Because implants can take a much higher load and are more mechanically stable than was ever imagined possible, there is no longer an indication for the hexagonal head (Fig 5-51). It was meant to provide a predetermined breaking point in case of overload to spare the implant; only the screw was meant to break.

Mechanically speaking, when two parts are connected, there is a difference between positive locking and friction locking. Positive locking is achieved when two precisely fitting parts are connected via an internal hexagonal connection or with a tube-in-tube system. Other internal systems have also been developed in the meantime (Figs 5-52 to 5-56). They all aim at transmitting the force from the abutment to the endosseous implant via this precise fit. The vertical screw, which acts as a friction lock because it is tightened with a defined torque (as discussed previously), protects the abutment from vertical forces that might cause it to dislodge and keeps it in position.

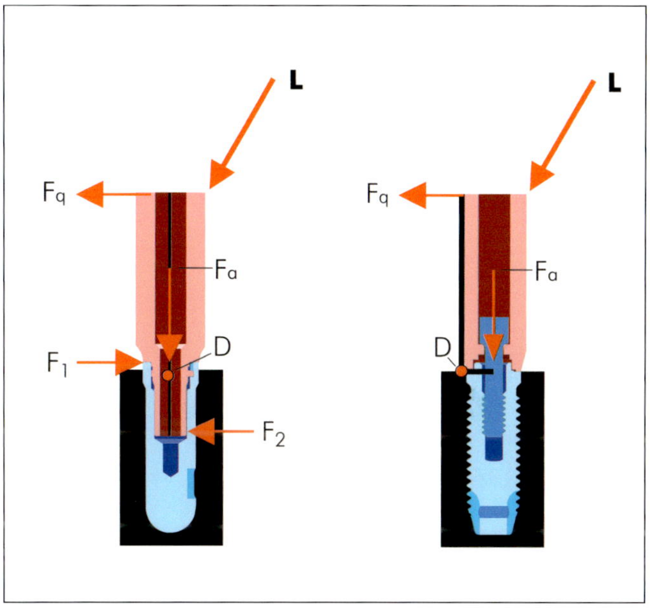

Fig 5-52 Internal versus external hexagon systems.

Length

The following implant lengths have proven useful: 9 mm, 11 mm, 13 mm, and 15 mm. Some systems also offer intermediate sizes and longer implants. According to the finite element analyses conducted by Vizethum,[6] implant lengths of more than 13 mm are unnecessary, because the greatest load is in the cervical cortical bone and not in the apical region, as was formerly assumed (bicortical support). A longer implant offers next to no increase in stability.

The failure rates for implants shorter than 9 mm are very high, which is why implant specialists have largely abandoned this concept. Moreover, 9-mm implants should be splinted with the superstructure, because the ratio between crown length and implant length is of great importance, especially for short implants (see Figs 5-31a and 5-31b).

Diameter

Much more important than the length of the implant is its diameter in the cervical region, in the bearing area for the abutment ($P = F/A$ also applies here). The bearing

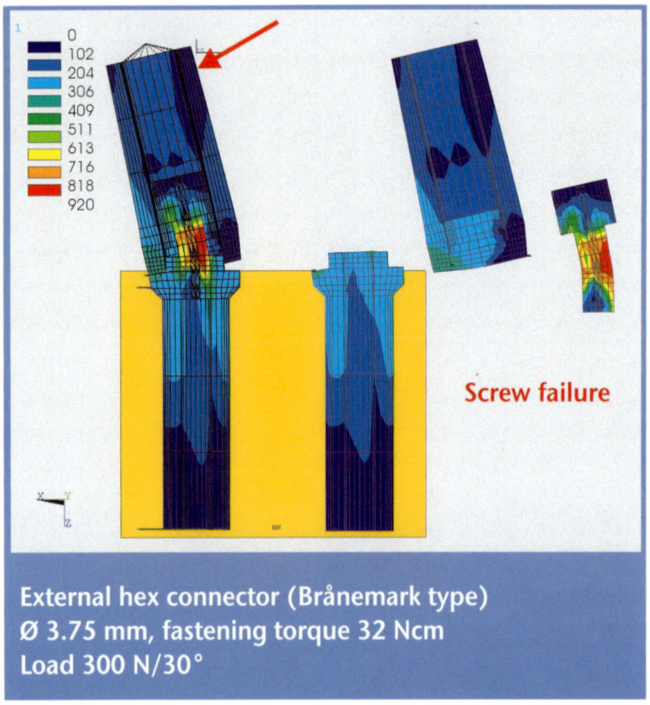

Fig 5-53a Finite element analysis of an external hexagon system (Brånemark).

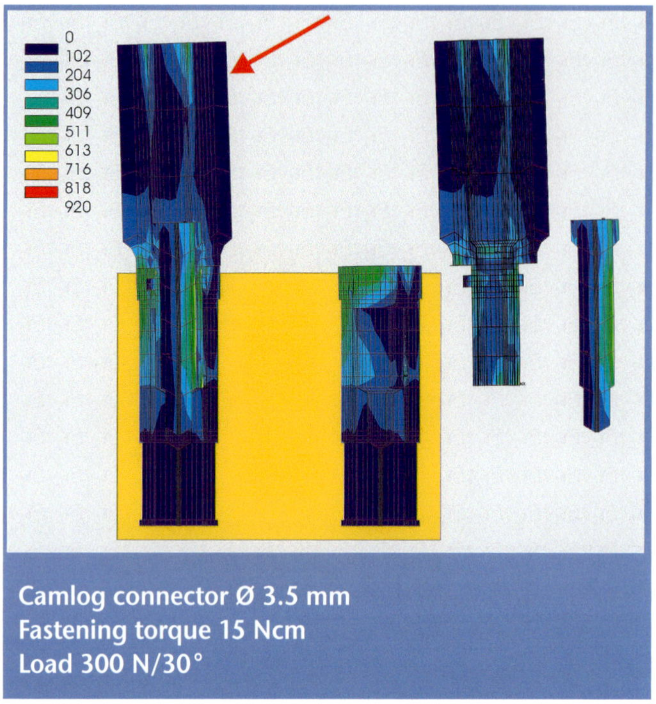

Fig 5-53b Finite element analysis of an internal hexagon system (Camlog).

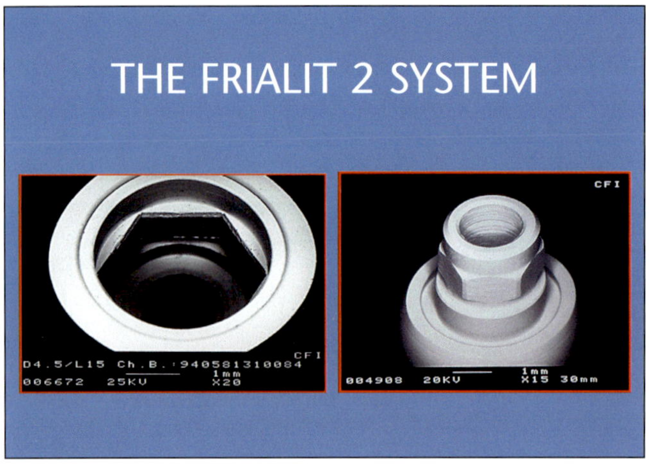

Fig 5-54 Frialit 2 hexagonal socket.

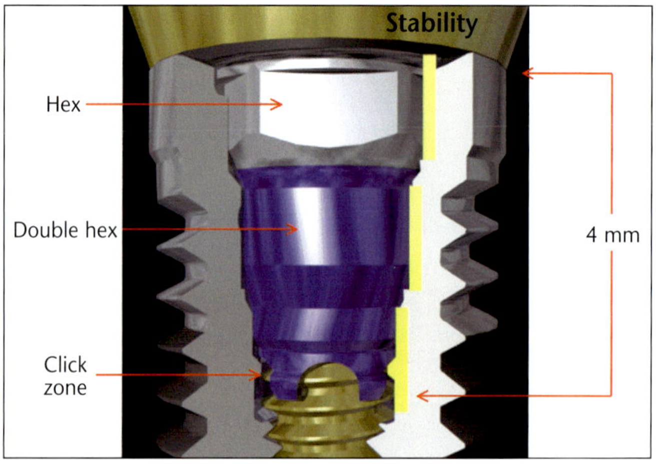

Fig 5-55 Osseotite Certain internal system (3i Implant Innovations).

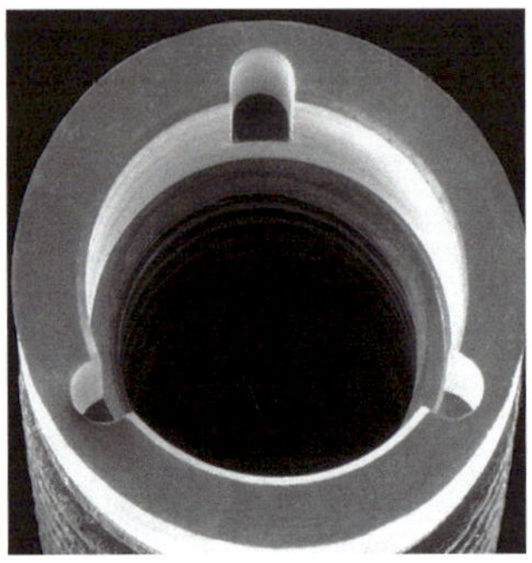

Fig 5-56a Camlog tube-in-tube system. Reflection electron microscopic image of the internal design of the implant body.

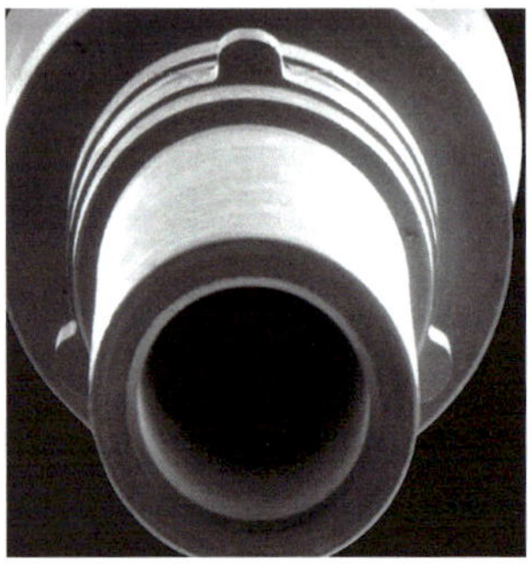

Fig 5-56b Reflection electron microscopic image of the external design of the Camlog implant abutment.

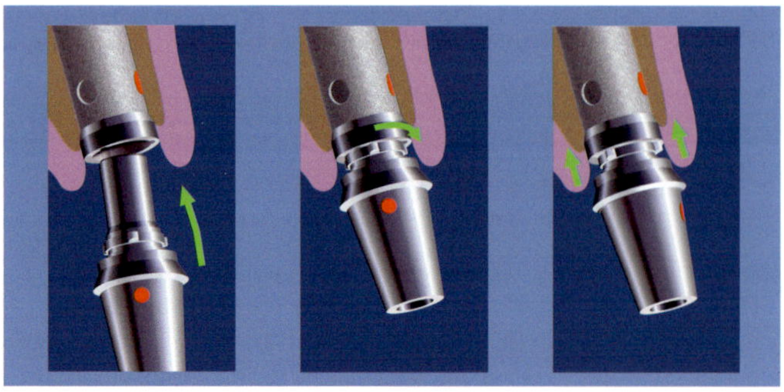

Fig 5-56c Placement of a Camlog abutment.

area for the abutment, ie, the implant diameter, should correspond to that of the tooth to be replaced at the height of the gingiva.

The following diameters corresponding to the teeth have proven successful: 3.0 mm, 3.4 mm, 3.8 mm, 4.3 mm, 5.0 mm, and 6.0 mm (see Figs 5-32a and 5-32b). These diameters are now offered by almost all implant systems with some variations. At the moment, the concept of "platform switching" is being discussed, in which a smaller diameter is chosen for the abutment than for the implant to allow better soft tissue management. There are, however, no conclusive research results to support this idea, to the author's knowledge.

Threaded implants versus press-fit cylindrical implants

There are arguments to support both kinds of designs. Threaded implants provide better initial stability and have a larger surface, but they are more difficult and take more time to insert. With excessive torques, pressure necrosis can occur when they are screwed in. They should therefore always be turned back one quarter to one half turn when they are screwed in with a torque of more than 20 Ncm.

Press-fit cylindrical implants should be tapered (to preserve blood supply of the cervical bone). These implants are faster to insert and are therefore very popular with dentists who perform many implantations. However, in the author's opinion, they lack sufficient primary stability, especially for immediate implantation.

For logistical reasons, it is recommended that the clinician choose only one of the systems. The author has decided to use threaded implants. To have both or more systems in one office is a great logistical problem for the dental team, and it requires the dentist to keep an expensive amount of stock (Fig 5-57).

Polished upper part with parallel walls and conical collar

The principle of the biologic width is also applicable (albeit in a modified form) to implants and the restorations supported by them. The implant has to project above the upper edge of the implant cavity by 1 mm with its parallel-walled upper body. Implants must therefore never be placed flush with the bone. To make sure that this is the case all around the implant, the bone cavity should be leveled. The parallel upper part of the implant should have a conical chamfer to ensure a tight seal of the implant cavity. This seal prevents connective tissue from growing into the cavity (Figs 5-58 and 5-59).

One-stage surgery versus two-stage surgery

One-stage surgical procedures are to be preferred, whenever possible. This eliminates the need for surgical exposure of the implant, which makes the implantation more economical. All two-stage implant systems can also be used in one stage. In the author's opinion, two-stage procedures are necessary only for concomitant augmentation.

The fastest way to place an implant, provided the gingiva is wide enough, is with the following procedure: The pilot hole is drilled with a 2-mm drill via the drill guide in a customized surgical template. The gingiva is punched out to the bone with a mechanical tissue punch. The 3-mm hole is drilled. The final hole is drilled to the desired length and diameter. The implant is placed, and a 4-mm healing abutment is screwed in. This procedure avoids sutures, postoperative complications, surgical exposure, and the risk of gingival recession.

A one-piece implant system can also be used but is not strictly necessary, because it makes keeping parts in stock and logistics more complicated.

Immediate implant placement

The implant system of your choice should allow immediate and delayed-immediate implantations as well as delayed implant placement. For immediate and delayed-immediate implant placement (after 8 weeks), the implant has to have a sharp thread in the apical part to achieve enough primary stability beyond the alveolus. The alveolus is rarely congruent with the implant. Implants will only heal if they are initially stable (Figs 5-60a to 5-60d).

Defined torques with manual and power tools

The implant system must allow handling of all parts with a defined torque, both manually as well as via a machine. This was discussed in detail in the earlier section on screws, screwdrivers, and torques.

Exchangeable depth stops

All implant drills must have an exchangeable depth stop, simply because this will reassure the dentist. Numerous risks—injury of the inferior alveolar nerve, entry of the maxillary sinus, drilling through the floor of the nose, etc—are all minimized or even eliminated by a defined depth stop. This component is a must, especially for beginners, but more advanced users need it just as much (Fig 5-61).

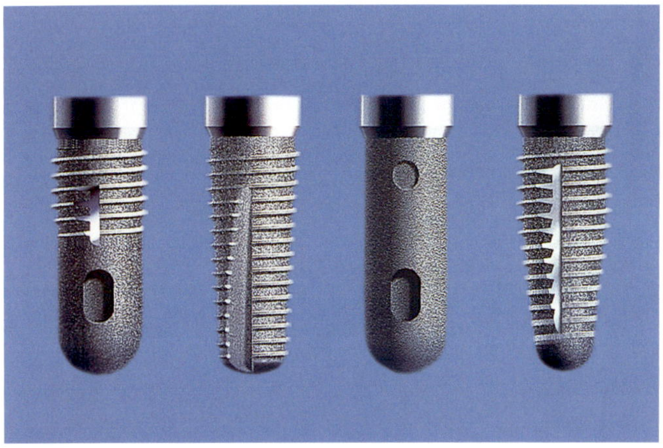

Fig 5-57 *(left to right)* Press-fit cylindrical implant with additional partial thread, conical threaded implant, press-fit implant, root-shaped threaded implant.

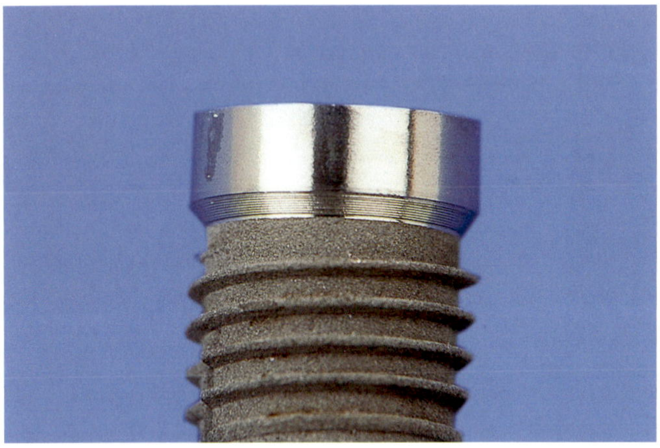

Fig 5-58 Polished upper part to seal the bone cavity.

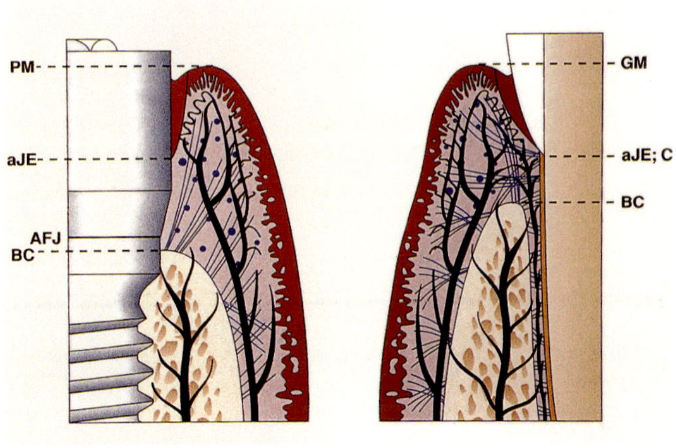

Fig 5-59 Comparison of the biologic widths of teeth and implants.

Color-coded parts

No matter whether a beginner or a pro, everyone is grateful for a consistent color coding of all parts. This makes handling of the parts logical, fast, and reliable. Most companies use more or less the same color codes:

1. Silver = 3.0 to 3.4 mm in diameter.
2. Gold = 3.8 mm in diameter.
3. Red = 4.0 to 4.3 mm in diameter.
4. Blue = 5.0 mm in diameter.
5. Green = 6.0 to 6.5 mm in diameter (Fig 5-62).

Implant tray with logical sequence of drills and screwdrivers

Almost all the implant systems offer sterilizable implant trays with a logical sequence of drills and screwdrivers. For beginners and advanced users alike, this allows easy, efficient, fast, and reliable use of the instruments (Fig 5-63). Dentists who perform many implantations should buy a second tray.

Implantation drive unit with three settings

An implantation drive unit with three different settings is recommended for the following procedures: preparing the bone cavity, screwing in the implant, and screwing in the healing caps or healing abutments.

Dentists in Germany are now legally obliged to document the torques that they use in an implantation. The drive unit should therefore offer the ability to save and print the torques that were applied during the implantation (Fig 5-64). It is recommended that the dentist not cut corners when it comes to this feature. It is useful to have a second sterilizable micromotor so that two implantations in a row can be scheduled if the need arises.

Surgical templates with steel and titanium drilling guides

The field of implant prosthodontics is prosthetic dentistry with a surgical component. Therefore, to be successful functionally and esthetically, the implant has to be placed exactly where it was planned in prosthetic planning (Fig 5-65). An implant-retained prosthetic restoration can only be successful if this requirement is fulfilled, even though it may often involve compromise.

The very expensive titanium guides are only needed for computed tomogram–based diagnosis. In other cases it is sufficient to use inexpensive, high-grade steel jackets (2.0-mm diameter) from a building supply store, where they are sold as wire end sleeves for a few dollars.

Reliable information about the height, width, profile, and quality of the bone where the implants are to be placed is essential for the implantation (see chapter 3).

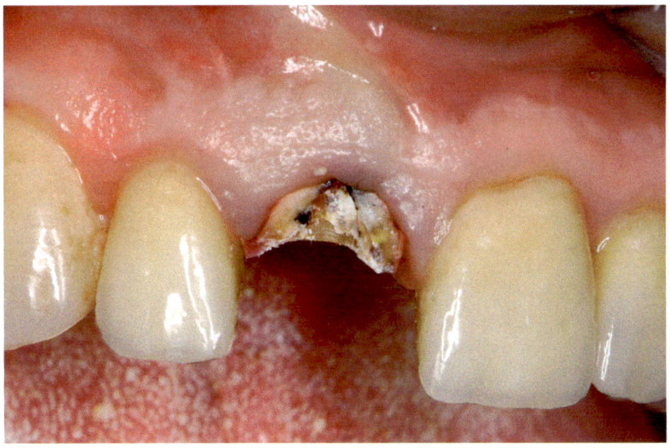

Fig 5-60a Immediate implantation. The root remnant of the maxillary right central incisor is shown prior to extraction.

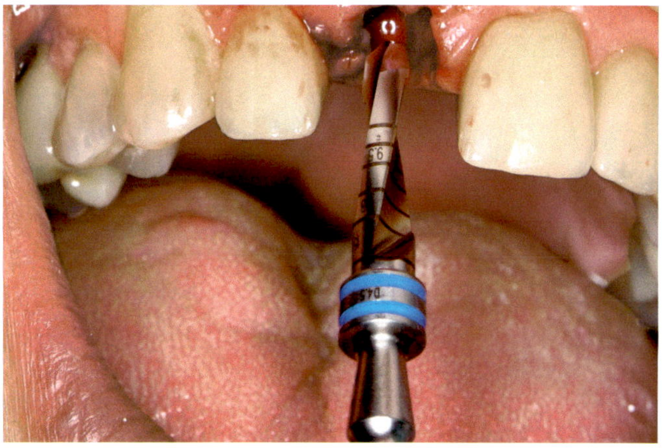

Fig 5-60b The hole is drilled to the final size of 4.5 mm.

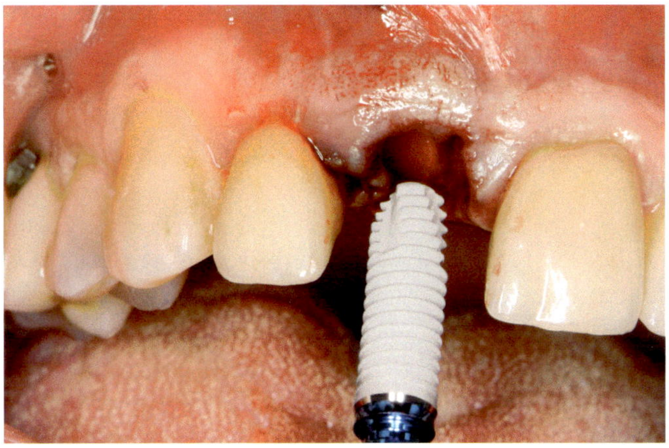

Fig 5-60c The implant is carefully inserted.

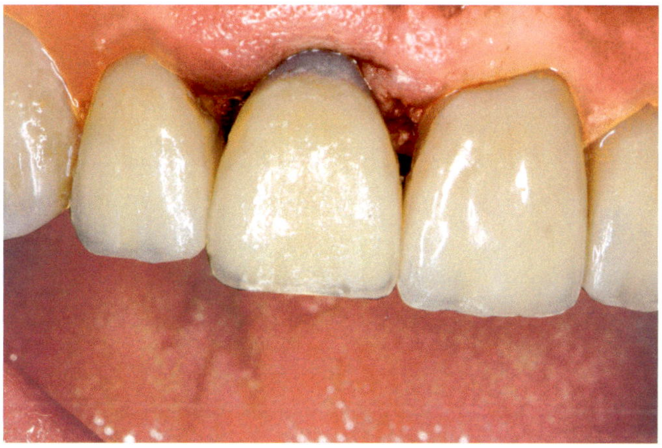

Fig 5-60d The crown has been cemented with temporary cement.

Vertical screws with hexagonal sockets that grip the screwdriver

These vertical screws can be put in place with a defined torque. Not all types of screws are suitable for use in implantology:

1. Slotted screws absolutely do not belong in the mouth, because they do not keep a good grip on the end of the screwdriver.
2. The same is true of Phillips screws.
3. Allen screws are very well suited for dental use.
4. Square socket screws are not suitable, because they do not grip as well when they are inside the deep shaft.
5. TORX screws are the best choice in terms of engineering, but only one implant system uses them.

The author does not see an indication for horizontal screws for crowns anymore, because he almost exclusively cements crowns (see Figs 5-35 and 5-36).

Two-part impression posts and impression sleeves

If several implants have to be cast, internal systems require two-part impression posts (Fig 5-66), because it is not possible to cast divergent abutments with the pick-up or window technique. In the author's opinion, it is impossible to make an impression of several posts with a closed tray, even with impression caps.

Customizable healing abutments for immediate and delayed implant placement

Designing an esthetically satisfactory restoration with respect to the soft tissue, the gingiva, is incomparably

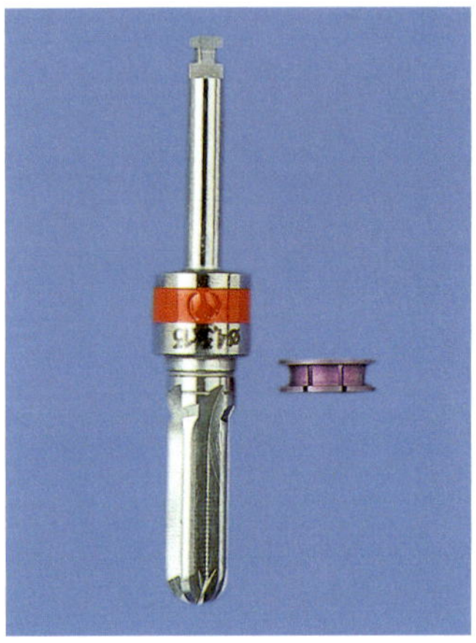

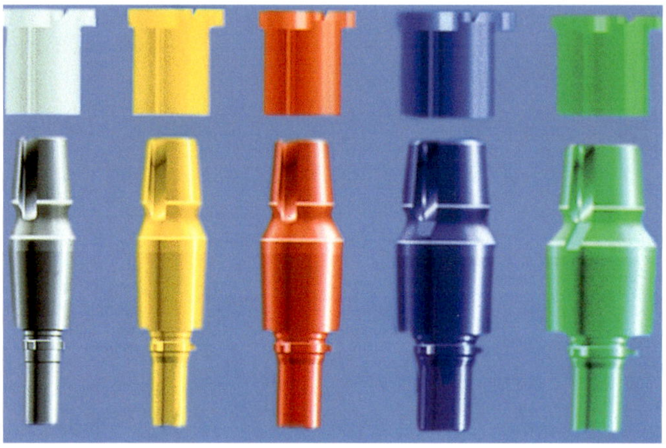

Fig 5-61 *(left)* Depth stop.

Fig 5-62 *(right)* Color coding.

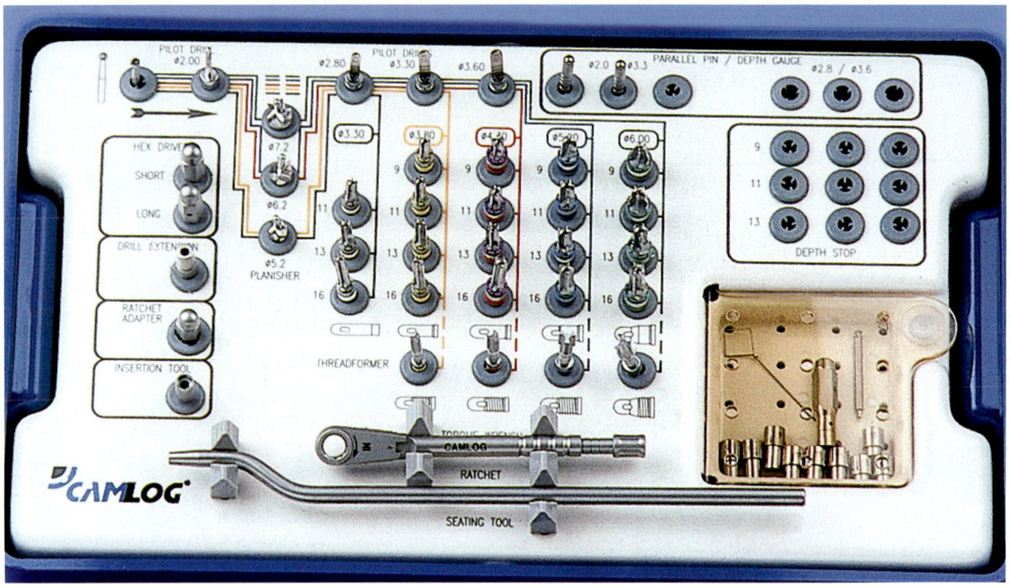

Fig 5-63 Implant tray.

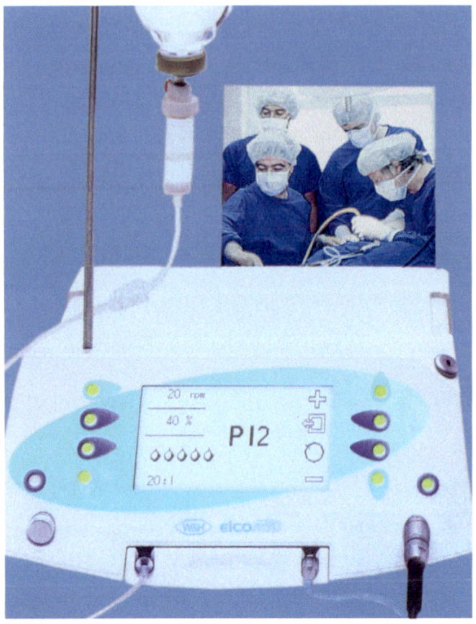

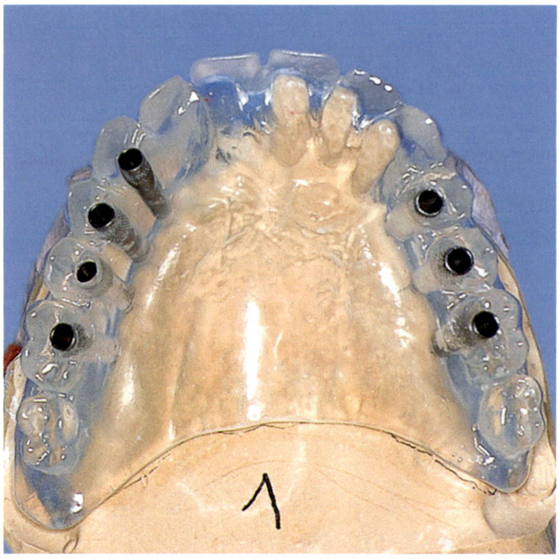

Fig 5-64 *(left)* Implantation driver unit.

Fig 5-65 *(right)* Surgical template with guide sleeves.

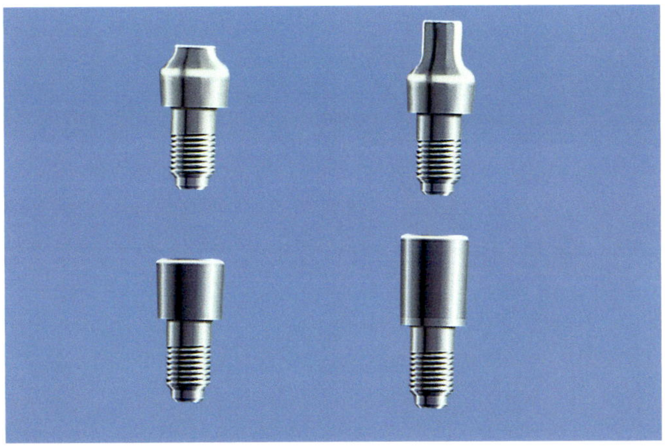

Fig 5-66 Two-part impression post.

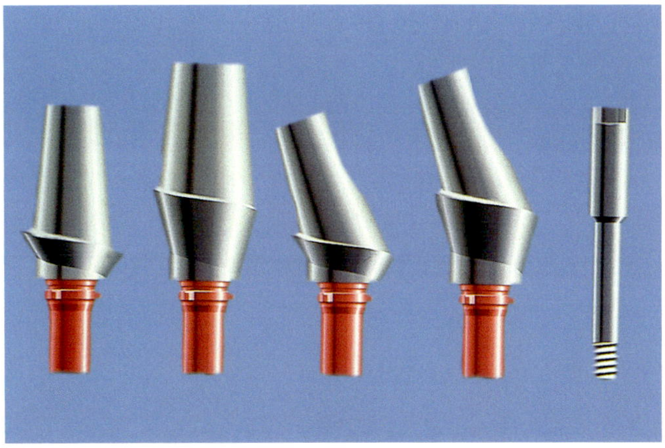

Fig 5-67 Assortment of healing abutments.

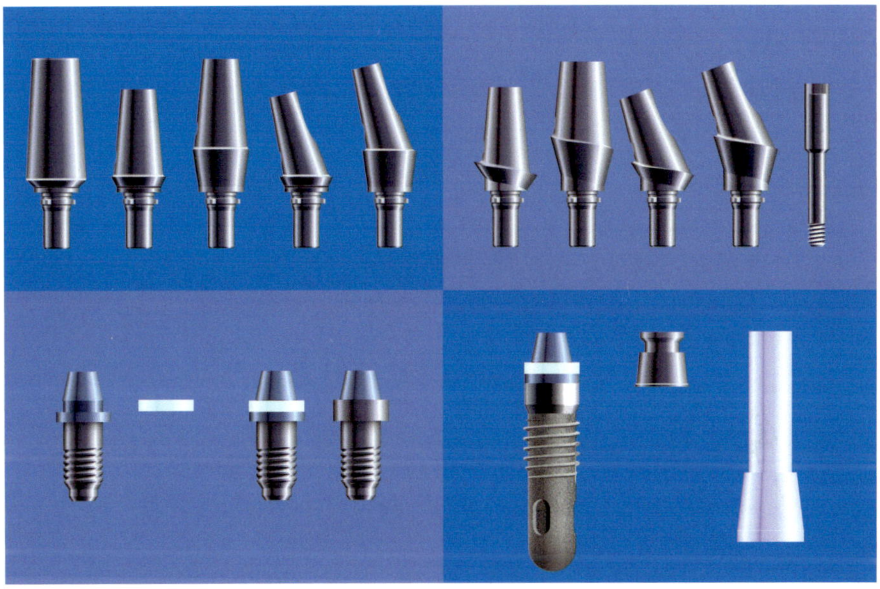

Fig 5-68 Well-assorted prosthodontic system. This is but a small selection; many more components (such as all-ceramic and telescopic abutments and magnetic and ball attachments) are needed to make a prosthodontic system complete.

more difficult in implant prosthodontics than in normal prosthodontics, where it is already troublesome enough. The anterior maxilla is the benchmark of success here: Dentists who manage to create "invisible" restorations even under difficult conditions with respect to the soft tissues are masters of implant prosthodontics. For these cases, the dentist needs the appropriate customizable gingiva formers or healing abutments in the implant system, for both immediate and delayed implantations (Fig 5-67).

Well-assorted prosthodontic system for all indications

In a prosthodontic system, it is essential that all parts be fabricated with great precision. The system requires color coding and a systematic structure (Fig 5-68). It has always been very interesting to observe how newly introduced systems always promised and attempted to make everything easier, but in the end they all were retrofitted very quickly to meet the real requirements of implant prosthodontics.

Materials

A list of materials is not included in this section, in order to give readers the opportunity to form their own opinions without prejudice.

6

Esthetic Dentistry

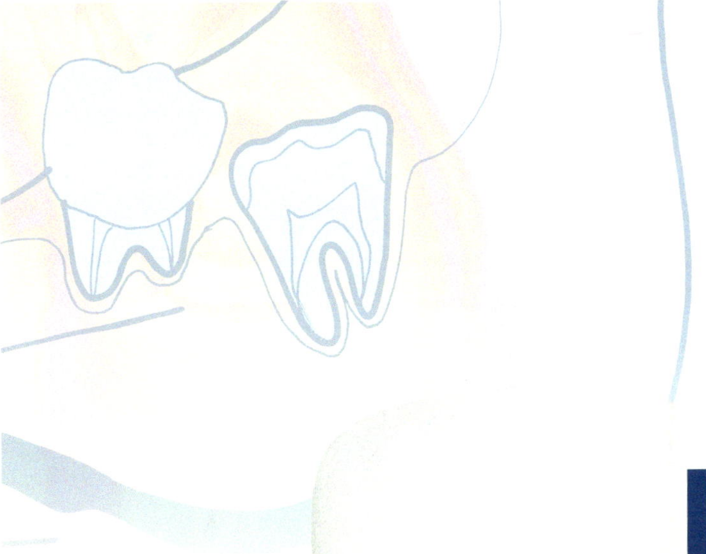

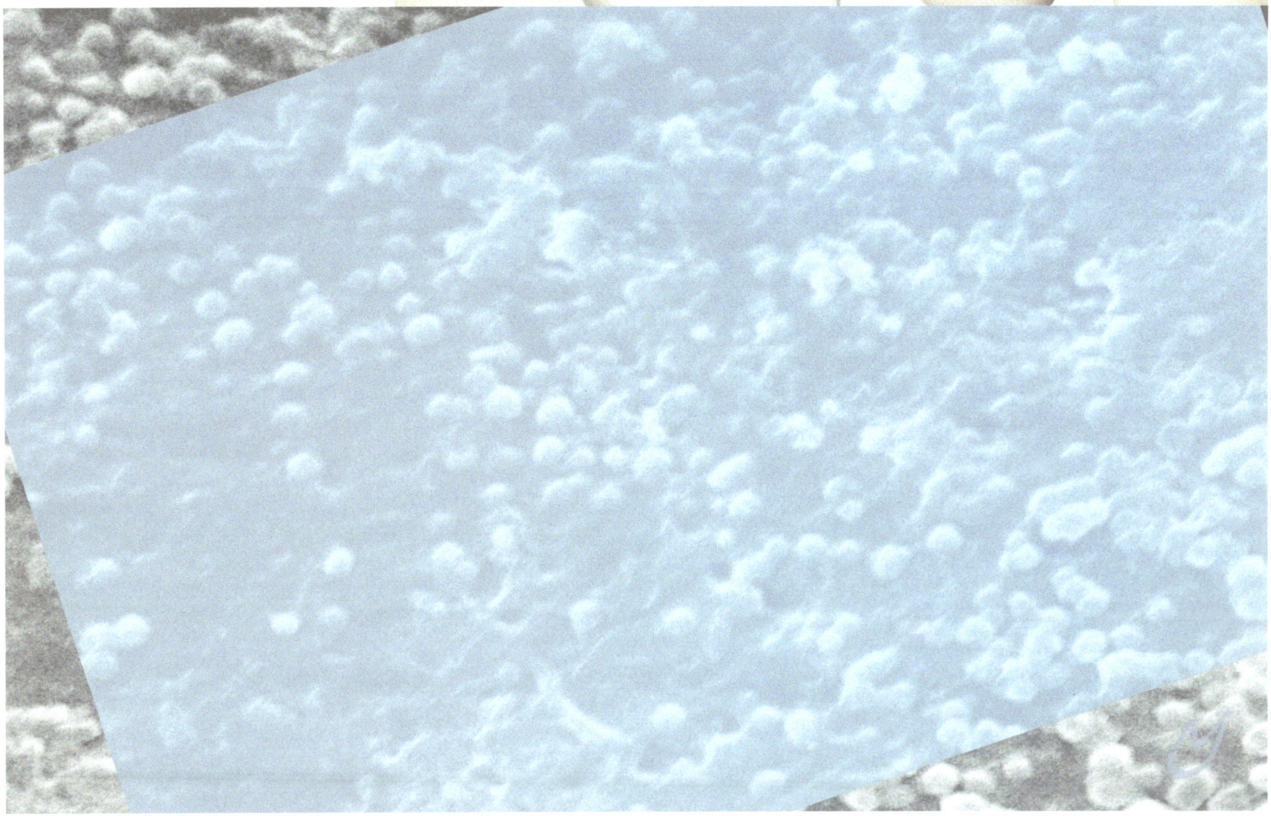

6

Functional Analysis of Lateral Cephalograms: Planning Prosthodontic Treatment

Functional Analysis of Lateral Cephalograms: Reestablishing the Vertical Dimension

Facial Profile Analysis

Mock-up: Dental Imaging Directly on the Patient

Determination and Reconstruction of Correct Anterior Tooth Length

Shade Matching

Analysis and Transfer of the Midline

Horizontal Facial Planes

Functional Analysis of Lateral Cephalograms: Planning Prosthodontic Treatment

Common problem: Unknown factors in the planning of complex restorations

When planning complex and major restorations for patients, dentists are often faced with uncertainties. There are many factors about which dentists have to make an educated guess, albeit uneasily, or about which they just have to do what they can while relying on opinions or schools of thought that might have become outdated. In this context the following questions arise:

1. How can the appropriate occlusal height be determined?
2. What influence does the setup of the teeth have on the profile of the face?
3. Can a setup for the teeth be created that ensures a biomechanically correct load along the functional axis?
4. What is the best way to plan treatment for patients with dysgnathia, eg, with a distal occlusion, mandibular prognathism, or a deep overbite?
5. Can the desired implant position for an esthetic setup be realized with respect to the function of the stomatognathic system?
6. Are there reliable values for the horizontal and vertical dimensions, tooth positions, tooth axes, occlusal plane, etc?

In short: How can the dentist achieve more safety and predictability in prosthetic planning?

Proven solution: Functional analysis of cephalometric radiographs

In orthodontics, the analysis of cephalometric radiographs is an integral part of the orthodontic treatment planning. A higher degree of certainty in the planning and treatment of orthodontic cases is attained when these radiographs are used in conjunction with the oral findings and the analysis of the casts mounted to an articulator.

Clinicians should also take advantage of this tool in prosthodontics: The functional analysis of cephalometric radiographs should become an integral part of planning, treatment, and check-up procedures.

In other words, three equally important sources of information are available, and they must be integrated and used together: the patient, the cephalogram, and the casts in the articulator. Only after all the required parameters of the patient, the casts, and the cephalogram have been analyzed and used in planning can an extensive prosthetic treatment begin.

Figures 6-1a to 6-1c show the initial dental situation of a patient whose anterior maxilla is to be restored in an esthetic and functional way with the help of an implant-supported partial denture. A functional analysis of the cephalogram will be performed to facilitate prosthetic planning.

To ensure that the cephalogram will be suitable for functional analysis, the patient has to be prepared carefully. To ensure that the image is taken while the mandible is in a centric position, the patient may have to wear an anterior jig while the radiograph is being taken to "lock" the mandible in this position. This jig is made in the articulator with light-curing tray material or self-curing acrylic resin. The finished jig should be examined in the patient's mouth and corrected if necessary. The anterior jig can also be included in a provisional restoration or an existing prosthesis.

To enhance the visibility of the anterior tooth contours in the sagittal section, lead foil should be wrapped along the contours of the maxillary and mandibular left central incisors. The lead foil from the back of a single-tooth radiographic film is removed (Fig 6-1d) and cut into 3-mm-wide strips with a pair of scissors (Fig 6-1e). These strips are bonded along the contour of the maxillary and mandibular left central incisors with light-curing bonding material used without tooth etching (Figs 6-1f to 6-1h).

The patient is ready for the image to be taken. Because most dental offices have no cephalometric unit, patients can be sent to an orthodontist's office to have the image taken there. The patient will return with the developed image.

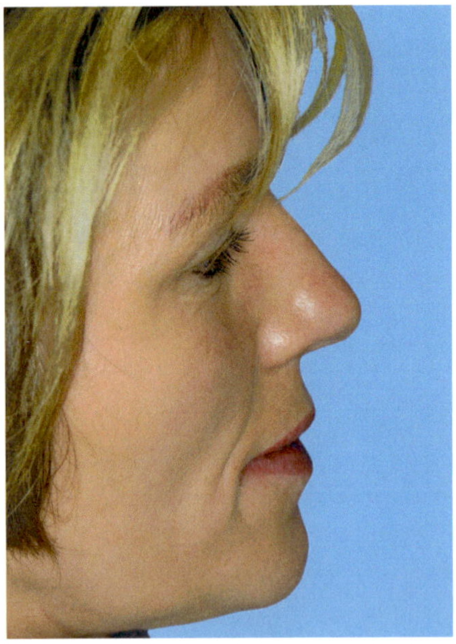

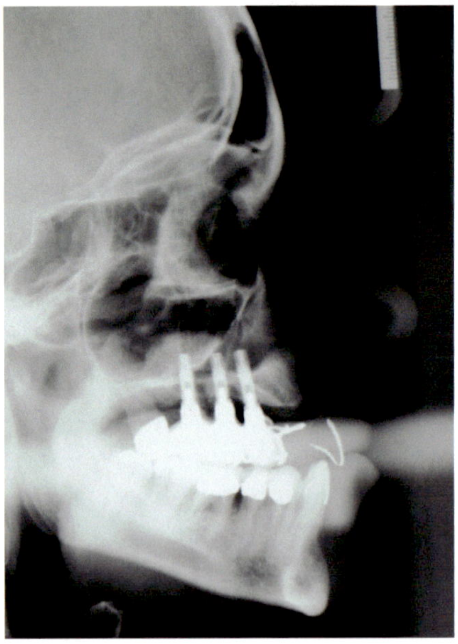

Fig 6-1a *(left)* Patient's profile.

Fig 6-1b *(right)* Patient's lateral cephalogram.

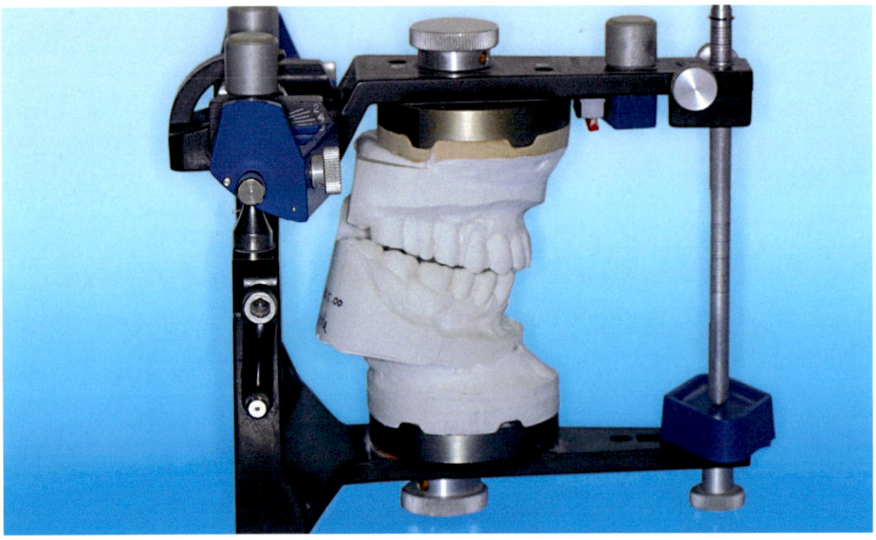

Fig 6-1c Patient's casts mounted on the articulator.

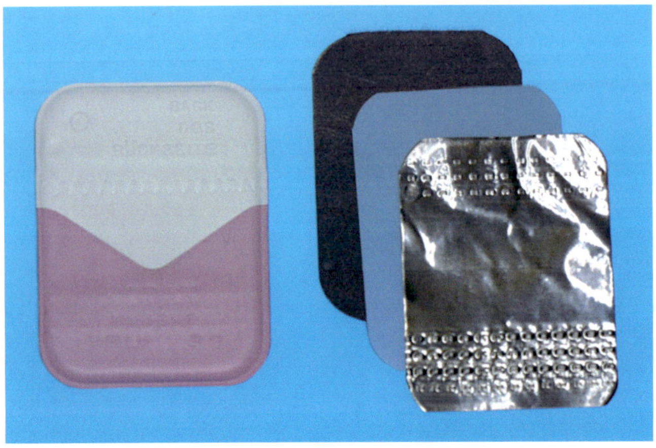

Fig 6-1d Different layers of a single-tooth radiographic film.

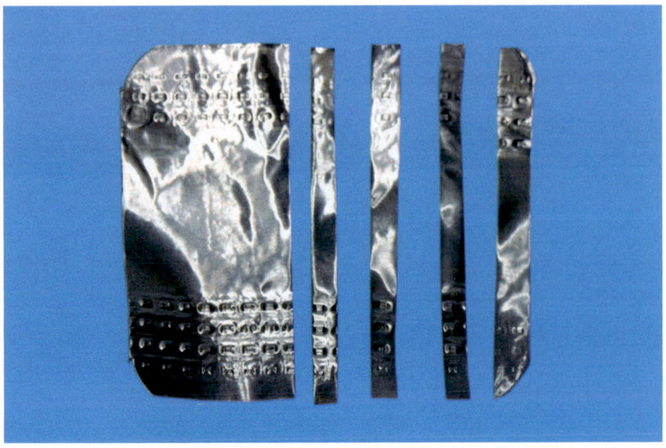

Fig 6-1e Lead foil cut into strips.

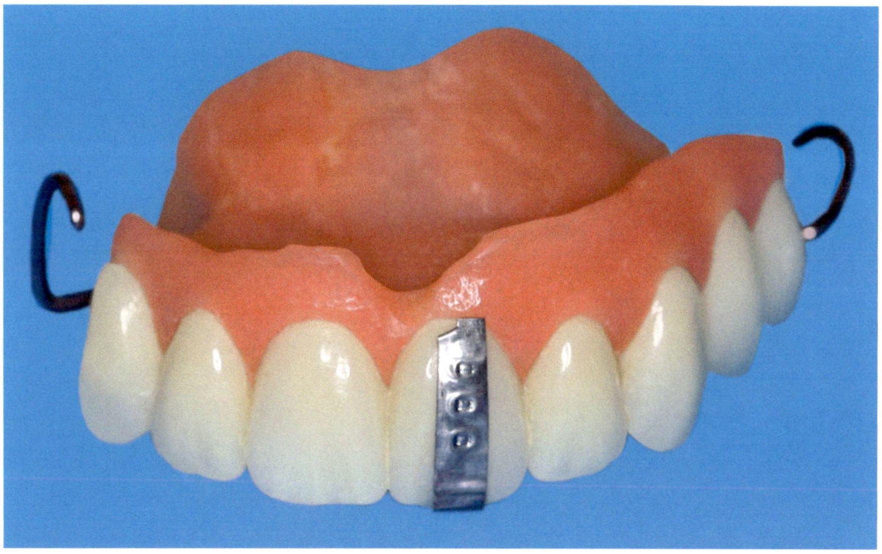

Fig 6-1f Labial view of the lead foil wrapped around the tooth on the maxillary partial denture.

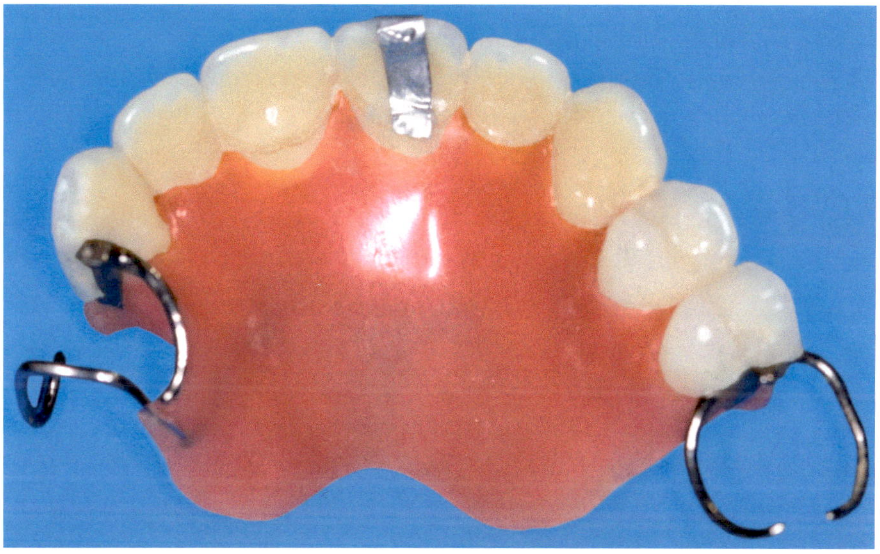

Fig 6-1g Palatal view of the lead foil wrapped around the tooth.

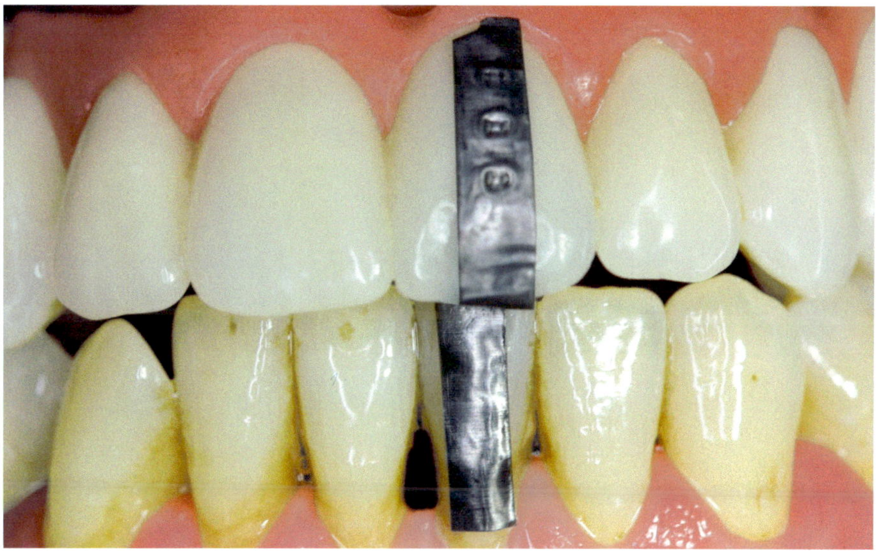

Fig 6-1h Lead foil in the patient's mouth; the contours of the maxillary and mandibular left central incisors are marked with foil strips.

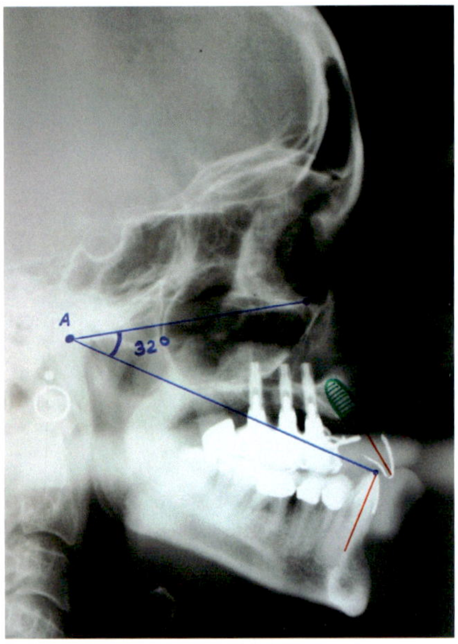

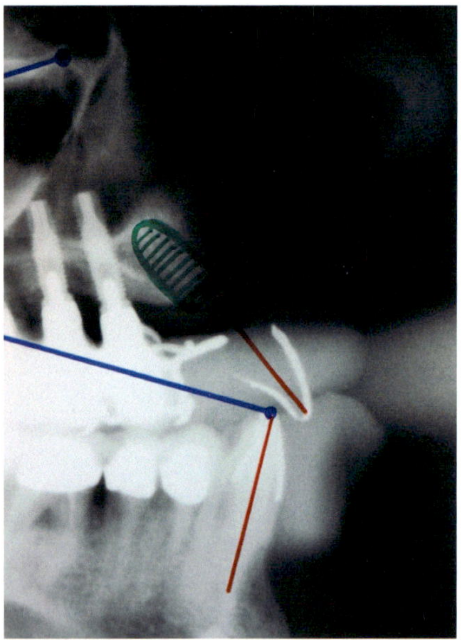

Fig 6-1i *(left)* Functional analysis of the cephalogram.

Fig 6-1j *(right)* Marking the implant position (magnified view of the anterior region).

Planning prosthodontic measures

A photograph of the patient's profile is taken. Casts are mounted on an articulator. Then the functional analysis of the cephalometric radiograph is performed. The positions of the maxillary anterior teeth and the inclination of the implants are determined by analyzing the available bone. The cephalometric radiograph serves as midsagittal tomography. For all measurements, the viewer must be aware that the factor of magnification is 1:1.10. This magnification is shown on the image on the nose-rest, like on a nautical chart.

The following procedure is used to analyze the cephalogram (Figs 6-1i and 6-1j). First, the cephalogram is placed in a transparent slip cover and labeled. Then, the lowest point of the orbital cavity is determined as the infraorbital point. The center of the visible condyloid process is determined as the axis point. The axis orbital plane is drawn. The coupling plane, the connecting line between the incisal edge of the mandibular anterior tooth and the axis point, is drawn.

The tooth axis of the maxillary anterior tooth is drawn. The individual interincisal angle is determined. The angle between the axis orbital plane and the coupling plane is measured. In the patient shown in the figures, the angle was 32 degrees. The vertical dimension was therefore correct.

The angle of inclination of the planned implant is determined according to the prosthetic position required. A surgical template with guide sleeves is made in the laboratory according to the analysis.

This example shows the use and purpose of a functional analysis for prosthetic planning.

The next section will discuss how to determine the occlusal height and the vertical dimension of occlusion as well as how to position the anterior teeth and secure the centric position of the temporomandibular joints (TMJs). The functional analysis of cephalometric radiographs can also yield very useful values for these parameters.

Materials

Proline 2000 cephalometric x-ray unit (Planmeca)
Kodak cephalometric radiographic film (Eastman Kodak)
Lead foil from Kodak single-tooth radiographic film (Eastman Kodak)
Jig from a light-curing tray material (Ivoclar Vivadent)
Radiograph viewer (obtained from dental wholesalers)

Functional Analysis of Lateral Cephalograms: Reestablishing the Vertical Dimension

Common problem: Determination of the vertical dimension or the occlusal height

Reconstructing the vertical dimension is one of the greatest problems in prosthodontics. The normal course of everyday prosthodontics involves trying out and cutting wax rims and shifting the artificial teeth around again and again.

The following principles are taught at dental schools:

1. The vertical dimension is a life-long constant. Is this true?
2. The normal occlusion is 2 mm less than the resting position (Fig 6-2a). Is this true?
3. The occlusal height must not be greater than the resting position. Is this true?

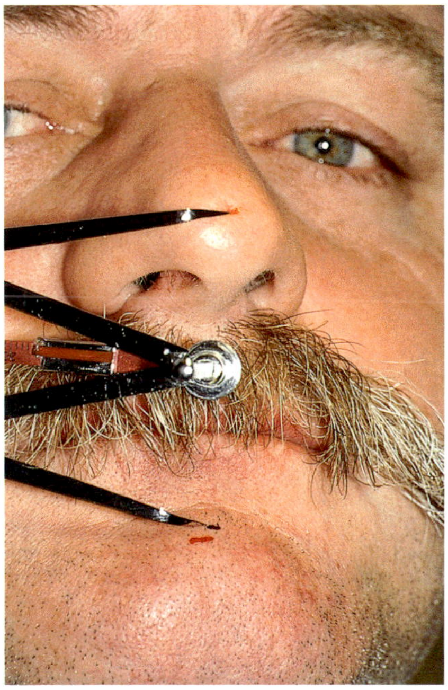

Fig 6-2a This is what was once taught to dentists: The normal occlusion minus 2 mm is the patient's vertical dimension.

From time to time, dentists should question everything they have learned in their dental training and investigate whether the things learned in school are still valid today. Most dentists would prefer a reliable measurement over a statistical value or just "trying". Which options do dentists have when determining the exact vertical dimension? In order to find a precise method for measuring the occlusal height, the author has tried the following possibilities:

1. Assuming that a patient who smiles slightly adopts a resting position of the jaw, the author measured the interpupillary distance (distance *x*) on a photograph and the midsagittal perpendicular line through the tip of the patient's chin (distance *y*). Then the true interpupillary distance (x') was determined on the patient, and the midsagittal perpendicular line was calculated with the formula $y' = x/x' \times y$. This approach produced results with an accuracy of ± 1 mm. This was not satisfactory, and moreover the results were strongly dependent on the angle from which the photograph was taken (Figs 6-2b to 6-2d).
2. In the cephalometric analysis according to Hasund[1] (known in Germany as the *Bergen technique*), the different types of faces are classified as prognathic, orthognathic, and retrognathic in a pattern of even proportions. Orthodontic treatment aims at creating linear harmony within this classification. The example in Figs 6-3a and 6-3b shows the cephalometric measurements before and after treatment. After treatment, the measurements became linear. The last column shows the mandibulolabial-nasolabial angle, which is relevant for the vertical dimension. It is within the classification of orthognathic at 25 to 27 degrees. This is another indicator, but the range is too large to obtain an exact value that is reliable enough to be used for a prosthetic restoration.

Proven solution: Functional analysis of cephalometric radiographs

Kubein-Meesenburg et al[2] tried to determine the center of growth of the viscerocranium in adolescents. They took standardized lateral cephalograms at regular intervals; the growth of the viscerocranium could be illustrated quite impressively when the images were projected onto one another.

From its center in the posterior region of the skull, the viscerocranium grows radially in the anterior direction with the coupling plane as the central axis of the growth.

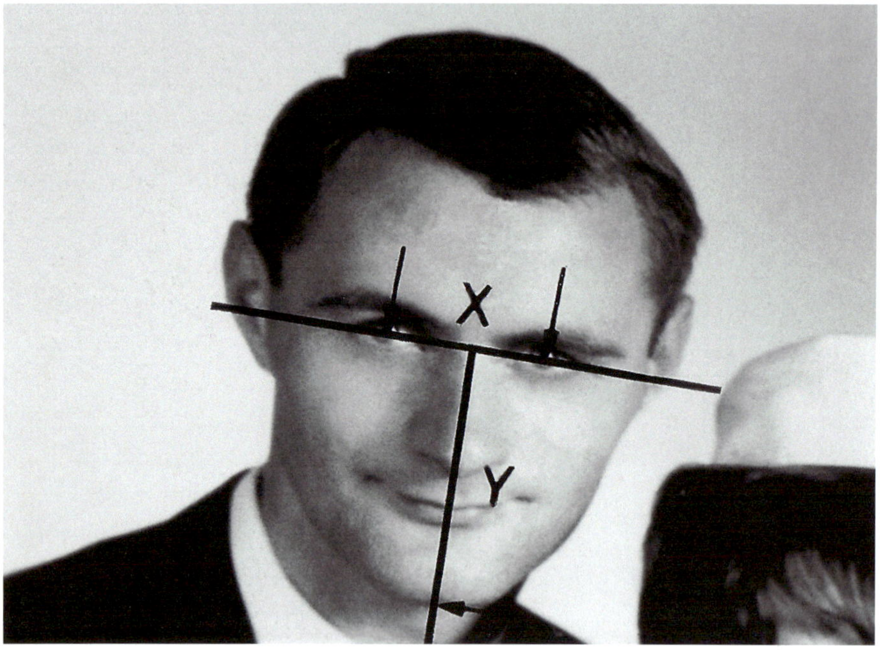

Fig 6-2b Photograph of the patient as a young man. The interpupillary distance *(x)* and a midsagittal perpendicular line to the tip of the chin *(y)* are marked.

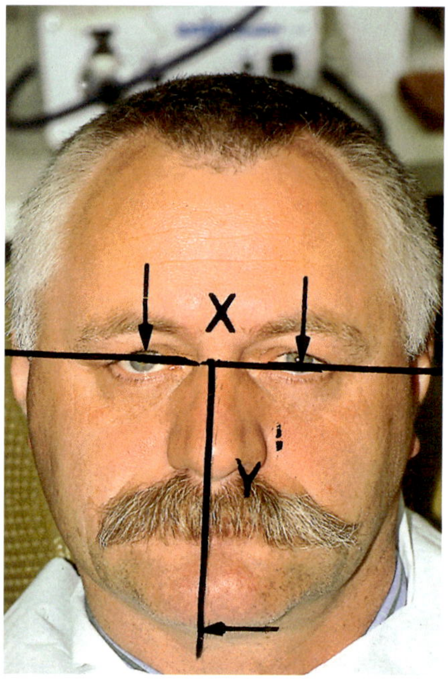

Fig 6-2c Recent photograph of the patient. The interpupillary distance *(x)* and a midsagittal perpendicular line to the tip of the chin *(y)* are indicated.

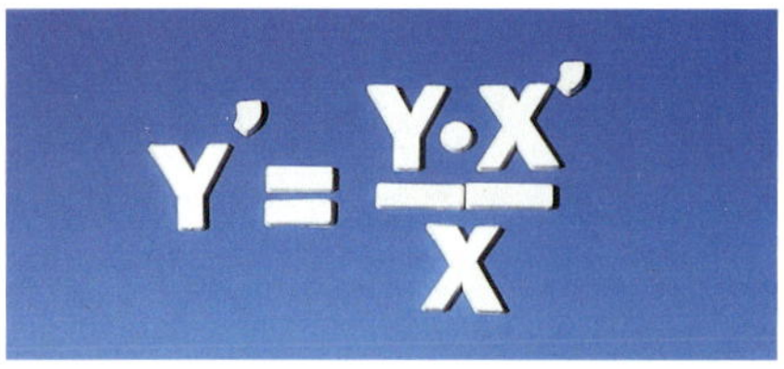

Fig 6-2d Formula for determining the occlusal height.

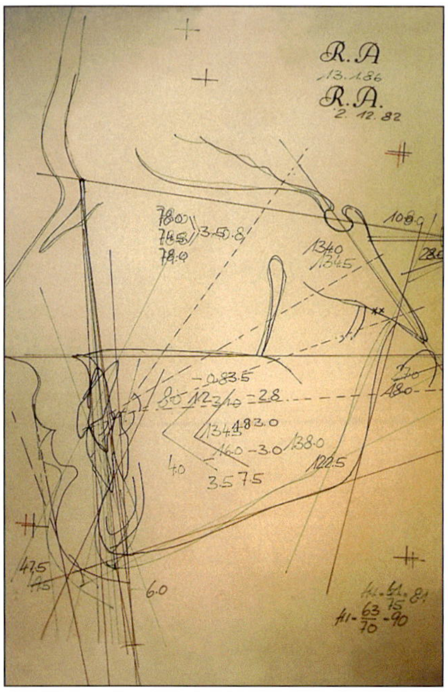

Fig 6-3a Cephalometric tracing.

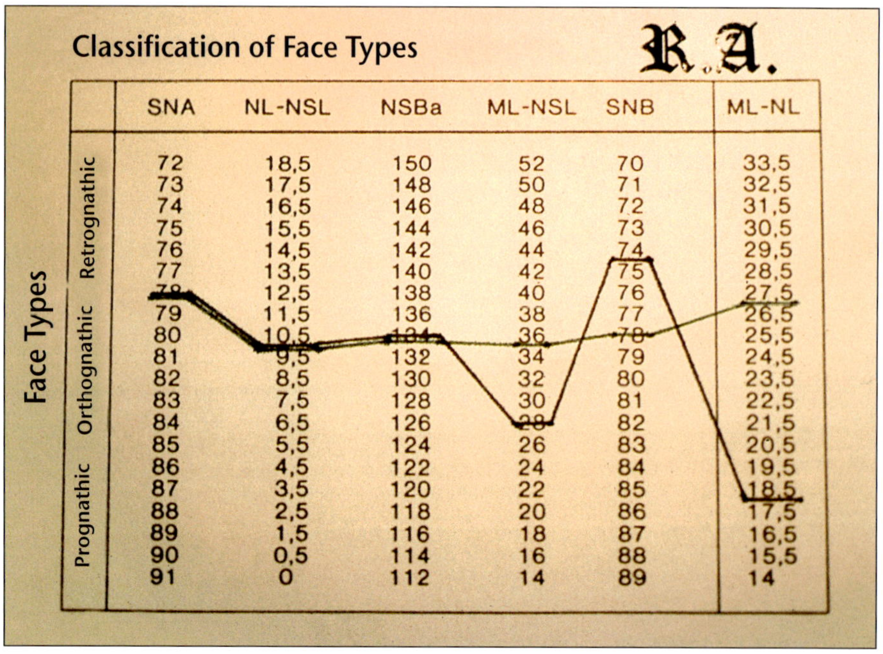

Classification of Face Types — R.A.

Face Types	SNA	NL-NSL	NSBa	ML-NSL	SNB	ML-NL
Retrognathic	72	18,5	150	52	70	33,5
	73	17,5	148	50	71	32,5
	74	16,5	146	48	72	31,5
	75	15,5	144	46	73	30,5
	76	14,5	142	44	74	29,5
	77	13,5	140	42	75	28,5
Orthognathic	78	12,5	138	40	76	27,5
	79	11,5	136	38	77	26,5
	80	10,5	134	36	78	25,5
	81	9,5	132	34	79	24,5
	82	8,5	130	32	80	23,5
	83	7,5	128	30	81	22,5
	84	6,5	126	28	82	21,5
	85	5,5	124	26	83	20,5
Prognathic	86	4,5	122	24	84	19,5
	87	3,5	120	22	85	18,5
	88	2,5	118	20	86	17,5
	89	1,5	116	18	87	16,5
	90	0,5	114	16	88	15,5
	91	0	112	14	89	14

Fig 6-3b Formula for even proportions; Hasund's cephalometric analysis (the Bergen technique)[1] showing the patient's values *(black)* before and *(green)* after orthodontic treatment. (SNA) Sella-nasion–point A; (NL-NSL) nasolabial-naison-sella–point L; (NSBa) naison-sella-baisón; (ML-NSL) mandibulolabial-naison-sella–point L; (SNB) sella-nasion–point B; (ML-NL) mandibulolabial-nasolabial angle.

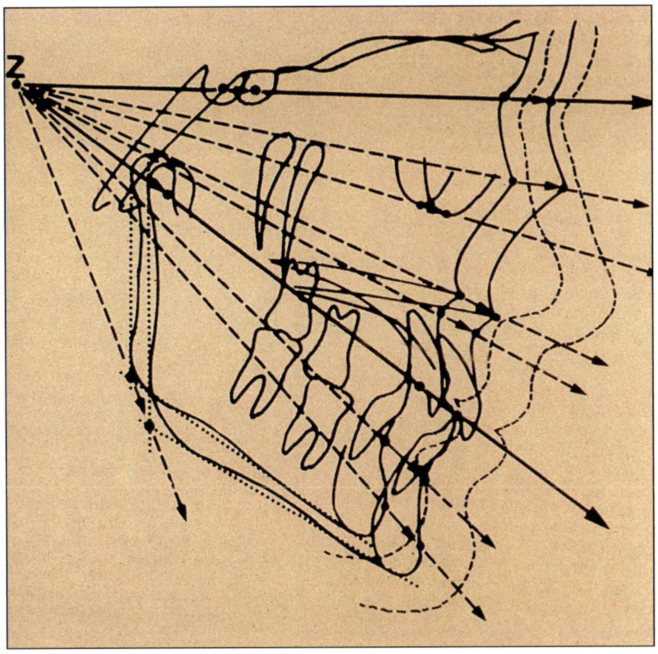

Fig 6-4a Determining the center of growth in the skull.

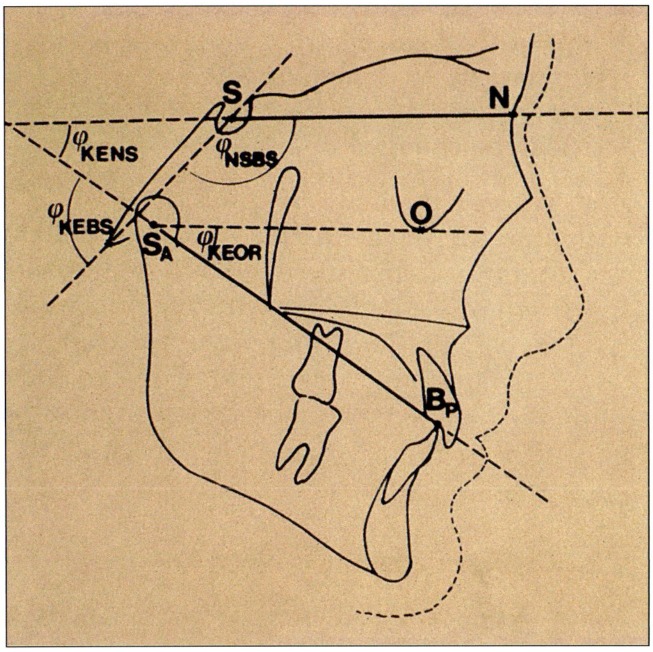

Fig 6-4b Angle between the coupling plane and the axis orbital plane.

Table 6-1 Maxillary angles after bone growth is completed

Angle	Mean (degrees)	Standard deviation (degrees)
Coupling plane–sella-nasion	34.45	3.59
Coupling plane–BS	84.95	5.95
Coupling plane–orbital axis plane	32.25	3.13

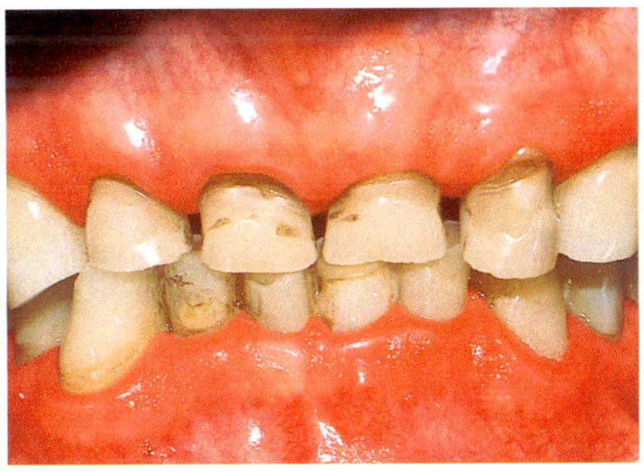

Fig 6-5a Severely abraded dentition.

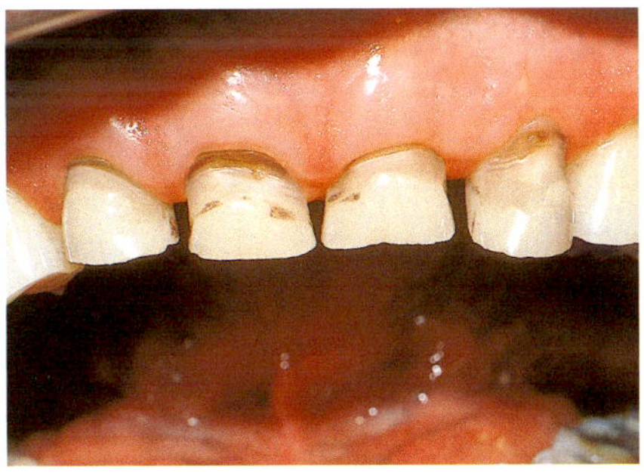

Fig 6-5b Abrasion of the maxillary teeth.

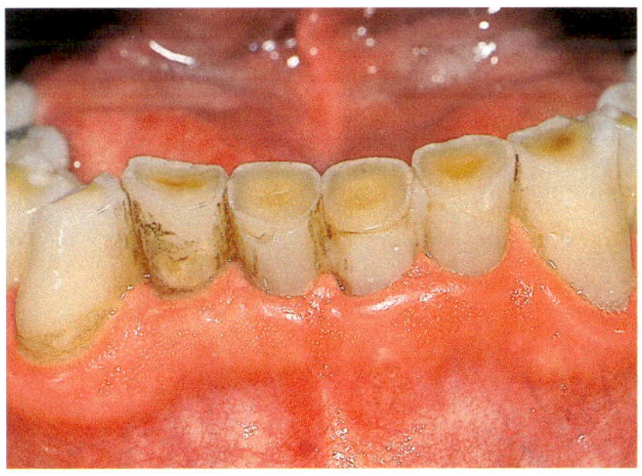

Fig 6-5c Abrasion of the mandibular teeth.

The coupling plane is the connecting plane between the hinge axis of the TMJs and the incisal edges of the mandibular anterior teeth. Kubein-Meesenburg et al[2] reported that this angle between the coupling plane and the orbital axis plane (CP-OP) remains almost constant because of the central direction of growth in relation to the coupling plane. It is 31.3 degrees for adolescents and 32 degrees in adults. This is the key to an exact measurement of the vertical dimension that can be transferred to the articulator (Figs 6-4a and 6-4b and Table 6-1).

Case report

A 55-year-old patient presented with severe bruxism and a loss of tooth substance in the vertical dimension (Figs 6-

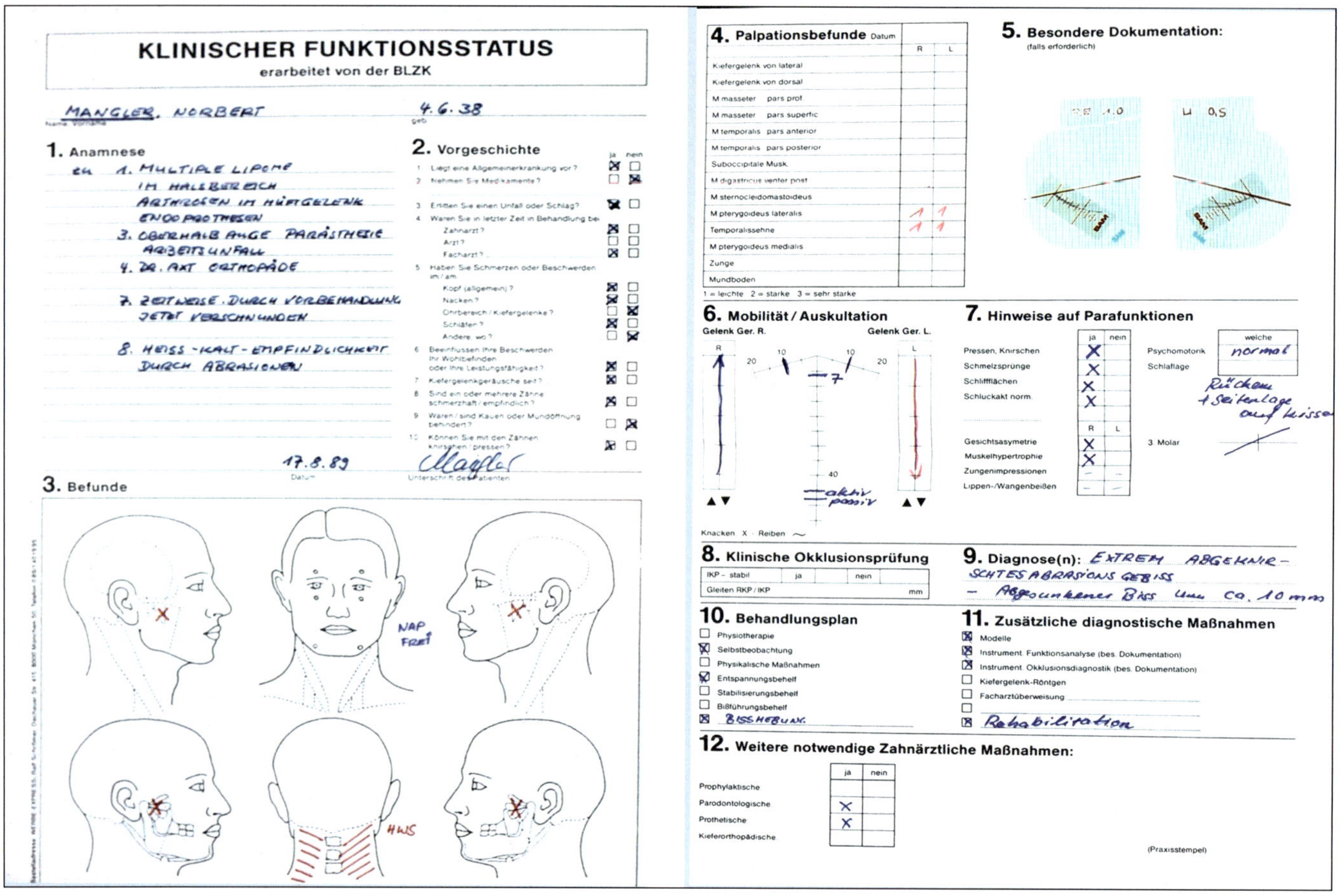

KLINISCHER FUNKTIONSSTATUS
erarbeitet von der BLZK

MANGLER, NORBERT — Name, Vorname
4.6.38 — geb.

1. Anamnese
zu 1. MULTIPLE LIPOME IM HALSBEREICH
ARTHROSEN IM HÜFTGELENK
ENDOPROTHESEN
3. OBERHALB AUGE PARÄSTHESIE
ARBEITSUNFALL
4. DR. AXT ORTHOPÄDE
7. ZEITWEISE. DURCH VORBEHANDLUNG JETZT VERSCHWUNDEN
8. HEISS-KALT-EMPFINDLICHKEIT DURCH ABRASIONEN

2. Vorgeschichte

		ja	nein
1	Liegt eine Allgemeinerkrankung vor?	X	
2	Nehmen Sie Medikamente?		X
3	Erlitten Sie einen Unfall oder Schlag?	X	
4	Waren Sie in letzter Zeit in Behandlung bei		
	Zahnarzt?	X	
	Arzt?		
	Facharzt?	X	
5	Haben Sie Schmerzen oder Beschwerden im/am		
	Kopf (allgemein)?	X	
	Nacken?	X	
	Ohrbereich / Kiefergelenke?		X
	Schläfen?	X	
	Andere, wo?		X
6	Beeinflussen Ihre Beschwerden Ihr Wohlbefinden oder Ihre Leistungsfähigkeit?	X	
7	Kiefergelenkgeräusche seit?	X	
8	Sind ein oder mehrere Zähne schmerzhaft / empfindlich?	X	
9	Waren / sind Kauen oder Mundöffnung behindert?		X
10	Können Sie mit den Zähnen knirschen / pressen?	X	

17.8.89 — Datum
Unterschrift des Patienten

3. Befunde
NAP FREI
HWS

4. Palpationsbefunde Datum

	R	L
Kiefergelenk von lateral		
Kiefergelenk von dorsal		
M masseter pars prof		
M masseter pars superfic		
M temporalis pars anterior		
M temporalis pars posterior		
Suboccipitale Musk.		
M digastricus venter post		
M sternocleidomastoideus		
M pterygoideus lateralis	1	1
Temporalissehne	1	1
M pterygoideus medialis		
Zunge		
Mundboden		

1 = leichte 2 = starke 3 = sehr starke

5. Besondere Dokumentation: (falls erforderlich)
1.0
0,5

6. Mobilität / Auskultation
Gelenk Ger. R. — Gelenk Ger. L.
R L 20 10 10 20 7 40
aktiv
passiv
Knacken X · Reiben ~

7. Hinweise auf Parafunktionen

	ja	nein
Pressen, Knirschen	X	
Schmelzsprünge	X	
Schliffflächen	X	
Schluckakt norm.	X	
	R	**L**
Gesichtsasymetrie	X	
Muskelhypertrophie	X	
Zungenimpressionen	–	–
Lippen-/Wangenbeißen	–	–

	welche
Psychomotorik	normal
Schlaflage	Rücken + Seitenlage auf Kissen

3. Molar

8. Klinische Okklusionsprüfung

IKP – stabil	ja		nein	
Gleiten RKP / IKP				mm

9. Diagnose(n): EXTREM ABGEKNIRSCHTES ABRASIONS GEBISS
– Abgesunkener Biss um ca. 10 mm

10. Behandlungsplan
- [ ] Physiotherapie
- [x] Selbstbeobachtung
- [ ] Physikalische Maßnahmen
- [x] Entspannungsbehelf
- [ ] Stabilisierungsbehelf
- [ ] Bißführungsbehelf
- [x] BISSHEBUNG

11. Zusätzliche diagnostische Maßnahmen
- [x] Modelle
- [x] Instrument. Funktionsanalyse (bes. Dokumentation)
- [x] Instrument. Okklusionsdiagnostik (bes. Dokumentation)
- [ ] Kiefergelenk-Röntgen
- [ ] Facharztüberweisung
- [ ]
- [x] Rehabilitation

12. Weitere notwendige Zahnärztliche Maßnahmen:

	ja	nein
Prophylaktische		
Parodontologische	X	
Prothetische	X	
Kieferorthopädische		

(Praxisstempel)

Fig 6-5d Clinical functional analysis.

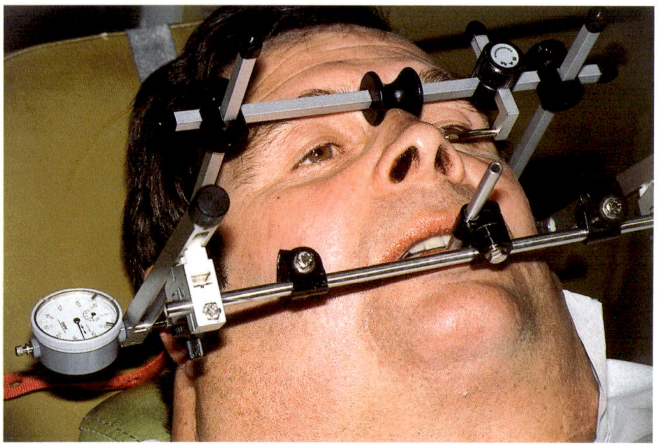

Fig 6-5e Technical functional analysis.

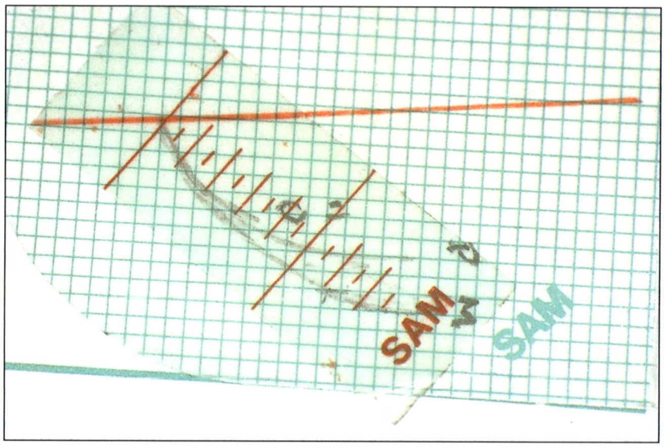

Fig 6-5f Axiography.

5a to 6-5c). All the teeth had to be restored with crowns because of the substantial loss of calcified tooth structures and the exposed, hypersensitive dentin. The patient wished to look good and to be able to chew properly.

The central question in such cases is: How far should the lost vertical dimension be restored? A prerequisite for successfully raising the occlusion is that the muscles and the TMJ have to be symptom-free. This must be confirmed with a clinical and technical functional analysis (Figs 6-5d to 6-5f).

A lateral cephalogram for functional analysis was taken with the patient's dentition in a centric position and with

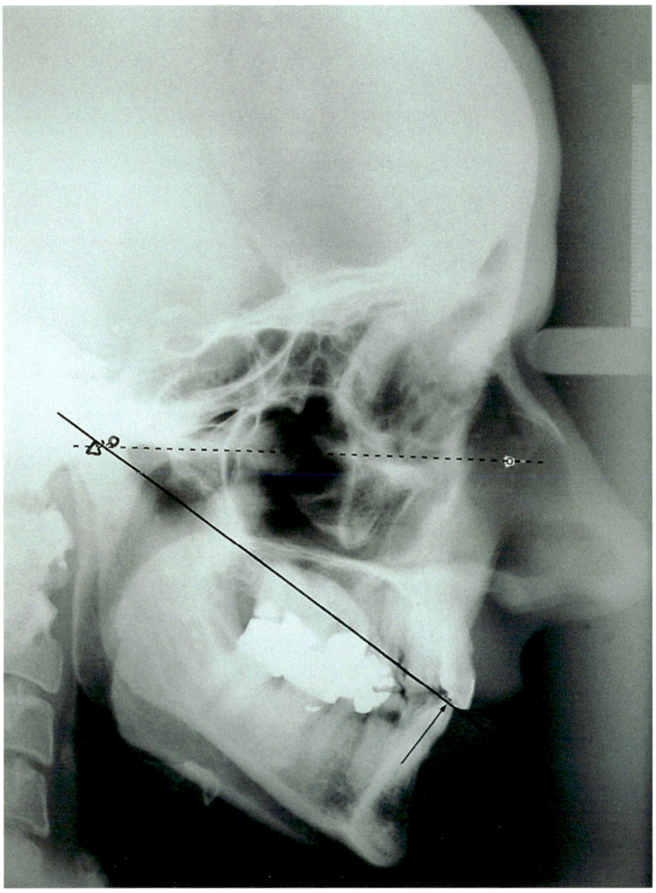

Fig 6-5g Functional analysis of the cephalogram.

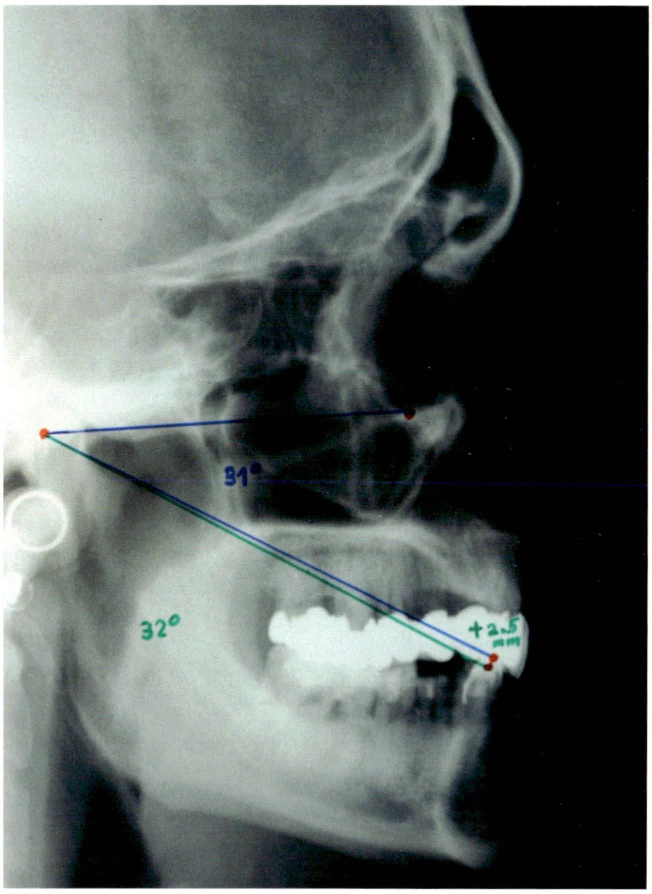

Fig 6-5h Vertical dimension.

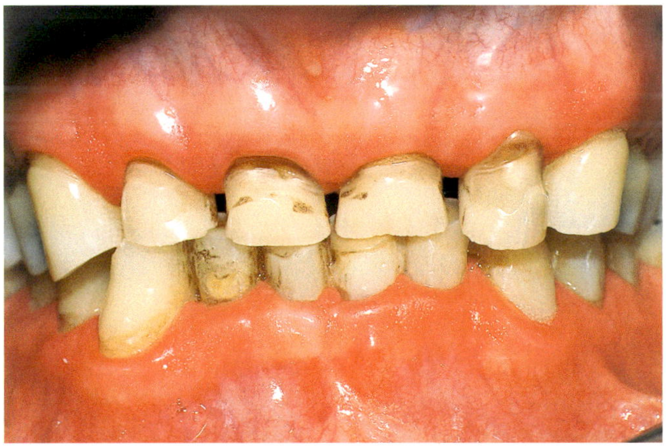

Fig 6-5i Appearance before restoration of the maxillary and mandibular teeth.

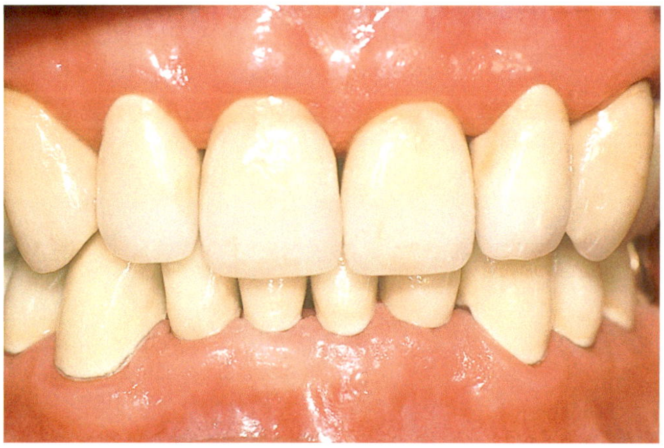

Fig 6-5j Appearance after restoration.

a slightly raised occlusion (Fig 6-5g). After the occlusion was raised, the angle CP-OP was drawn and measured. In this case, the angle was 31 degrees. Therefore, the occlusion had to be raised by 1 degree.

To transfer this measurement to the articulator, the coupling plane was drawn with the required angle of 32 degrees (Fig 6-5h). The distance between the two angles was measured along the tooth axis of the mandibular anterior tooth with a divider. In this patient, the distance was 2.5 mm.

As could be seen on the nose-rest, the cephalometric radiograph had a magnification of 1:1.10. This scale was used to measure off the raised occlusion to which the divider was adjusted (4 mm). This was performed in a manner similar to the use of a nautical chart. The value thus gained was transferred to the articulator as the degree to which the occlusion should be raised, and the incisal pin was adjusted to the raised occlusion.

If no muscle or TMJ symptoms are present, this new vertical dimension can be tested in the patient's mouth with splints or provisional restorations. In this case, after a trouble-free trial period of 6 months, this new vertical dimension was transferred to the patient's permanent crowns (Figs 6-5i and 6-5j).

The functional analysis of cephalometric radiographs should not be understood as a mathematical analysis with an accuracy to a hundredth of a millimeter but as a guideline that can help the clinician to determine the vertical dimension, which of course has to be tested clinically.

Facial Profile Analysis

Common problem: Change of the facial profile after placement of partial or complete dentures

A patient's profile may change when fixed or removable partial dentures or complete dentures are placed in the anterior region of the mouth. Despite good occlusion and good anterior esthetics, the resulting facial profile may be unattractive. The face may look sunken, or the mouth may appear too prominent. This is primarily a result of the occlusal height but also may be caused by the tooth setup and the design of the arch form (Fig 6-6).

Proven solution: Facial profile analysis

In orthodontics, soft tissue analysis performed with the help of a lateral cephalogram—an analysis of the facial profile—is an integral part of treatment planning (Fig 6-7). This concept could also be useful in prosthetic dentistry to create predictable facial profiles for the benefit of patients. Are there any guidelines for creating an esthetic profile?

Two methods for analyzing lateral cephalograms (and variations thereof) are used in orthodontics: cephalometric analysis according to Ricketts and cephalometric analysis according to Hasund[1] (Bergen analysis). Both methods also include soft tissue analysis and, in particular, both use an "esthetic line" to analyze the facial profile (Fig 6-8).

Ricketts' esthetic line is defined as the tangent from the tip of the nose to the most prominent point of the chin, pogonion. The lower lip is supposed to be a distance of 2 mm from this esthetic line; the upper lip is supposed to be 4 mm from this esthetic line. This can be verified very easily, directly on the patient, with a ruler or something similar and without analyzing a cephalogram.

Holdaway's esthetic line, based on a concept by Leonardo da Vinci, is defined as the connecting line from the transitional point at the underside of the nose (where the line of the nose changes from convex to concave) to the most prominent part of the chin, pogonion. The upper and lower lips should both make contact with this esthetic line.

Both esthetic lines will be demonstrated with a practical example: The orthodontic treatment of a young man was

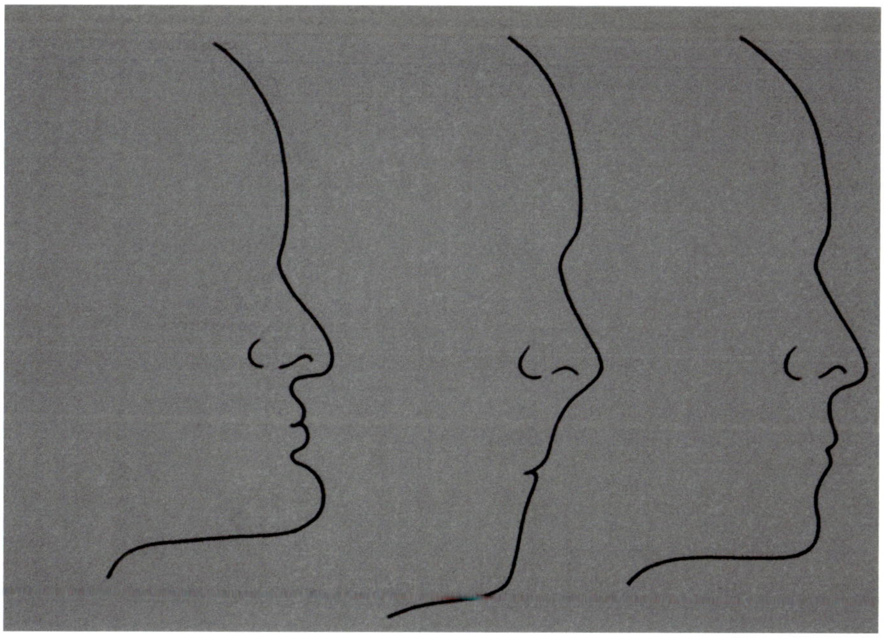

Fig 6-6 Traced facial profiles.

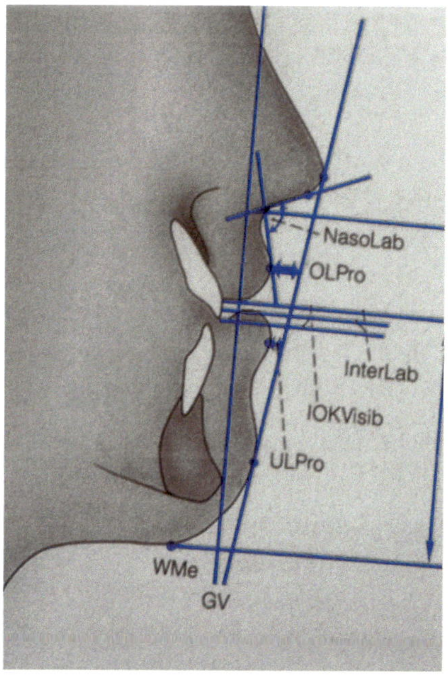

Fig 6-7 Soft tissue analysis.

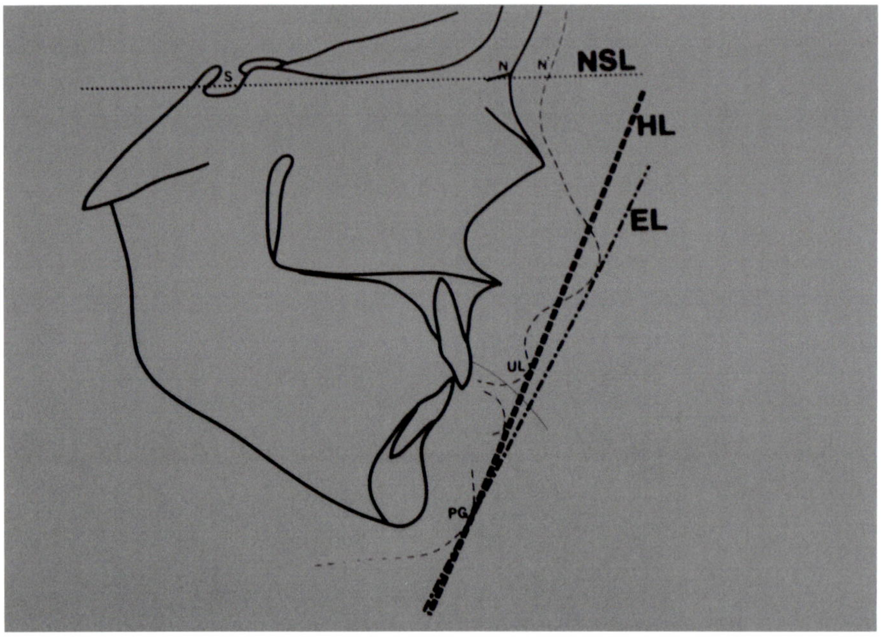

Fig 6-8 The esthetic lines according to Ricketts and Holdaway. (S) Sella; (N) nasion; (NSL) nasion-sella line; (HL) Holdaway's esthetic line; (EL) Ricketts' esthetic line; (UL) upper lip; (PG) pogonion.

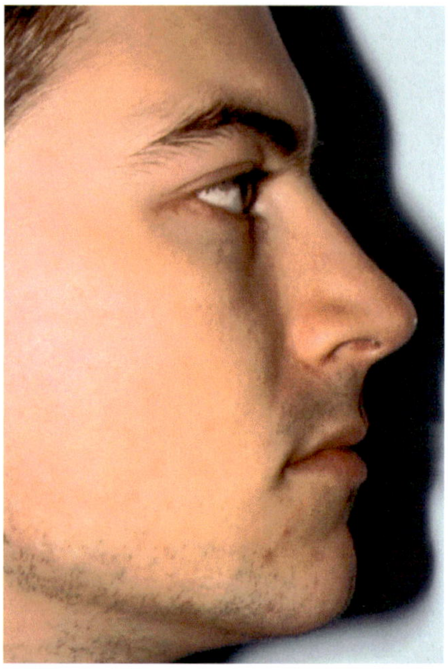

Fig 6-9a Young patient after the completed orthodontic treatment.

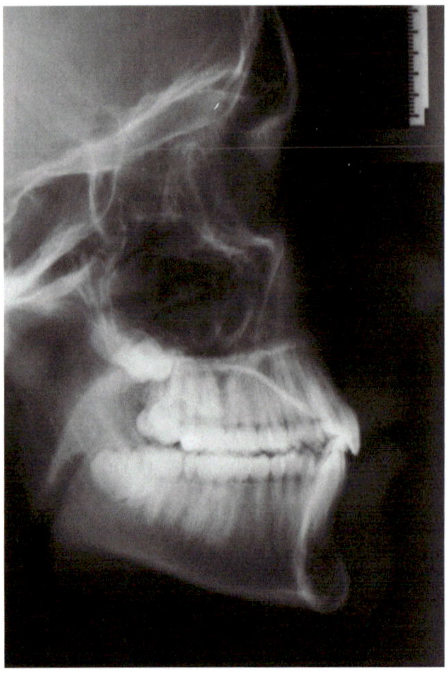

Fig 6-9b Patient's lateral cephalogram.

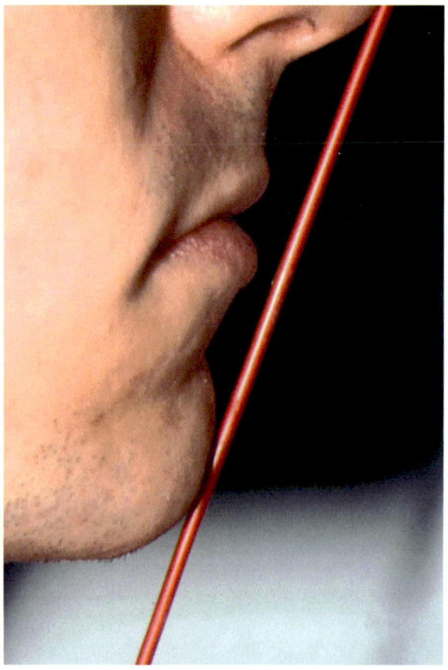

Fig 6-9c Facial profile analysis with the Ricketts esthetic line.

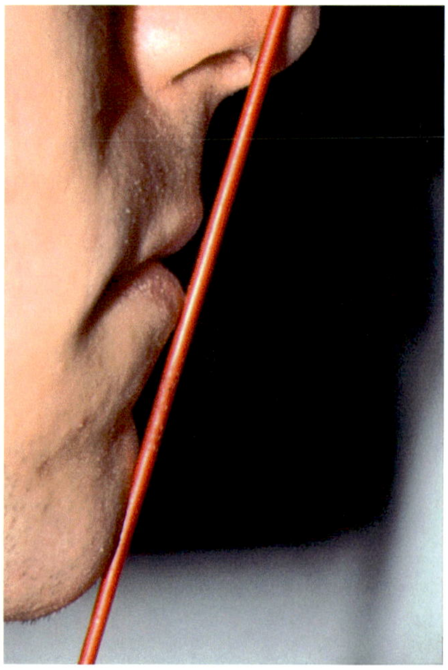

Fig 6-9d Facial profile analysis with the Holdaway esthetic line.

successfully completed 10 years ago (Figs 6-9a and 6-9b). A ruler was placed on the patient's face, and the facial profile was assessed with both the Ricketts esthetic line (Fig 6-9c) and with the Holdaway esthetic line (Fig 6-9d). The profile analyses revealed that the distance between the upper lip and both esthetic lines was 1 mm too long. Examination of the casts (Fig 6-9e) reveals that the maxillary incisors of the patient are somewhat too steeply inclined, thus causing the retrusion of the upper lip.

Which of the esthetic lines is more useful? Because the size of the nose varies widely and the nose can be prominent in many patients, the esthetic line described by

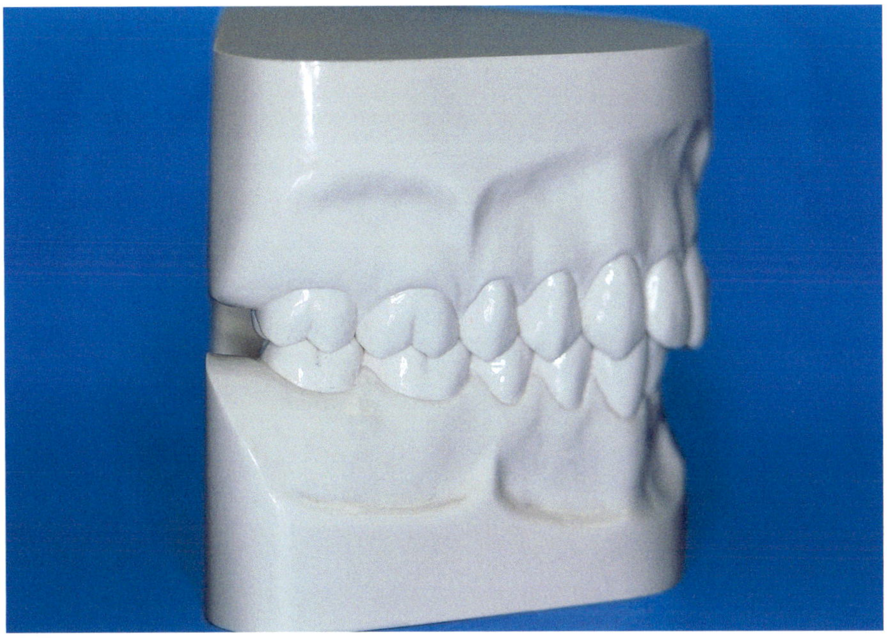

Fig 6-9e Patient's casts.

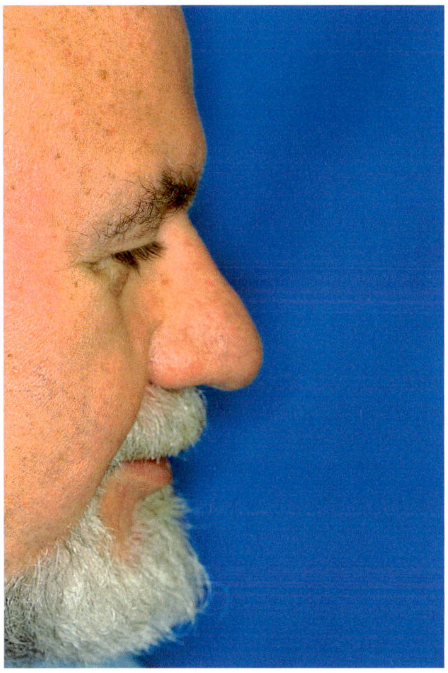

Fig 6-10 Profile of a bearded patient.

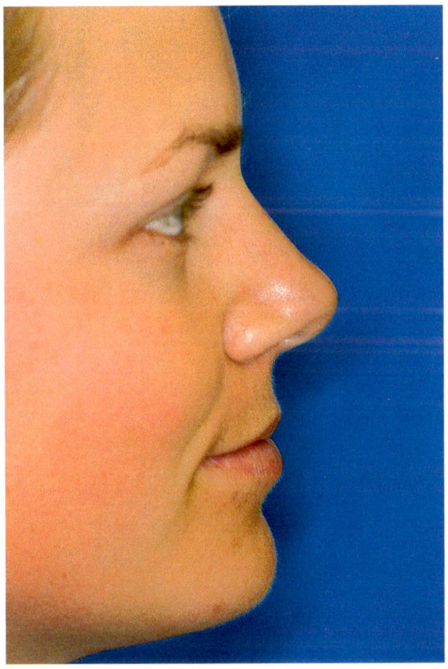

Fig 6-11a Patient photograph for practicing facial profile analysis.

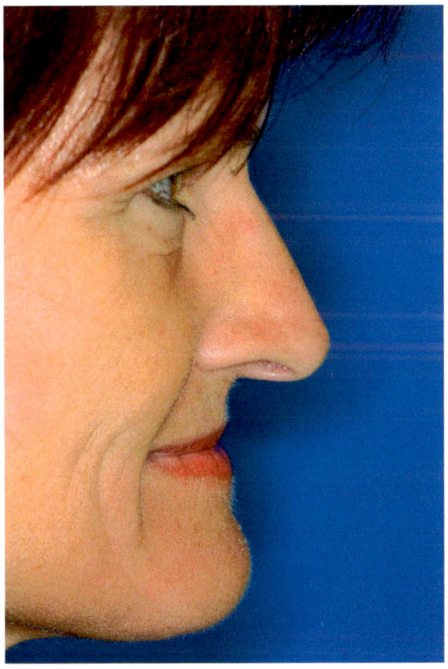

Fig 6-11b Profile for practice.

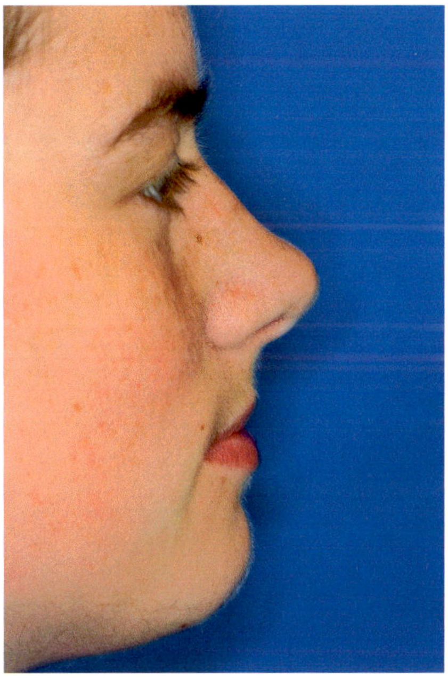

Fig 6-11c Profile for practice.

Ricketts often is not a great help. Surprisingly, though, the transitional convex-to-concave point of underside of the nose is relatively constant, leading to good results with use of the esthetic line defined by Holdaway. With this line, no matter how prominent the nose, this point on the underside is constant in relation to the facial profile.

A simple profile analysis using a ruler is not possible if the patient is wearing a beard (Fig 6-10). There are only two options: Either the patient will have to shave, or a soft tissue analysis will have to be performed on the lateral cephalogram.

Three different patient profiles for practicing profile analysis are shown in Figs 6-11a to 6-11c. The esthetic lines can be drawn in with a ruler and a light pencil. Interested readers can consider possible corrections for the patients in these examples.

Soft tissue analysis does offer far more opportunities to predict the facial profile in orthodontics, eg, the classification of skeletal angles. It is also an integral part of planning procedures for plastic surgery.

Mock-up: Dental Imaging Directly on the Patient

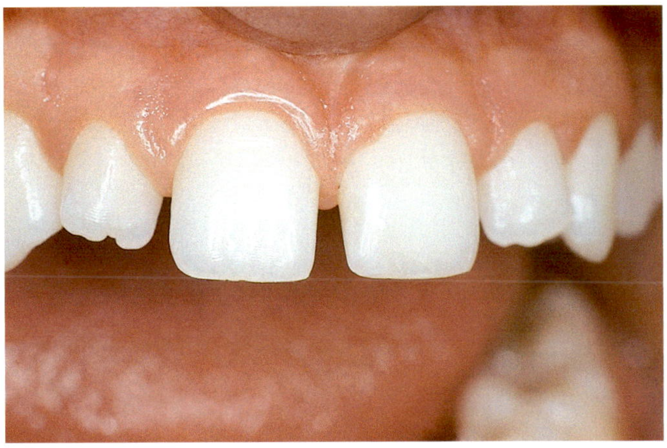

Fig 6-12a Initial situation. Spaces are present in the maxillary anterior teeth.

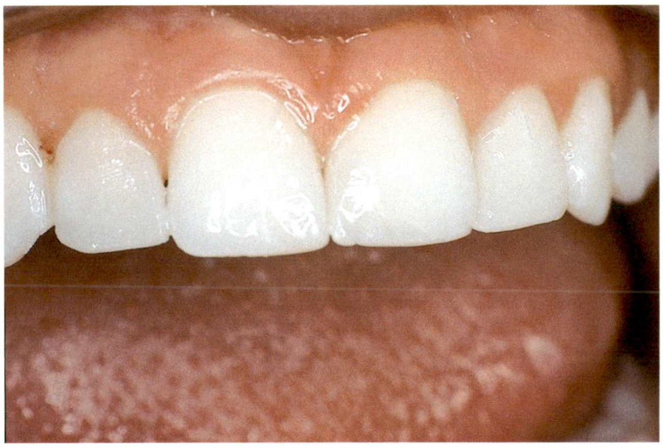

Fig 6-12b After a mock-up, the direct method of dental imaging.

Common problem: Simulation of an adhesive restoration for patient education and treatment planning

In everyday practice, a dentist is faced with the same challenge over and over again—providing the patient with a vivid picture of the achievable treatment outcome. On the one hand, this serves to let the patient know what to expect; on the other hand, it allows the dentist and the dental technician to develop a clear vision of what is feasible with respect to the shape and color of the restorations. This should be done without any preparation of the teeth, ie, noninvasively; if the teeth are prepared before both parties agree on an esthetic concept and the result differs largely from the patient's expectations, the dentist will be in trouble.

Everything a clinician may tell a patient prior to a restorative procedure can be considered patient information, whereas whatever the dentist says afterward amounts to an excuse—or to testimony in front of some commission or even in court.

What noninvasive options do the dentist and dental technician have when it comes to informing the patient about the achievable treatment outcome? The following tools are available for dental imaging:

1. Waxup on the patient's casts. This procedure is of little informative value for the patient.
2. Computer imaging on a digital photograph. This option is very expensive, very complex, and has to be practiced constantly.
3. Mock-up—diagnostic veneering directly in the patient's mouth. With some practice, this method leads to great success (Figs 6-12a and 6-12b).

Proven solution: Direct veneering in the patient's mouth for diagnostics

A 14-year-old girl and her mother visited the dental office after the girl's orthodontic treatment had been completed. They inquired about the possibilities for closing the space in the girl's anterior maxilla (Figs 6-12c to 6-12e). The orthodontist had found that the teeth in the maxilla were too narrow, had indicated that orthodontic space closure was not possible in this case, and had recommended a restorative solution through the dentist.

An oral examination confirmed the orthodontist's assessment. The anterior region had spaces and the lateral incisors were rotated. The mother requested use of an adhesive technique instead of crowns to protect the tooth substance.

The mother and daughter were informed that treatment was possible both in a direct technique with resin composite and in an indirect technique with ceramic veneers. The problem, however, was the achievable result. Before the actual treatment began, a cost projection

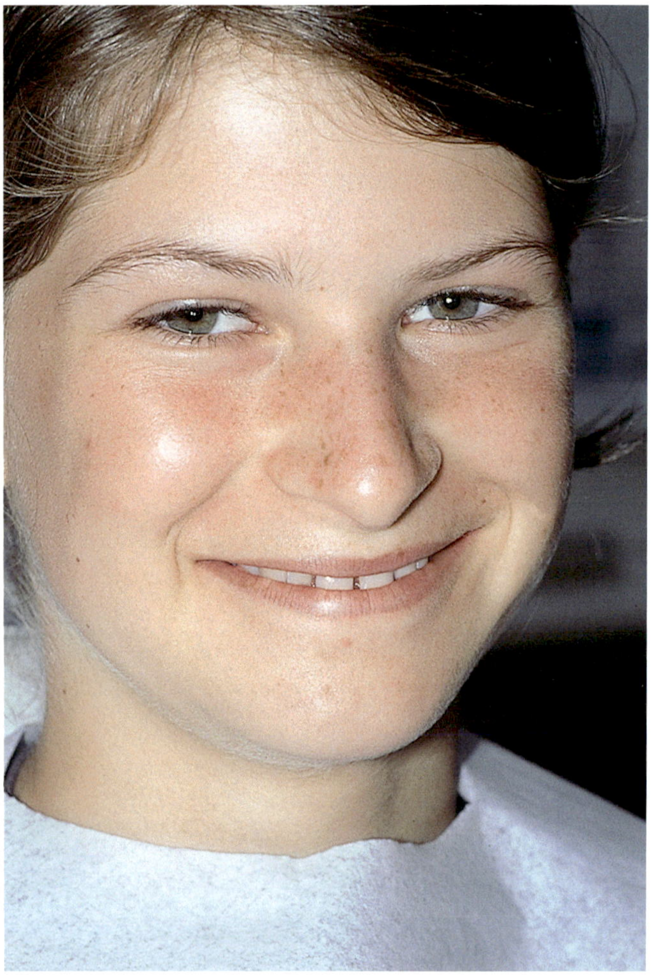

Fig 6-12c Full-facial view of the 14-year-old patient .

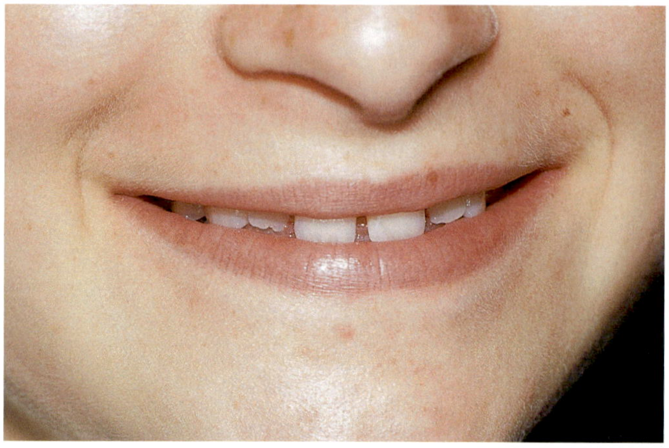

Fig 6-12d Patient's smile.

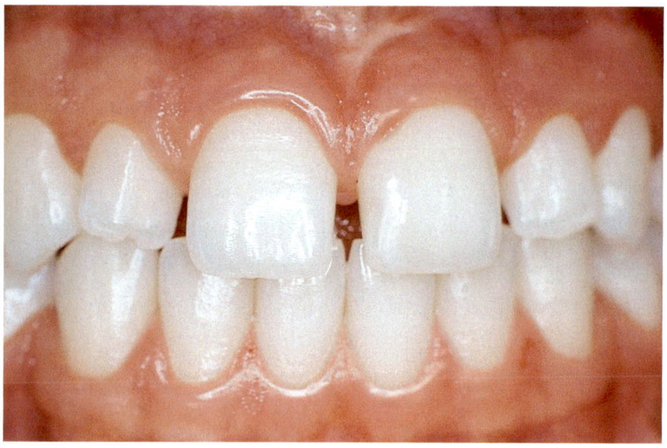

Fig 6-12e Maxillary anterior region with spaces.

would have to be reviewed with the patient. Direct diagnostic veneering without damage to the teeth was the ideal tool for this purpose.

The patient's teeth were carefully dried with air, and a cheek retractor was inserted to gain a better view (Fig 6-12f). The appropriate shade was chosen with the help of a shade guide. In most cases, one color for the tooth body and one color for the cervical area are sufficient. For this young patient, one color was sufficient.

The dentist should always sit behind the supine patient and look down on the teeth from above and behind the patient. The width of the patient's teeth was measured with a small ruler and the available space was divided. Because the work should always start from the midline and then proceed to the sides, in this patient, the maxillary central incisors had to be broadened and elongated first.

A matrix band was contoured to proximally shape the broadened part of the tooth and to separate the teeth (Figs 6-12g to 6-12i). The matrix band was adapted to the tooth and the resin composite was applied (Fig 6-12j). To facilitate flat application, resin composite was used in an application syringe whose opening was flattened with pliers (Figs 6-12k to 6-12m).

The resin composite was given the appropriate tooth shape with the help of rubber modeling instruments (Fig 6-12n). The advantage of these instruments is that they do not stick if they are slightly moistened with bonding agent. The elastic rubber instruments allow flexible modeling of the teeth, which permits development of a good tooth shape very quickly. These instruments for dentists and dental technicians, which are available in various shapes, were especially developed to contour strong and nonflowable resin composite materials (Fig 6-12o). Rubber instruments like these were originally used as cuticle sticks in manicures. The different shapes of the rubber tips and their applications are listed in Table 6-2.

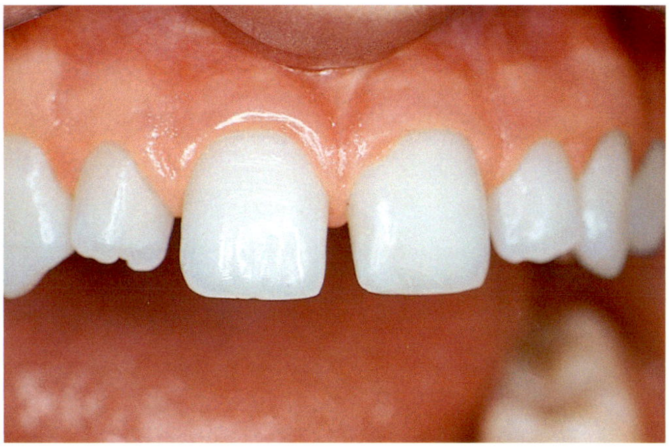
Fig 6-12f Maxillary incisors after drying, ready for the mockup.

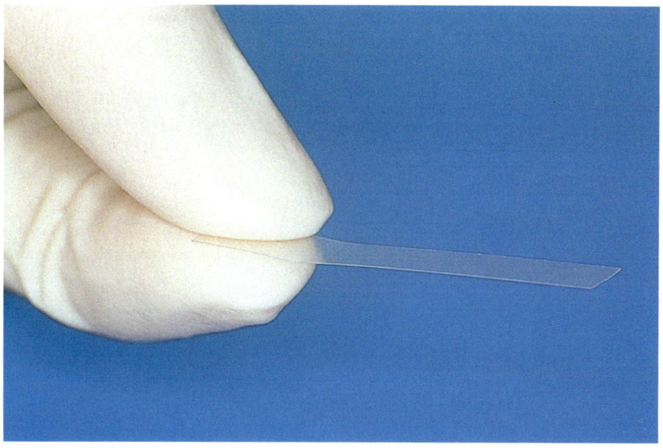
Fig 6-12g Clear matrix band.

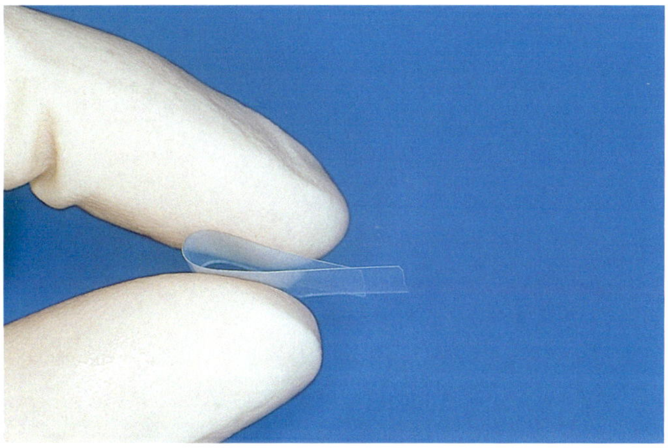
Fig 6-12h Rolling the matrix band without creasing it.

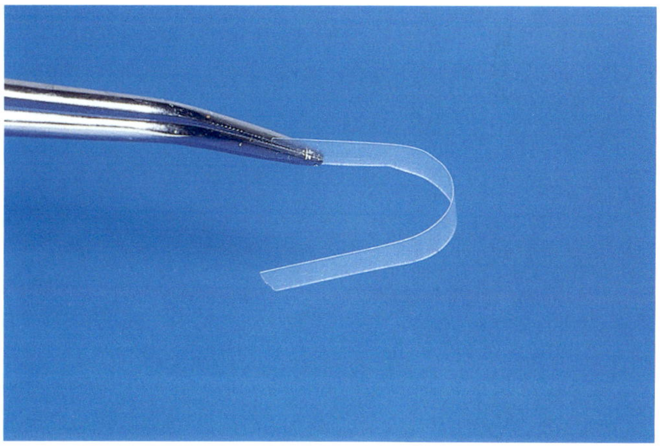
Fig 6-12i Contoured matrix band.

The central incisors were shaped (Fig 6-12p). The individual layers were polymerized briefly with a curing light for 20 seconds, to keep the previous layer from being deformed when the next layer was applied. Finally, the surface was smoothed with a fine watercolor brush. Then the lateral incisors were reshaped with resin composite (Figs 6-12q and 6-12r). The application of the resin composite was completed with a final light-curing step (Fig 6-12s).

The tooth contours were carefully polished and finished. Care was taken to avoid damaging the natural tooth substance (Figs 6-12t to 12x). The mock-up must be reversible; therefore, the dentist can add material but not remove tooth substance.

A final inspection was made from behind the supine patient and from the anterior perspective (Fig 6-12y). The biggest mistake that could have been made at this point would have been to simply give the patient a hand mirror and ask, "So what do you think?" The effect of the teeth on the entire appearance should always be tested in a full-length mirror. The patient should walk up to this mirror, and the dentist can gauge the effect of the direct dental imaging by the patient's reactions. In this case, the patient was amazed and very pleased with the simulated outcome (Figs 6-12z and 12aa).

Subsequently, photographs with and without the mock-up were taken. It is also recommended that impressions be taken to allow the vision of the desired outcome to be communicated to the dental technician.

At this point, the treatment options were discussed with the patient and her mother. Orthodontic closure of the diastema between the central incisors did not make sense from an esthetic point of view, because the lateral incisors would have become too wide. The tooth eruption process and the alveolar growth were not completed in the 14-year-old patient; thus, placement of a permanent restoration did not make sense. Therefore, the following treatment plan was developed: The space would be eliminated through immedi-

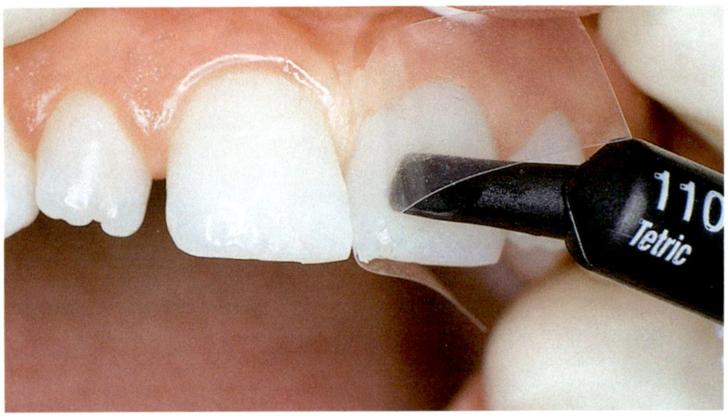

Fig 6-12j Application of resin composite.

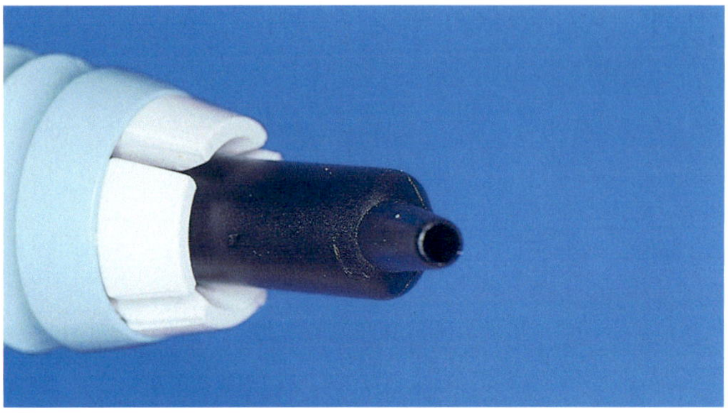

Fig 6-12k Round opening at the tip of the application syringe.

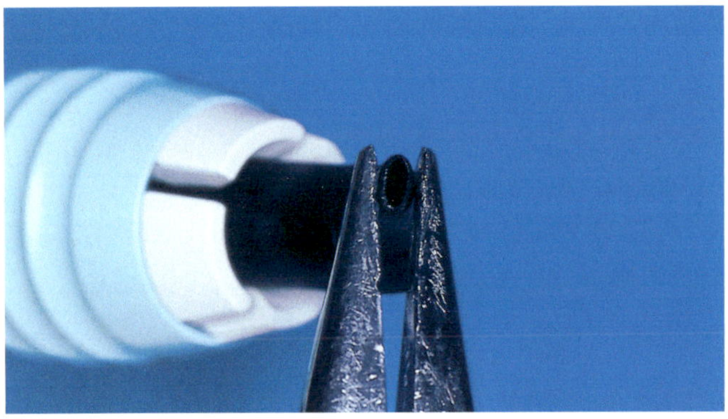

Fig 6-12l Opening pressed flat with flat-nose pliers to give it an oval shape.

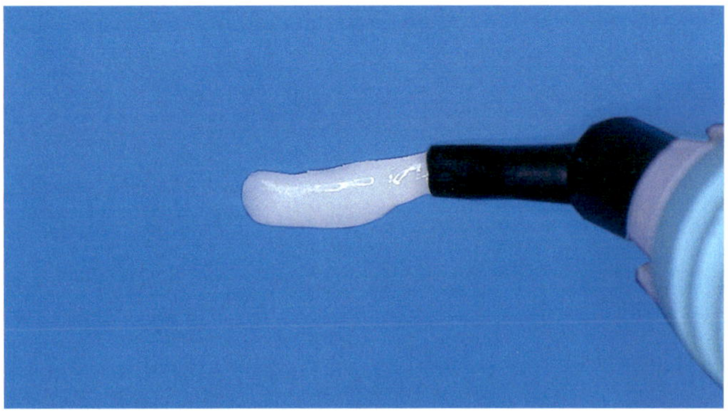

Fig 6-12m Syringing a flat stripe of resin composite.

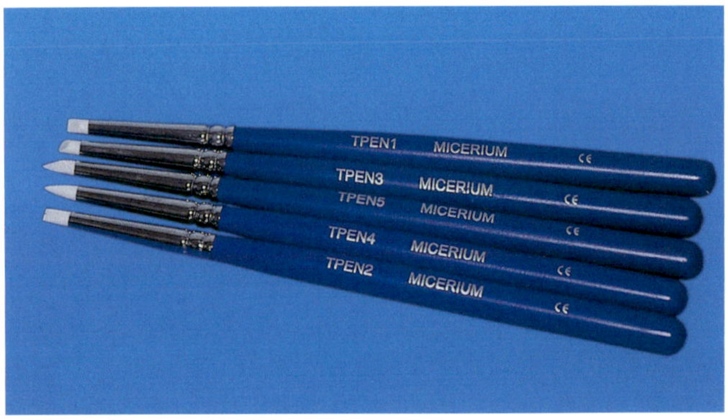

Fig 6-12n Modeling instruments with rubber tips (Micerium).

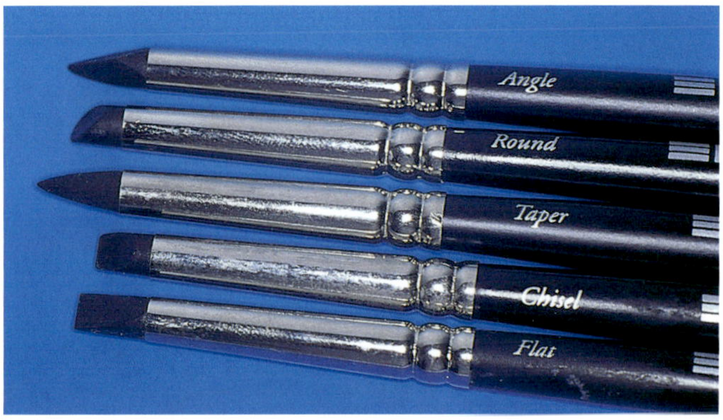

Fig 6-12o Various shapes of rubber instrument (Ivoclar Vivadent).

Modeling instrument	Application
Chisel	Universal instrument for spreading resin composite and modeling larger surfaces
Round	Modeling and shaping of the cervical region
Flat	Lamination, shaping, and structuring of the surface
Taper	Formation of occlusal surfaces
Angle	Application of opaquers and tints and shaping

Table 6-2 Application for the different shapes of rubber tools

ate restoration with direct resin composite veneers and minimally invasive preparation. Permanent restoration with indirect ceramic veneers of minimal extent would occur when the patient reached the age of 18 to 20 years. The cost was discussed with the patient and her mother, a treatment plan and cost projection were developed, and the necessary appointments were made.

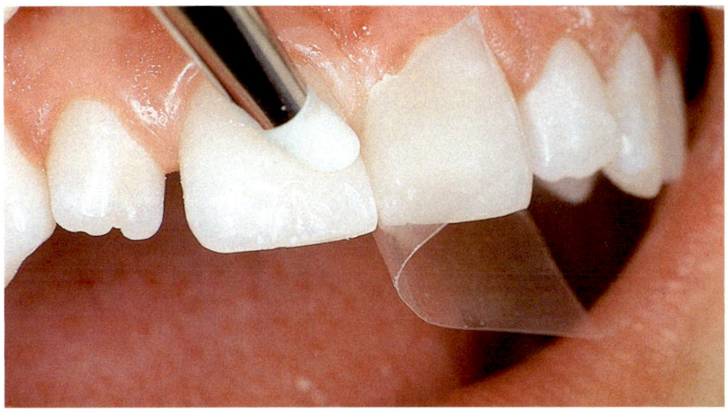

Fig 6-12p Shaping of the central incisors.

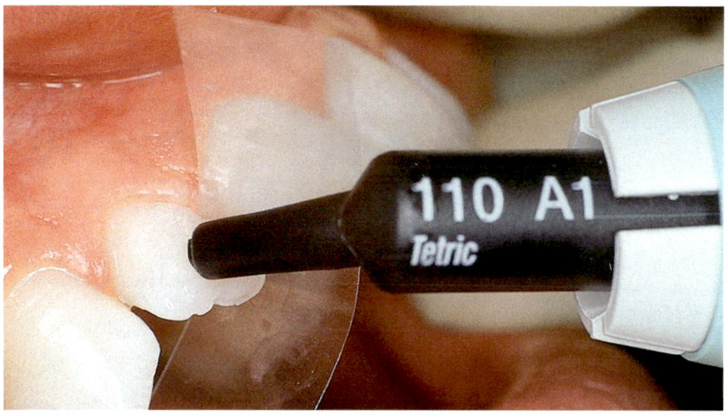

Fig 6-12q Modeling of the lateral incisors. Application of resin composite.

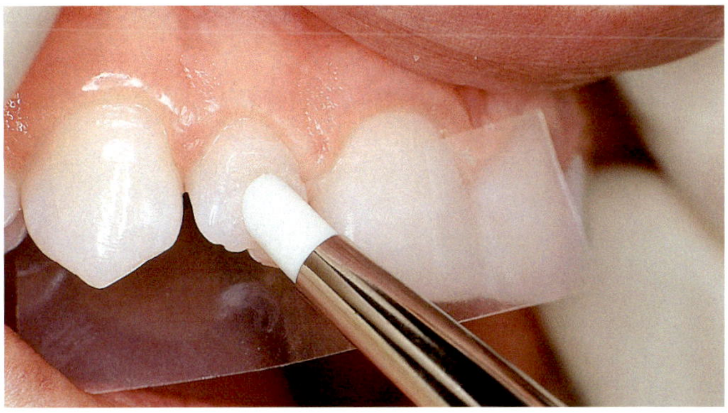

Fig 6-12r Shaping with the modeling instrument.

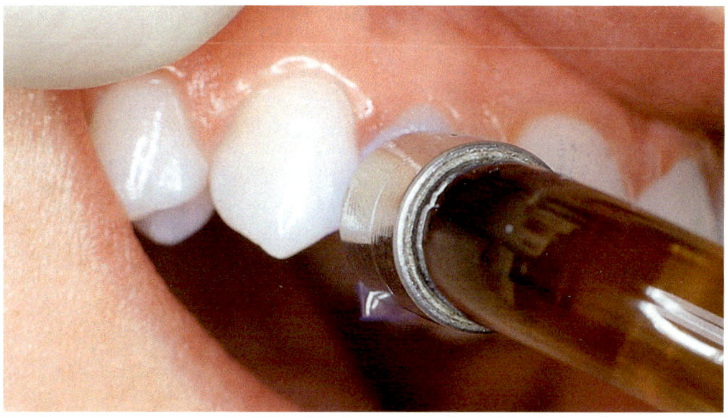

Fig 6-12s Polymerization of the resin composite.

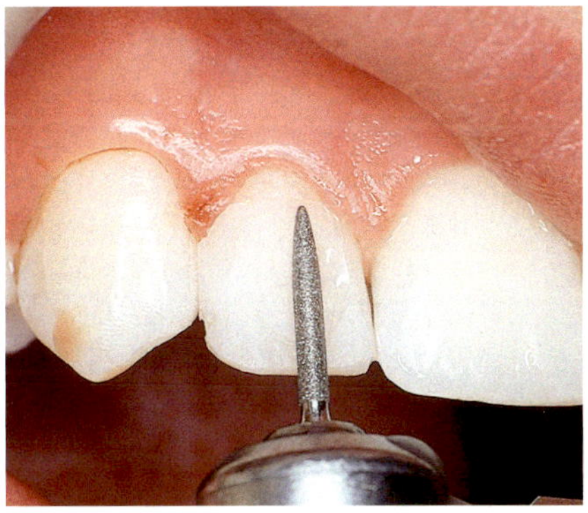

Fig 6-12t Careful finishing of the tooth contours.

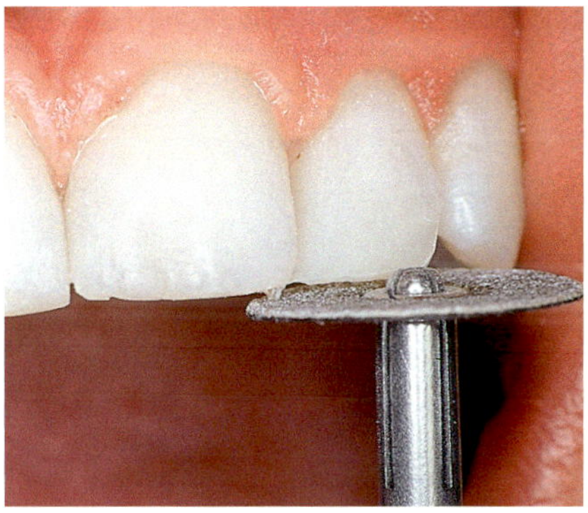

Fig 6-12u Finishing with an abrasive wheel.

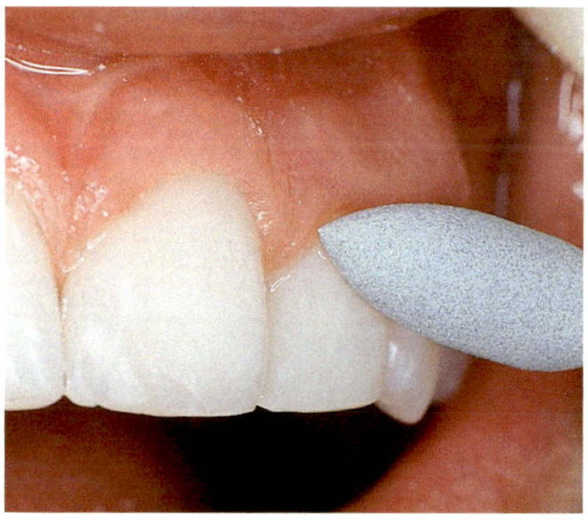

Fig 6-12v Finishing with an abrasive point.

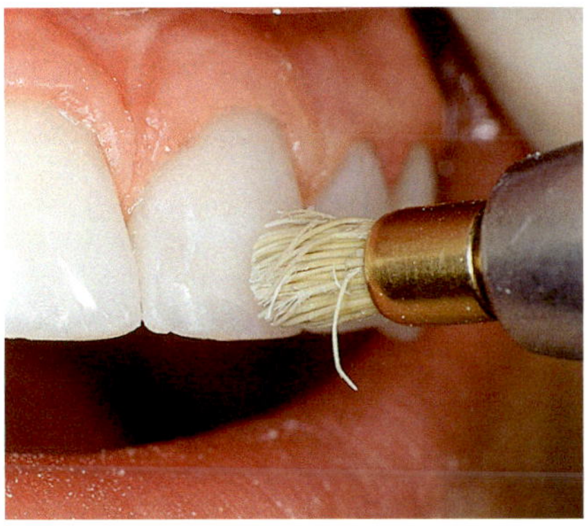

Fig 6-12w Polishing with a brush.

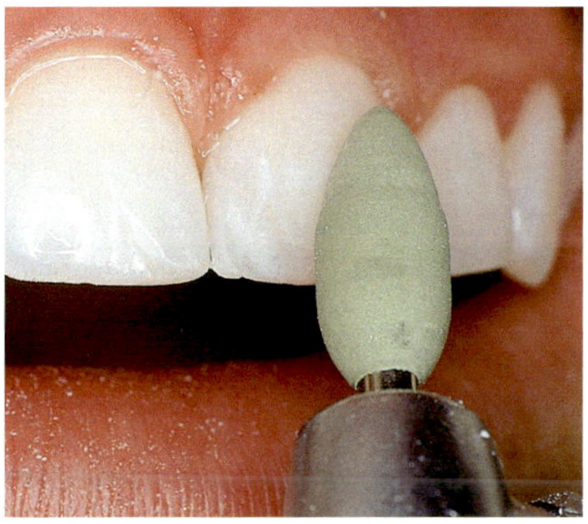

Fig 6-12x Polishing with a rubber point.

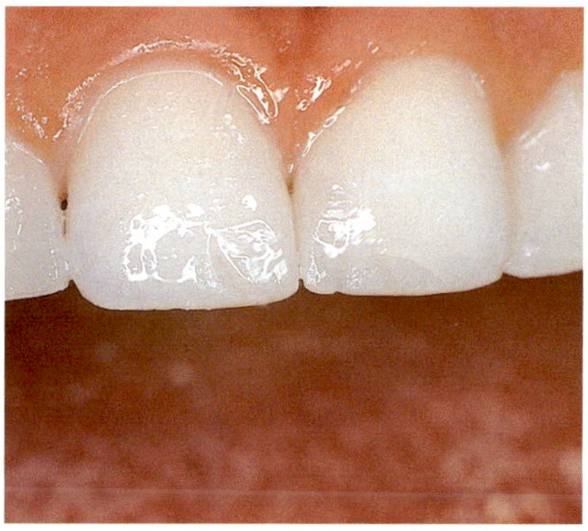

Fig 6-12y Final inspection of the mock-up.

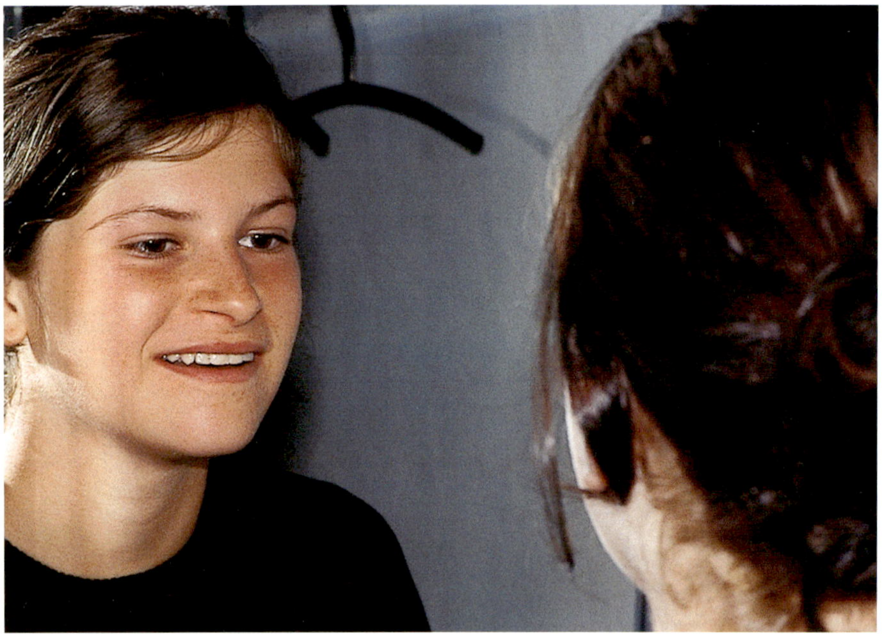

Fig 6-12z Patient examining the new appearance of her anterior teeth in a large mirror.

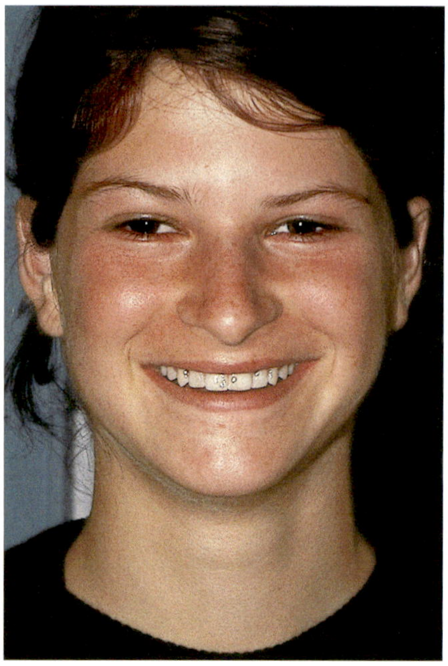

Fig 6-12aa Beaming patient. The restorations have met her expectations.

In the author's opinion, obtaining the patient's consent by using the mock-up method as a means of direct dental imaging is the most effective way to give the patient an idea of the final restorative result. Moreover, it is really enjoyable for a dentist to experience the positive reactions of the patients.

Materials

Tetric resin composite in application syringes (Ivoclar Vivadent) or any other high-quality resin composite in an application syringe
Modeling instruments with rubber tips (Girrbach; Ivoclar Vivadent; or, as used in the case report, Micerium)
Matrix bands, clear (Frasaco)
Watercolor brush C 2 (Ivoclar Vivadent)

Determination and Reconstruction of Correct Anterior Tooth Length

Common problem: Reconstruction of abraded anterior teeth

Reconstruction of severely abraded maxillary and mandibular anterior teeth is often a great challenge, as is determination of the correct tooth length. In many cases, this is problematic for everyone involved—the dentist, the dental technician, and especially the patient, who is given a totally new (or maybe the old) appearance through the reconstruction (Figs 6-13a to 6-13d).

A reconstruction with the correct tooth length results in a completely new appearance, a new smile, a new coordination of the lips, tongue, and facial muscles, and a change of phonation. The following problems can also occur, however: The patient may feel disfigured, have

Fig 6-13a *(left)* Patient's smile before reconstruction of her anterior teeth.

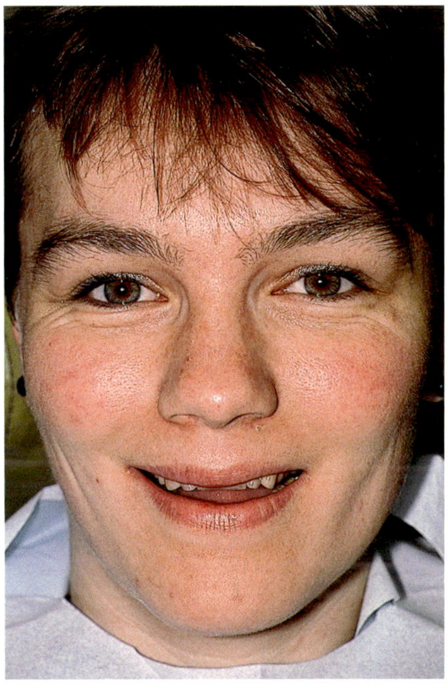

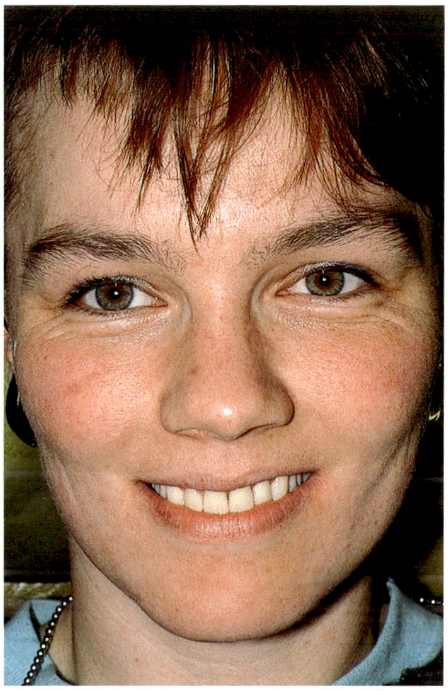

Fig 6-13b *(right)* Posttreatment smile.

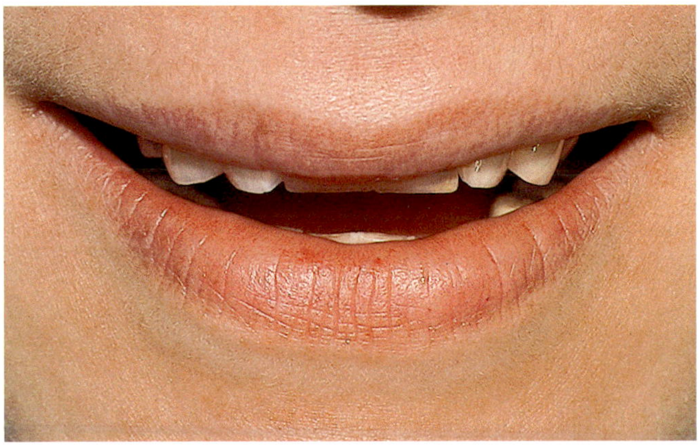

Fig 6-13c Patient's smile line before reconstruction of her anterior teeth.

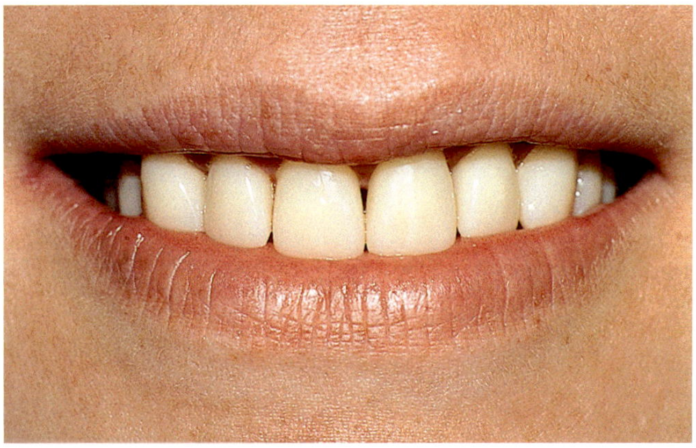

Fig 6-13d Posttreatment smile line.

Table 6-3 Relationship between body height and the length of maxillary anterior teeth

Body height (m)	Central incisor (mm)	Lateral incisor (mm)	Canine (mm)
1.90	13.0	-2.0	13.0
1.80	12.0	-2.0	12.0
1.70	11.0	-2.0	11.0
1.60	10.0	-2.0	10.0

pronunciation difficulties, or have problems with eating, or the patient's friends and relatives may not accept the new look.

There are two prerequisites for a successful reconstruction of anterior teeth: The patient has to be willing and able to accept a new appearance, and the dentist and dental technician have to be skillful and knowledgeable. In this context, it is necessary to know how to determine the correct length for the anterior teeth. The following options are feasible: attempts with provisional restorations, an older photograph of the patient as a young man or woman or the judgment of a relative. The biggest problem is often the preconceived notions of the patient: "Listen, Doc, in our family we've always had small (or white) teeth, so don't make me look like Count Dracula!"

So where do dentists obtain points of reference for successful reconstruction of tooth length? In fact, how long are human incisors and canines? Are there any measurements that could be used? What can be found in the relevant literature?

Proven solution: Determining the length of anterior teeth with individual measurements

The literature reports average lengths of 11.0 to 12.0 mm for maxillary incisors and 9.0 to 10.0 mm for mandibular incisors[4–8] (Figs 6-14 and 6-15). If dentists apply these average values to all patients, they will encounter the same problem as with all statistical averages; the measurements may be a perfect fit for many patients but not work at all for a large number of other patients. Basically, this is the same difficulty found with buying clothes. For example, a certain group of 20 people may have an average height of 5 feet 9.7 inches (1.8 m), but it is unlikely that a single pair of pants will fit each member of the group properly.

Hans Naegerl, a physicist and physician from the University of Göttingen, has pointed out the solution to this problem. He postulated that most body measurements are proportional to body height. He claimed that, in most cases, a tall person will have long arms and large hands, whereas a short person will have short arms and small hands, with some exceptions.

Therefore, the author conducted a measurement of the tooth length in his own office with 100 young patients between 20 and 25 years of age. The requirements for inclusion were that the anterior teeth had erupted entirely, were not abraded, and showed no gingival recession. The measurements were taken from the gingival crest to the unabraded incisal edge. The values were correlated to the patient's body height. This yielded the values listed in Table 6-3. For maxillary anterior teeth, it can be deduced that, for every 10.0 cm of body height, 1.0 mm of tooth length must be added.

The maxillary lateral incisors are 1.0 mm shorter than the canines and the central incisors in both directions—measured from the gingival crest and measured from the incisal edge (Fig 6-16). Thus they are 2.0 mm shorter in total. The mandibular anterior teeth vary far less—lengths of 9.0 to 10.0 mm, as cited in the literature, can usually be found.

These numbers are not to be viewed as absolute mathematically defined values, but they are meant to serve as a guide for waxing up the teeth and for making provisional restorations. If no other information about the original length of the teeth is available, the values in Table 6-3 are a useful guide to achieving good function and esthetics. Another point of reference is the proportion of tooth length to tooth width (Table 6-4 and Fig 6-17).

Application

New lengths for the anterior teeth should be tried using a mock-up with resin composite (see the previous section and Fig 6-18). If the abrasion is already greatly advanced, laboratory-made provisional restorations are better.

Length (%)	Width (%)	Ratio
100	80	1.25 (ideal)
100	95	1.05 (wide)
100	65	1.53 (narrow)

Table 6-4 Relationship between the length and the width of teeth

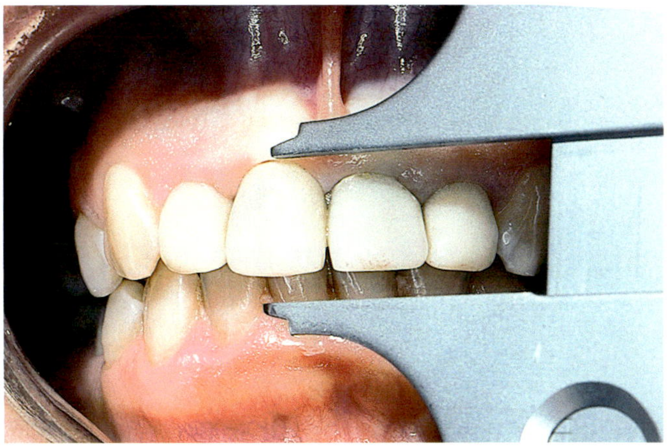

Fig 6-14 How long are maxillary incisors?

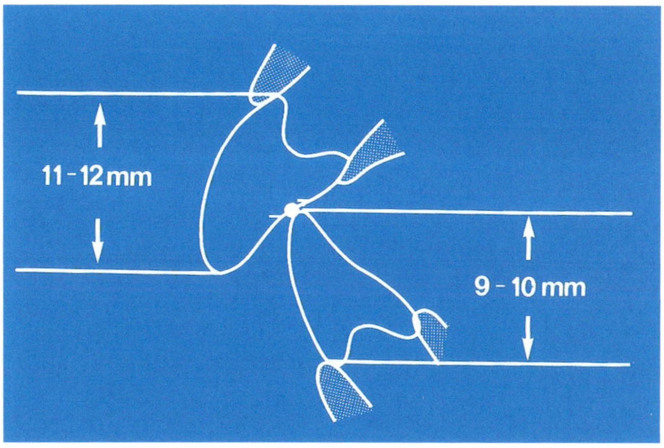

Fig 6-15 According to Wheeler's atlas of anatomy.

Fig 6-16 The lateral incisors are 1.0 mm shorter than the canines and central incisors in both directions—from the gingival crest and from the incisal edge (2.0 mm shorter in total).

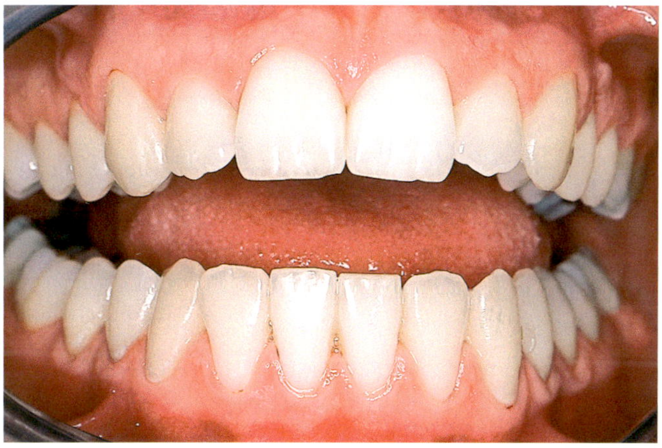

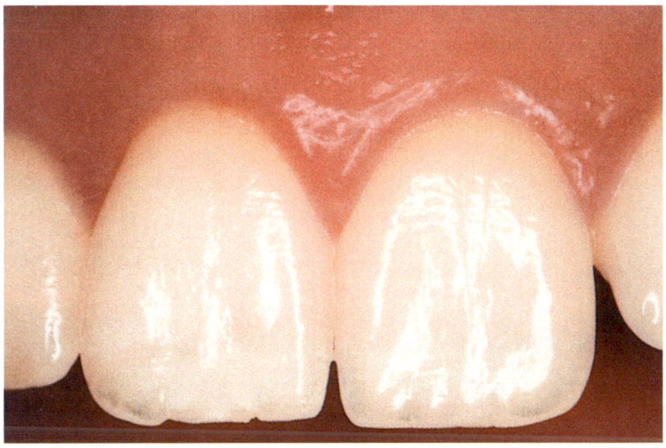

Fig 6-17 Relationship between the length and the width of teeth.

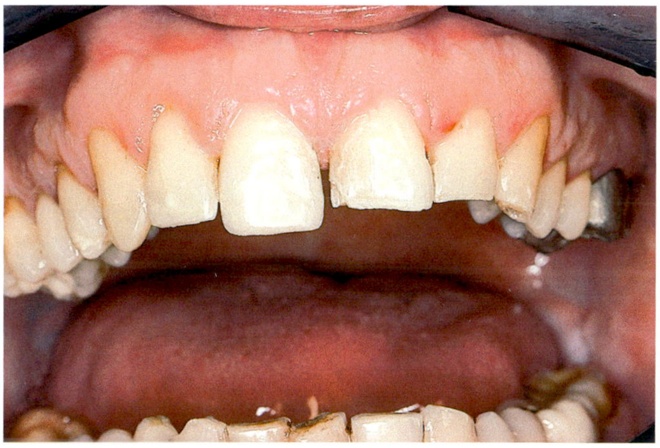

Fig 6-18 Resin composite mock-up on the maxillary right side (canine and lateral and central incisor) in a 28-year-old patient.

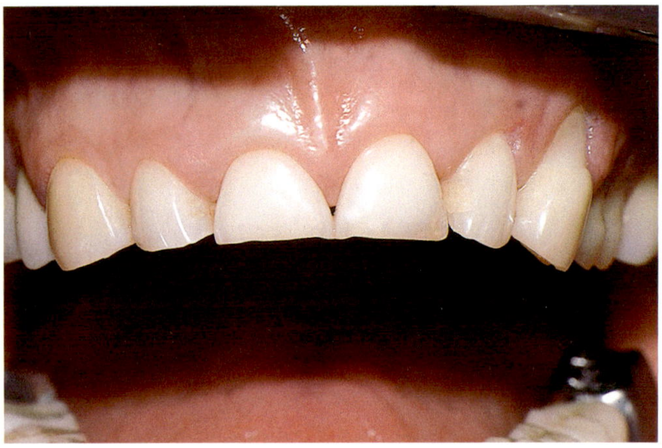

Fig 6-19a Patient with advanced abrasion.

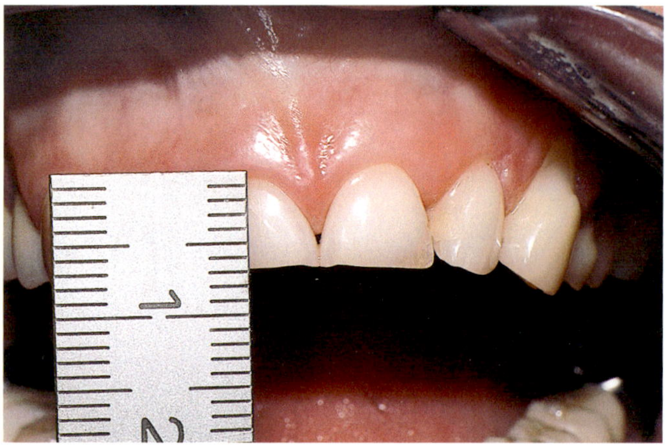

Fig 6-19b Measurement of the length of the abraded teeth in the maxilla.

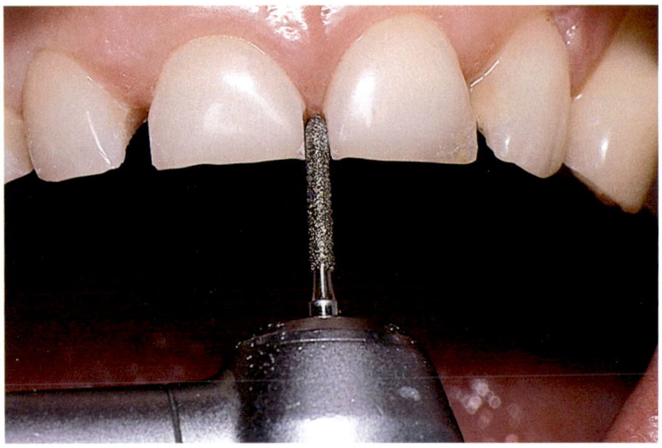

Fig 6-19c Separation of the anterior teeth.

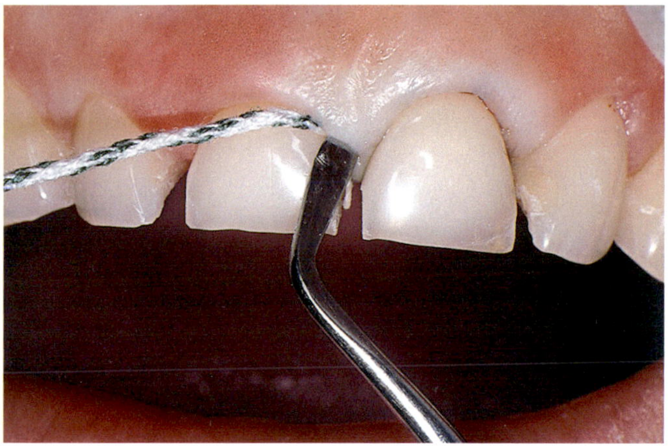

Fig 6-19d Placement of the retraction cords.

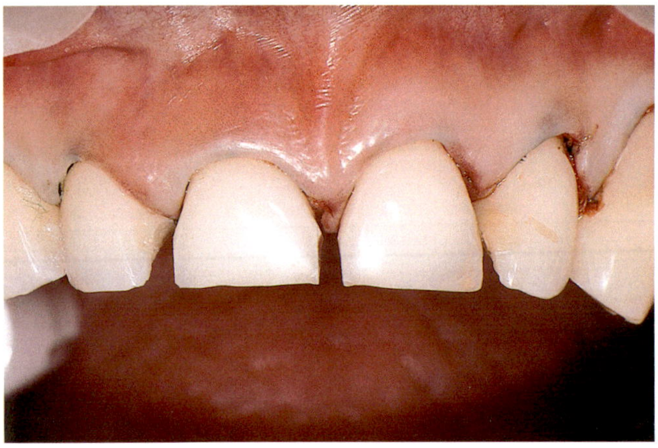

Fig 6-19e Retracted gingiva with cords in place.

Case report

A 35-year-old woman had severely abraded anterior teeth. This bothered her immensely, and she asked for restoration of the abraded teeth.

Treatment with a occlusal guard had been successful, and her muscles and TMJ were in fine shape. The remaining crown length was measured with a steel ruler and recorded (Figs 6-19a and 6-19b) to demonstrate to the patient how much tooth substance had been lost. The central incisors were only 7.0 mm long. In relation to the patient's body height of 1.7 m, the target value for the central incisors (11.0 mm) was taken from Table 6-3. She had lost 4.0 mm of tooth length.

It was decided to place provisional crowns on the abraded anterior teeth as a test. After administration of local anesthesia, the teeth were separated and the gingiva was retracted with nonimpregnated retraction cords

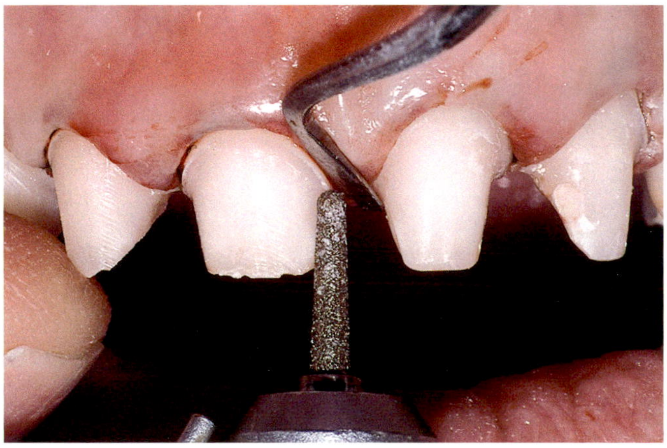

Fig 6-19f Careful preparation of the anterior teeth.

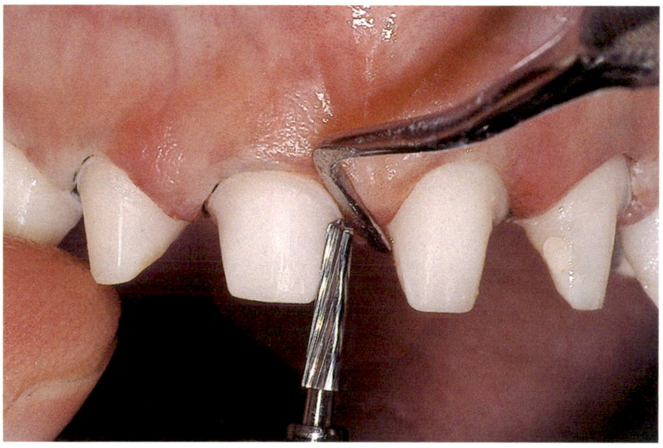

Fig 6-19g Careful finishing of the anterior teeth.

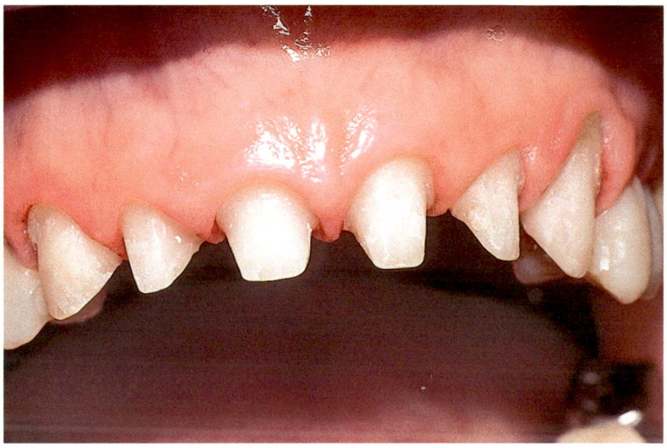

Fig 6-19h Finished preparations.

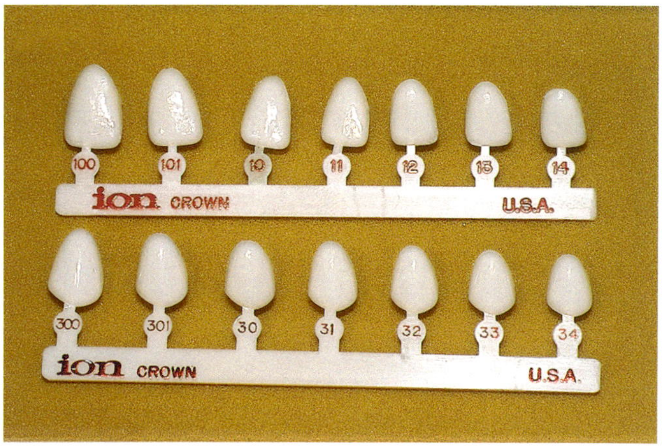

Fig 6-19i Set of prefabricated provisional crowns.

(Figs 6-19c to 6-19e). During the subsequent preparation and finishing stages, the gingival margin was held away and protected with a spatula (Figs 6-19f and 6-19g).

After the preparation (Fig 6-19h), the appropriate sizes from a set of prefabricated provisional single crowns (Fig 6-19i) were chosen symmetrically. The crowns were relined with self-curing acrylic resin (Fig 6-19j), finished, and provisionally cemented (Figs 6-19k and 6-19l).

The patient was thrilled with the result, and the dentist's reward was the patient's radiant smile (Figs 6-19m and 6-19n).

All alterations to anterior teeth have to be checked with respect to their effects on phonation, particularly */f/*, */s/*, */sh/*, and */t/* sounds, and their effects on facial expressions involving the lower lip line (smile line). The incisal edges of the anterior teeth should follow the curve of the lower lip when the patient is smiling and should touch

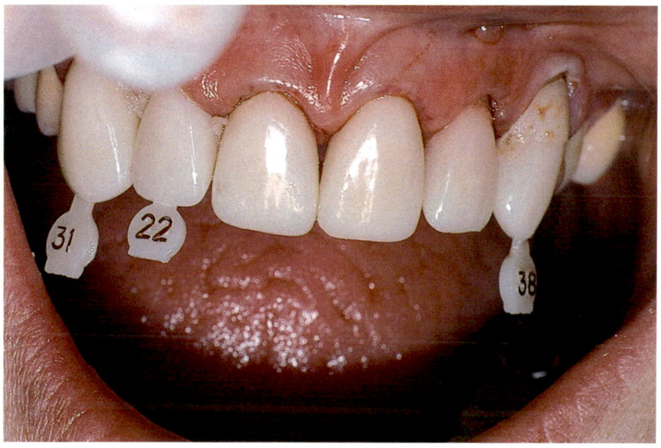

Fig 6-19j Relining of the selected crowns.

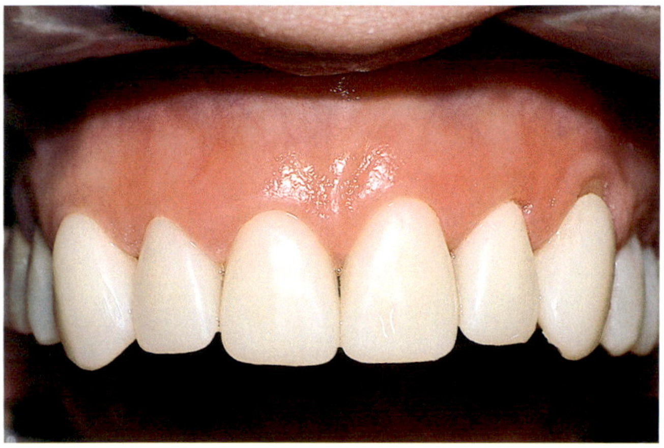

Fig 6-19k Labial view of the provisional crowns in place.

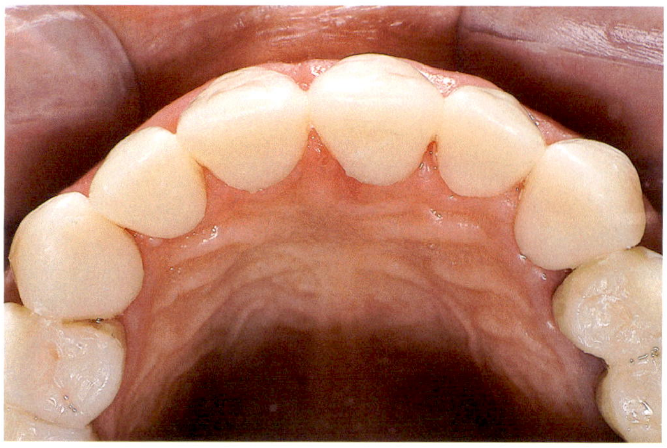

Fig 6-19l Palatal view.

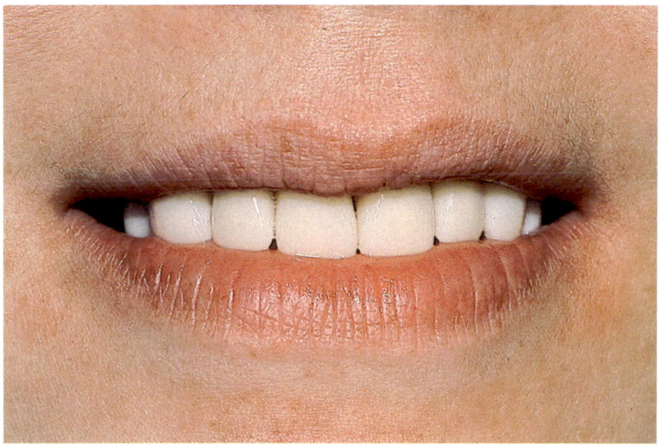

Fig 6-19m Patient's lip line after the provisional restoration.

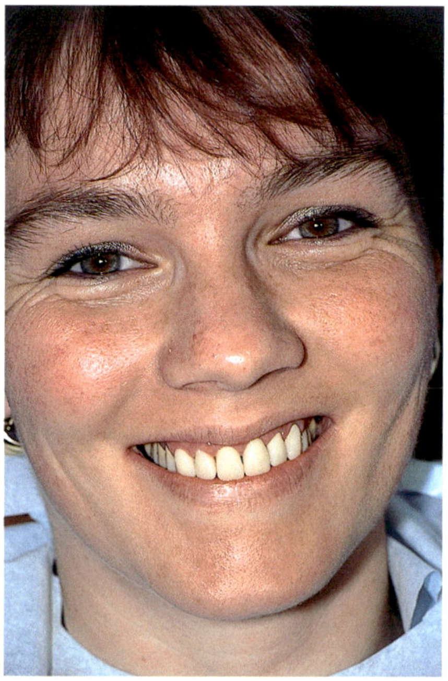

Fig 6-19n Patient's radiant smile.

the lower lip in the area where the wet and dry parts of the labium meet.

Materials

Steel ruler (Sam Dental)
Customary precision calipers from hardware stores or the orthodontic section of dental wholesalers
Mock-up with resin composite (eg, Tetric, Ivoclar Vivident; Miris, Coltène Whaledent; or Herculite, Kerr Dental)
Pocket calculator for calculating the ratio between length and width
Preparation diamonds (Brasseler)
Ultrapak retraction cords (Ultradent)
Ion crowns, prefabricated single-tooth provisional restorations (3M ESPE)
Dentalon Plus self-curing acrylic resin for relining (Heraeus Kulzer)
Durelon temporary cement (3M ESPE)
Phonetic test (developed by Master Dental Technician, Jürg Stuck, Singen, Germany)

Shade Matching

Common problem: Selection of correct tooth shade

The question of how to determine the correct tooth shade (or rather, shades) for patients is and probably always will be a matter of much dispute in restorative dentistry (Fig 6-20). Figure 6-21 shows the success rates of shade matching as reported in statistical research. The diagram suggests that, for 65% of prosthetic restorations, the restoration should or must be redone and the patient should or must return to the office more than once. As a result, the dentist and dental technician both lose a fair amount of time, patients will lose confidence in their dentist, and the office's image may suffer. In the context of tooth shade matching, the following questions arise:

1. Does everyone perceive color in the same way?
2. Is it possible to communicate colors or shades?
3. Is it possible to physically measure tooth shades?
4. How many dentists or dental technicians actually know whether their color vision is without deficiencies?
5. Who should determine the tooth shade—the dentist, the dental technician, or even the dental assistant?
6. Should the patients make this choice themselves, thus assuming the responsibility?

Proven solution: Systematic shade matching

Prerequisites

When dentists or dental technicians place tooth-colored restorations or make metal-ceramic crowns, all-ceramic crowns, or porcelain veneers in the laboratory, they are the ones to choose the tooth colors. If the two parties have to communicate about tooth colors, there is always the general problem that, under most circumstances, a color cannot be effectively described without special tools.

Color vision

Statistically, 8.0% of men and 1.5% of women have a color perception deficiency or are color-blind. Knowing this, every dentist and dental technician should have his or her color vision tested. This test can be considered a kind of "driver's license" for esthetic dentistry.

Color vision can be determined with the Ishihara color charts (Figs 6-22a and 6-22b),with the Farnsworth color sequence test, and with the Nagel Anomaloscope.

All three tests are suitable, but the Anomaloscope is the most reliable.

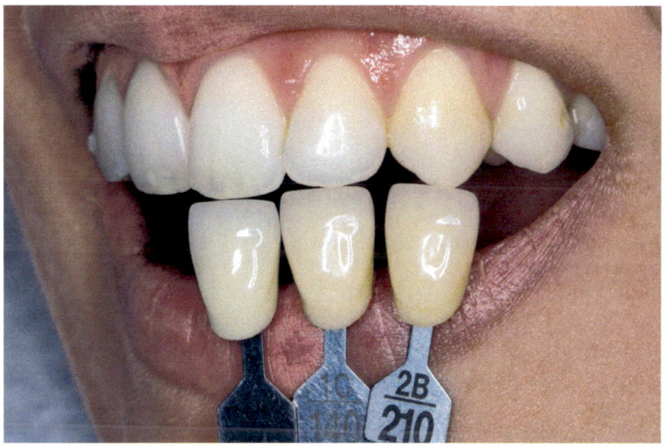

Fig 6-20 Shade matching on the patient.

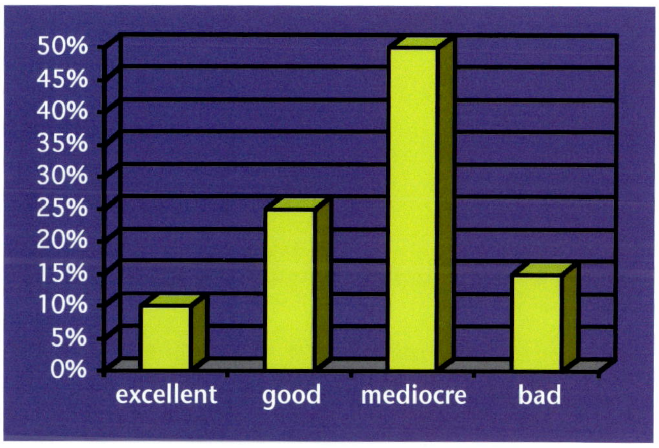

Fig 6-21 Success rates in tooth shade matching. (Adapted from the chart by Henning).

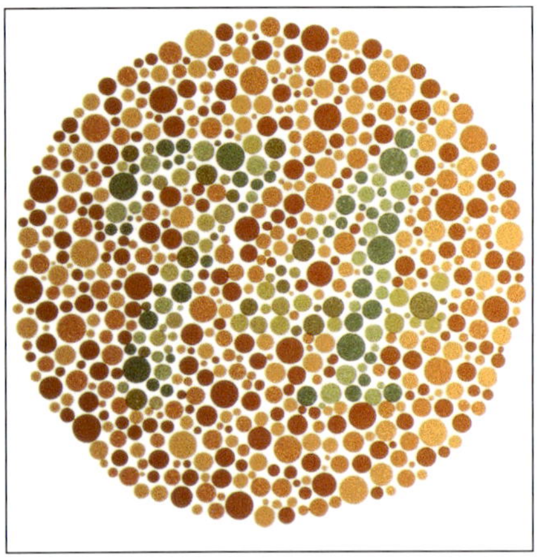

Fig 6-22a *(left)* Ishihara chart for color vision testing.

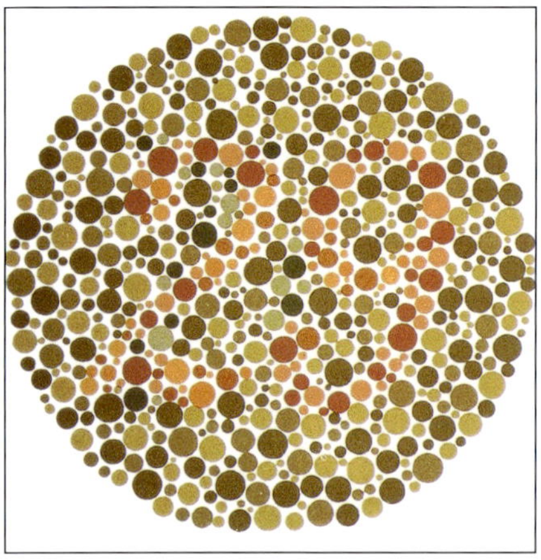

Fig 6-22b *(right)* Another Ishihara color vision test.

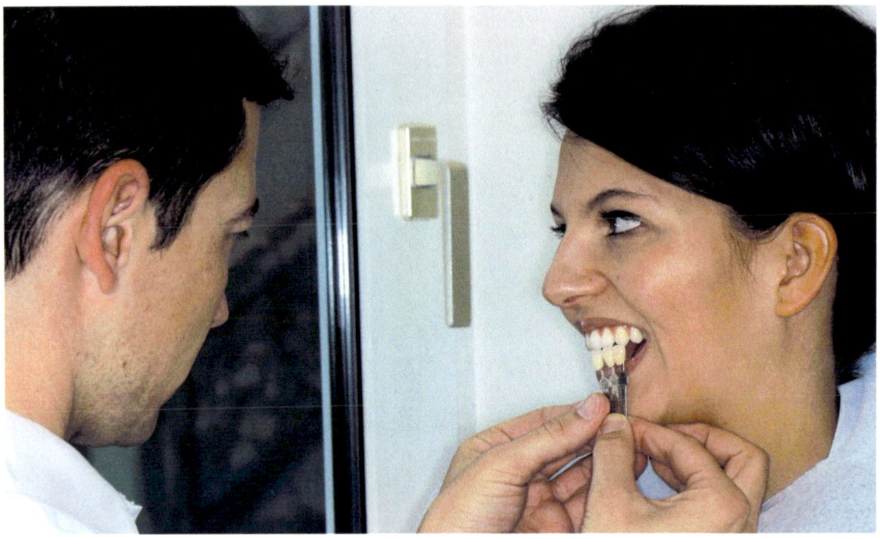

Fig 6-23 Selecting a shade at a north window.

If a dental professional's color perception is found to be limited, he or she need not give up working as a dentist or dental technician. The clinician should, however, acknowledge the situation, have others perform the shade matching, and then change working methods accordingly.

Constant lighting conditions

The ideal light for determining tooth shades is the diffuse daylight between 10 AM and 12 PM, at a window facing north, with a clouded, white sky (Fig 6-23). In the morning before that time, the shades tend to be blue-tinged, whereas in the late afternoon the proportion of red is too high. The shade should never be selected in direct sunlight or when the sky is clouded and dark.

Because color matching in natural sunlight is subject to too many variations, constant lighting conditions with a fluorescent lamp should be given preference over natural sunlight. The operating light in the dental office is only suitable if the brightness can be dimmed and its light corresponds to daylight. All the light sources in the office or laboratory can be checked with the Kodak View Card to make sure they are equivalent to daylight (Figs 6-24a and 6-24b). In artificial light, it is possible to see vertical stripes on the View Card that are not visible in daylight.

In other words, light sources in the dental office and laboratory must provide a constant and standardized illumination for shade selection. The ideal physical values for this purpose are a color temperature between 5,000 and 5,500 K and a brightness between 1,200 and 1,500 lux. The bandwidth is defined in the German standard DIN 67505. The dental industry offers lights that meet these

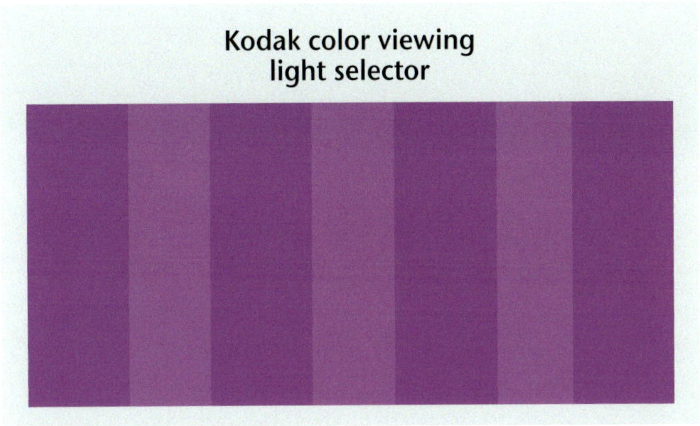

Fig 6-24a Testing card for daylight and suitable artificial light. Stripes are visible in artificial light.

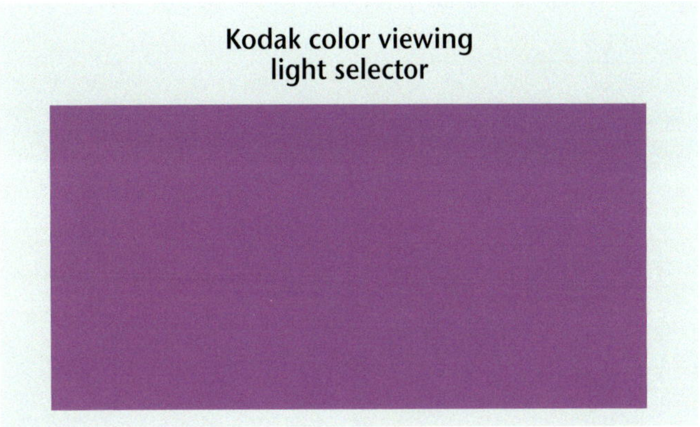

Fig 6-24b Stripes are not visible in daylight or suitable artificial light.

specifications; one example is the Waldmann shade selection light for dental offices that comes with a mirror for the patient and a loupe for the dentist. The illuminated loupes on laboratory lights also create ideal conditions. Illuminated mirrors like the ones used in color and fashion makeovers are suitable as well.

Relative color perception

The human eye is incapable of judging one shade beside another one. It is the same as in music; only a trained ear can tell the single notes in a chord apart. The eye, however, is prone to optical illusions because of the characteristics of vision. It is therefore absolutely essential that no intense colors be in close proximity to the patient or on the patient when the dentist is selecting a shade. For example, lipstick (Fig 6-25), strong makeup, colorful clothing (Fig 6-26a), or colorful surroundings (walls, pictures, plants, etc) would interfere with accurate shade selection. If the patient is wearing colorful clothes, a light gray or blue drape should be used as a neutral background (Figs 6-26b and 6-26c).

According to Henning,[9] the human eye tires after 5 to 7 seconds. This fatigue leads to a color shift. If the clinician looks at a bright white or light gray surface for a while (and not at a blue surface, as is often claimed), the eyes will be neutralized much in the same way that the white balance with a videocamera is adjusted. The dentist's eyes will then be ready again for shade matching.

Color systems

The following systems are most commonly used for shade matching: Vita Classic shade system (Vita, Fig 6-27) and Chromascop shade system (Ivoclar Vivadent, Fig 6-28).

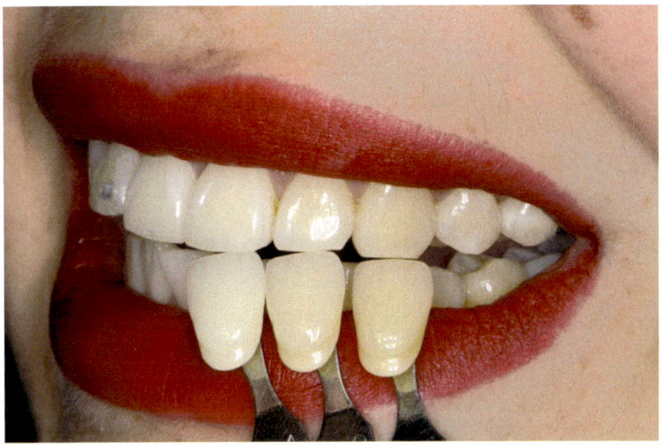

Fig 6-25 Difficulty in shade matching when lipstick is too intense.

The Vita Classic shade system is the international standard. Most manufacturers around the globe match their materials with this system. The Biodent system (Fig 6-29) used to be in widespread use but has become obsolete. There are many other shade systems of lesser importance, because these systems are all bound to the materials of one particular company or another. The pervasiveness of a shade system determines how much it will be used.

This is indeed a major issue for dentists and dental technicians; there is no standardized shading system. For example, a new shade system may seem useful, but it cannot be used unless the dentist is willing to switch all materials. Hence, it would be more than desirable if the individual manufacturers could agree on one system and standardize their materials accordingly.

The Vita Classic and Chromascop systems have similar structures. The samples are grouped with respect to the dominant colors in the group: white, yellow, reddish-brown, brown, and gray.

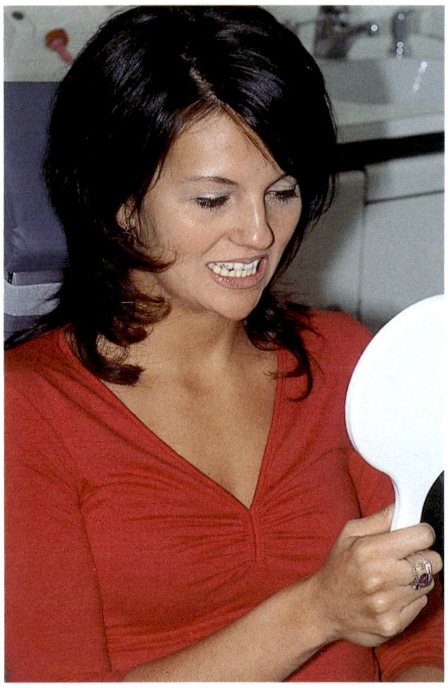

Fig 6-26a Patient with a colorful top.

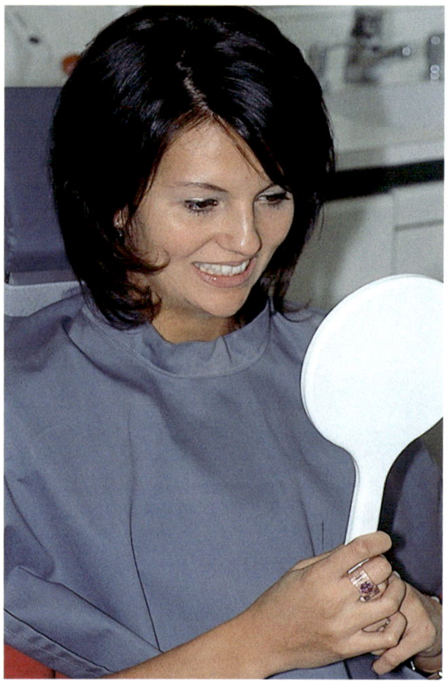

Fig 6-26b Patient with light gray drape.

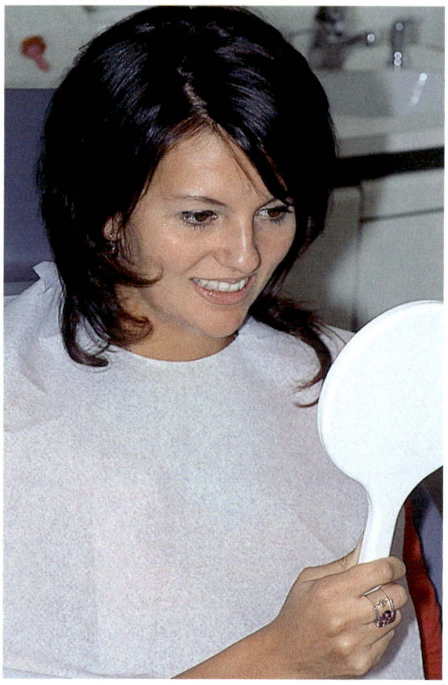

Fig 6-26c Patient with protective napkin.

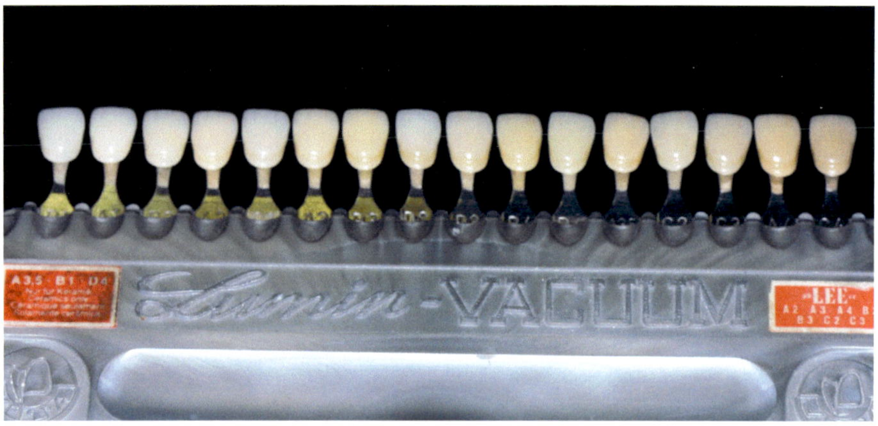

Fig 6-27 Vita Classic shade system.

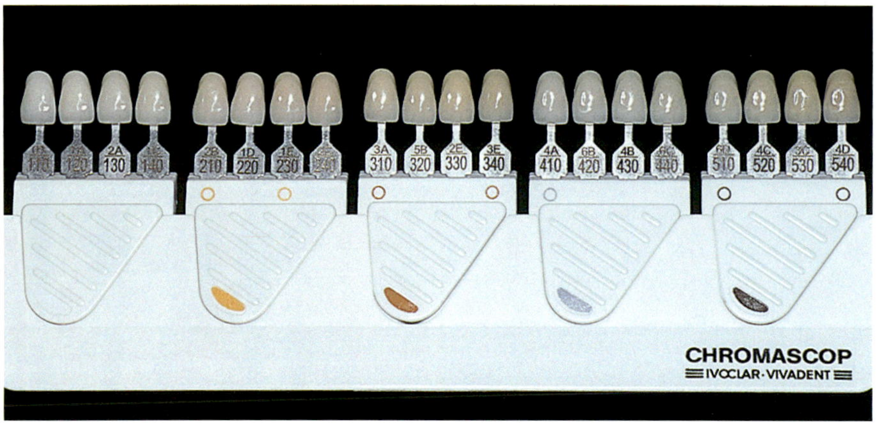

Fig 6-28 Chromascop shade system.

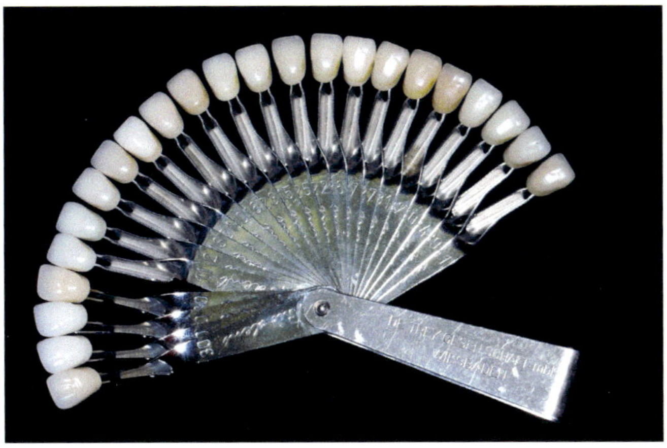

Fig 6-29 Biodent shade system.

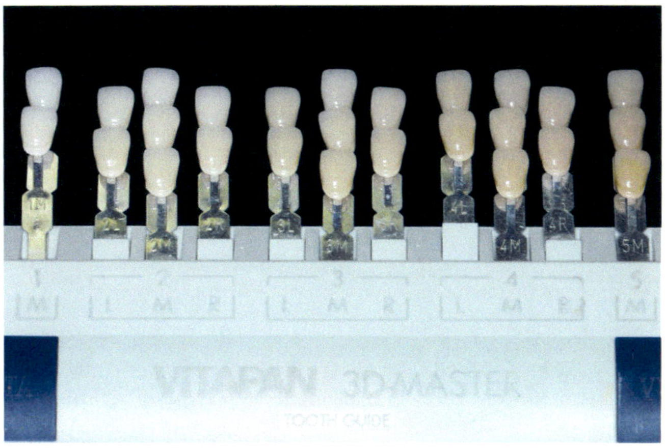

Fig 6-30 Vita 3D-Master shade system.

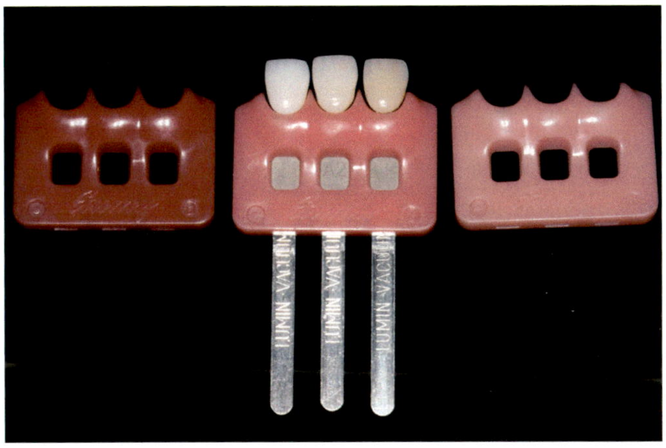

Fig 6-31 Gingiva GUMY shade system.

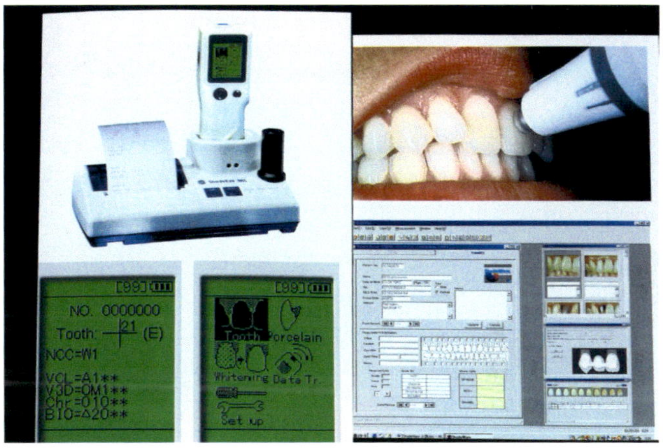

Fig 6-32 ShadeEye NCC shade system.

With the 3D-Master (Fig 6-30), Vita is pursuing a more intelligent approach in terms of physics and optics by determining the brightness first, then the color intensity, and subsequently the hue (whether it is more yellow or red). So far this shade system, with its logically correct sequence in a three-dimensional color space, only works for Vita products; thus, it is correspondingly limited in its use.

The tooth shade matching systems have undergone further improvement through the possibility of additionally determining the color of the gingiva, thus combining tooth and soft tissue esthetics to create a good overall impression (Fig 6-31). The GUMY gingiva shade matching system (Shofu Dental) is the only one on the market to date, to the author's knowledge. This system, however, can be combined with any other tooth shade matching system. The following shade matching systems are novelties:

1. Color scanners, such as ShadeEye NCC (Fig 6-32). After the tooth has been scanned, the color can be analyzed so that the data can be processed by computer. This device is expensive and system-oriented; furthermore, it is reportedly complicated to use. The Sigma system has a similar design.
2. The Ikam digital shade system uses digital photographs and computer analysis with a shade analysis application.

Electronic systems are still being tested in daily practice.

Procedure for shade matching

Vita Classic and Chromascop systems

The following procedure should be used with the color groups and color intensity scales of the Vita Classic and Chromascop systems[10]:The shades should be selected before treatment is initiated, because the natural teeth dry out during treatment (especially with rubber dam) and can thus become up to two shades brighter. The person fabricating the restoration (dentist or dental technician) chooses the color.

The person selecting the shade should sit at a distance of 50 to 70 cm from the patient. The light should come from the side at an angle of 45 degrees. The color group (white, yellow, etc) is selected first. It may prove helpful to squint slightly to be able to perceive the color group more as a color and less as individual teeth (Fig 6-33a).

The color group is selected and the exact color intensity within this group is determined (Fig 6-33b). The selected color sample is taken away from the group and checked against the almost dry tooth, which is slightly moistened with saliva (Fig 6-33c).

While matching shades, now and again the individual should look at something further away, preferably in light gray, for 10 seconds to give the tired eyes a chance to regenerate.

Subsequently the characteristics of the teeth (layering, transparency, opalescence, shape, and texture) are determined and sketched on a form (Fig 6-33d).

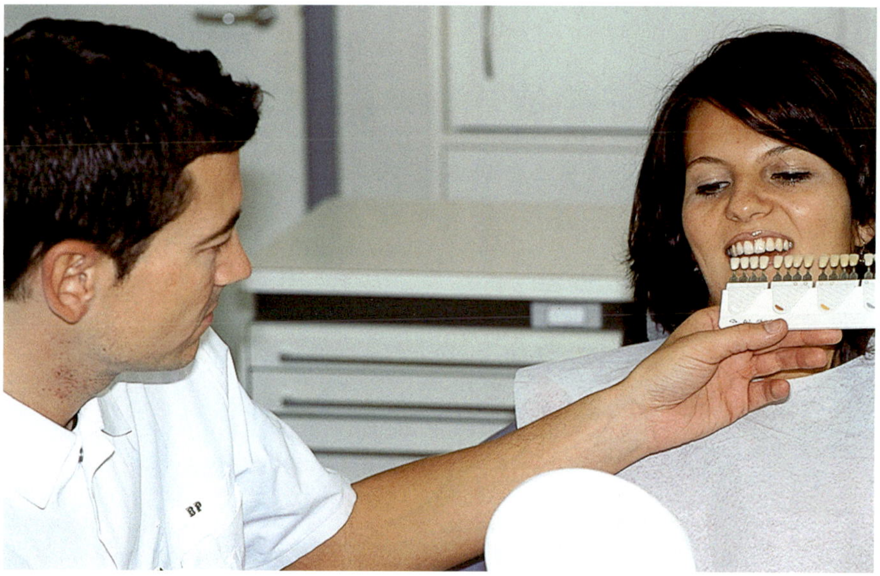

Fig 6-33a First step of shade matching from a distance.

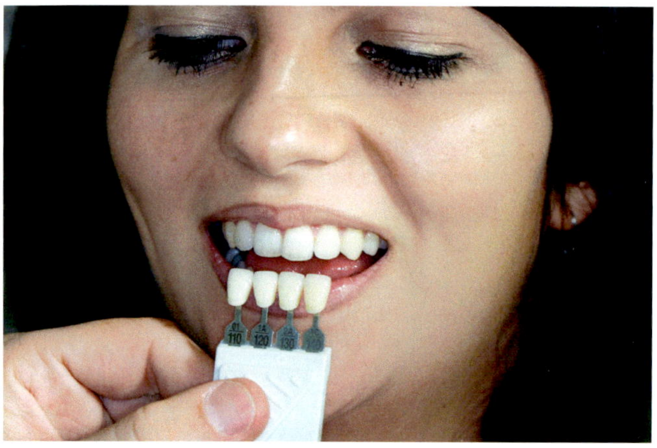

Fig 6-33b Determining the color intensity within the color group.

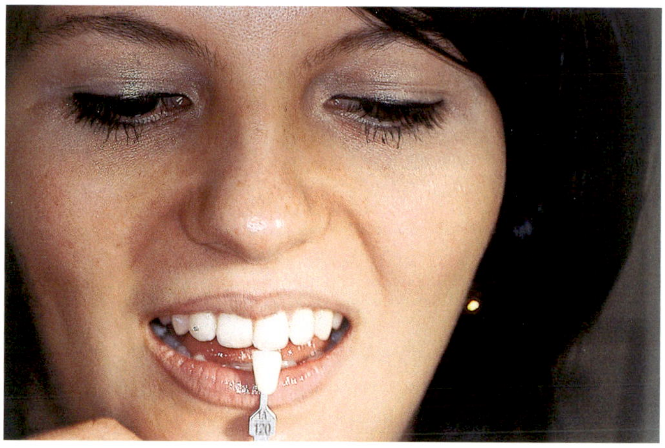

Fig 6-33c Checking the shade sample.

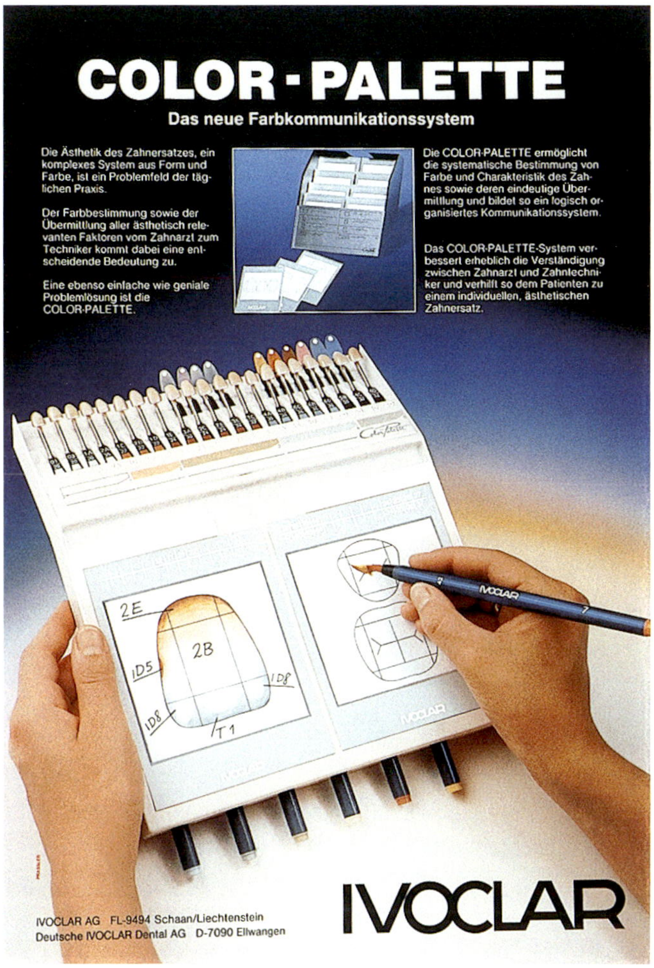

Fig 6-33d Sketching the findings on a form.

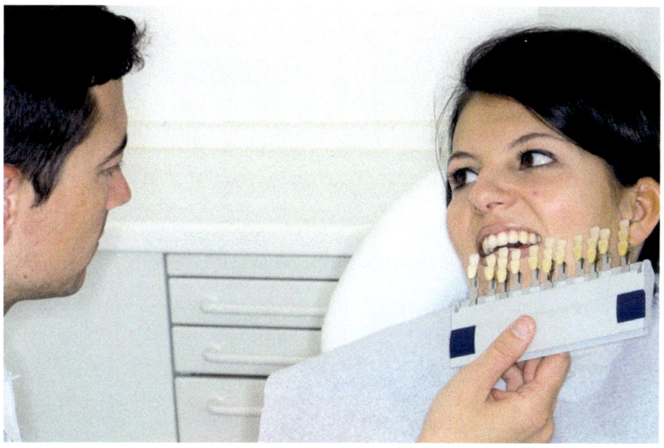

Fig 6-33e Vita 3D-Master shade system: Choosing the color value.

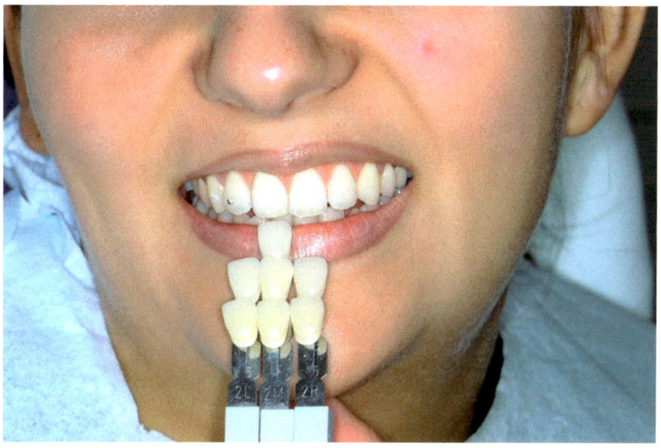

Fig 6-33f Vita 3D-Master shade system: Choosing the color hue (in this case, L, M and R, reddish/yellowish).

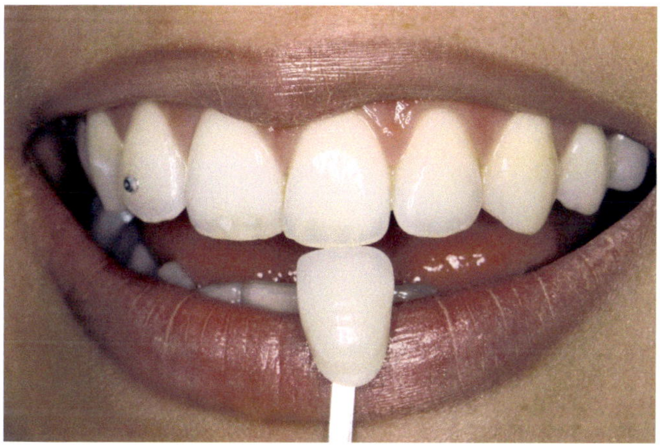

Fig 6-33g Vita 3D-Master shade system: Choosing the color intensity.

Vita 3D-Master system

The following procedures are used to assess the value, hue, and intensity with the Vita 3D-Master system. With this system, the shades should also be selected before the treatment commences, because the natural teeth dry out during treatment (especially with rubber dam) and can thus become up to two shades brighter. The person fabricating the restoration (dentist or dental technician) chooses the color.

The person selecting the shade sits at a distance of 50 to 70 cm from the patient. The light should be coming from the side at an angle of 45 degrees. The color Value (brightness) is selected. It may prove helpful to squint slightly to be able to perceive the color group more as a color and less as arrangement of individual teeth (see Fig 6-33a).

The required value is selected from among the five brightness levels (Fig 6-33e). Then the hue is selected (Fig 6-33f). As the third step, the color intensity (pale to saturated) is selected from groups 1, 1.5, 2, 2.5, and 3 (Fig 6-33g).

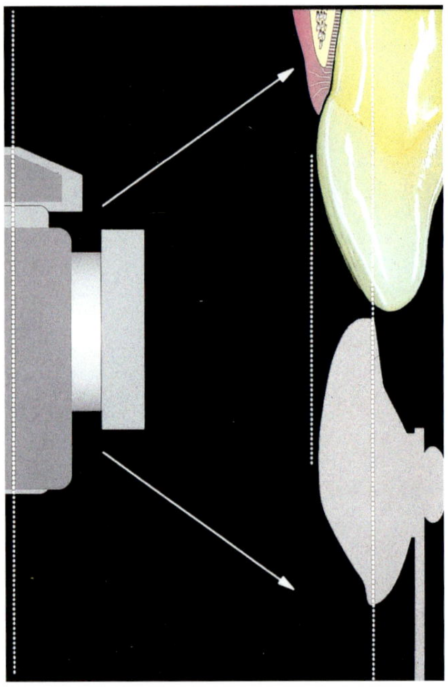

Fig 6-33h Photograph of the surfaces in the same plane.

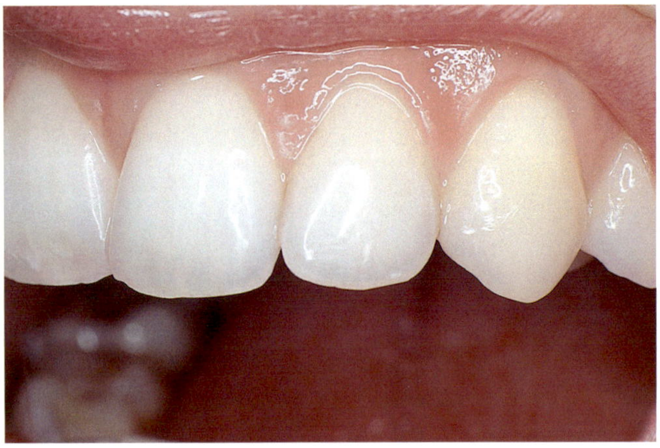

Fig 6-33i Differing shades of the maxillary anterior teeth.

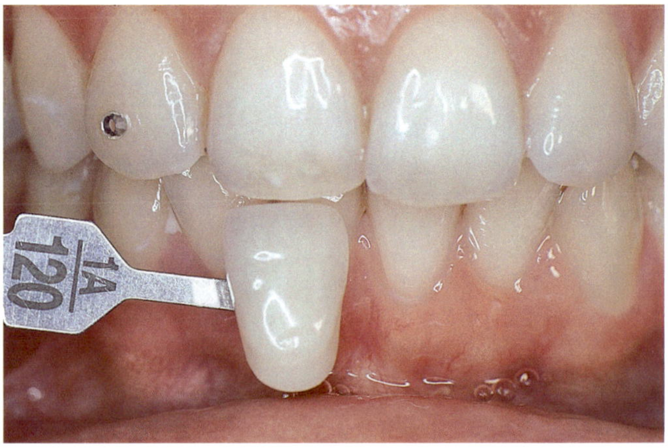

Fig 6-33j Checking the shades, edge to edge.

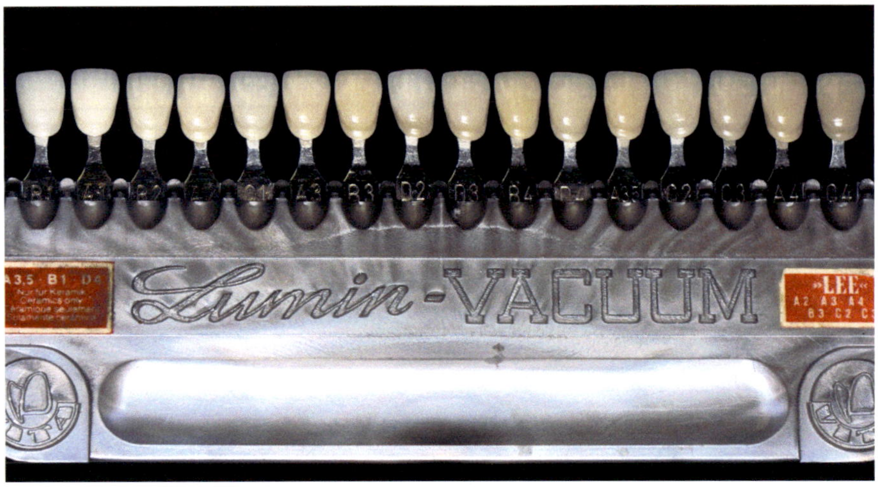

Fig 6-34 Vita Classic shade system arranged according to brightness (value). (See Fig 6-27 for traditional arrangment.)

The selected color sample is removed from the set and turned around so that the sample and the tooth in question are edge to edge. This puts the surfaces of the tooth and the sample in the same optical plane (Fig 6-33h). While matching shades, now and again the individual should look at something farther away, preferably in light gray, for 10 seconds to give tired eyes a chance to regenerate.

The shade of the anterior teeth is never the same for all teeth; it shifts towards the warmer hues in the region of the canines (eg, incisors A2, canines A3.5) (Fig 6-33i).

Subsequently, the characteristics of the teeth are determined with the tooth slightly moistened with saliva and a slightly moistened color sample. Moistening the tooth and sample brings out the texture, shape, layering, and highlights. Check the sample again against the dry tooth. The important characteristics are layering, transparency, opalescence, shape, and texture. Determine these traits and sketch them on a form.

Regardless of the shade matching system used, a photograph taken with the selected tooth shade for the dental technician is a must (Fig 6-33j). The author recommends Kodak Ektachrome EPP 100 or EPN 100 film.

Tip

The Vita Classic System can also be arranged in such a way that the shades can be determined according to value, hue, and intensity. The colors are arranged according to their values: The order is B1, A1, B2, A2, C1, A3, B3, D2, D3, D4, A3.5, C2, C3, A4, and C4, according to measurements conducted by Henning[10] (Fig 6-34).

Materials

Vita Classic and Vita 3D-Master shade systems (Vita Zahnfabrik)
Chromascop shade system (Ivoclar Vivadent)
Kodak Color Viewing Light Selector (Eastman Kodak)
Lighting systems (eg, Waldmann)
Ishihara Test for Color Deficiency (available from medical supplies stores)
Farnsworth Test, Anomaloscope (for further information, please contact Dr Gerd Henning, Lörrach, Germany)
GUMY Gingiva shade system (Shofu Dental)
ShadeEye NCC color scanner (Shofu Dental)
Sigma systemlkam digital shade system (Metalor)
Kodak Ektachrome films (Eastman Kodak; available photography shops)

Analysis and Transfer of the Midline

Common problem: Shifted, tilted, or unidentifiable dental midlines

Patients' standards with respect to esthetics are far higher now than they were only a few years ago. Beauty, wellness, and, increasingly, dental esthetics are the focus of interest of many magazine articles. An impressive, immaculate smile with bright teeth is a part of most individuals' desired facial esthetics. The last few years have seen the development of very sophisticated and long-lasting methods to restore both the "white" and "pink" eshtetics of a smile in an amazingly natural fashion. In dentistry and general medicine alike, this has led to discussions about whether there is a medical indication for esthetic restorations and at what point these changes should be considered merely a cosmetic improvement. It is the task of dentists and dental technicians to draw clear lines.

Esthetics is defined as the study of the perfect natural beauty—a state which each individual is entitled to pursue to counteract the flaws of their outward appearance as well as the emotional effects these flaws have. Figure 6-35 depicts the correlation among the emotions, function, and facial esthetics; there is a dynamic equilibrium among these three components. In terms of dentistry, this means that a restoration that does not look good will also not work well in most cases; this in turn leads to psychological distress. To distinguish a dentist's work from that of mere cosmetology and thus sustain credibility, dental professionals need to clearly mark this indication as separate from cosmetics, the art of adornment.

An esthetic analysis is an indispensable tool for achieving the goal of successful and attractive restorations. How else would it be possible to find solutions for cases such as those shown in Figs 6-36 and 6-37? Every analysis and treatment plan begins with the foremost esthetic parameter—the analysis of the midline. The midline is the vertical symmetry axis of the face. If a face is symmetric, the two halves of the face appear well-balanced, with evenly spaced eyes and ears, a straight nose and chin, clearly defined cheekbones, and so on (Figs 6-38a and 6-38b). This type of symmetry, however, is not characterized by the precise symmetry that would be created with a ruler and a micrometer gauge; such a face would appear stereotypical and boring. Rather, it is characterized by a relaxed symmetry that leads to a well-balanced overall esthetic impression. Figure 6-39 shows what happens when each half of the face is mirrored.

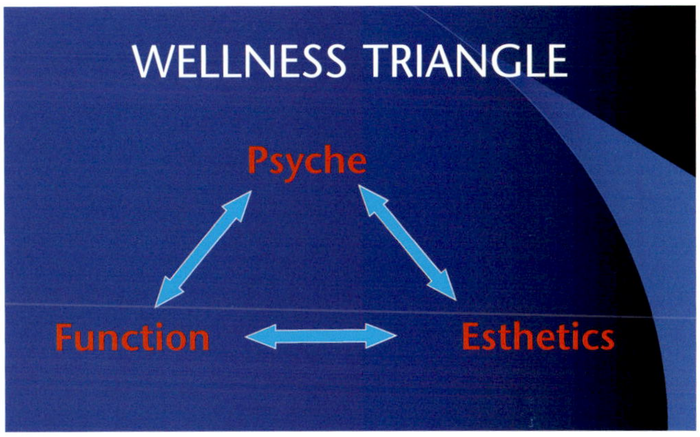

Fig 6-35 Triangle of well-being: the dynamic equilibrium among mind, function, and esthetics.

It is necessary to find the midline to correctly position the teeth in relationship with the face. But how can the midline be defined?

Proven solution: Analysis and transfer of the midline

The following reference points are available to determine the exact middle of the face (Fig 6-40a): *(1)* the middle of the bridge of the nose, *(2)* the interpupillary distance, *(3)* the tip of the nose, *(4)* the philtrum, *(5)* the maxillary labial frenum, *(6)* the midline of the teeth in the maxilla and mandible, *(7)* the mandibular labial frenum, and *(8)* the tip of the chin.

In the author's experience, the most reliable points are the interpupillary distance (Fig 6-40b) and the maxillary labial frenum (Fig 6-40c). When the middle of the face is determined, however, all the reference points have to be considered to gain an overall impression as to precisely where the middle of the face can be found. There is probably not a single person in whom all the reference points actually are on the midline.

Apart from that, every individual has a face that is slimmer on one side and fuller on the other (Fig 6-41d).

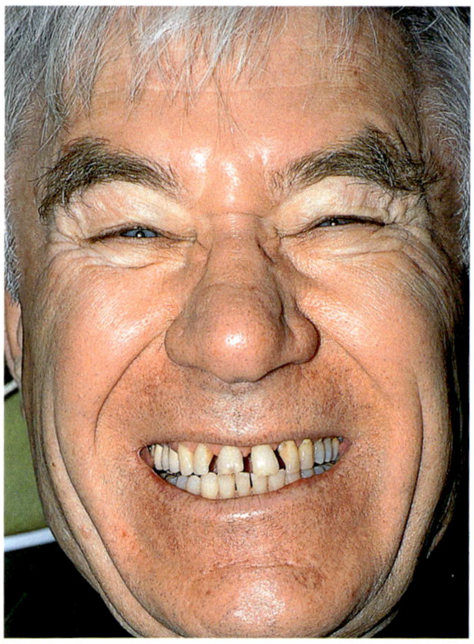

Fig 6-36a Patient with spaced and "fanned out" maxillary anterior teeth.

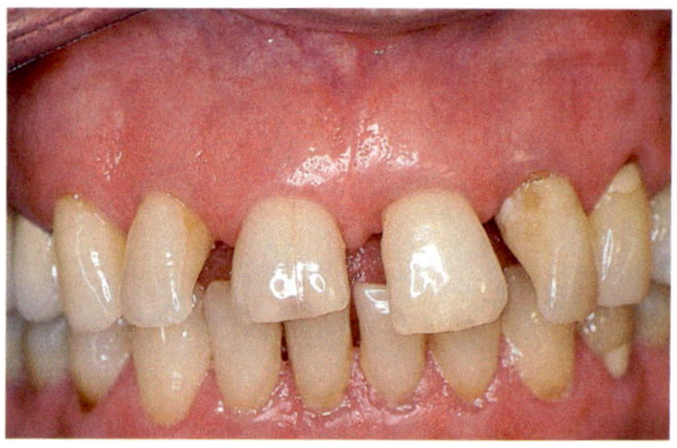

Fig 6-36b Discrepancy of tooth sizes and arch form with displaced midline.

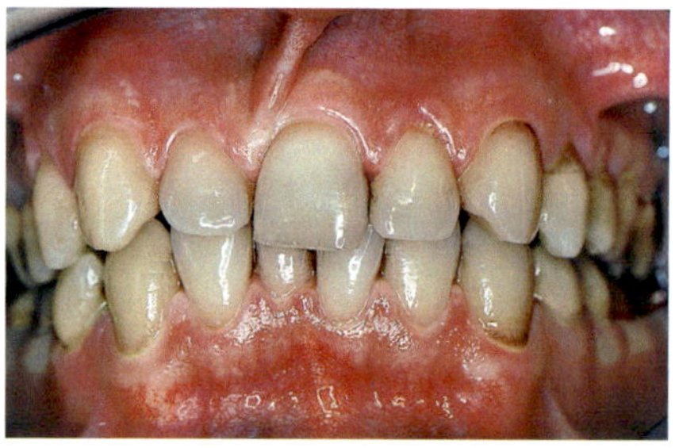

Fig 6-37a Congenitally missing maxillary right central incisor.

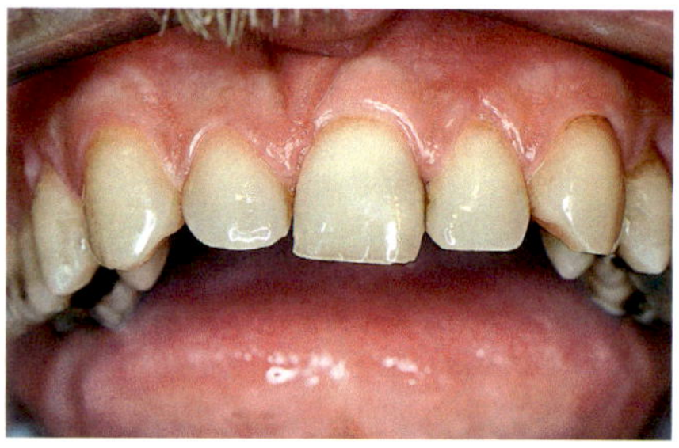

Fig 6-37b Where in the world is the midline?

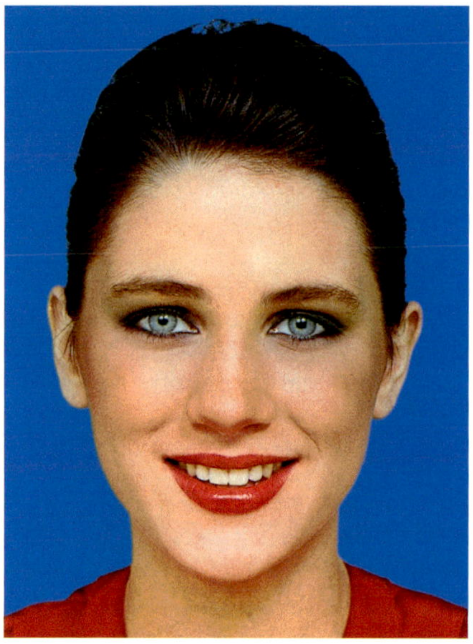

Fig 6-38a *(left)* Face photographed from the exact front (From Goldstein.[11] Reprinted with permission.)

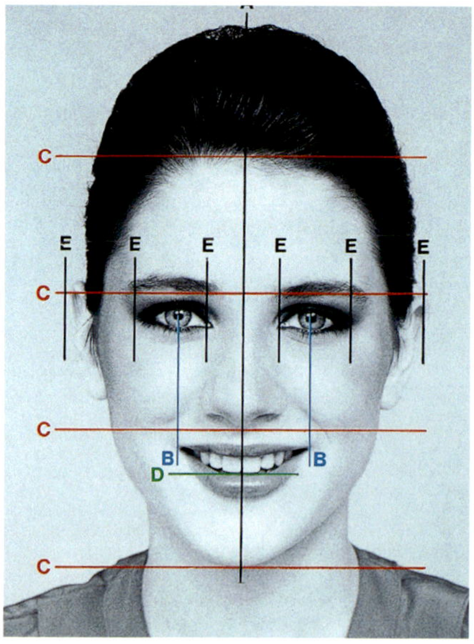

Fig 6-38b *(right)* Same image shown in Fig 6-39a, with analysis lines (From Goldstein.[11] Reprinted with permission.)

Embryologists and anatomists assume that this phenomenon goes all the way back to the lateral position of the embryo in the womb when the viscerocranium is formed from the three main branchial arches; laying an infant on its side may also play a part in this process. When making crowns, dental technicians can work with this phenomenon to either correct a symmetric imbalance (by following the facial contour) or create balance (by working against it).

Procedure

The midline can be examined with a ruler into which the dentist has carved a midline. It is also recommended that the patient's face be viewed from behind and above, so as not to be distracted by the effect of the facial features. This will facilitate the assessment of the location of the midline.

As soon as a discrepancy is found between the midlines of the face and of the teeth, a more detailed analy-

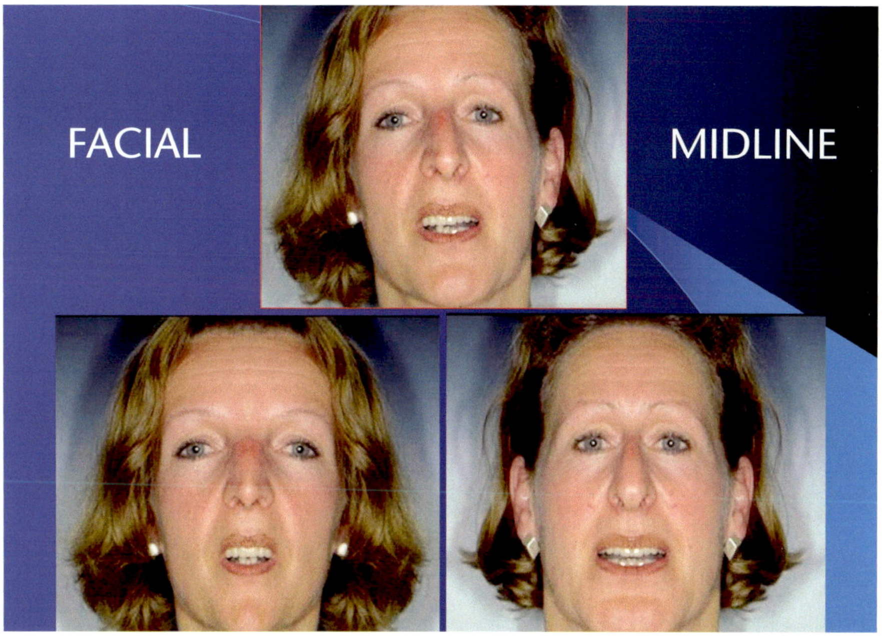

Fig 6-39 Mirrored images of one half of the face. *(upper middle)* Original picture; *(lower left)* mirrored left side of the face; *(lower right)* mirrored right side of the face. (Courtesy of Master Dental Technician Stefan Schunke.)

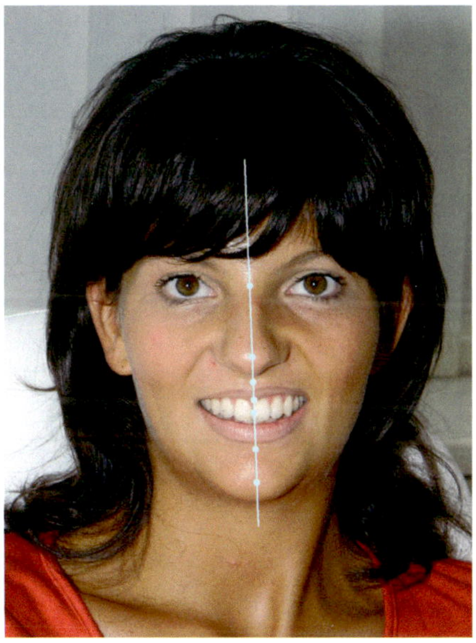

Fig 6-40a Reference points required to determine the midline.

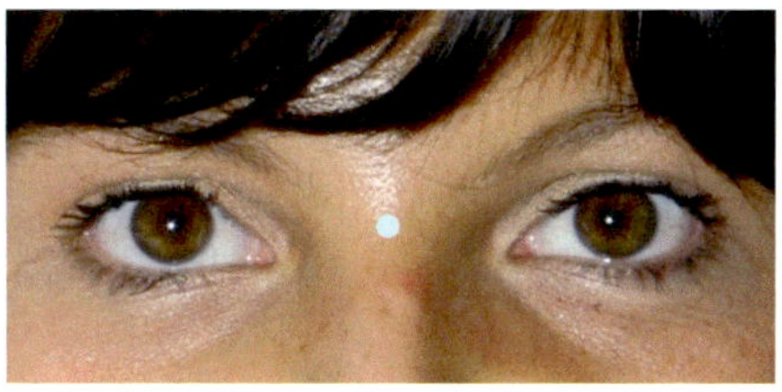

Fig 6-40b Midpoint between the pupils.

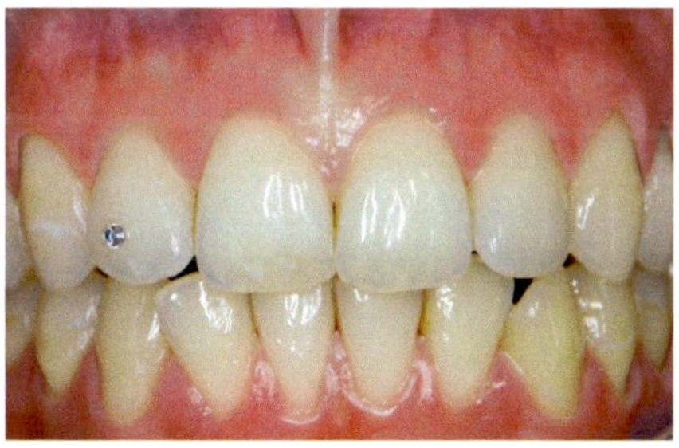

Fig 6-40c Maxillary labial frenum.

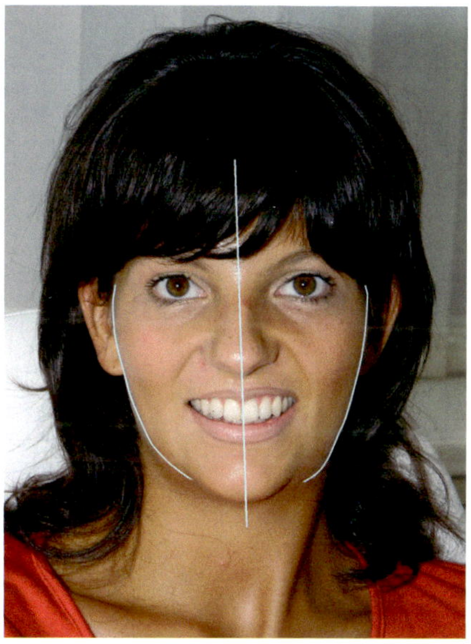

Fig 6-40d Slim and round sides of the face.

sis becomes necessary. Photographic documentation is always recommended. It is best to use a reflex camera with crosshairs to enable the picture to be correctly aligned with the middle of the face.

To transfer the midline from the face to the casts mounted on the articulator, the aforementioned centric reference points should be drawn on the patient with a felt-tip pen. Then the bitefork of the Langner Linefinder with the silicone putty should be adapted in a centric position (Figs 6-41a to 6-41d). The alignment rod, which is held on the bitefork with a magnet, is adjusted (Figs 6-41e and 6-41f). The upper part of the articulator is turned around, and the bitefork is put on the mounted cast of the maxilla. Finally, the alignment rod is replaced with the midline indicator from the articulator and fixed with autopolymerizing acrylic resin in the shoe attachment mounted to the upper part of the articulator (Figs 6-41g to 6-41j).

The midline indicator can be removed and remounted at any time. The dentist or the dental technician can thus

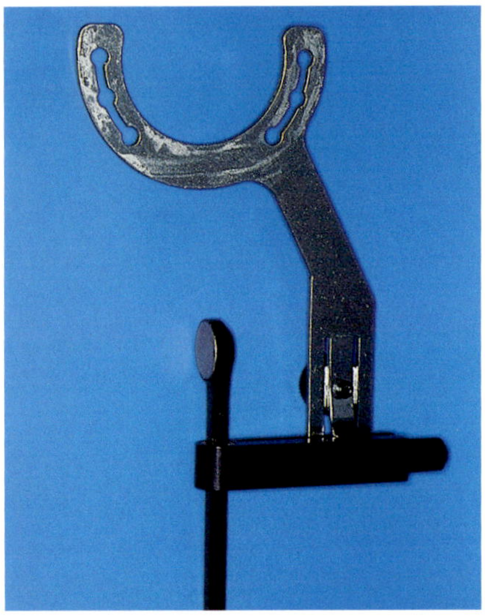

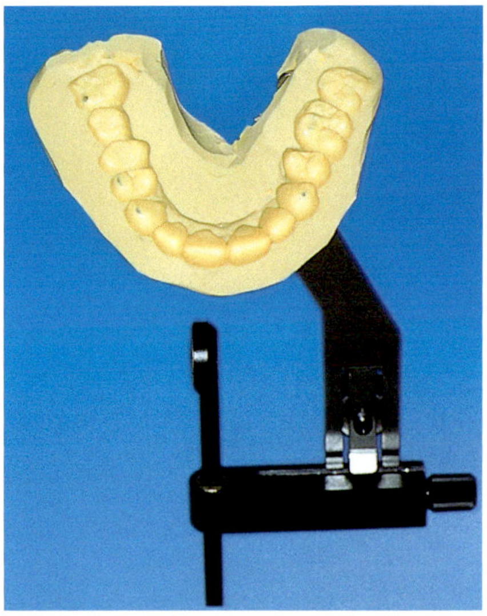

Fig 6-41a *(left)* Bitefork from the Linefinder.

Fig 6-41b *(right)* Bitefork with the silicone putty.

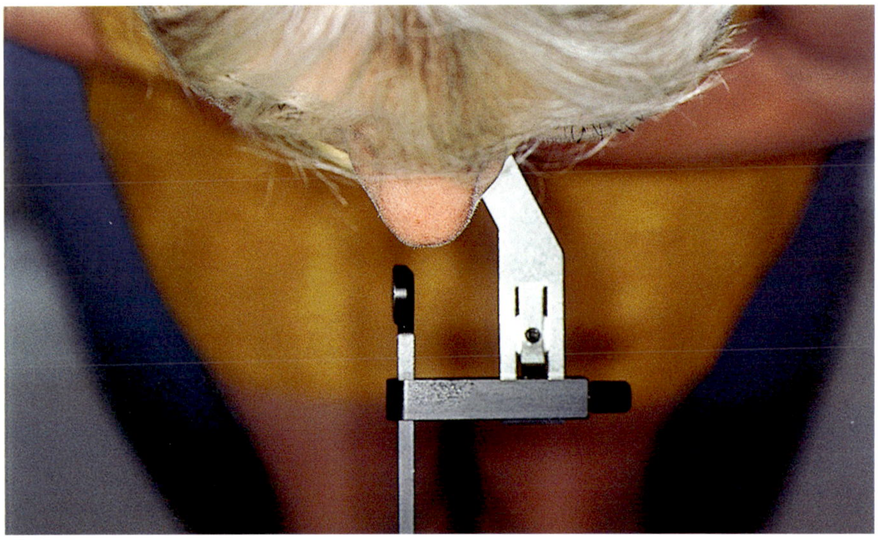

Fig 6-41c Top view of the bitefork in a centric position.

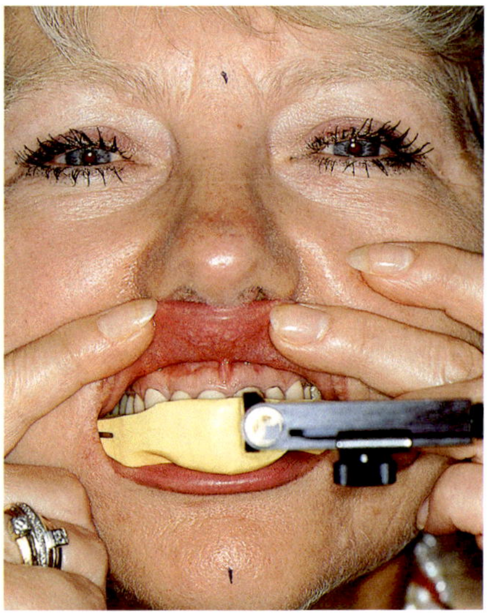

Fig 6-41d Front view of the bitefork in a centric position.

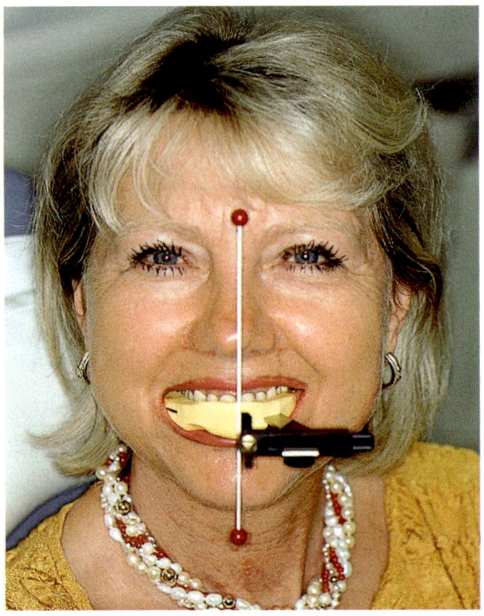

Fig 6-41e *(left)* Adjustment of the magnetically fixed alignment rod.

Fig 6-41f *(right)* Alignment rod from the Linefinder system.

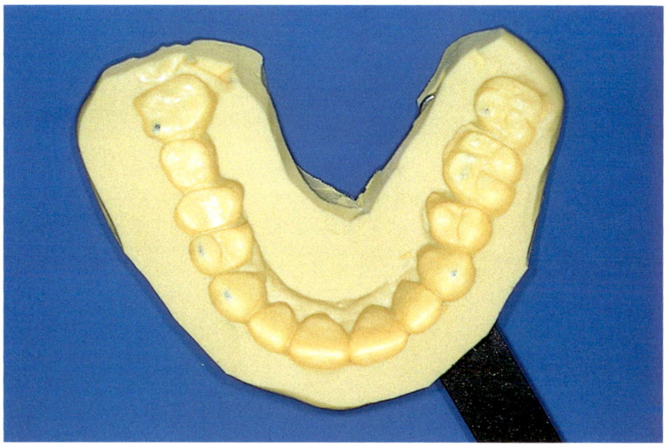

Fig 6-41g Bitefork after removal.

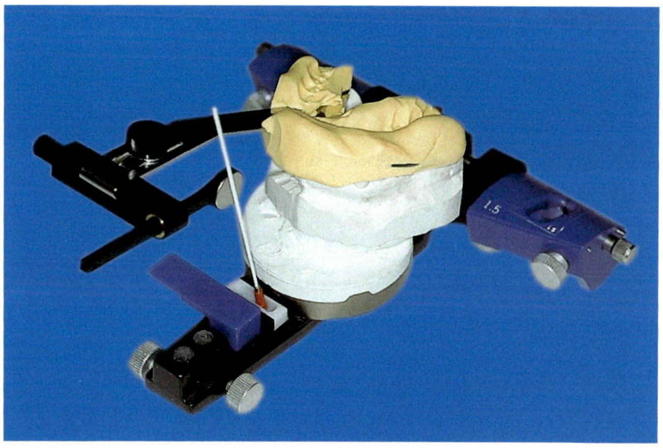

Fig 6-41h Bitefork on the mounted maxillary cast.

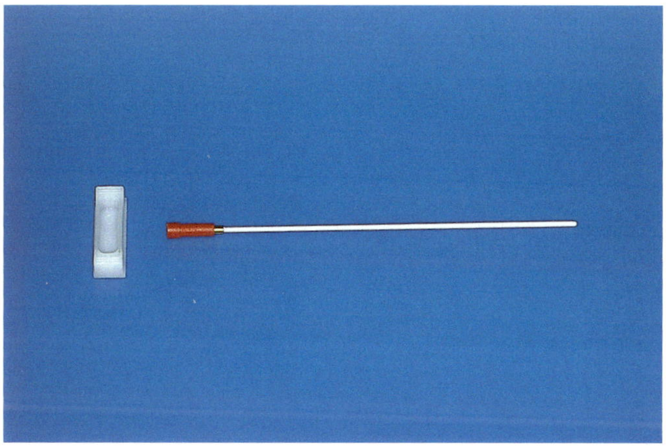

Fig 6-41i Midline indicator for the articulator.

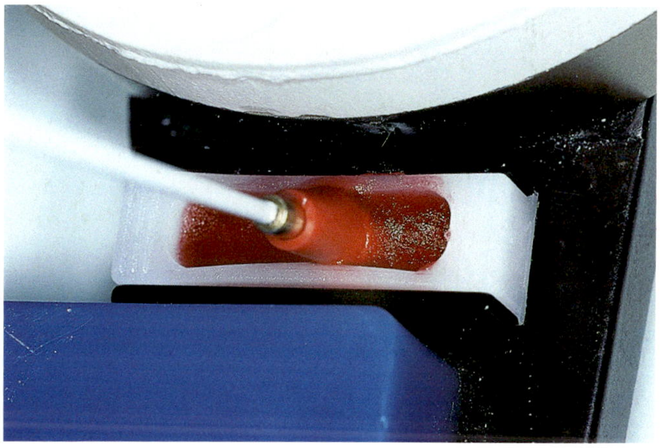

Fig 6-41j Midline indicator fixed in the shoe attachment on the articulator.

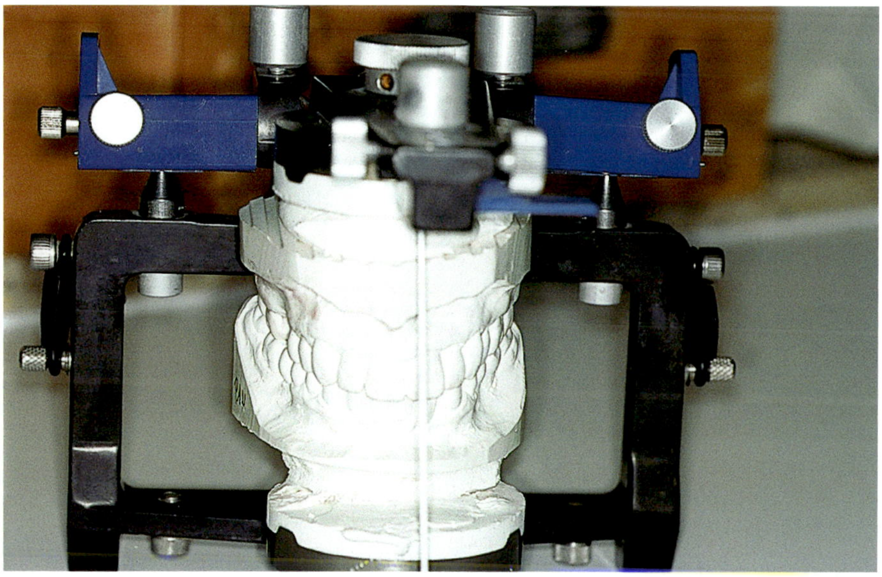

Fig 6-41k Midline analysis on the articulator.

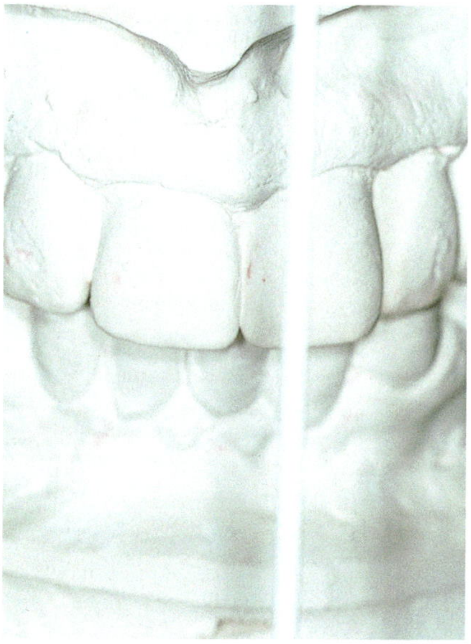

Fig 6-41l Close-up of the anterior maxilla during midline analysis on the articulator.

measure the displacement of the midline on the casts and correct it in the permanent restoration (Figs 6-41k and 6-41l).

The next section will discuss the horizontal planes which, together with the midline, allow a more complete esthetic assessment of the position of the teeth within the face.

Materials

Transparent ruler (use a scalpel to carve a middle line) and felt-tip pen (available from a stationery shop)
Linefinder (Langner)
Pattern Resin (GC America)

Horizontal Facial Planes

Common problem: Unparallel horizontal facial planes

The horizontal facial planes play an important part in the esthetic arrangement of the teeth, much like the midline, which is the vertical axis of symmetry in the face. The facial planes are made up of the following points of reference (Figs 6-42a to 6-42c):

1. The interpupillary plane is the horizontal plane through the pupils. It is a very reliable parameter, because asymmetry of the pupils on the horizontal plane is rare.
2. The horizontal plane through the corners of the mouth is a "muscular" plane, defined by the activity of the orbicularis oris during facial expressions, and depends strongly on the patient's age and habits.
3. The horizontal anterior occlusal plane is the plane through the eminences of the canines. The incisors should be symmetrically aligned in a harmonious curve following the contour of the lower lip. It is not identical with the "glass slab plane" that dentists know from making complete dentures, in which the canines and central incisors are supposed to be in contact with the slab while the lateral incisors should stand 1.0 mm above, often resulting in the notorious "piano key" appearance.
4. The gingival plane is the horizontal plane cutting through the gingival level of the anterior teeth. The canines and the central incisors should be on the same level, whereas the gingiva of the lateral incisors is 1.0 mm lower.

In most cases, these facial planes are in harmony, ie, parallel with the horizontal plane and each other, so that they are usually not a problem for the esthetic appearance of the mouth. If, however, there are larger discrepancies between the facial planes, it becomes very difficult to correctly position the teeth in a restoration and achieve a good esthetic outcome. Dentists can only influence the look of the gingiva and the teeth but cannot directly influence other facial features. Only through plastic surgery can the parameters of the face be permanently altered.

The following problems can be encountered in facial esthetics: an asymmetric midline (eg, a bent nose or an off-center chin); a disharmonious interpupillary plane (eg, if one eye is higher than the other); an inclined plane

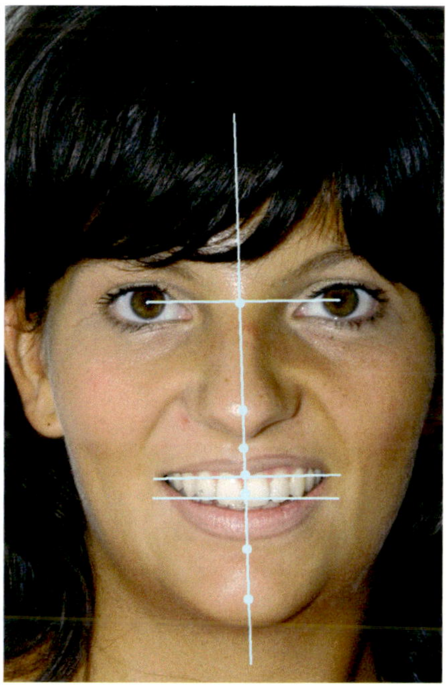

Fig 6-42a *(left)* Horizontal facial planes (interpupillary plane, plane through the corners of the mouth, and frontal occlusal plane).

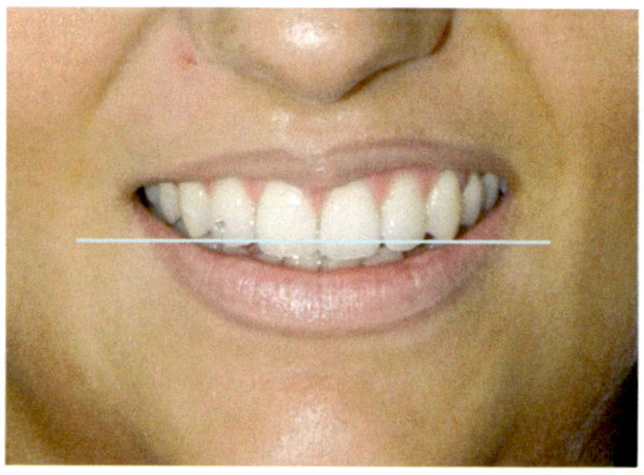

Fig 6-42b *(top right)* Anterior occlusal plane through the eminences of the canines.

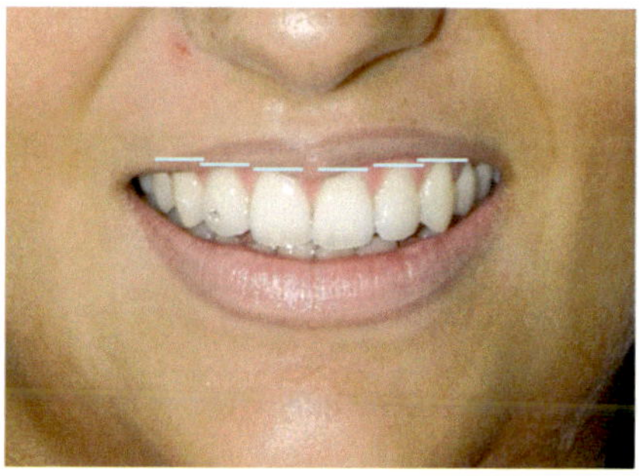

Fig 6-42c *(bottom right)* Gingival planes.

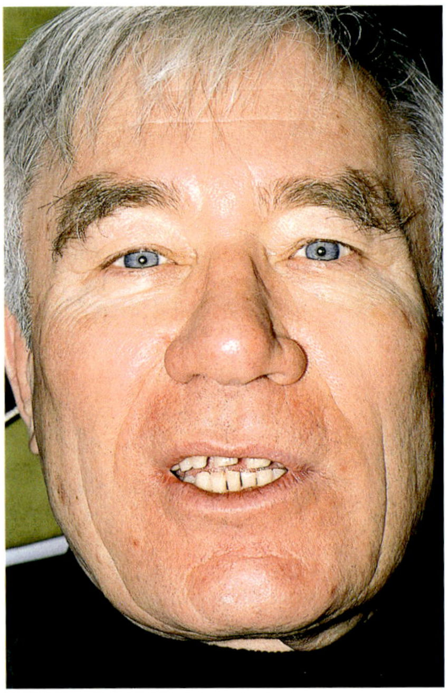

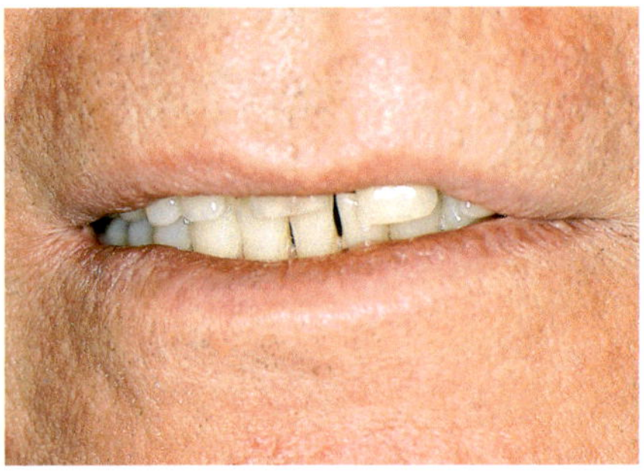

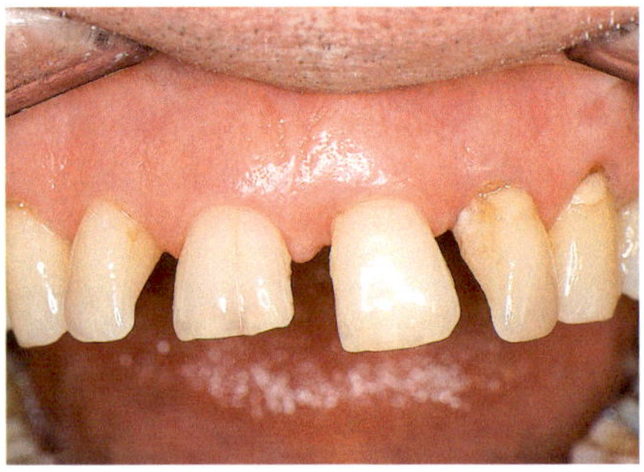

Fig 6-43a *(left)* Neither the midline nor the horizontal lines are harmonious in this patient.

Fig 6-43b *(top right)* The plane through the corners of the mouth is not horizontal.

Fig 6-43c *(bottom right)* The positions and inclination of the anterior teeth are hard to integrate in an esthetic concept.

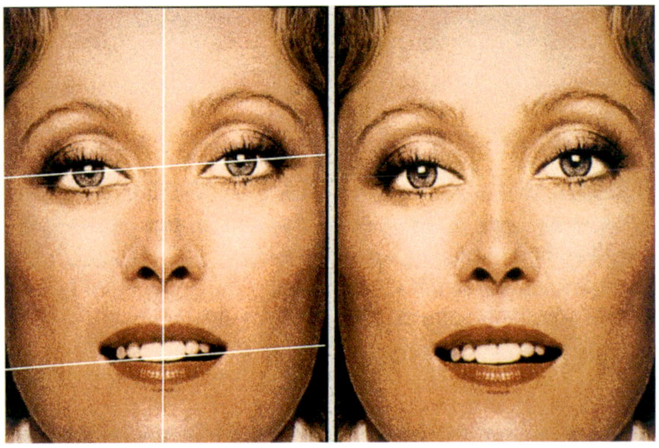

Fig 6-44 If the interpupillary plane is not parallel with the horizontal plane, should the teeth be aligned with the interpupillary plane or with the horizontal plane?

through the corners of the mouth (eg, if one corner is pointing downward or the corners of the mouth are asymmetrically shaped); and deformation of the lips through occlusal habits (eg, lip biting).

The following problems can be encountered in the esthetics of the mouth (Figs 6-43a to 6-43c): an inclined occlusal plane; an asymmetric midline; inclined tooth axes; diastemas; anterior crowding; protruding teeth; retruding teeth; and dramatically varying gingiva (especially problematic with "gummy" smiles).

How can the dentist position the teeth esthetically in a restoration (Fig 6-44)?

Proven solution: Facial analysis with the Dento-Facial Analyzer

The Dento-Facial Analyzer, developed by Kois,[12] consists of a facebow, a magnetically positionable level, and a bitefork connected to the facebow, on which an adjustable Index Tray can be snapped (Figs 6-45a and 6-45b). The system also features a Golden Ruler, which allows the dentist to measure the facial proportions, tooth lengths, tooth positions, and so on, according to the golden ratio (Fig 6-45c).

The Dento-Facial Analyzer is based on the following principles:

1. The bow uses the horizontal plane as its reference plane and not the Frankfort horizontal as is the case with facebows with arbitrary or individual registration. This is done with the help of a level in the transverse and sagittal directions (Fig 6-45d and 6-45e).
2. The position of the casts mounted on the articulator according to this method of analysis is absolutely identical to the results or the variations of arbitrary mounting versus mounting with reference to the hinge axis. This has been confirmed in extensive research[12] (Fig 6-45f).

3. Based on these data, the distance to the condyles is 100 mm (Fig 6-45g).

Recording process

The compound Bite-Tabs on the index tray of the bitefork are immersed in hot water for 3 minutes to be warmed (Figs 6-45h to 6-45j). The facebow is aligned on the patient so that the maxillary incisors bite down exactly behind the incisal stop of the index tray (Figs 6-45k and 6-45l). The facebow is aligned with the horizon, both sagittally and transversely, with the help of the magnetically adaptable level, while the patient is sitting upright without leaning against anything. The midline is adjusted with the vertical rod (Figs 6-45m and 6-45n). The rubber rings on the vertical rod are adjusted to the various facial planes (Fig 6-45o).

The facebow is removed and the index tray is released (Fig 6-45p). The index tray is snapped onto the platform screwed into the articulator (Figs 6-45q and 6-45r). In this example, a Panadent articulator was used. The Dento-Facial Analyzer system can also be used with other articulators. The patient's maxillary cast is seated on the index tray and the cast is prepared as usual (Figs 6-45s and 6-45t).

Analysis

The patient's lip line and smile line for the upper lip are transferred to the cast (Figs 6-45u and 6-45v). The teeth and gingiva are revealed furthest not when the patient smiles but when he or she makes a long /e/ sound. The symmetry of the gingiva must be examined.

The index tray is replaced with the analysis and waxing guides, which are chosen according to the size of the dental arch. The set comes with waxing guides in six different sizes (Figs 6-45w and 6-45x).

The proportions of the teeth relative to the face can be examined with the Golden Ruler (Fig 6-45y). This is especially useful for determining the tooth lengths and widths that would correspond to the facial proportions.

Esthetic treatment plan

The original or esthetically desirable tooth lengths and widths can be determined in the following ways: *(1)* tooth length proportional to body height (see Table 6-3); *(2)* ratio between tooth length and width (see Table 6-4);

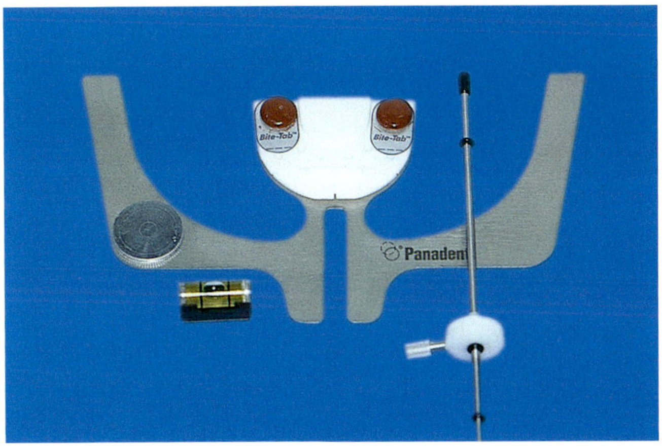

Fig 6-45a Individual parts of the Kois Dento-Facial Analyzer.

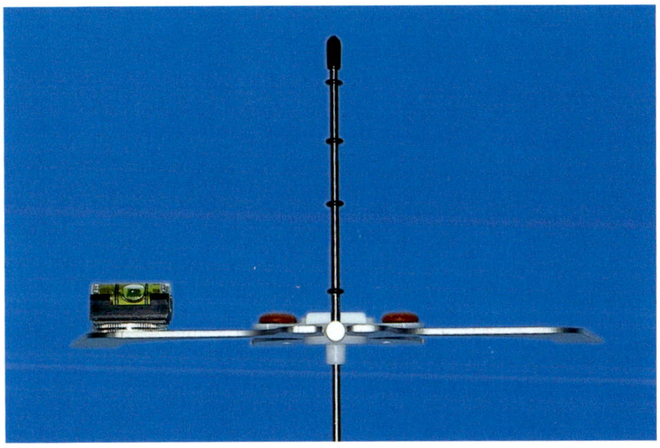

Fig 6-45b Dento-Facial Analyzer with parts mounted for recording.

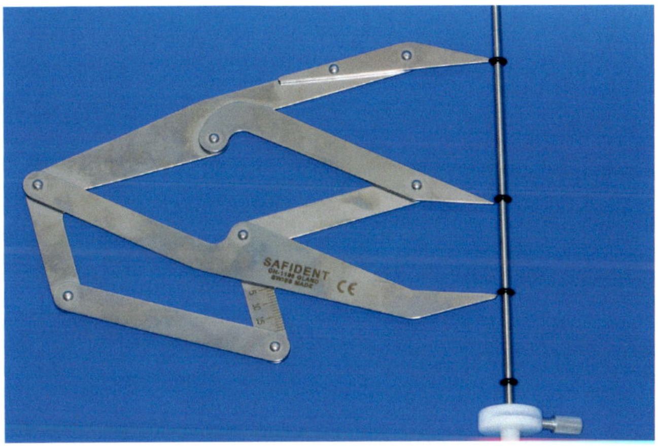

Fig 6-45c Golden Ruler.

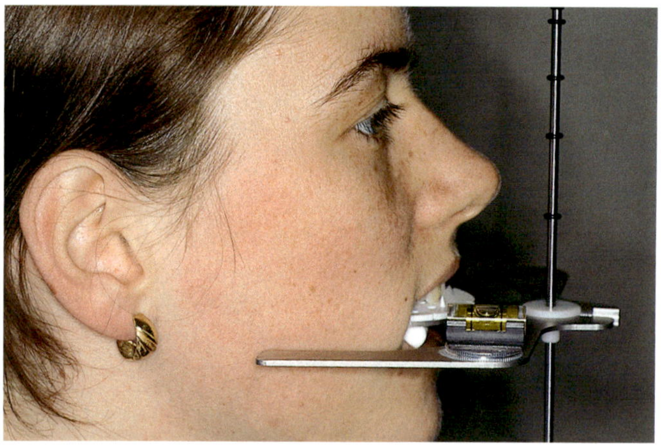

Fig 6-45d Sagittal alignment of the facebow.

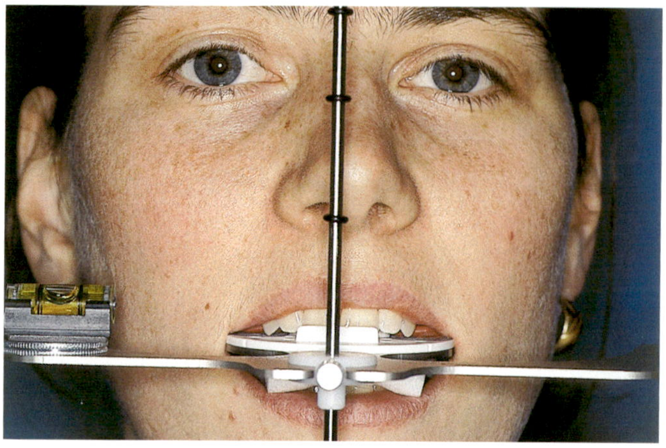

Fig 6-45e Transverse alignment of the facebow.

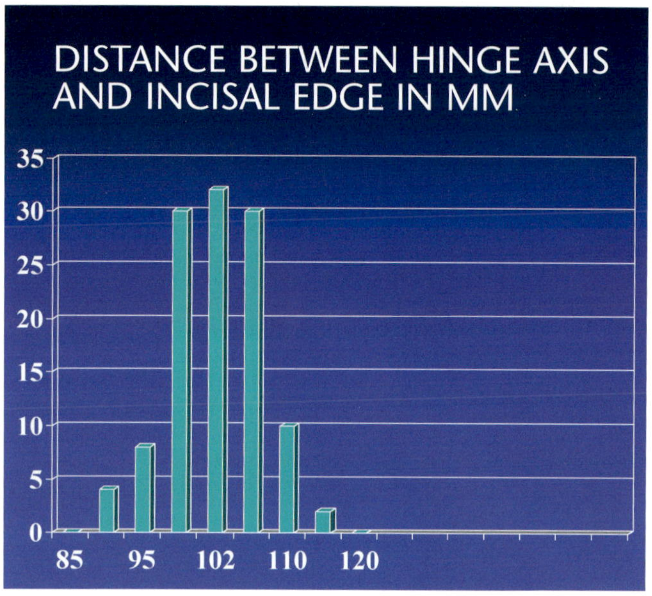

Fig 6-45f *(left)* Average distances between the condylar hinge axis and the incisal edge of the mandibular central incisor.

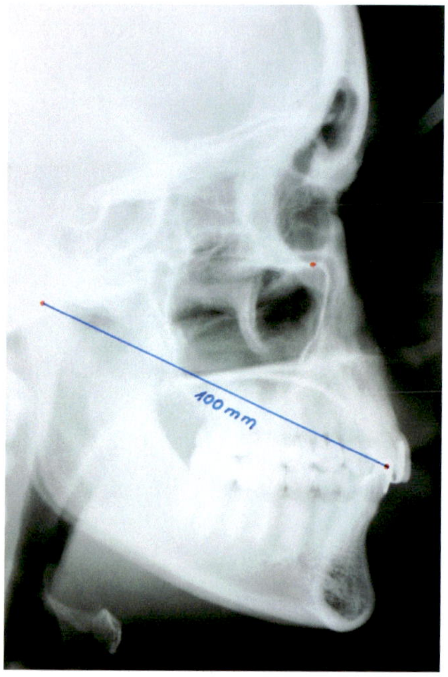

Fig 6-45g *(right)* Average distance of 100 mm on a radiograph.

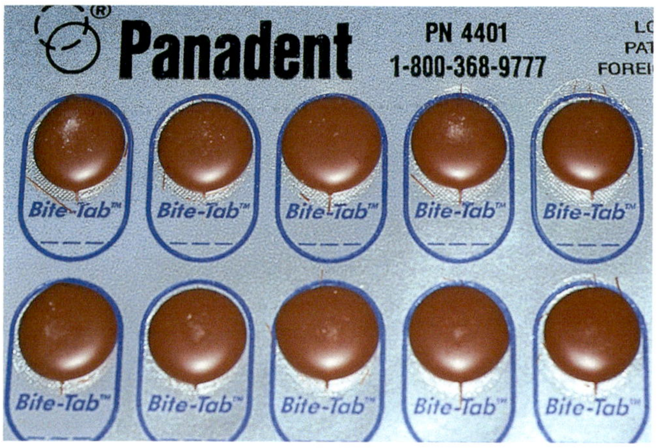

Fig 6-45h Bite-Tabs are self-adhesive compound tablets.

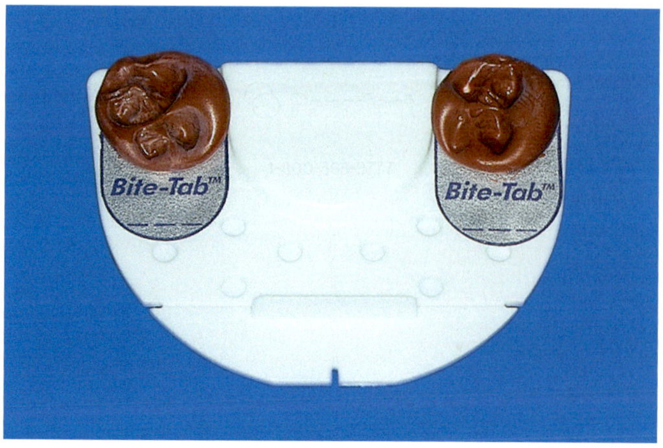

Fig 6-45i The Bite-Tabs are in place on the index tray.

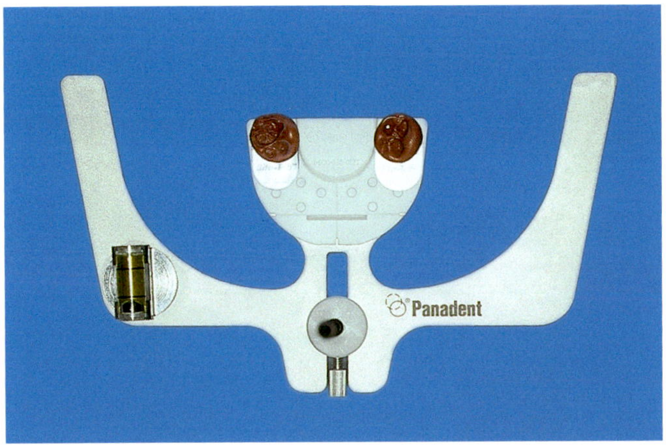

Fig 6-45j The Dento-Facial Analyzer is ready for recording.

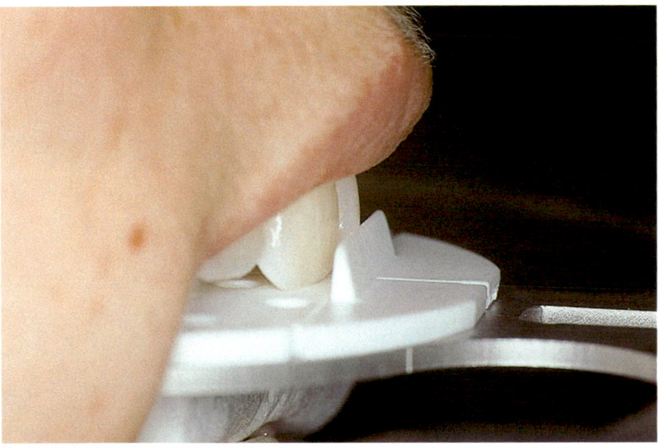

Fig 6-45k The maxillary incisors bite down exactly behind the incisal stop.

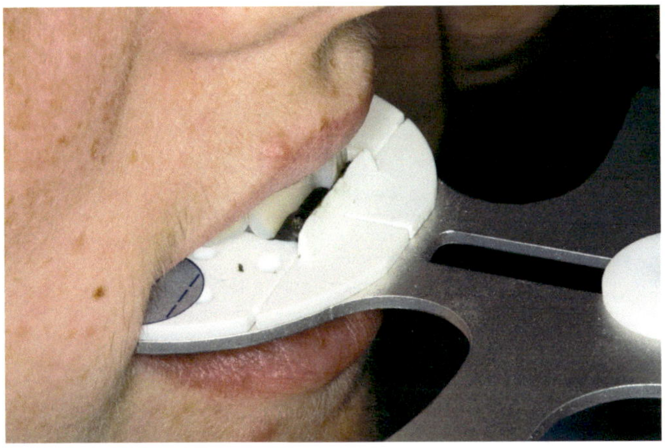

Fig 6-45l The patient bites down behind the incisal stop. If the occlusal plane is inclined, compound can be applied for horizontal adjustment.

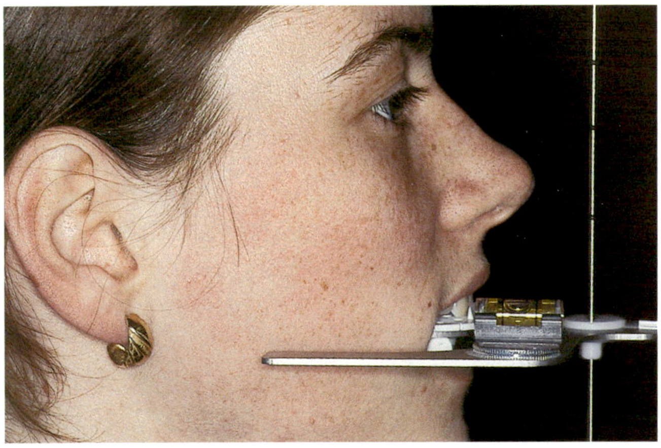

Fig 6-45m The level is used to determine sagittal adjustment.

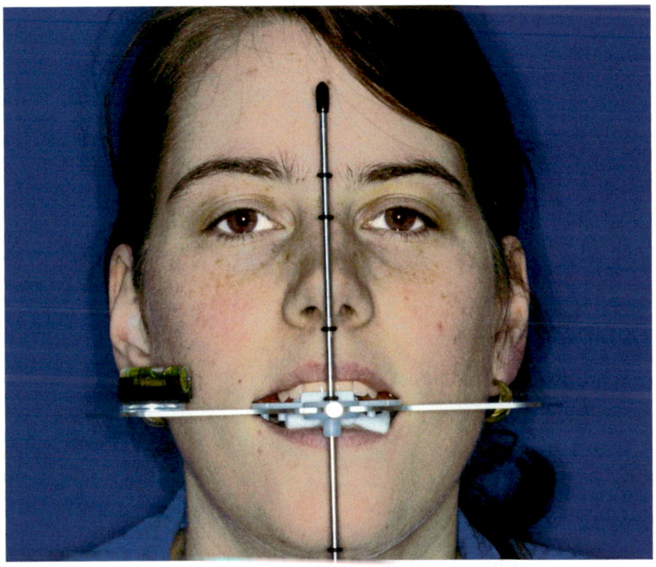

Fig 6-45n The level is used for adjustment of the transverse plane and the midline.

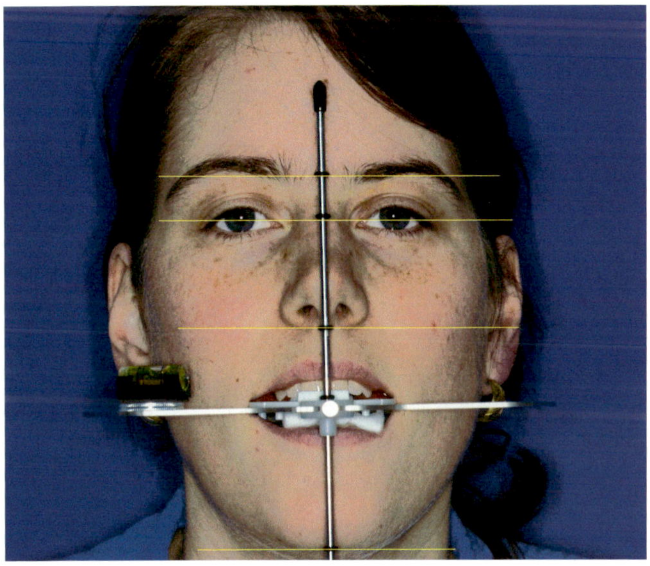

Fig 6-45o The adjustable rubber rings on the vertical rod are aligned with the horizontal facial planes.

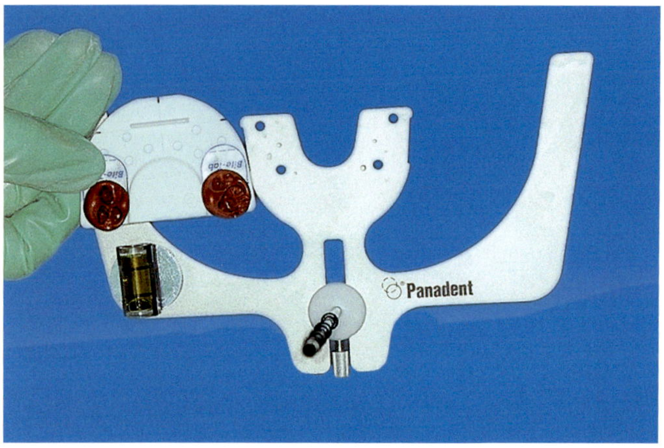

Fig 6-45p The facebow is removed and the index tray is released.

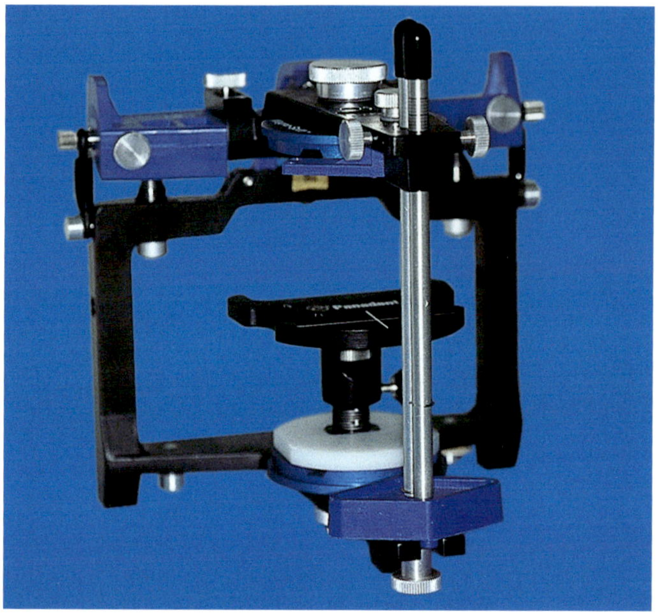

Fig 6-45q The platform is attached to the articulator.

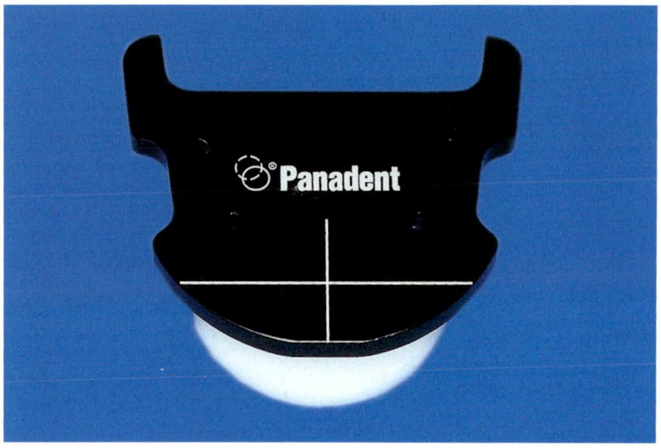

Fig 6-45r The index tray is snapped on the platform.

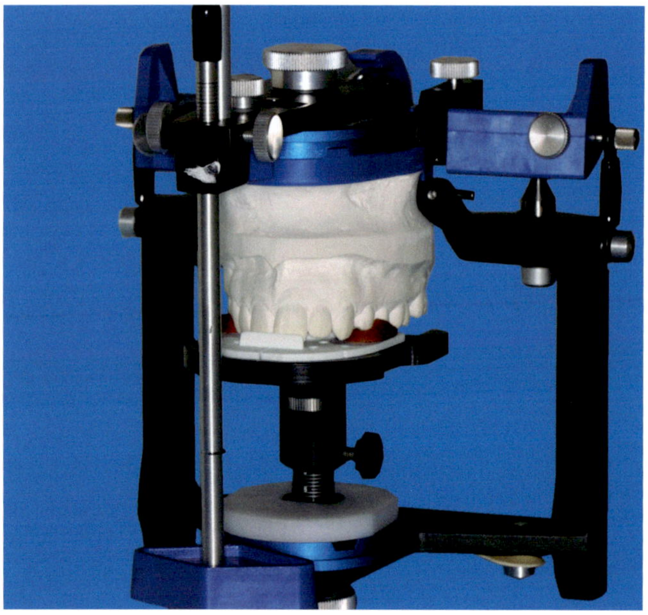

Fig 6-45s The maxillary cast is placed on the index tray.

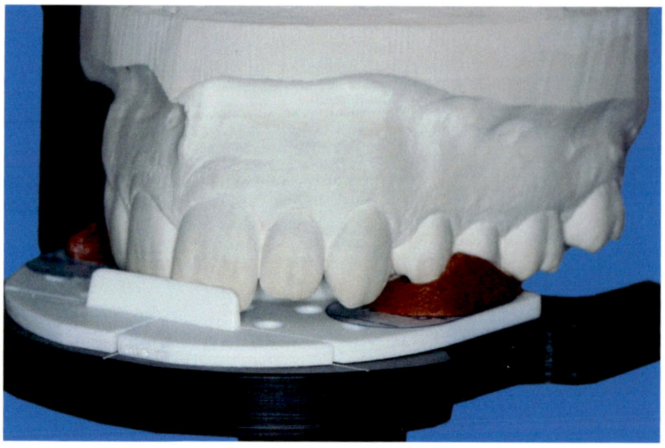

Fig 6-45t Close up view of the position of the cast on the index tray.

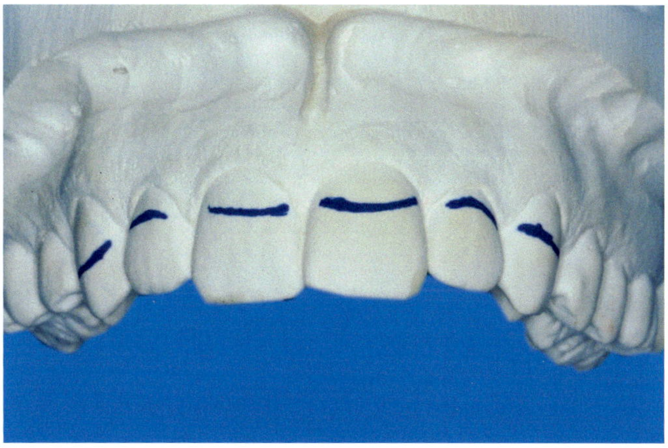

Fig 6-45u The lipline (*blue*) is transferred to the maxillary cast.

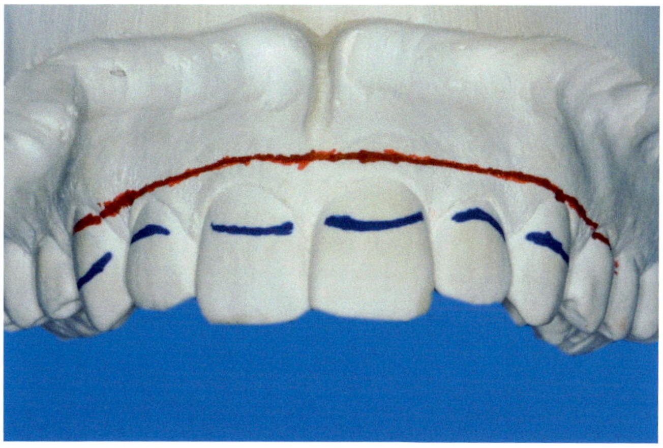

Fig 6-45v The smile line (*red*) is transfered to the maxillary cast.

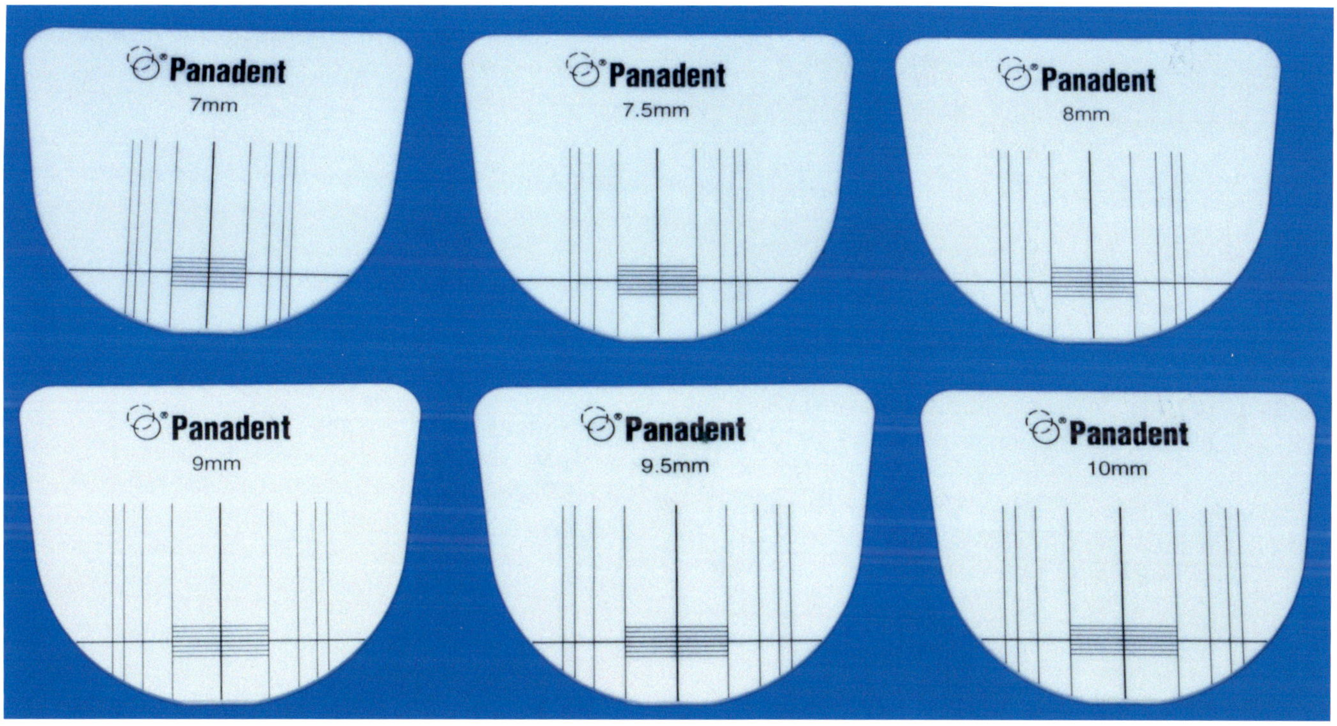

Fig 6-45w The waxing guides are available in six sizes.

and *(3)* distribution of tooth widths as stated by Levy[23] (Fig 6-46). The waxing guides are engraved with these proportions, which correspond to the respective arch size. They help in analyzing and reconstructing teeth, for the setup, for the waxup, or for making permanent restorations.

The gingiva is drawn on the individual anterior teeth: the original or esthetically desirable course, level, and apex. This can be used as a basis to plan the appropriate mucogingival corrections (Fig 6-47).

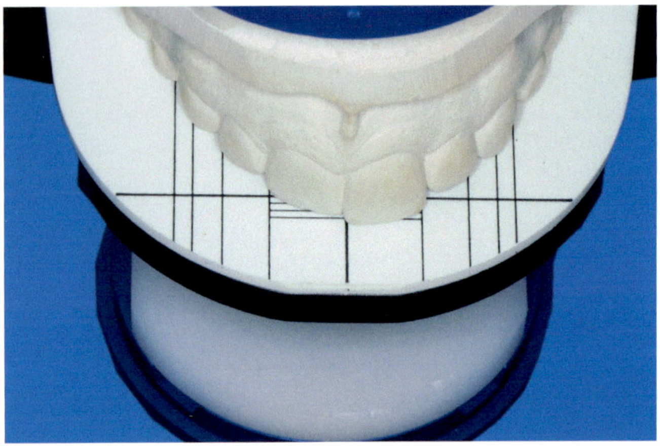

Fig 6-45x The correct arch size is selected.

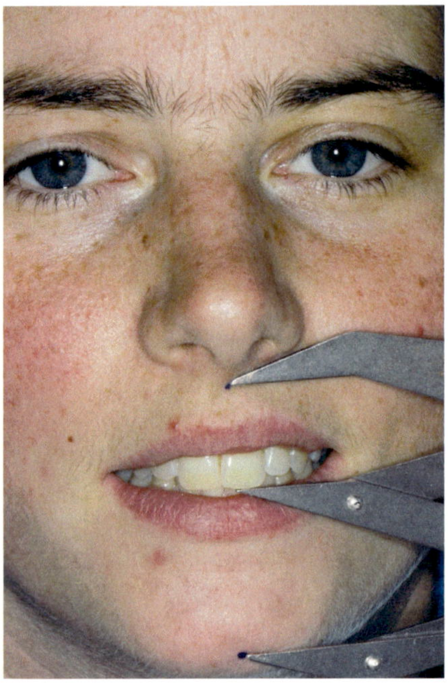

Fig 6-45y The teeth are assessed in relation to the face with the Golden Ruler.

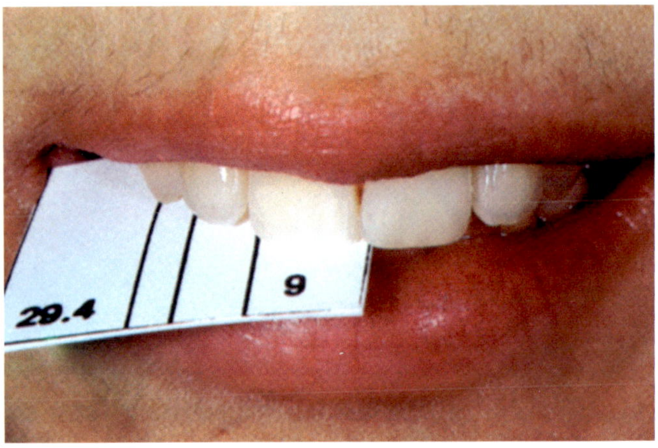

Fig 6-46 Distribution of tooth widths according to Levy.

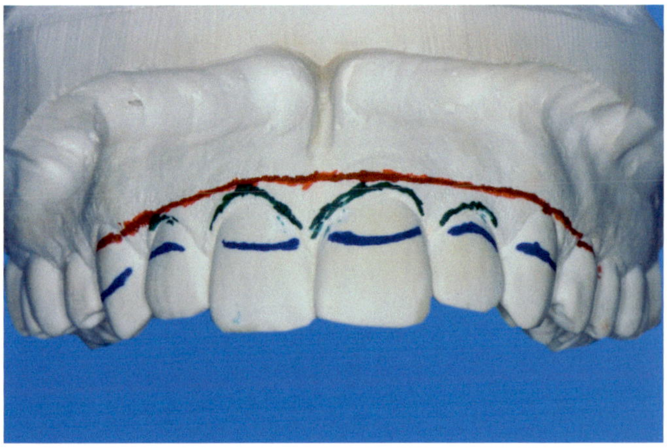

Fig 6-47 The mucogingival corrections (*green line*) are planned.

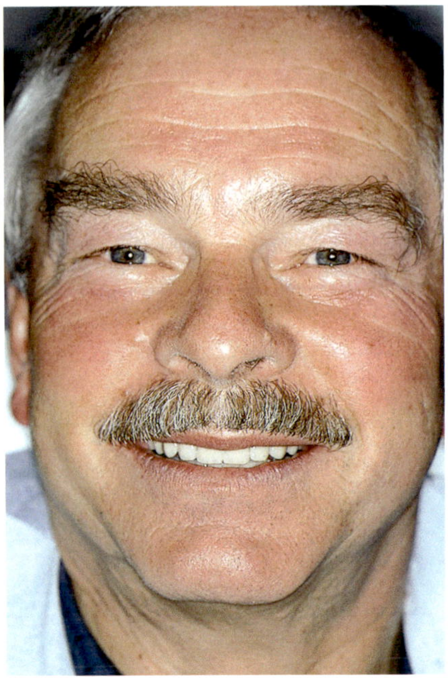

Fig 6-48 The esthetic restoration in this patient is successful.

Conclusion

The Kois Dento-Facial Analyzer[12] is a logical, self-contained system for analysis and restoration that has been scientifically proven to be accurate and has become an indispensable tool in restorative dentistry and in the dental laboratory (Fig 6-48).

Materials

Kois Dento-Facial Analyzer (Panadent)
Panadent articulators (Panadent)
Golden Ruler (comes with the Dento-Facial Analyzer kit; can also be purchased from Safident)

7

Orthodontics

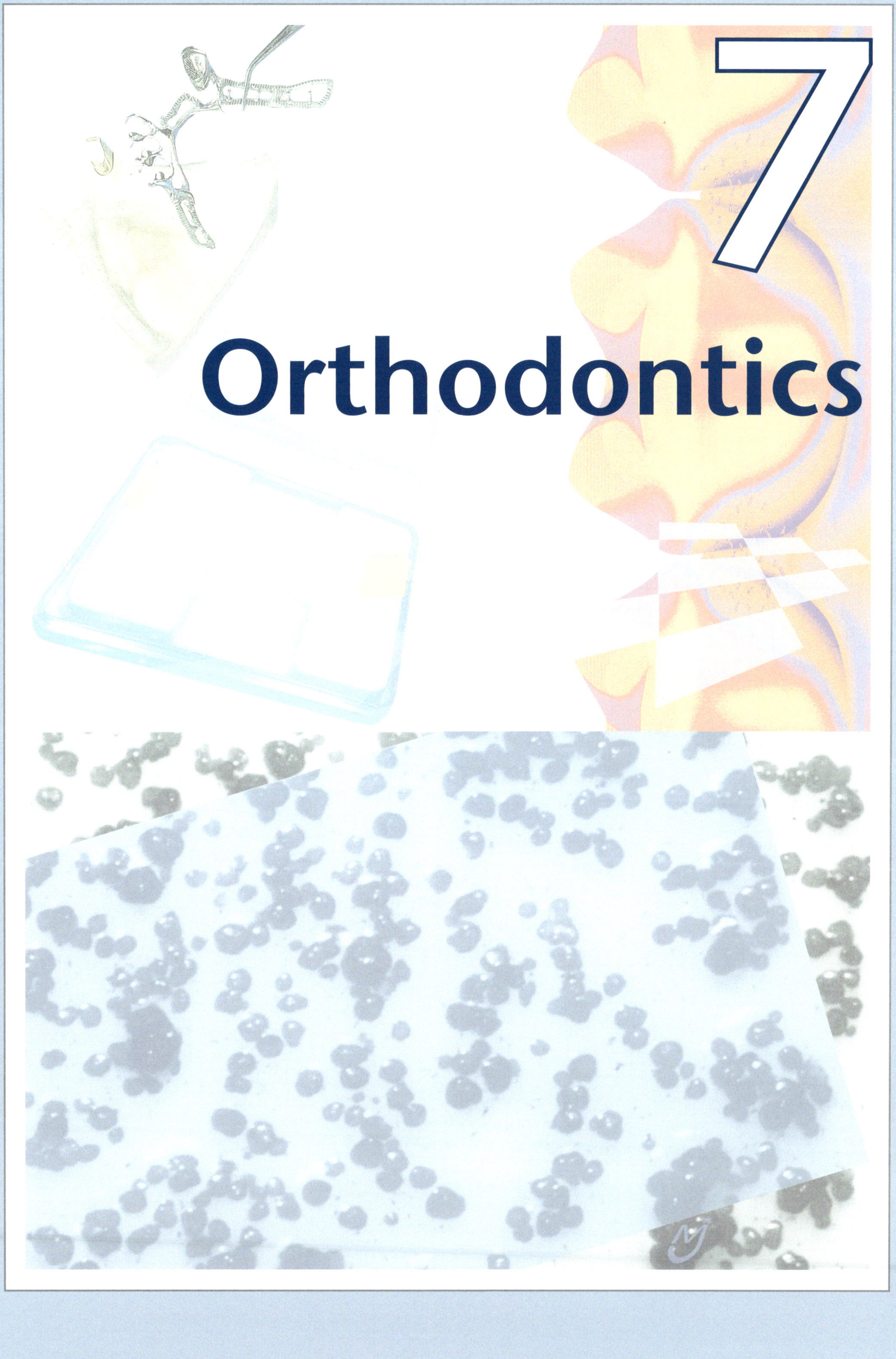

7

Orthodontic Retainers

Correction of Mandibular Anterior Crowding

Orthodontic Retainers

Common problem: Functional and esthetic retention after orthodontic treatment

The final retention period is an integral part of any orthodontic treatment. It is the only means of ensuring the long-term stability of the treatment outcome. The following options are available for retention:

1. Removable retainers with positioners, if further fine adjustment of the occlusion is planned
2. Removable retainers of cold-cure acrylic or vacuum-formed retainers, both of which are worn mainly at night and thus may involve the risk of a relapse
3. Fixed retainers with wires, which can cause pronunciation difficulties, interfere with oral hygiene, and encourage occlusal parafunctions

Proven solution: Adhesive fixed retainer with glass fiber resin composite

Adhesive retainers are a considerably more comfortable way of providing fixed retention for the patient, especially because they are functional and esthetic. The procedures will be demonstrated through some case reports.

Direct retainers

Correction of retrusion and anterior crowding in the maxilla of a 42-year-old woman had been completed. She was to wear a fixed retainer for 1 year (Figs 7-1a and 7-1b).

The teeth that were to be retained were cleaned and etched (Figs 7-1c to 7-1e). Wedjets (normally used with rubber dam) were placed in the interproximal spaces to block out the spaces and to form "channels" for Superfloss and interdental brushes (Figs 7-1f and 7-1g).

The length of the retainer was measured with a calibrated periodontal probe in the patient's mouth (Fig 7-1h). The bundle of Vectris Pontic fibers was thinned with a scalpel and cut to the required length (Figs 7-1i to 7-1k). The trimmed fiber bundle was kept on a light-protected tray to prevent early polymerization. The Vectris Pontic fibers are silanized and coated with dimethacrylate, which means that care must be taken to ensure that they do not cure prematurely.

A thin layer of flowable microfine hybrid resin composite was applied to the palatal surfaces of the maxillary anterior teeth (Fig 7-1l). The fiber bundle was adapted to the tooth as flatly as possible and polymerized step by step, ie, tooth by tooth (Figs 7-1m and 7-1n). Subsequently, a thin covering layer of flowable microfine hybrid resin composite was applied, shaped, and polymerized completely with two curing lights (Fig 7-1o).

The occlusion was checked and the retainer was examined to ensure that the interproximal spaces could be cleaned (Fig 7-1p).

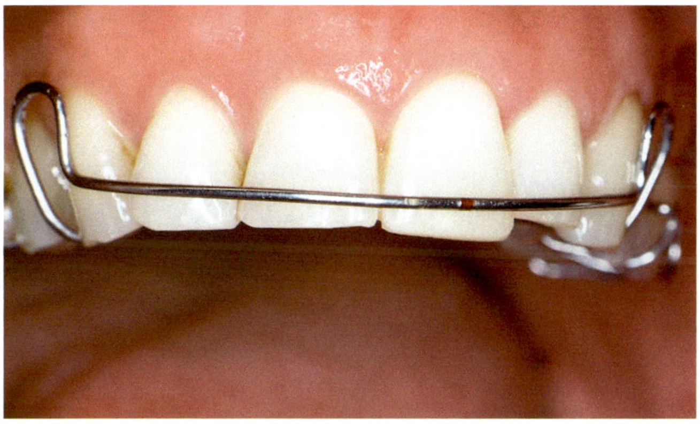

Fig 7-1a Orthodontic appliance in the patient's mouth. The anterior segment of the maxillary arch has now been completely rounded.

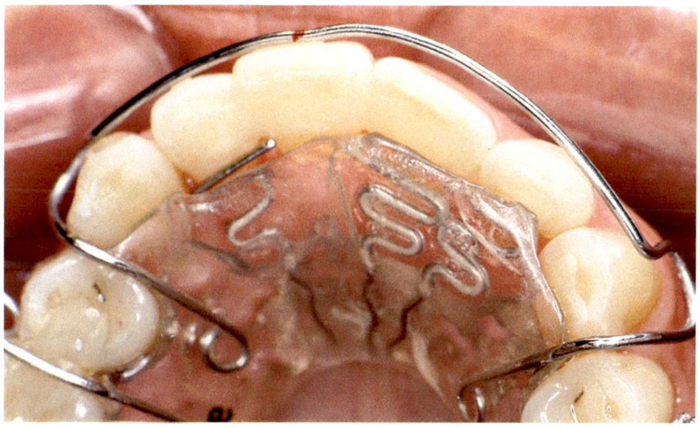

Fig 7-1b In the palatal view, the active elements of the appliance, the protrusive spring and the labial bow, are visible.

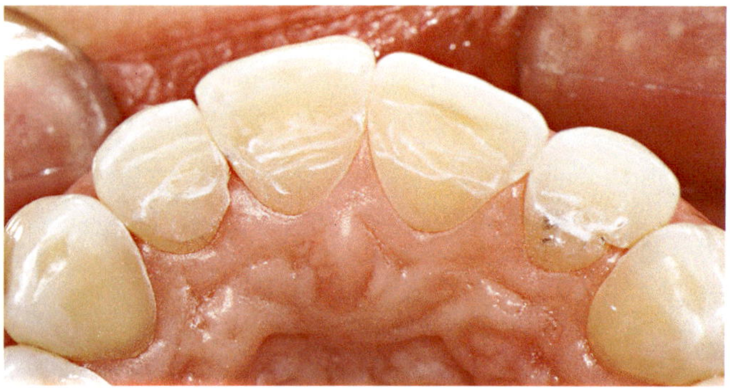

Fig 7-1c The surfaces are cleansed and slightly abraded for adhesive bonding.

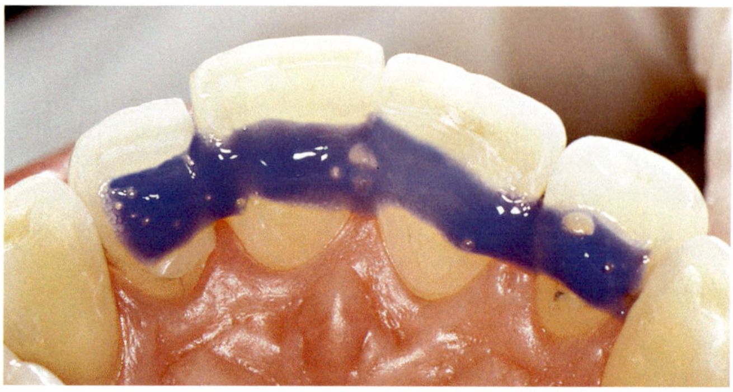

Fig 7-1d The surfaces are etched with phosphoric acid for 30 seconds.

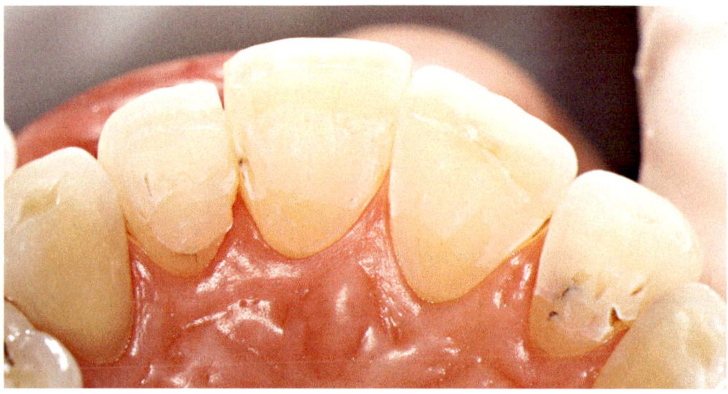

Fig 7-1e The etching pattern is examined.

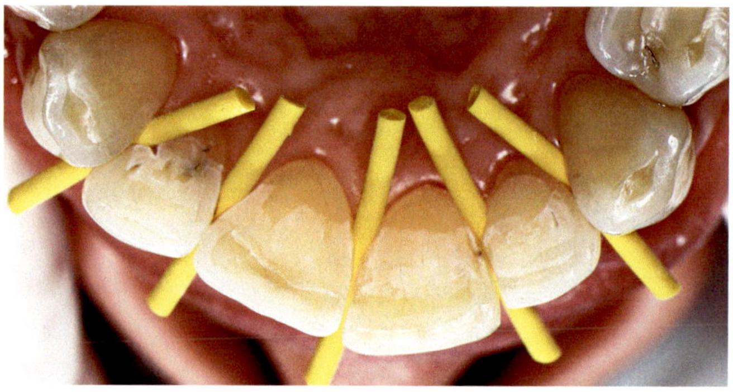

Fig 7-1f Wedjets are applied to block out the interproximal spaces and to form interdental channels for Superfloss and interdental brushes.

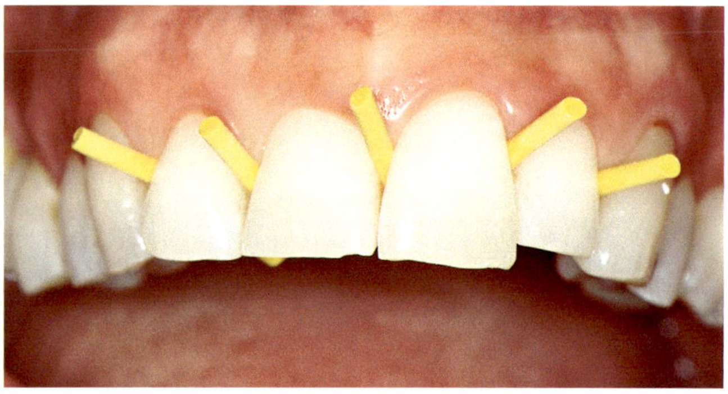

Fig 7-1g The Wedjets are in place.

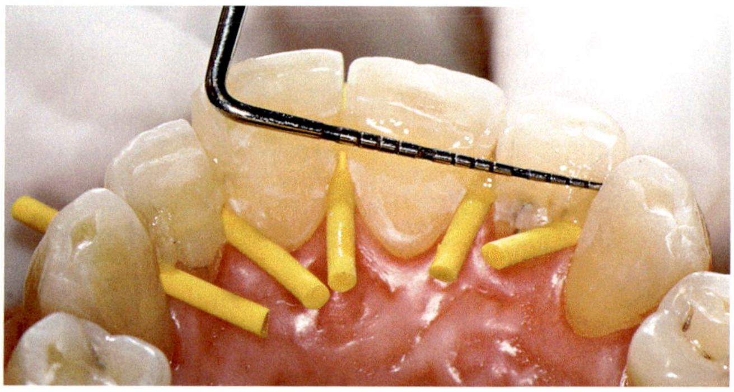

Fig 7-1h The length of the retention zone is measured with a periodontal probe.

Indirect retainers

Anterior crowding in a 20-year-old woman had been treated orthodontically. The orthodontically aligned teeth were to be retained over a period of 2 years, because substantial rotations had been corrected, and the risk of a relapse was correspondingly high.

Therefore, a long-term retainer was produced in the laboratory with the Targis/Vectris glass fiber resin composite system (Figs 7-2a to 7-2e). This retainer was cemented with an adhesive after a thorough try-in (Figs 7-2f and 7-2g). The procedure was completed with an examination of the occlusion and hygiene (Figs 7-2h and 7-2i).

Periodontal splinting

The splinting of periodontally compromised teeth is accomplished with the same method.

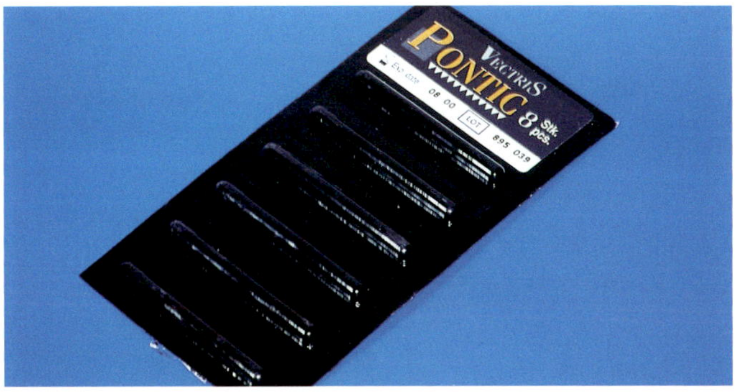

Fig 7-1i The long fibers from the Vectris System (Pontic fibers) are used for retainers and splints.

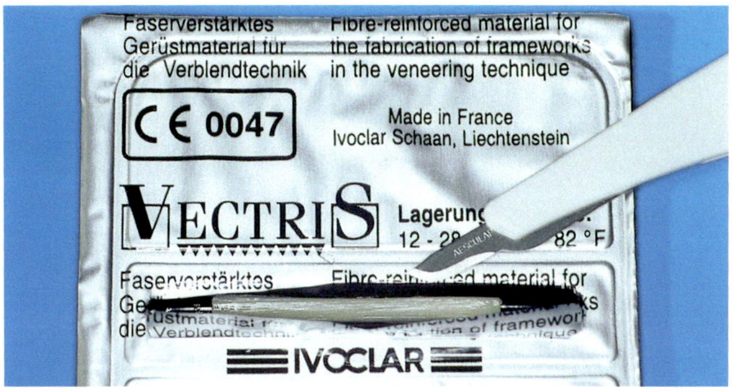

Fig 7-1j The silanized and dimethacrylate-coated fibers are removed from their pack.

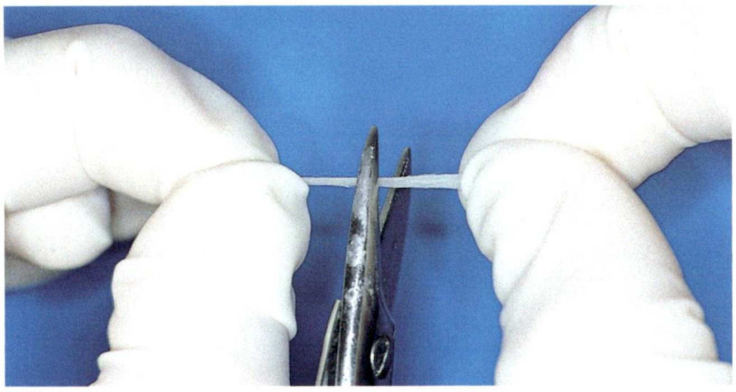

Fig 7-1k The fiber bundles are carefully thinned with a scalpel and trimmed with scissors. Because the fibers are very slick, the dentist should cut them while the assistant stretches them.

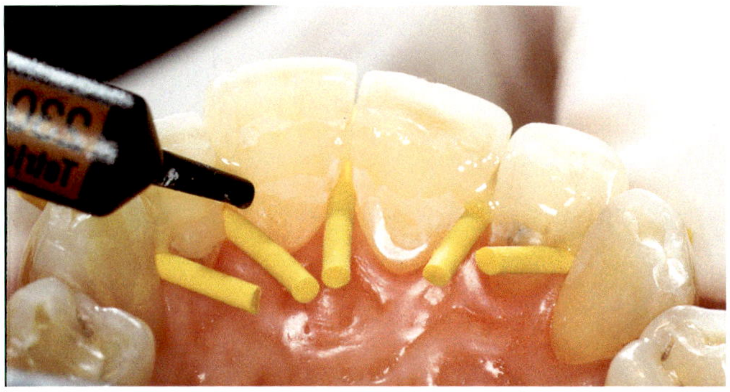

Fig 7-1l A base layer of flowable resin composite is applied, and interim curing is performed.

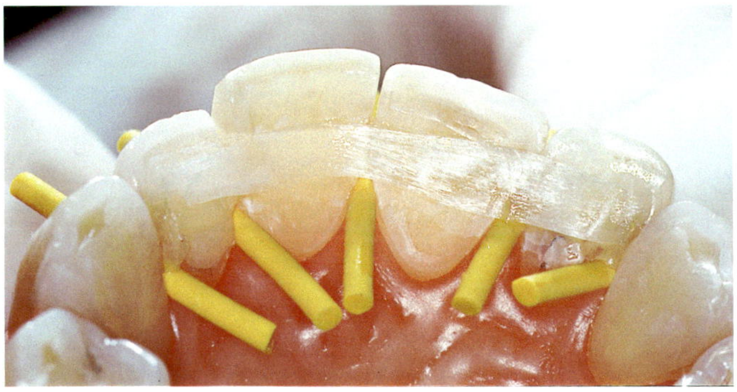

Fig 7-1m The glass fibers are adapted, pressed flat, and covered with resin composite.

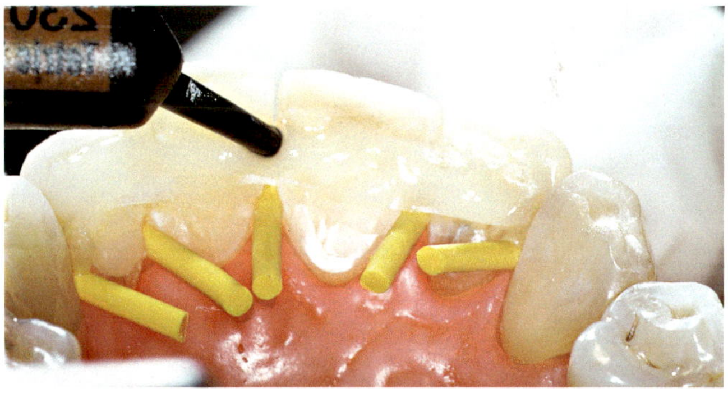

Fig 7-1n The flat glass fiber bundle is adapted and subjected to interim curing.

Fig 7-1o *(left)* After a last covering layer of resin composite is applied, it is carefully polymerized completely with two curing lights.

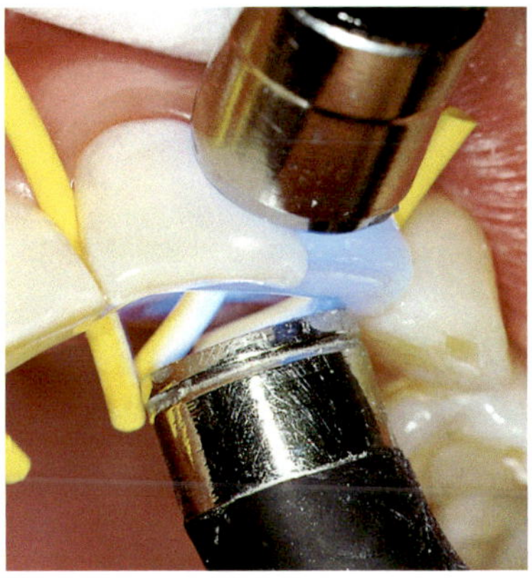

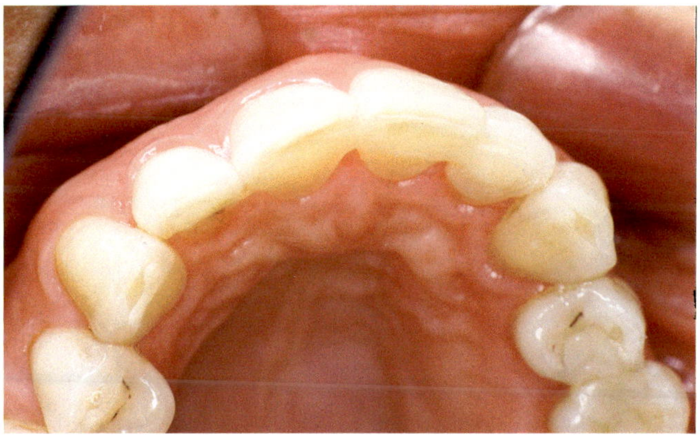

Fig 7-1p *(right)* The finished retainer is metal-free and esthetic.

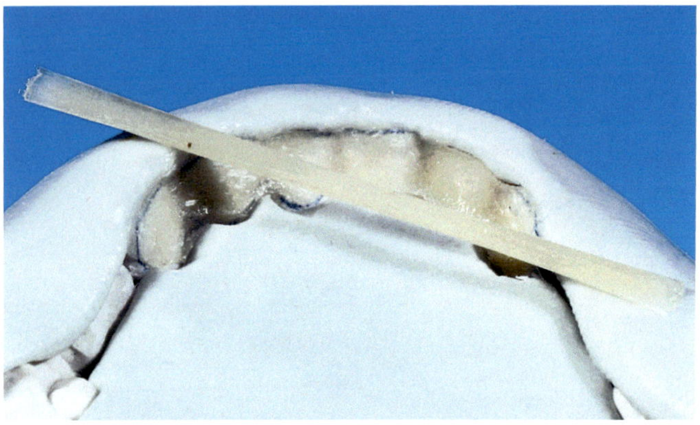

Fig 7-2a Laboratory-fabricated retainer. The base is applied and precured. The Vectris Pontic fibers are adapted.

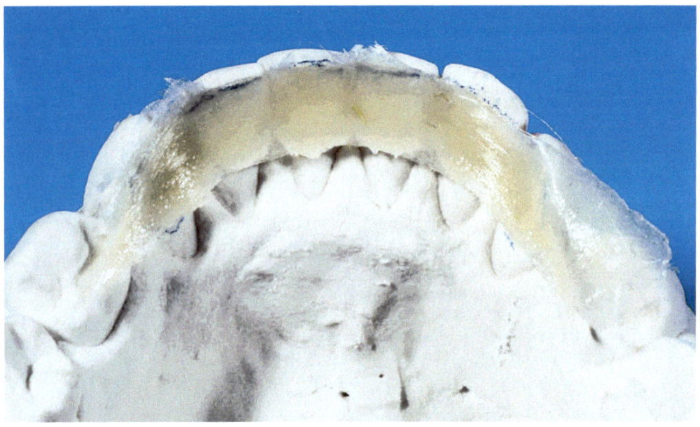

Fig 7-2b The glass fiber framework is finished. As a final step, the framework is covered with the Targis veneering material in a matching shade.

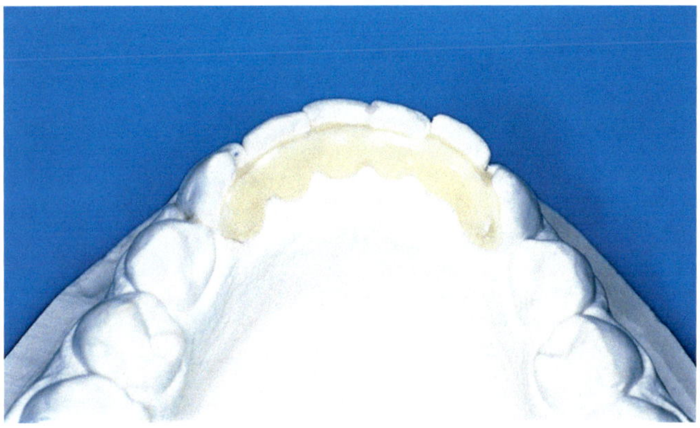

Fig 7-2c The finished orthodontic retainer is shown on the cast.

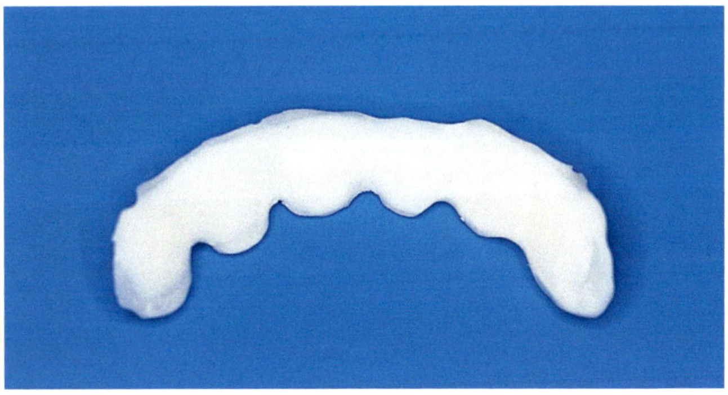

Fig 7-2d The orthodontic retainer is removed from the cast.

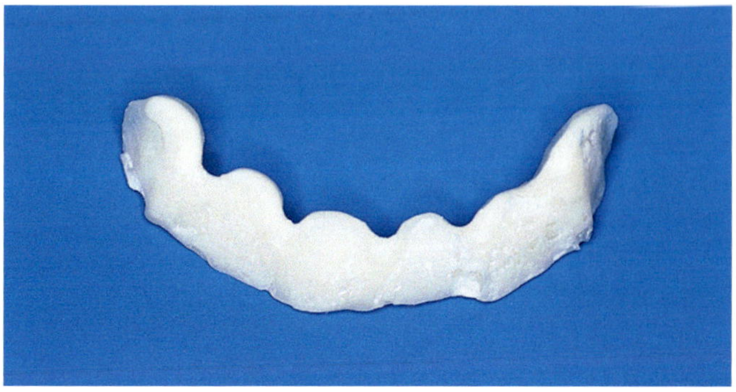

Fig 7-2e The orthodontic retainer is sandblasted, cleaned, and silanized. It is then ready to be cemented.

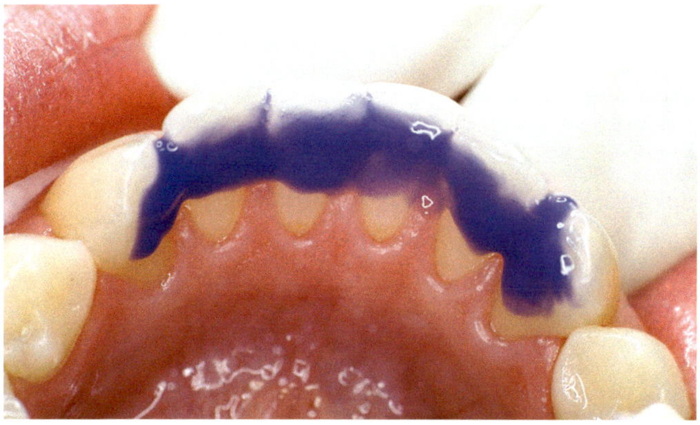

Fig 7-2f The enamel is etched after the surfaces have been cleaned.

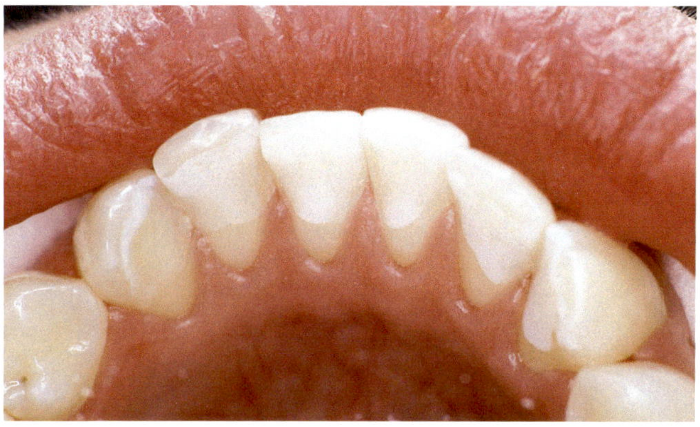

Fig 7-2g The etching pattern is checked.

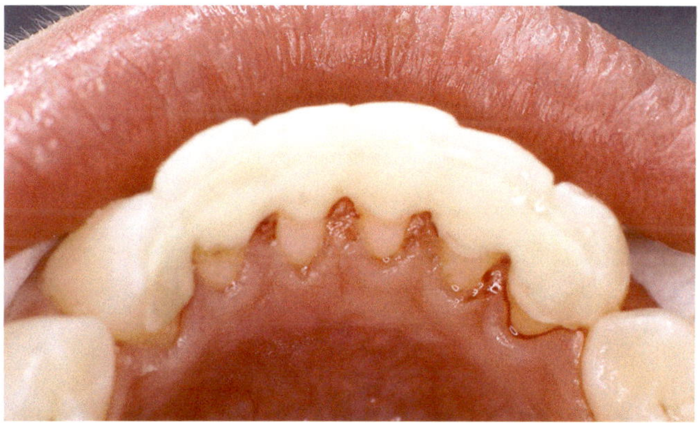

Fig 7-2h The adhesive orthodontic retainer is in place.

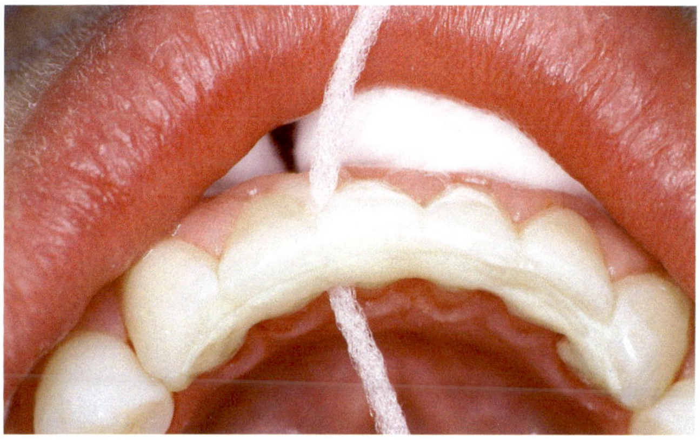

Fig 7-2i The retainer is checked to ensure that the interproximal spaces can be cleaned with Superfloss.

Materials

Ultra-Etch (Ultradent)
Wedjets (Coltène Whaledent)
Tetric Flow (Ivoclar Vivadent) or any other flowable, microfine hybrid resin composite
Vectris Pontic fibers from the Targis/Vectris System (now Adoro/Vectris, Ivoclar Vivadent)
Superfloss (Oral-B)
Stick Tech (Everstick Company)

Correction of Mandibular Anterior Crowding

Common problem: Functional, esthetic, and hygienic problems arising from crowding

Anterior crowding (Figs 7-3a and 7-3b), especially in the mandible, is associated with a number of problems and risks. The anterior guidance is usually heavily compromised by the presence of displaced, overlapping, and tipped teeth. The stomatognathic system usually responds with compensation through abrasion caused by dysfunction or with tooth mobility and recession. Minor malalignment can be functionally improved by selective grinding, whereas major malalignment has to be treated orthodontically.

The malalignment also compromises esthetics; some patients suffer considerably because of the poor esthetics. There is a widespread assumption that orthodontic treatment is only possible in children, and most patients have resigned themselves to the thought that their situation cannot be corrected.

Oral hygiene measures are severely restricted when the teeth are too crowded. The ensuing plaque accumulation further compromises esthetics, as do recessions and exposed roots. In many cases, periodontal problems are treated with mucogingival surgery, although this ultimately does not offer a solution to the actual problem—the crowding.

Because the patient is simply incapable of cleaning the teeth properly, there is also a higher risk of caries. For the dentist, the resulting caries lesions are very difficult to restore—again, because of crowding.

Proven solution: Orthodontic treatment

It is a sad fact that the average dentist has a meager knowledge of orthodontics. The extent of this knowledge usually begins and ends with the courses taken at dental school, where the dentist was very often instructed to stay away from orthodontic treatment in his or her own office. Dentists in training were simply told that any kind of tooth movement should be left to orthodontists. Orthodontists in turn have generally moved so far away from general dentistry that now the two professional groups might as well be on different planets. Dentists simply refer patients with malalignment or dysgnathia to an orthodontist. Neither of the parties involved really has a clear-cut idea of the treatment concept and, most importantly, of the common treatment goal.

Thus the general dentist refers the patient to the orthodontist, who then carries out the treatment to the best of his or her knowledge. However, no one defines a common treatment goal—which should be life-long preservation, function, esthetics, and periodontal health of the patient's teeth. In the end, the orthodontist takes the casts (initial and final casts, 4.8 to 5.2 cm high, with stable edges and a nice glossy talcum finish) and puts them on a shelf somewhere, convinced of having achieved a permanent success. The referring dentist, however, will usually see the patient for many years and can therefore track the success or failure in the long run.

If a patient is referred to an orthodontist for minor orthodontic measures, such as the correction of anterior crowding for future prosthodontic treatment, the orthodontist will usually want to initiate a complete orthodontic treatment. The confused patient, who by no means wants to endure a complete treatment over the course of several years, returns to the first office, telling the referring dentist that, according to the orthodontist, minor interventions are useless. This is why anterior crowding is corrected half orthodontically and half prosthetically in most offices, with the help of resin composite, veneers, or even full crowns and fixed partial dentures. To the author, this practice cannot be reconciled with a modern concept of dentistry.

It is therefore time for general dentists and orthodontics to enter into a dialogue, define common goals, and to catch up on each other's treatment options. Orthodontists should remember again that they are also dentists, while the dentists should integrate orthodontics into their treatment range as an integral part of dentistry. If a dentist enjoys "minor orthodontics," he or she should follow up with some continuing medical education or take classes from an orthodontist. The latter is only possible, though, if orthodontists who teach orthodontic practices to dentists are no longer stigmatized by their colleagues.

Many years ago, inspired by Dr Günter Staehle of Böblingen, Germany, the author began to integrate minor orthodontics into dental work, while fully acknowledging the possibilities and limitations. Through the cooperation with Kubein-Meesenburg's team from Göttingen University, the author especially realized the enormous functional importance of correcting mandibular anterior crowding by means of prosthetic rehabilitation with the Contour Curve Former (CCF).

Treatment of mandibular anterior crowding

In the author's office, the correction of anterior crowding is almost exclusively done in adult patients for the aforementioned reasons. In these patients, growth is complete, and widening of the arch via orthodontics is no longer possible.

Crowding means that the tooth widths and the arch width do not match; the dental arch is too small, causing the teeth to overlap. If the teeth are to be aligned correctly, it is necessary to work with the available space between the canines, because the distance between them cannot be changed in adult patients unless they wear a retainer for the rest of their life.

Therefore it is necessary to narrow the incisors laterally or to *strip* them, as orthodontists call this procedure. Before interproximal stripping of the incisors is performed, however, the dentist should calculate the exact amount of available space and the extent to which individual teeth can be reduced. A wax setup to simulate the planned treatment outcome is also recommendable. The patient should be informed about how minor the procedure is when only enamel is removed and the teeth are treated with fluoride afterward.

The following options are available for the correction of mandibular anterior crowding:

1. Treatment with a removable baseplate with spring arms and lingual arch. In the author's experience, adult patients usually decline this kind of treatment.
2. Treatment with a removable Crozat appliance. This appliance consists only of soldered wire (Fig 7-4) and is usually accepted by adults. For a dentist, this treatment is very easy to perform, because the spring arms allow clear and defined tooth movements. The appliance can only be made in specialized laboratories.
3. Treatment with a fixed appliance. The removable baseplate and Crozat appliances allow only tipping of the teeth, but cannot correct any other malpositions. Lateral tooth movement requires a fixed appliance with brackets. The "tin grin" look of metal appliances (Fig 7-5) is rarely tolerated by adults in the midst of their professional careers. Tooth-colored brackets of ceramic or acrylic resin, on the other hand, are usually readily accepted. Nowadays even tooth-colored ligature wires are available.
4. Treatment with a lingual fixed appliance. Lingual appliances have been in use for about 10 years. Because this treatment technique is not conspicuous to others, it has been very successful in treating adults. The device is implemented on the "back" of the teeth where it cannot be seen. Self-ligating brackets, which have been on the market for some years now, allow even orthodontically inexperienced dentists to quickly insert and fix the archwire.

Treatment with lingual appliances

A 26-year-old patient presented with minor anterior crowding in the mandible, which she wanted to have corrected for esthetic reasons (see Figs 7-3a and 7-3b).

The available space was measured and divided (a tooth setup was not necessary in this case). The brackets were placed using an indirect technique, which means that the brackets were applied in their exact positions on a working cast and subsequently transferred to the patient's mouth with a template. The position for the brackets was marked with a pencil, and the brackets were glued on the cast with ordinary glue (Figs 7-6a to 7-6g). Then a transparent silicone was applied and shaped (Figs 7-6h and 7-6i). After curing, the template with the brackets was removed from the cast. The template was examined, sandblasted, and cleaned (Figs 7-6j and 7-6k).

The enamel of the incisors in the patient's mouth was stripped interproximally by the calculated amount (Fig 7-6l). A diamond-coated metal strip clamped into a hemostat was used for stripping (Figs 7-6m and 7-6n). It is also possible to use a power tool. In this case, the oscillating Osada head for contra-angle handpieces was used with both diamond-coated metal strips and polishing strips (Figs 7-6o to 7-6s).

The teeth were cleaned with a pumice paste (Fig 7-6t) and rinsed. Then the template was checked for an exact fit (Fig 7-6u). The teeth were etched for 30 seconds with acid (Fig 7-6v) and rinsed for 15 seconds. The etching pattern was checked (Fig 7-6w). A light-curing bracket adhesive was applied to the teeth and to the brackets, which were still fixed in the template (Figs 7-6x to 7-6z). The template with the brackets was pressed against the anterior teeth (Fig 7-6aa). The adhesive was polymerized through the transparent template using two light sources

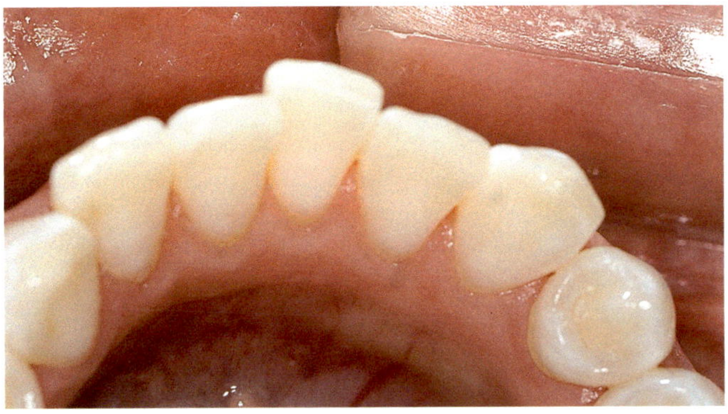

Fig 7-3a Lingual view of mandibular anterior crowding.

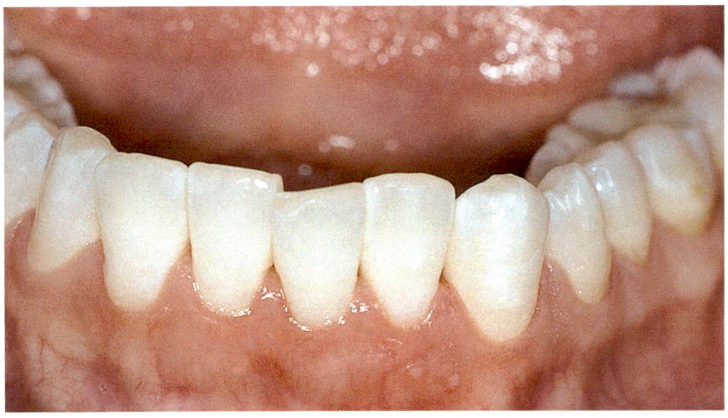

Fig 7-3b Labial view of mandibular anterior crowding.

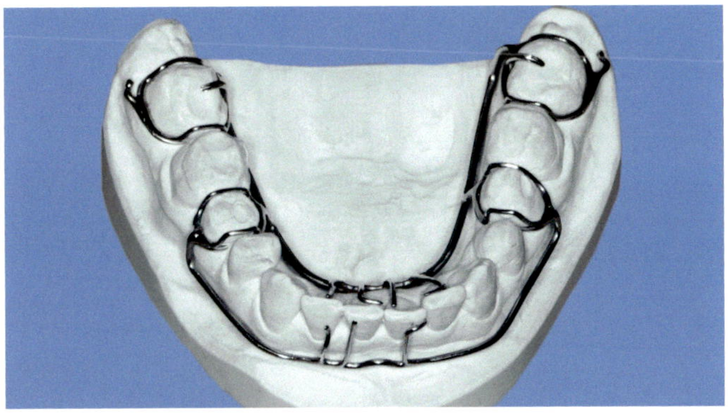

Fig 7-4 Crozat appliance on the cast.

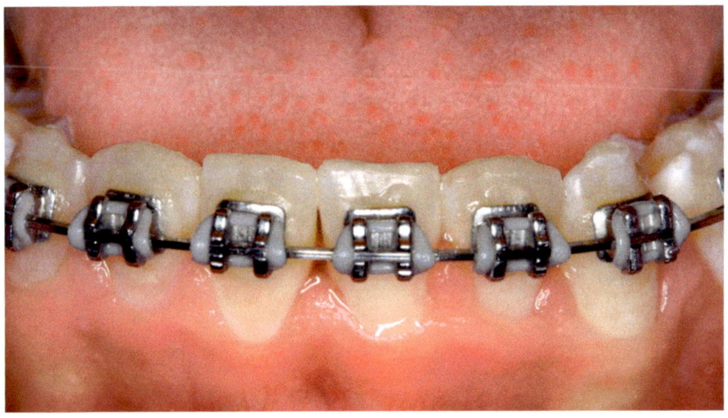

Fig 7-5 Metal appliances are very unpopular with adults.

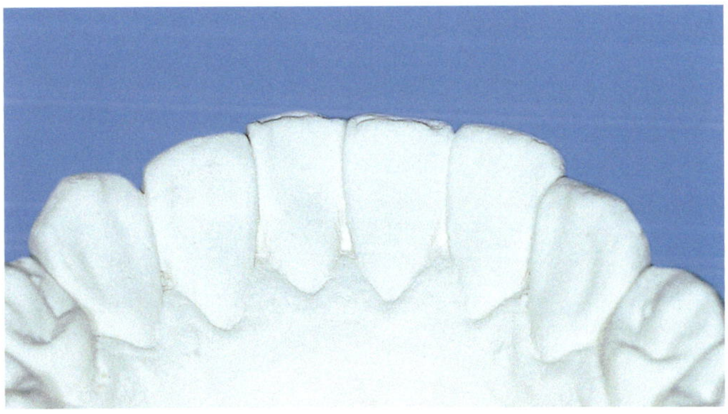

Fig 7-6a The working cast is used for indirect placement of brackets.

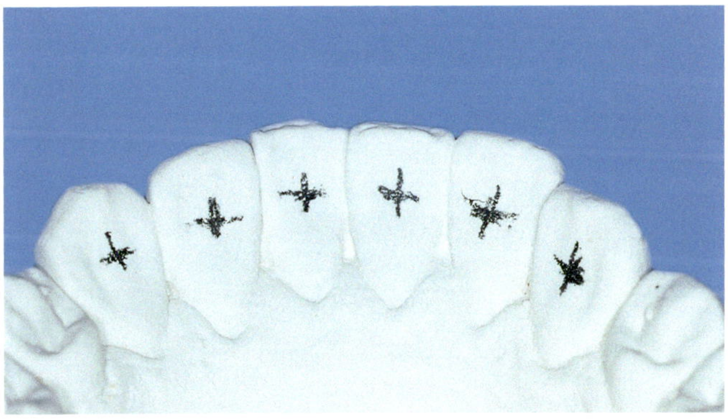

Fig 7-6b Positions for the lingual brackets are drawn on the cast.

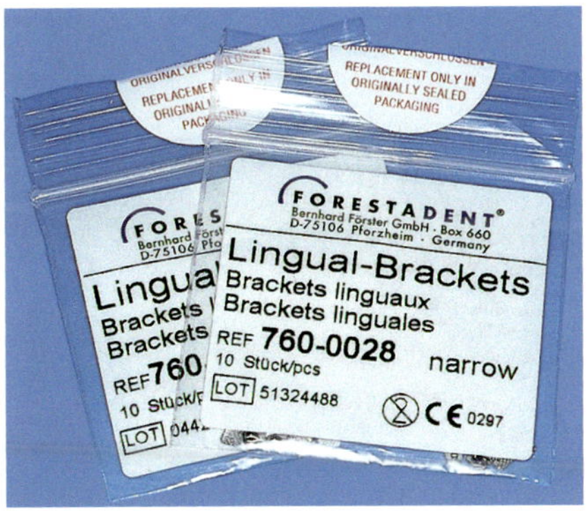

Fig 7-6c Lingual brackets in their package.

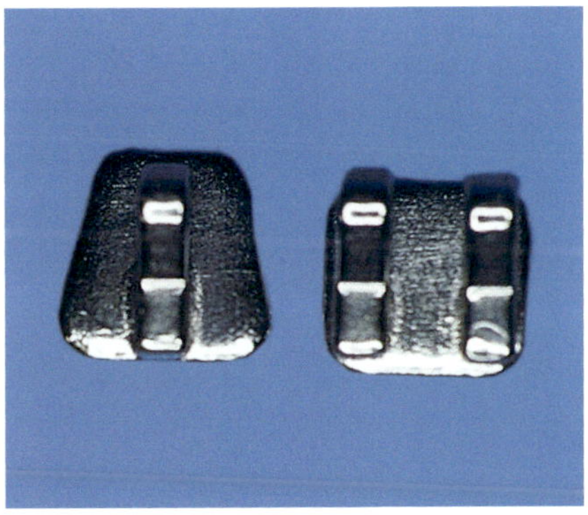

Fig 7-6d Self-ligating lingual brackets.

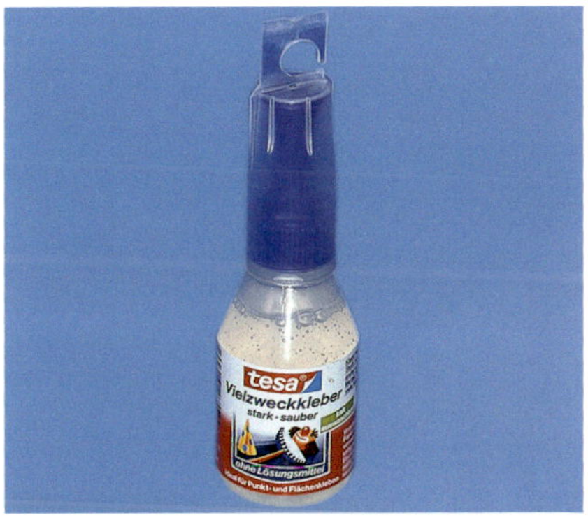

Fig 7-6e Paper glue.

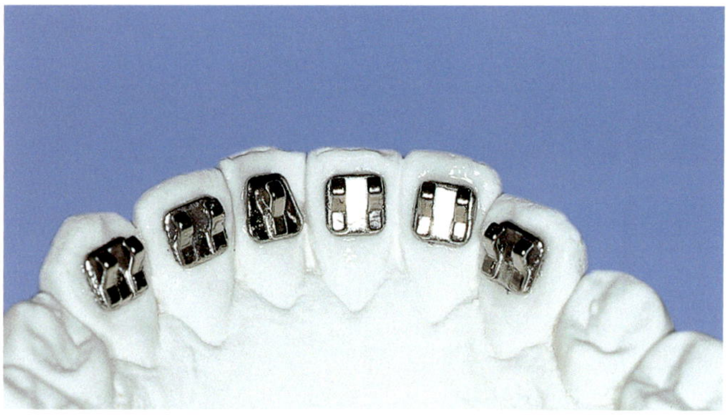

Fig 7-6f The brackets are glued to the cast.

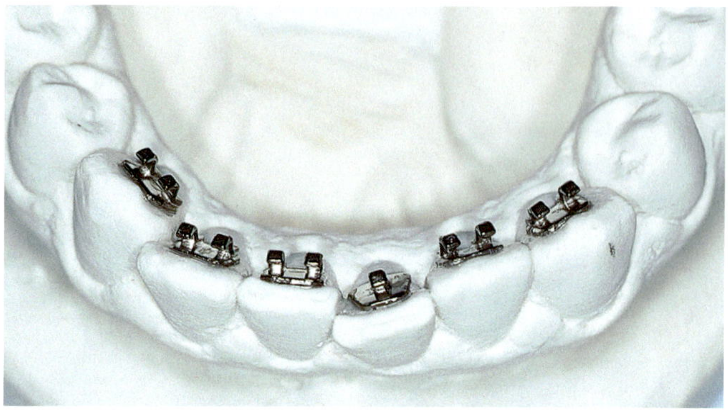

Fig 7-6g Occlusal view of the brackets.

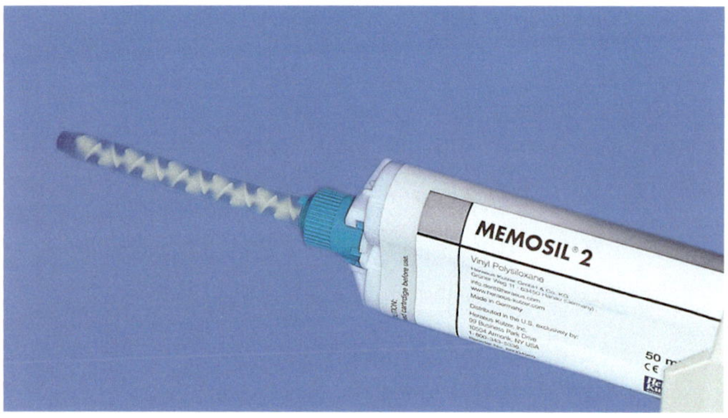

Fig 7-6h Transparent silicone is loaded in the mixing gun.

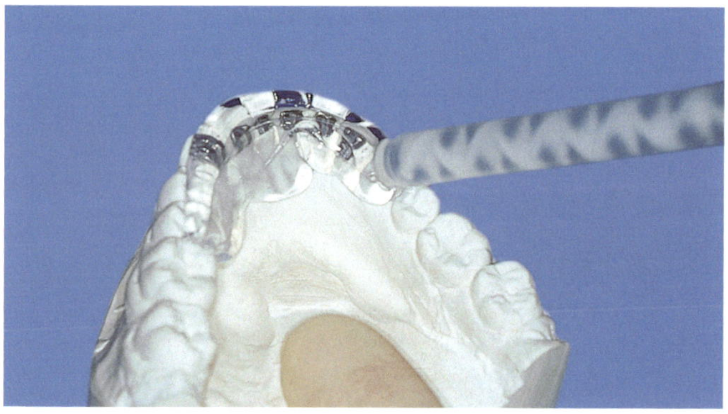

Fig 7-6i Transparent silicone is applied.

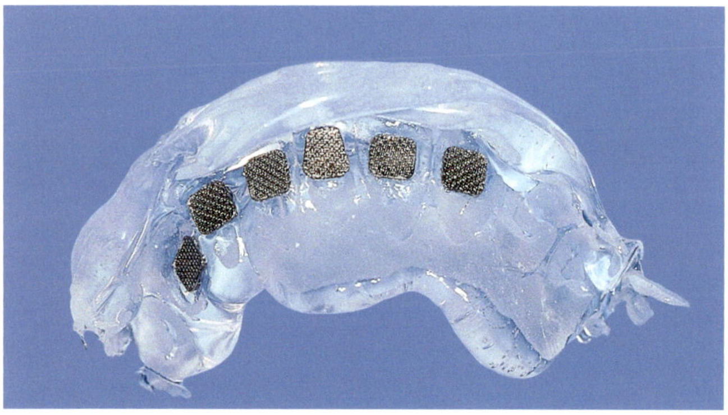

Fig 7-6j Positioning template with brackets.

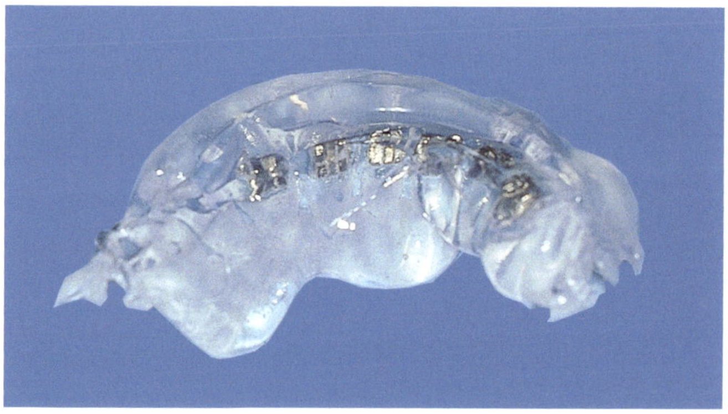

Fig 7-6k The positioning template with brackets is ready for try-in.

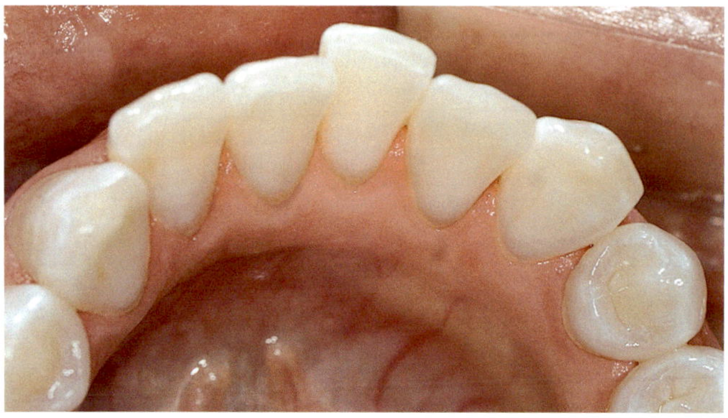

Fig 7-6l Available space in the mandibular anterior segment.

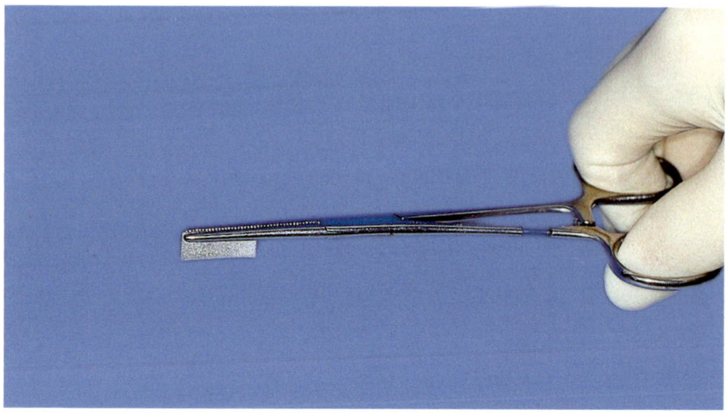

Fig 7-6m A diamond strip is clamped in the hemostat.

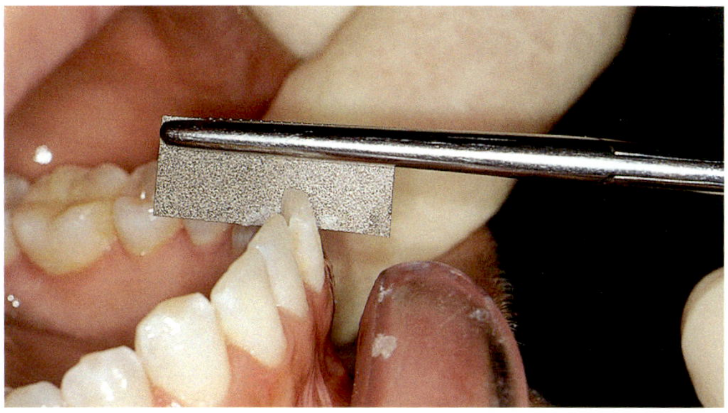

Fig 7-6n Interproximal stripping is carried out with a diamond strip.

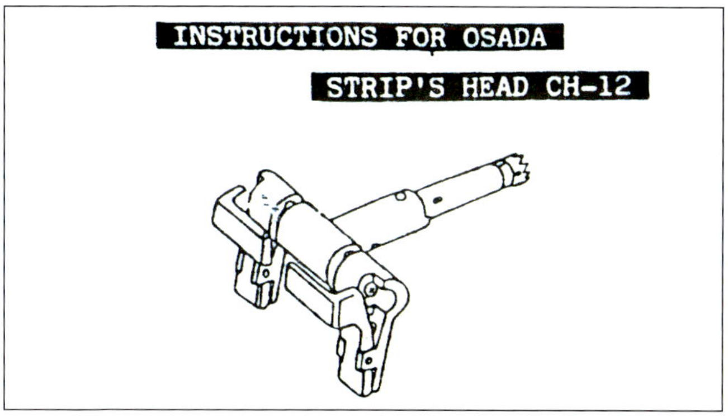

Fig 7-6o Osada Strip Head for contra-angle handpieces (no longer available).

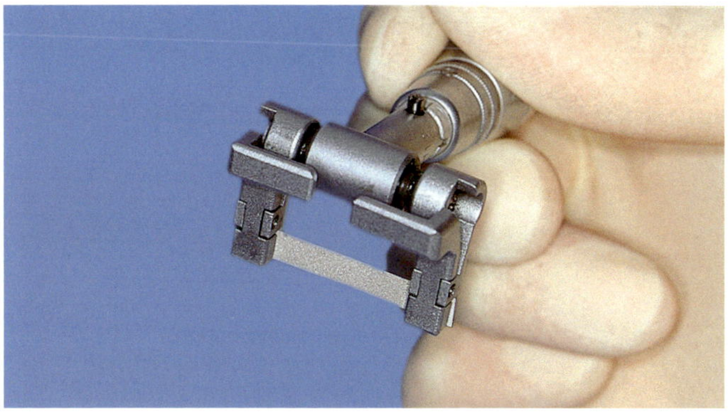

Fig 7-6p The Osada Strip Head is mounted in the handpiece.

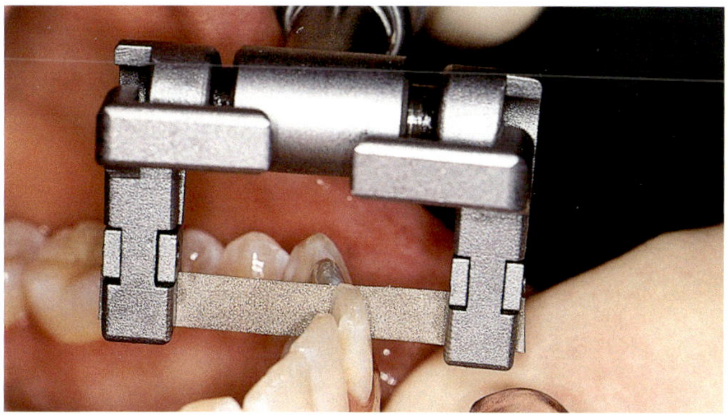

Fig 7-6q Straight stripping is performed with a diamond strip.

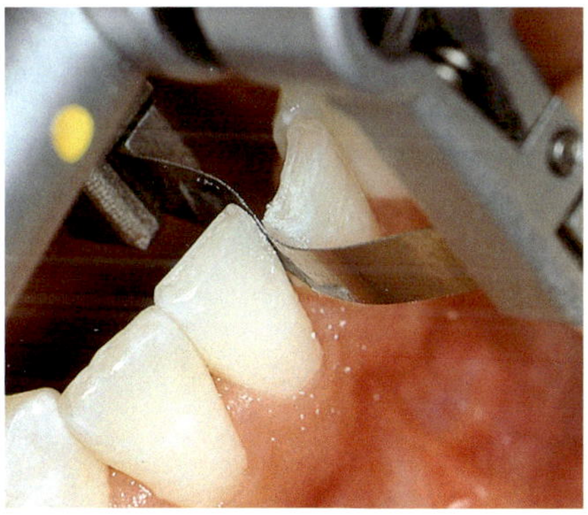

Fig 7-6r A loosely clamped strip is used for curved stripping.

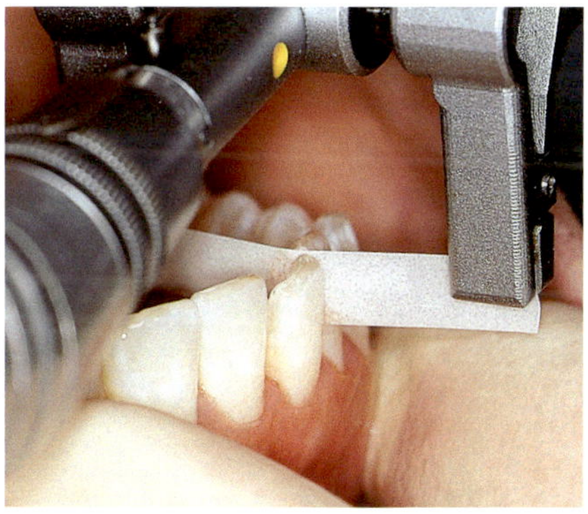

Fig 7-6s Finishing is accomplished with a polishing strip.

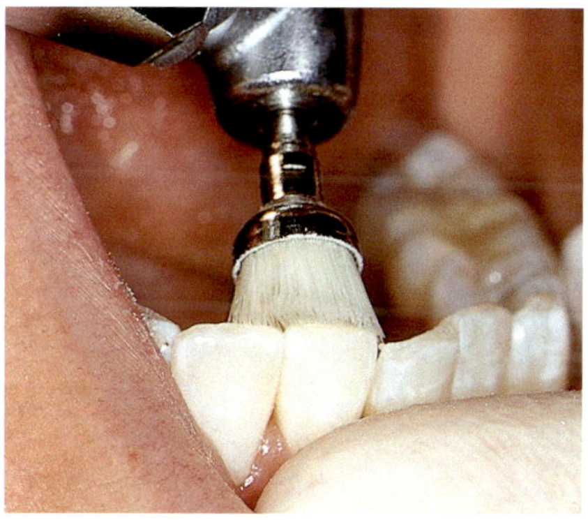

Fig 7-6t The teeth are cleaned with pumice paste.

(Fig 7-6bb). The template was carefully removed, and the position of the brackets in the patient's mouth was checked. Excess adhesive was removed (Fig 7-6cc).

The archwire (round wire) was cut with a ligature cutter, (Figs 7-6dd and 7-6ee) adapted, and inserted in the bracket slots. The bracket wings were closed with Weingart pliers, which are extremely practical, curved and pointed flat-nose pliers (Fig 7-6ff). They are the universal pliers for orthodontists, but they can also be used for many other purposes in general dentistry. Any irritating wire ends were covered with flowable resin composite (Fig 7-6gg).

The hygienist instructed the patient about the correct brushing technique. Recall appointments were scheduled for every 3 weeks to monitor the treatment progress, to repeat interproximal stripping, if necessary, or to activate the archwire (Fig 7-6hh). The treatment result shown in Fig 7-6ii was achieved after only 6 months.

At this point, the archwire with the brackets was removed. The residual adhesive was carefully removed

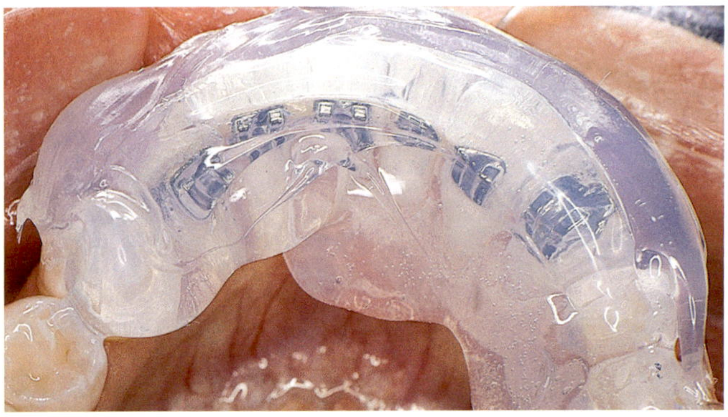

Fig 7-6u The template is tried in the patient's mouth.

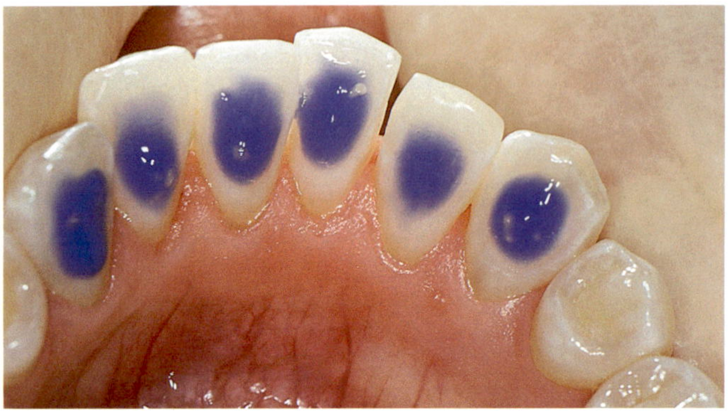

Fig 7-6v The areas where the brackets will be positioned are etched with phosphoric acid.

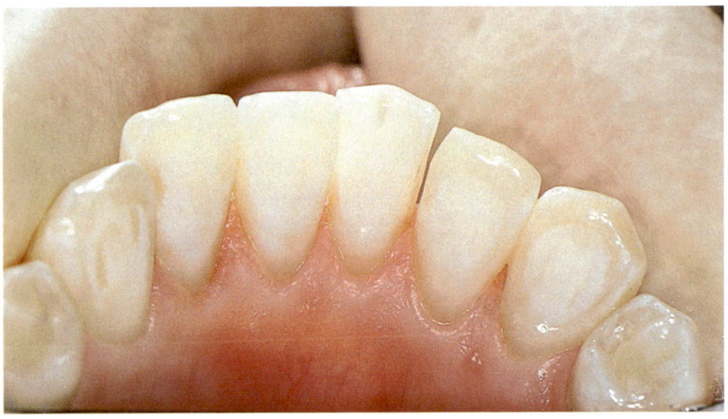

Fig 7-6w The etching pattern is examined.

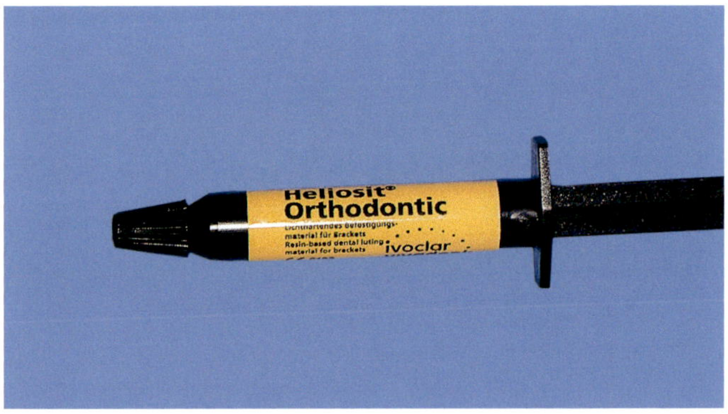

Fig 7-6x Bracket adhesive.

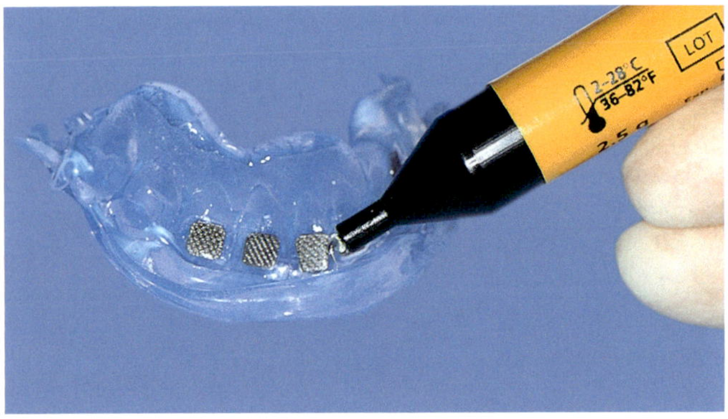

Fig 7-6y The bracket adhesive is applied sparingly.

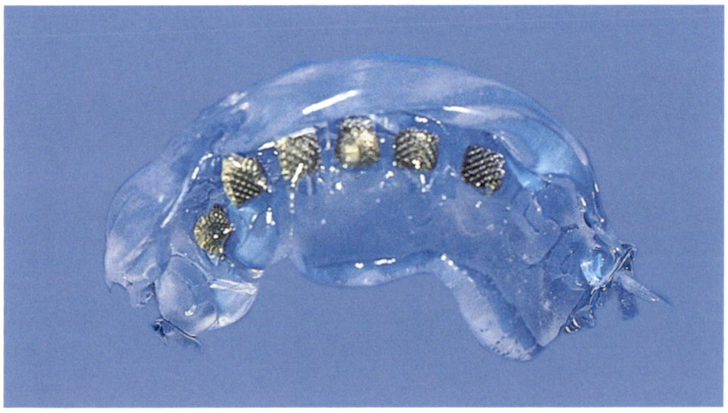

Fig 7-6z The brackets are covered with adhesive, ready for bonding.

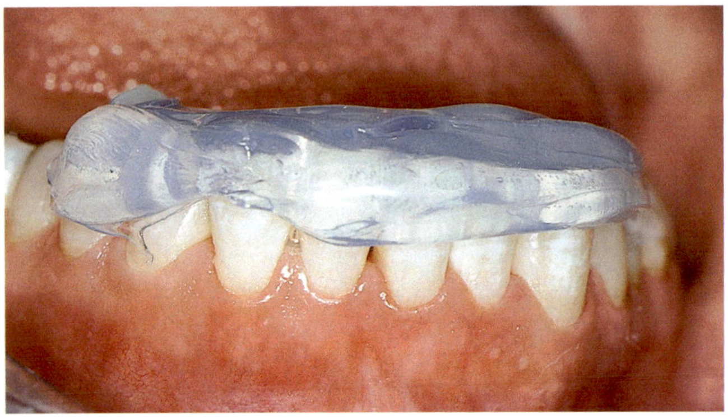

Fig 7-6aa The brackets are placed with a template.

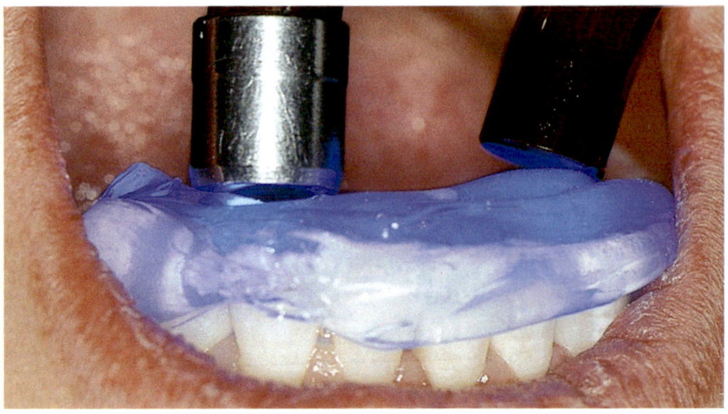

Fig 7-6bb Polymerization is accomplished with two light sources.

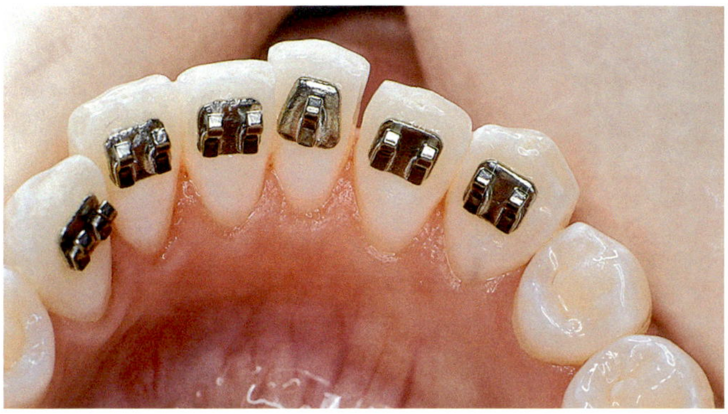

Fig 7-6cc Bonded brackets.

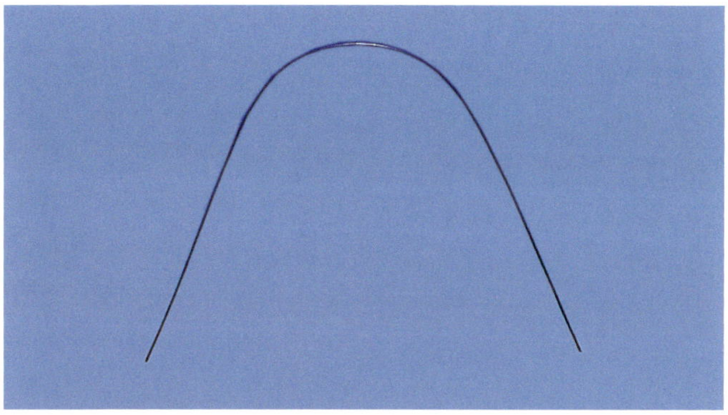

Fig 7-6dd Round memory wire.

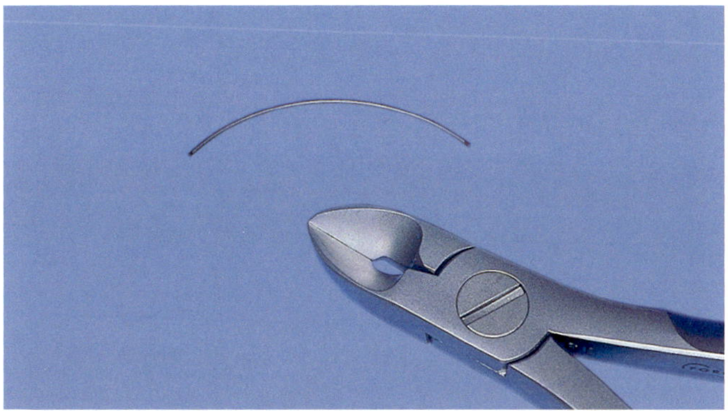

Fig 7-6ee The arch wire is cut to the exact length.

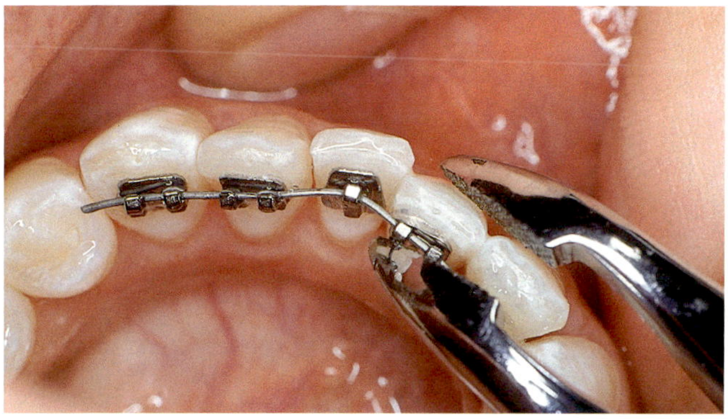

Fig 7-6ff The inserted arch wire is ligated by bending down the ends.

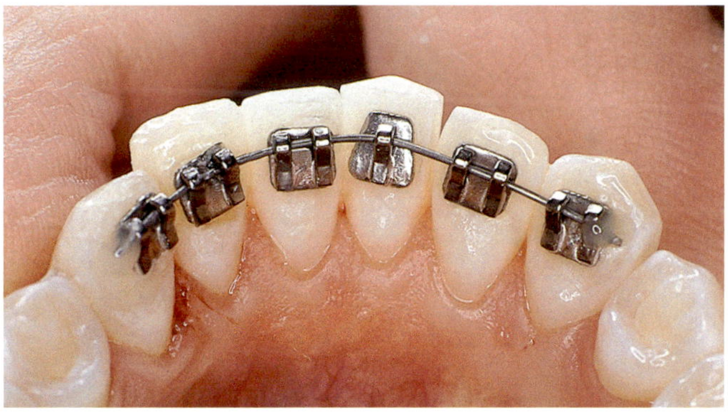

Fig 7-6gg Ligated arch wire. To protect the patient, the ends are covered with flowable resin composite.

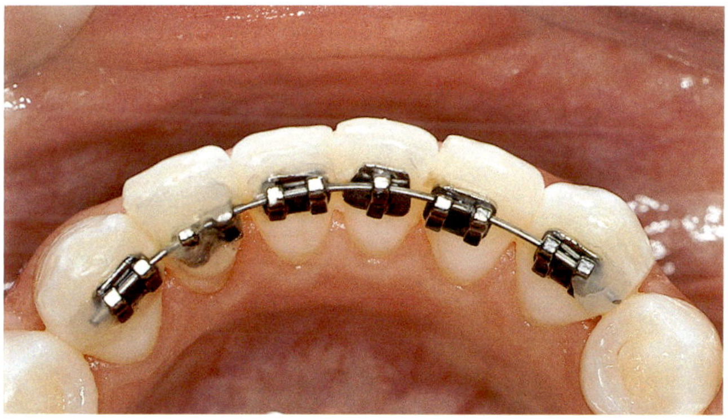

Fig 7-6hh Treatment progress.

with a semiblunt tungsten carbide spiral finishing bur. This was done using a magnifying loupe to prevent any damage to the enamel. It would be very useful if there were a bracket adhesive that changed color so that the residual adhesive could be seen more easily. The author is currently working with others to develop an adhesive with that property.

The slightly mobile teeth in the anterior mandible have a tendency to move back to their former positions and have to be retained for a period of about 1 year. For this patient, this was done with the help of flowable resin composite and with glass fibers that are already silanized and moistened with bonding agent. Wedjets were inserted in the interproximal spaces to ensure that they could be cleaned with a Proxabrush (Figs 7-6jj to 7-6nn) (see the earlier section on retention).

When the treatment was completed, the patient showed her gratitude for the outcome with a beaming smile (Fig 7-6oo and 7-6pp).

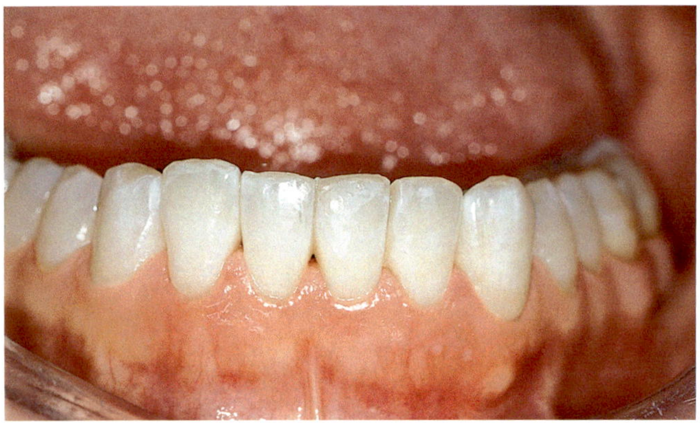

Fig 7-6ii Final result after 6 months.

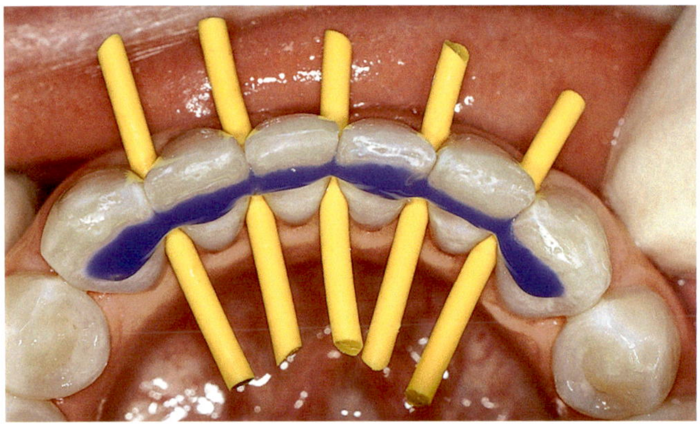

Fig 7-6jj The dentition is ready to receive the retainer; Wedjets are inserted and the lingual surfaces are etched.

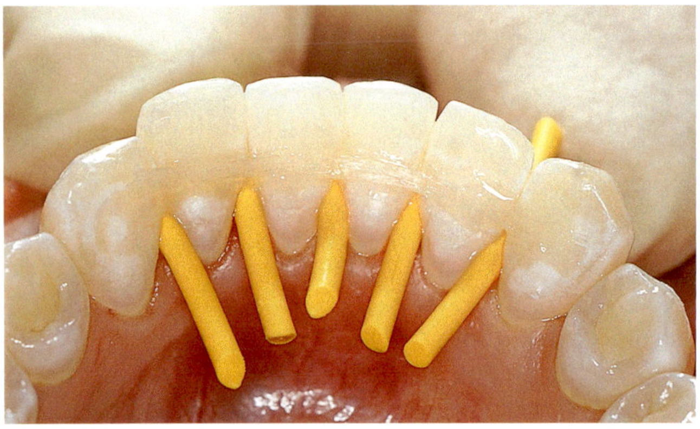

Fig 7-6kk The glass fibers are carefully adapted with flowable resin composite.

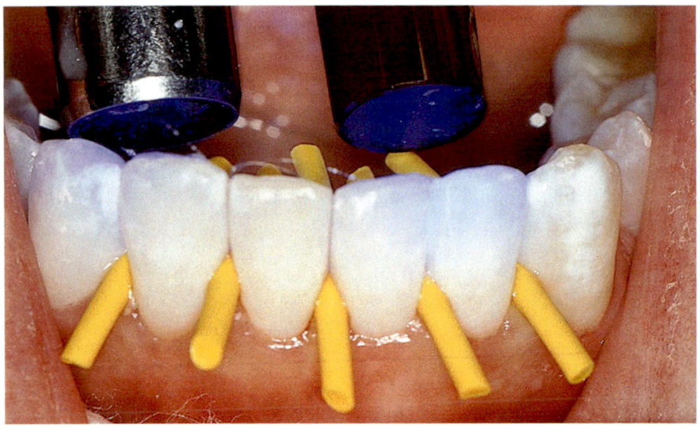

Fig 7-6ll The splint is polymerized with two light sources.

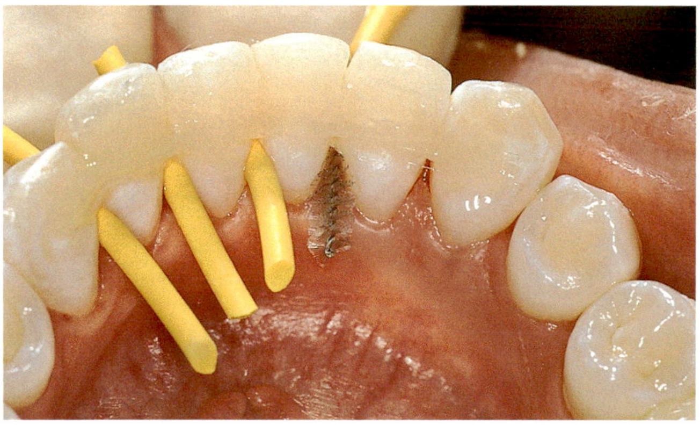

Fig 7-6mm Wedjets are used as placeholders for the Proxabrush.

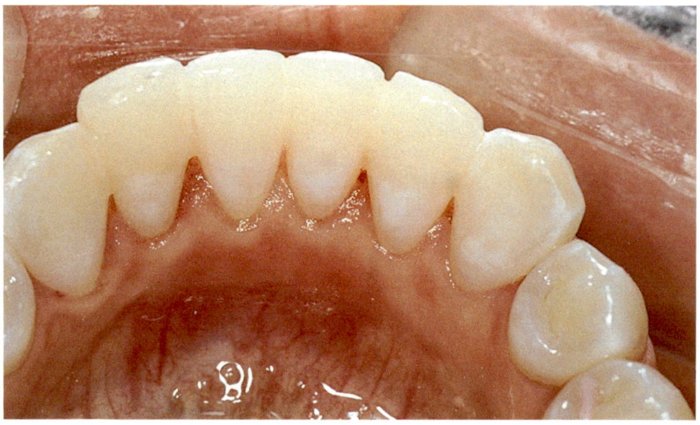

Fig 7-6nn The bonded retainer is finished.

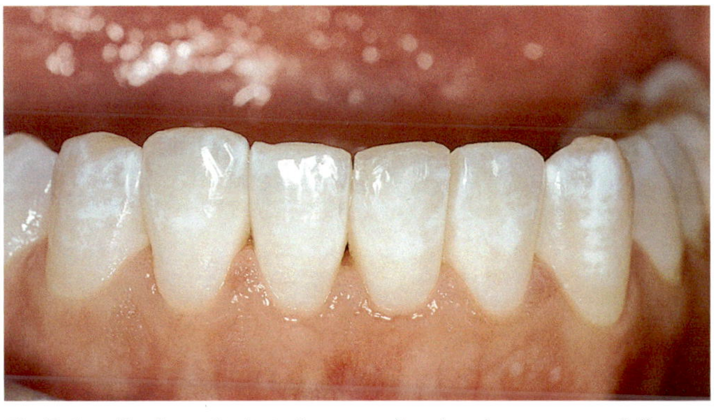

Fig 7-6oo Final result. Anterior crowding has been successfully corrected.

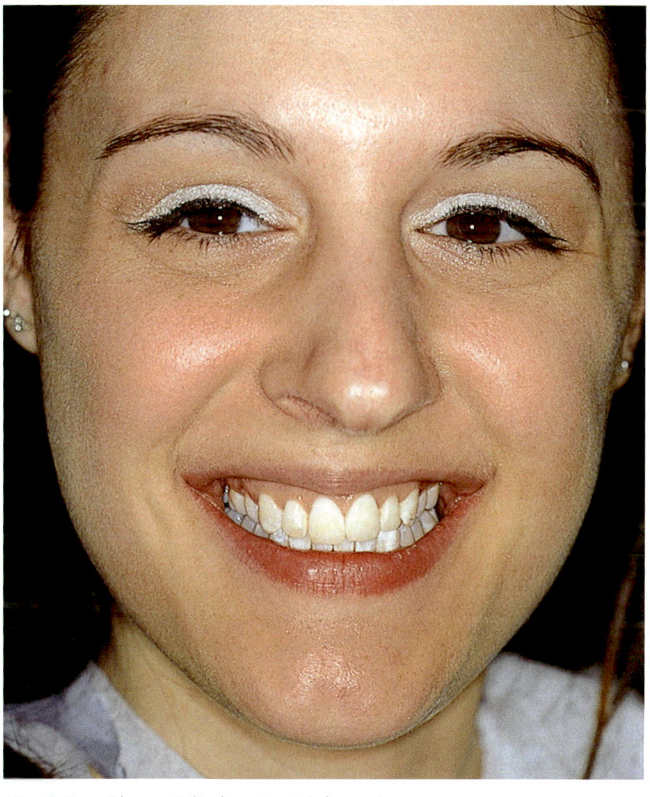

Fig 7-6pp The satisfied patient is beaming.

The author's intention in presenting this simple case was to encourage general dentists to carry out minor orthodontic treatment measures themselves. This thought is linked to the hope that orthodontists might become more open to the needs of practitioners of general dentistry. It would be beneficial to everyone for both groups to see each other as true colleagues.

Materials

Crozat appliances (specialized dental laboratories)
Lingual brackets (Forestadent)
All-purpose glue (eg, Elmer's)
Memosil transparent silicone for the template (Heraeus Kulzer)
Diamond strips (Horico)
Polishing strips (Kerr/Hawe)
Hemostat (Braun)
Osada Strip Head (no longer available; ask an orthodontist about comparable devices)
Heliosit Orthodontic bracket adhesive (Ivoclar Vivadent)
Nitinol Round Arch 0.016 mandibular round arch memory wire (3M ESPE)
Ligature cutter (Forestadent)
Weingart pliers (Forestadent)
Tetric Flow flowable resin composite (Ivoclar Vivadent)
Vectris Pontic (Ivoclar Vivadent) or other glass fibers (Stick Tech, Everstick)
Wedjets rubber cord (Coltène Whaledent)
Proxabrushes (Sunstar Butler)

8

Ergonomics

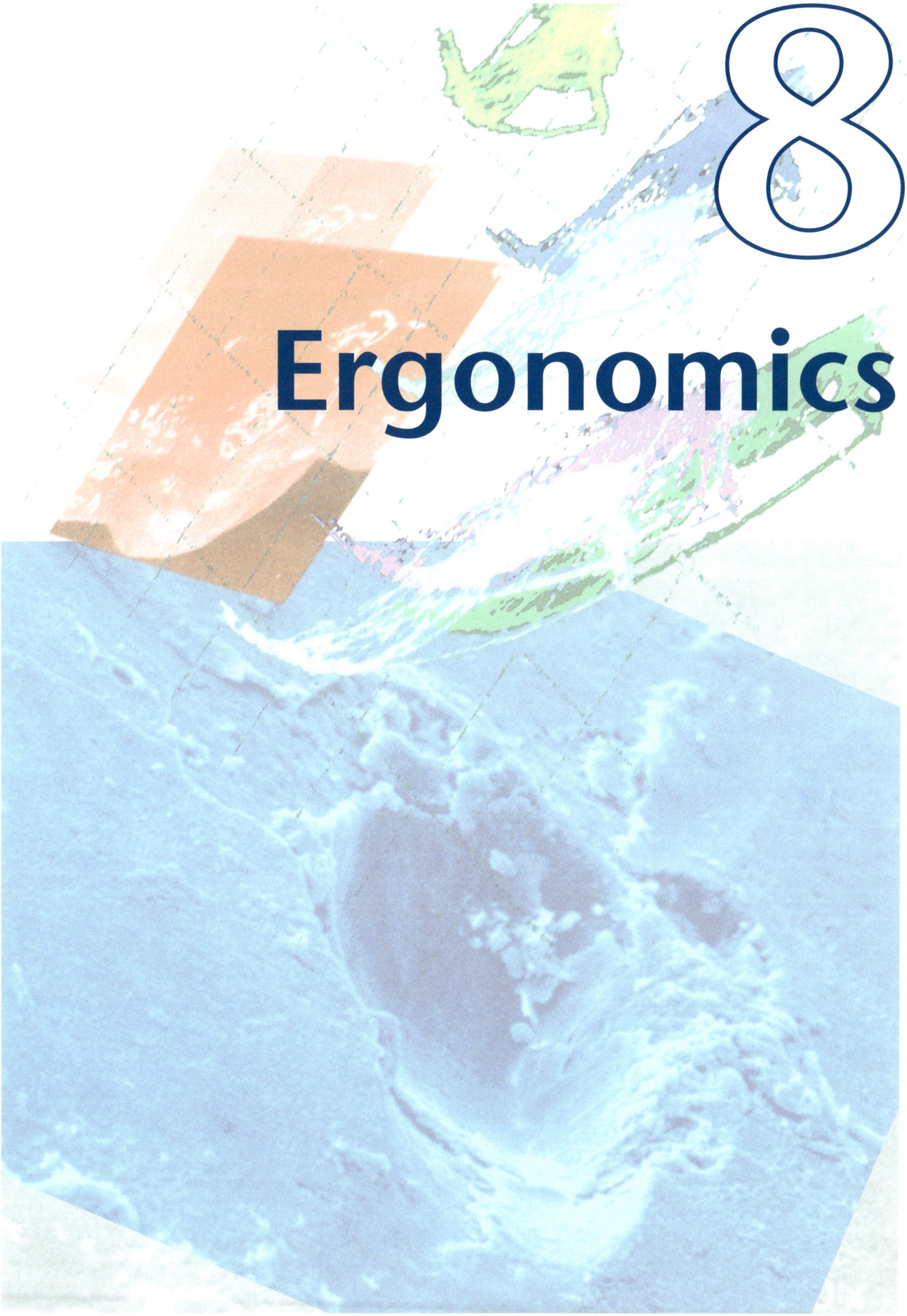

8

Dental Workspace

Dental Technique

Dental Workspace

Common problem: What makes dentists sick?

In their professional lives, dentists have to withstand high amounts of physical strain because of the intense concentration and stress they experience as well as the physical exertion they face every day (Fig 8-1). Hour after hour of sitting in unnatural positions and subjecting the muscles to isometric tension has a negative effect on the health of dental professionals. Many dentists experience such serious orthopedic problems in the early years of their careers that they have to endure pain, take medication, or perform physical therapy if they want to do their work.

In the mid-1960s, people first began advocating ergonomically healthy habits and workplaces for dentists. In Germany, Schön[1] (Fig 8-2), Kimmel,[2] Hilger,[3] and Neuhauser were the first proponents of ergonomics as a means of streamlining dentists' work and protecting their health. That was the time at which more and more dentists switched from working while standing over the seated patient to a more orthopedically friendly approach in which the dental team worked in a seated position around a reclining patient. Dentists' workplaces were redesigned and built to meet these needs as optimally as possible. At that time, this idea was revolutionary.

In the meantime, however, many of these ergonomic standards and demands have fallen by the wayside, while the layout of today's chairside station is most strongly influenced by marketing and esthetic appeal. It is difficult to detect the influence of any ergonomic principles. As a result, once again, dentists' offices are full of unnaturally crooked and uncomfortable practitioners and assistants who complain of pain and suffer health risks. These professionals believe that pursuing their work is making them age too quickly.

Proven solution: Back to the roots–Ergonomics

The core concept of physiologically healthy work was defined more than 30 years ago: four-handed dentistry practiced on a patient in a reclining position (Fig 8-3). When dentists select equipment for their offices, they should focus on this idea and take ergonomic and health considerations into account. Dentists should persuade the industry to pay more attention to their health when products are being developed. The 35 years or so of the professional life of a dentist should be viewed as a marathon that should be run in the best of health.

A dentist's workplace consists of the following components: the patient's chair with a cuspidor and shelf; the dental unit; stools for the dentist and assistant; the assistant's unit; including evacuation equipment; the tray

Fig 8-1 *(left)* What makes dentists sick? (Clipping of a cover page from *ZM* magazine.)

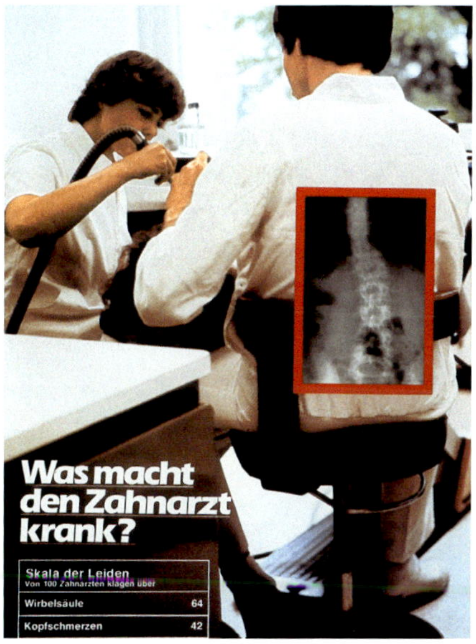

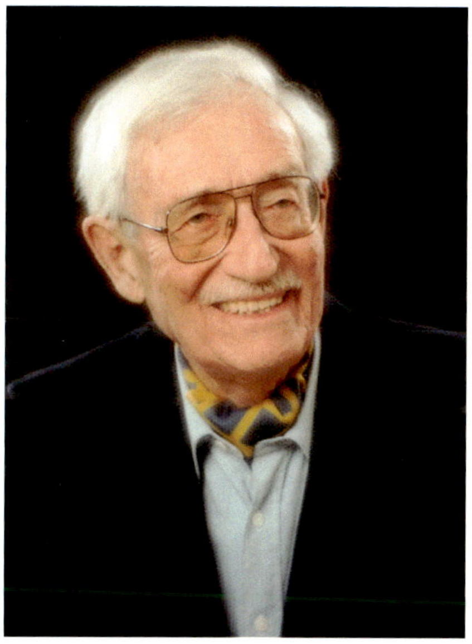

Fig 8-2 *(right)* Professor Fritz Schön, Bad Reichenhall, Germany.

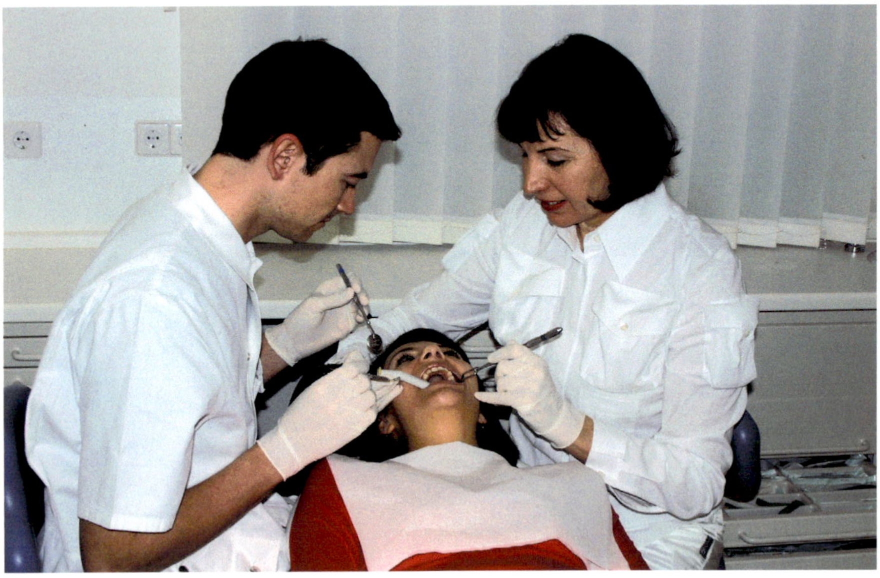

Fig 8-3 Four-handed dentistry, practiced on a patient in a lying position.

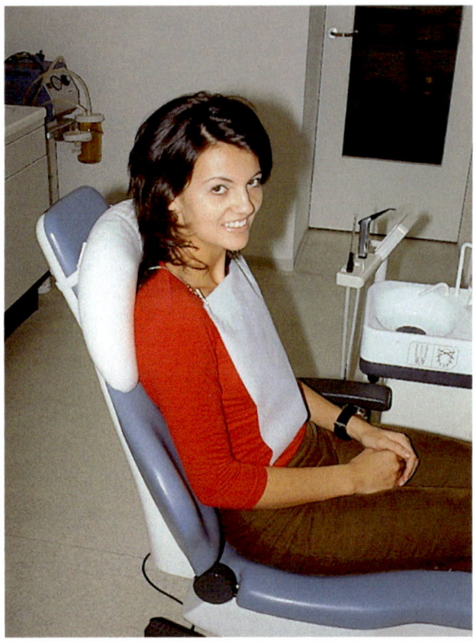

Fig 8-4a Patient chair.

table; the operating light; the dentist's zones (D1 and D2) on cabinets with the appropriate drawers; and the assistant's zones (A1 and A2) on cabinets with the appropriate drawers.

Patient's chair

The patient's chair should be comfortable, and the patient's body should be as relaxed as possible wherever it touches the chair (Fig 8-4a). The chair should permit a variety of sitting and lying positions. It must have programmable settings as well as hand and foot switches to adjust the various positions.

The head rest should be comfortable for the patient and firmly securable during treatment, especially in cases of longer sessions. Most of the head rests currently available are extremely uncomfortable (Fig 8-4b). The people who design dental equipment ought to undergo treatment while sitting on their own creations so they can see what they are inflicting on patients. The neck and shoulder roll designed by Schön can still be highly recommended (Fig 8-4c), because it supports both the neck and the shoulders. There are also other new kinds of cushions which support the head comfortably. If there is an armrest, it ought to be opposite the practitioner's side so that the practitioner can move in closer with the stool, as needed (Fig 8-4d). Foot rests, which were once standard equipment and can still be found here and there, are obsolete in today's equipment; with the much gentler methods used today, patients no longer need to "dig in" with their feet for additional support.

A cuspidor attached to the chair within reach of the patient allows the patient to rinse easily. Most offices feature basins with disposable cups that are filled with cold water. In the author's opinion, however, a proper glass with fresh water is more in keeping with the style of a good dentist's office (Fig 8-5). A fresh paper towel should always be placed next to this glass. There should also be a space for the patient's eyeglasses. Underneath the cuspidor, there should also be a hook so that patients can hang up their bags or purses within easy reach (Fig 8-6).

Dentist's unit

Ergonomically speaking, the best approach is the split unit, which creates separate working areas for the practitioner and the assistant (Fig 8-7). The dentist's side houses the turbines and the micromotors with the handpieces. There are different design concepts; in the author's opinion, the most recommendable one is the kind with the hanging tubes. The following sequence should be set up from left to right (Fig 8-8):

1. Turbine with a light
2. High-speed contra-angle handpiece with a light
3. Low-speed/polishing contra-angle or straight handpiece (as needed) with a light
4. Air/water syringe,

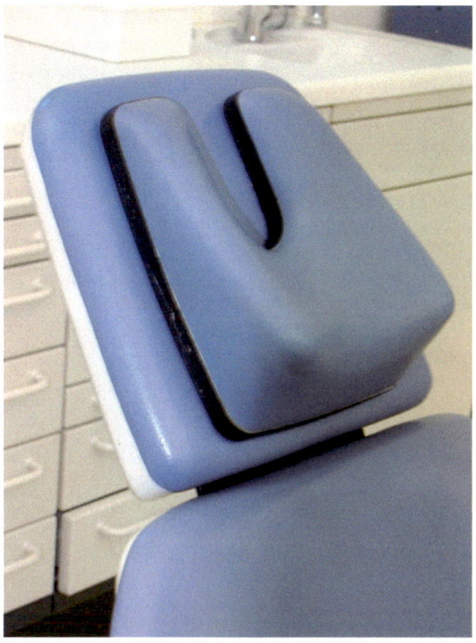

Fig 8-4b Standard neck rest.

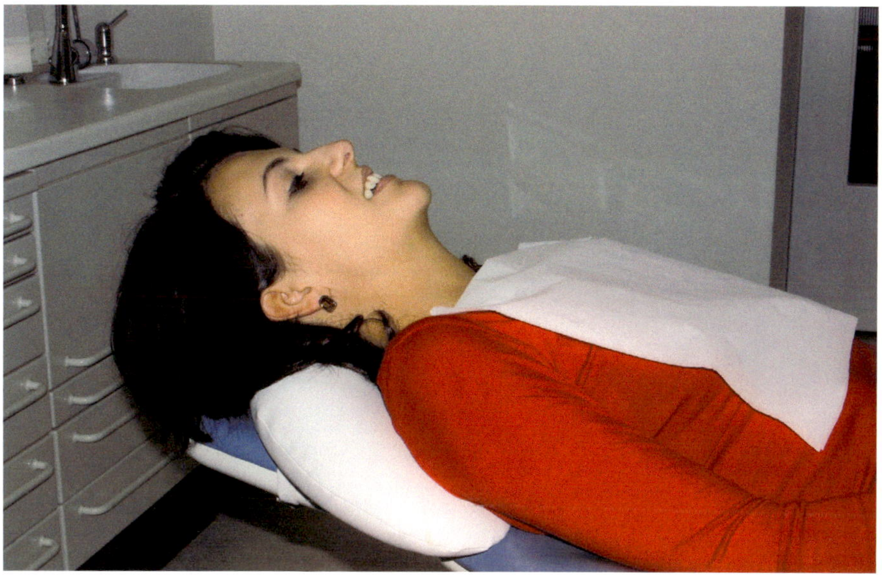

Fig 8-4c Shoulder and neck rest designed by Schön.

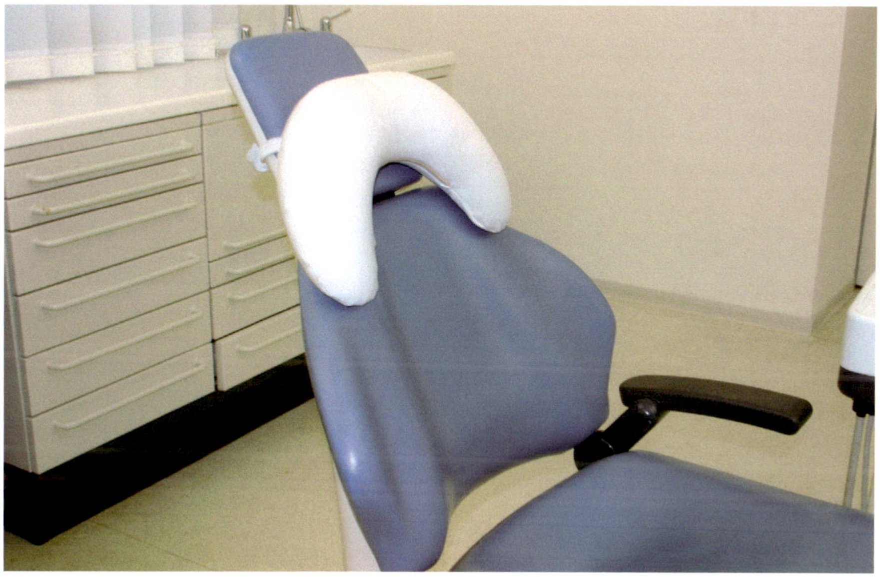

Fig 8-4d Arm rest on the left side only.

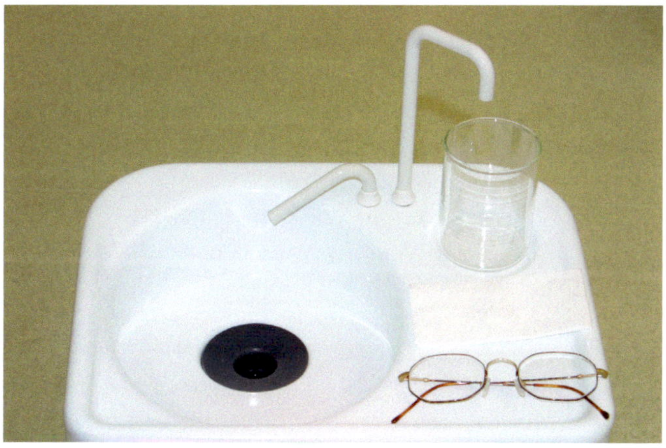

Fig 8-5 Cuspidor for rinsing, shown with tissues, a drinking glass, and a space for eyeglasses.

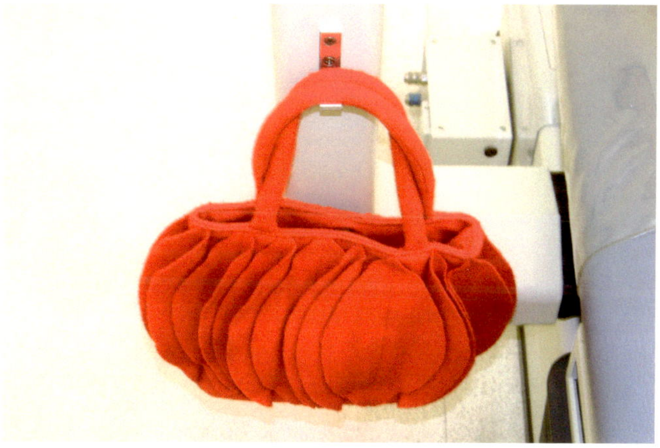

Fig 8-6 Hook for keeping the patient's bag or purse within reach.

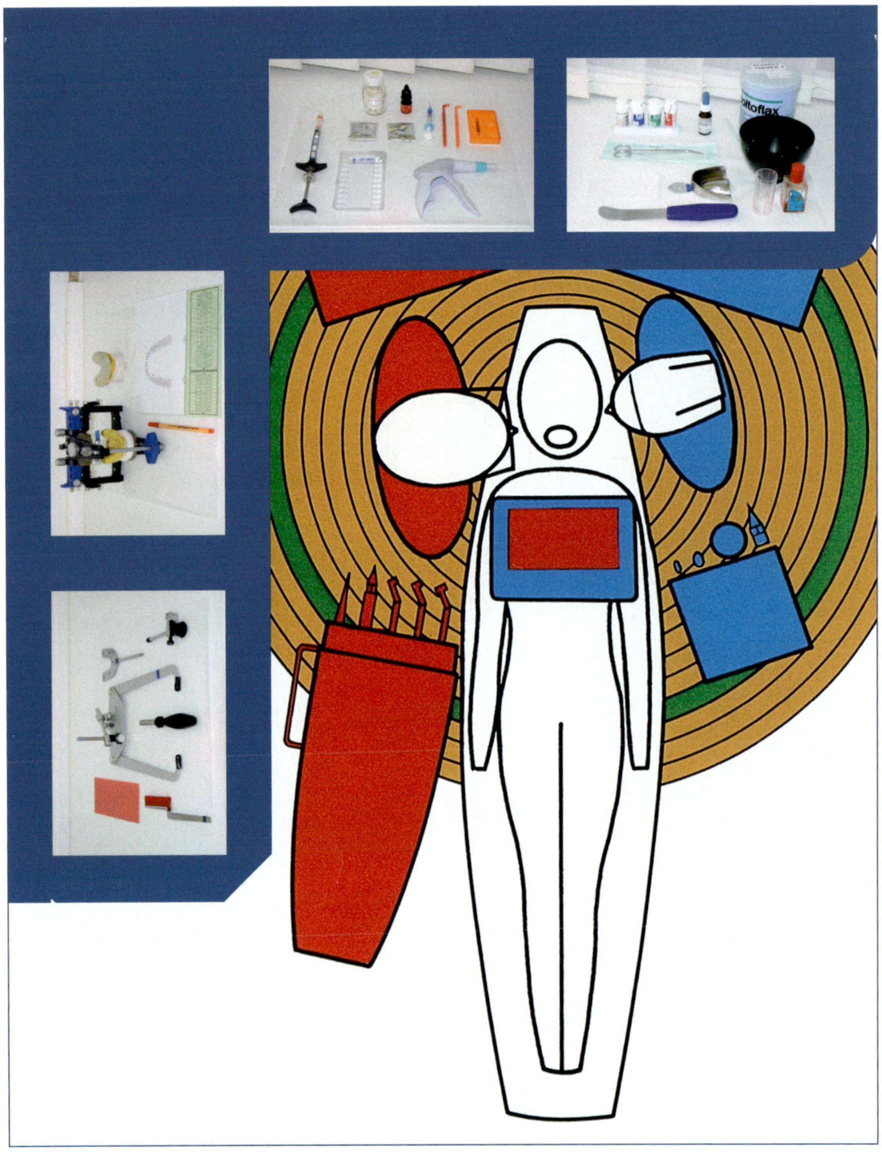

Fig 8-7 Split-unit concept. *(red)* Dental practitioner's zones; *(blue)* dental assistant's zones.

5. Multipurpose piezo system for removing calculus, inserting inlays, endodontic treatment, etc
6. Electrosurgery device
7. Buttons for adjusting the chair backward and forward, speed, etc

Above this unit, there should be a space to put preparation kits and similar tools. The author recommends a magnetic stand for placement of diamonds, finishers, and so on, and a basin for the rotary instruments that are not needed at the moment. This shelf for the dental unit is located in the area for the right hand.

The turbine and the micromotors are controlled via a foot pedal (speed, left/right, and on/off switch for water spray). Many foot pedals are too high and cannot be reached properly if they are put under the chair when the dentist sits. Most practitioners push the foot pedal off to the right, which makes them have to stretch out their right leg in a thoroughly unnatural position, creating strain (Fig 8-9). The ideal solution was an older model, which was flat and let the clinician work while both feet were under the chair; unfortunately, this model is no longer available (Fig 8-10).

Today, foot pedals serve as multipurpose switches, and they are usually too high and cannot be used comfortably (Fig 8-11). Dentists must be careful if different makes or models of pedals are present in the office, because this can often lead to unintentional and surprising settings.

No matter what is used, a separate control unit for adjusting the patient's chair is strongly recommended, so that precise adjustments can be made during treatment if necessary (Fig 8-12).

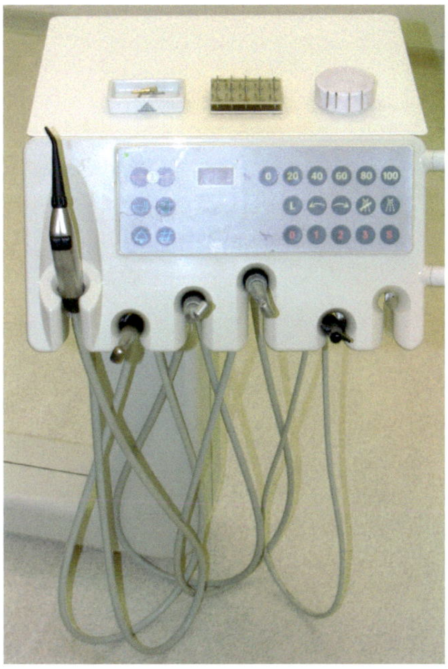

Fig 8-8 Dentist's unit.

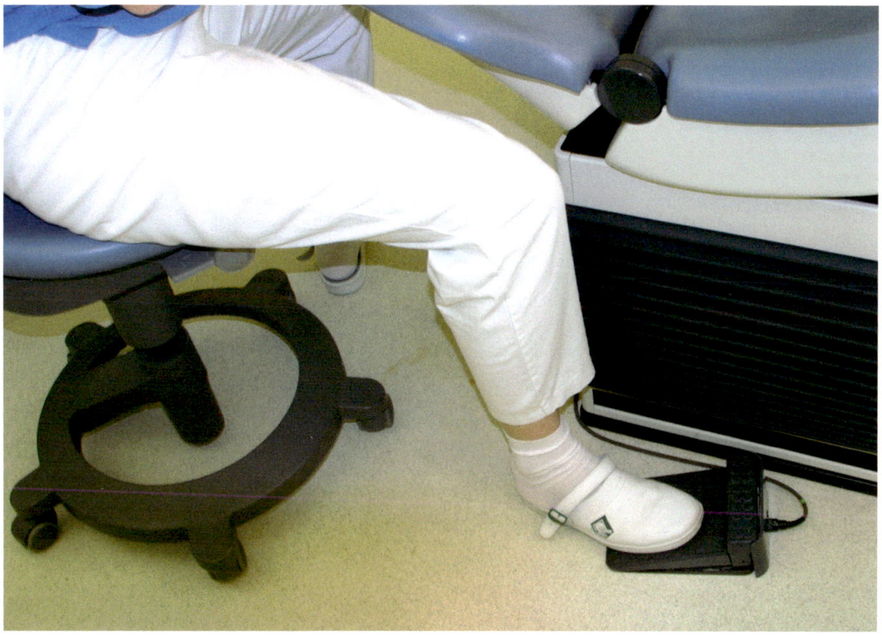

Fig 8-9 Stretching the right leg unnaturally to reach the foot pedal.

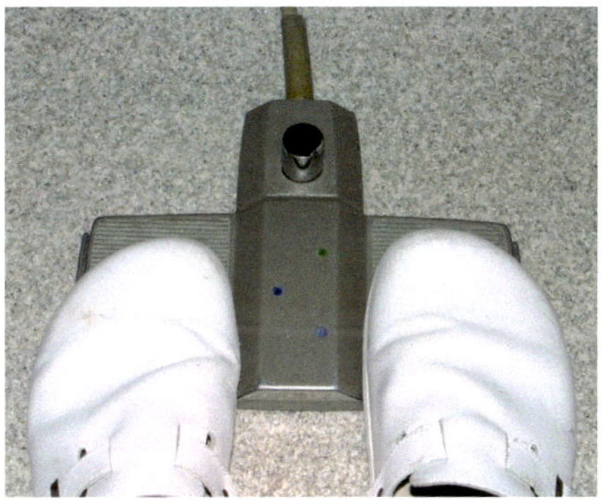

Fig 8-10 Older model of a flat foot pedal, which could be operated with both feet.

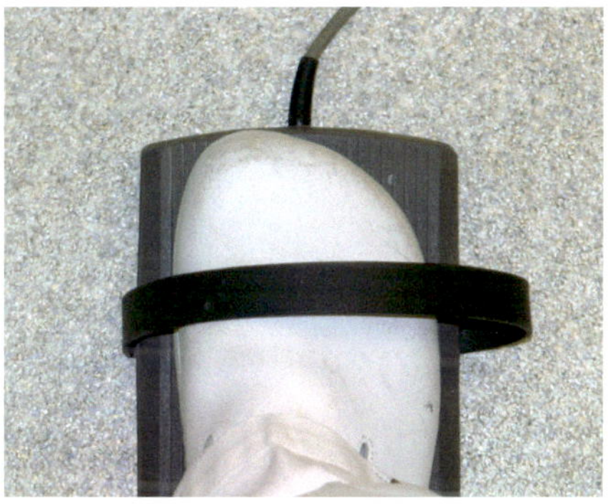

Fig 8-11 Modern multifunction foot pedal.

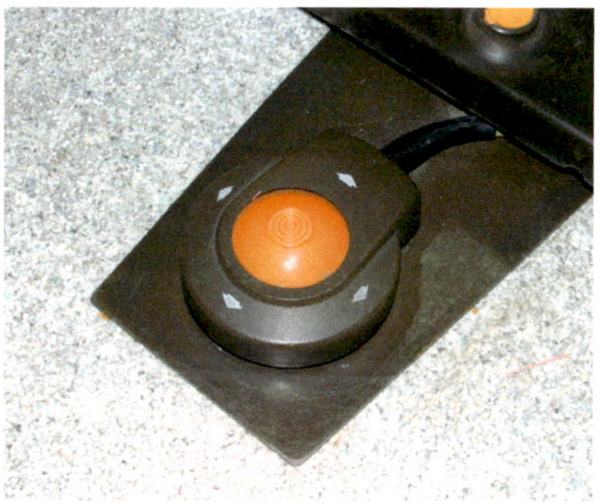

Fig 8-12 Multidirectional ball touchpad for hands-free adjustment of the chair.

Stools

Many kinds of different five-castered stools allow the members of the dental team to sit upright and securely. In terms of orthopedic and dental needs, the dentist may also wish to consider saddle stools and knee stools.

Assistant's unit

In most dental units, the assistant's unit is located on the left side of the chair. It consists of the following: evacuation equipment, air/water syringe, saliva ejector, and a control panel (Figs 8-13 and 8-15).

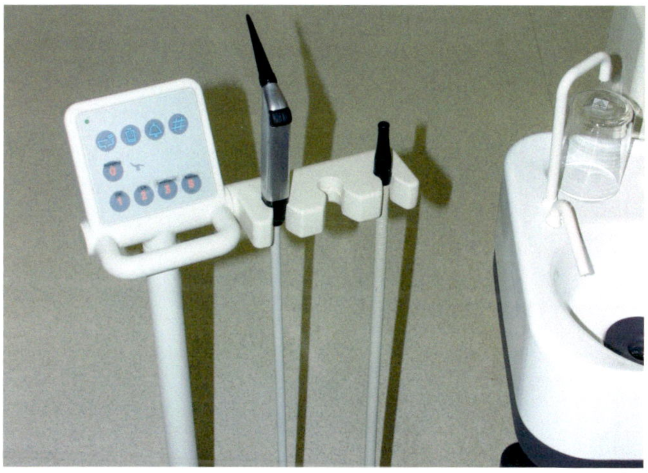

Fig 8-13 Assistant's unit

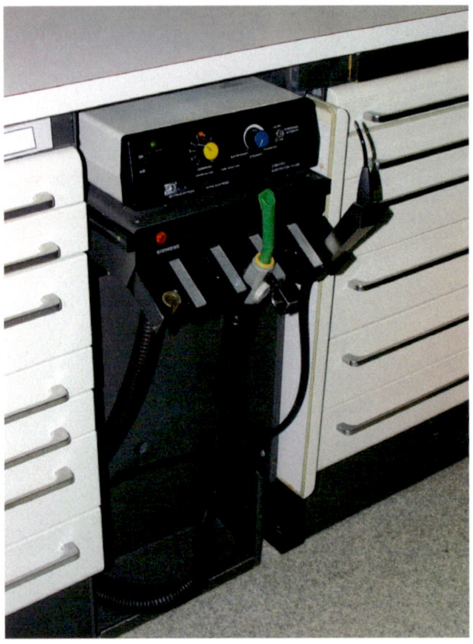

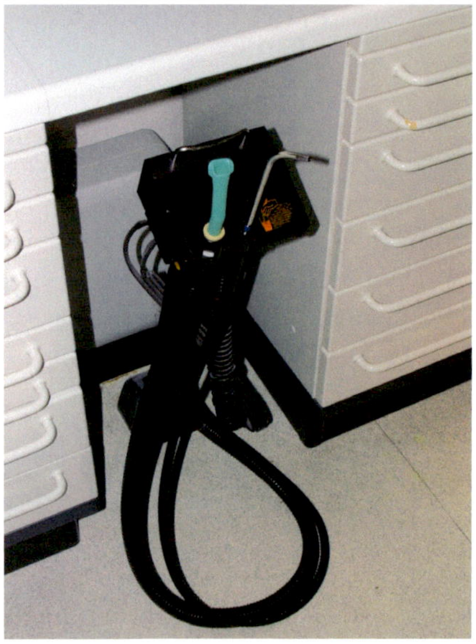

Fig 8-14 *(left)* Cabinet suction and evacuation module (Sironette E).

Fig 8-15 *(right)* Cabinet suction and evacuation module (Dürr).

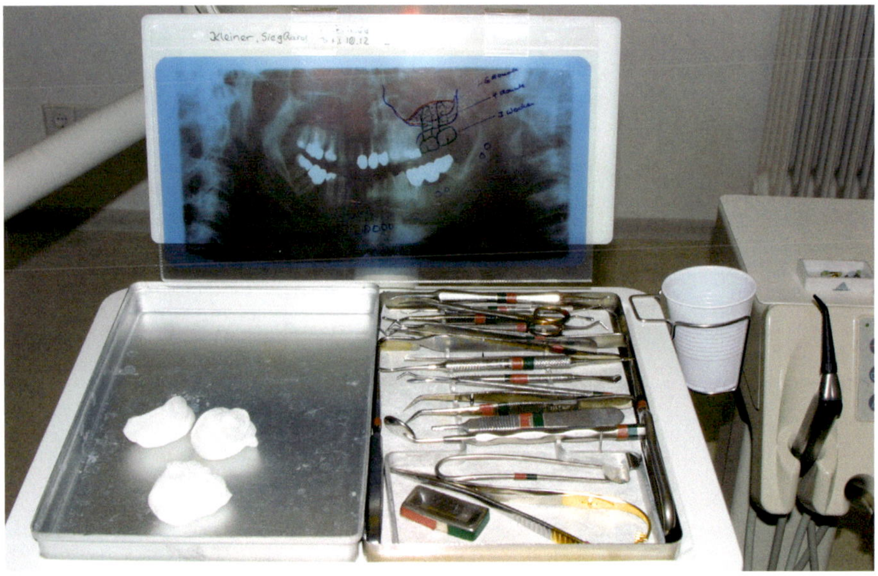

Fig 8-16 Tray table with a monitor and the open tray.

In the approach to four-handed dentistry described in the next section, a cabinet suction and evacuation module is the best way of working with a direct view of the patient. This keeps things equidistant to the patient on both the left and right.

Cabinet suction and evacuation modules are only available from a very few manufacturers for a very high price, unfortunately.

Tray table

The central working area should be a tray table that can swing out over the patient. An open tray should fit perfectly on top of the tray table (Fig 8-16).

The author also recommends a vertically mounted radiograph viewer for panoramic radiographs. Newer models often feature a monitor and an intraoral camera so that the dentist can show the patient the findings directly. This proves to be especially useful when the monitor is bright enough to serve as a radiograph viewer as well. The split unit was originally designed in such a way that the tray table could be lowered as far as the dentist wanted, which is usually not possible with currently available units; nowadays, the dentist has to work while sitting next to the supine patient and more or less has to stand up to reach the tray table.

The tray table is in the area the dentist can access by reaching forward with the right hand without turning his or her body.

Operating light

The operating light should be as bright as daylight and be dimmable (Fig 8-17). It should be programmable to certain lux settings so that various procedures can be done under optimal lighting conditions without having to spend time adjusting the light. These settings include examination, color selection colors, restoration with light-curing materials, grinding and contouring, and transillumination.

Most of today's setups do not allow the dentist to move the light close enough to be able to illuminate the inside of the patient's mouth.

Working areas in the split-unit concept

In the split-unit concept, everything is within easy reach of the dentist and the assistant (Figs 8-18a and 8-18b). The working areas for the dentist and the assistant are located on top of cabinets with designated drawers and can be classified as follows (Figs 8-19a to 8-19d):

1. D1 is located at the patient's head. It is the working area for the instruments, and the practitioner can reach it with the left hand without having to turn.
2. D2 is located behind the practitioner on the right and is accessible by reaching to the left with the left hand.
3. A1, at the right of the patient's head next to the cabinet suction and evacuation module, is the most important working area for the assistant and can be reached with the assistant's right hand without turning the body. The curing lights and mixing equipment are usually found here; there is a pull-out surface for writing or using a keyboard.
4. A2 is to the right of A1 and serves as an additional area for keeping instruments within reach.

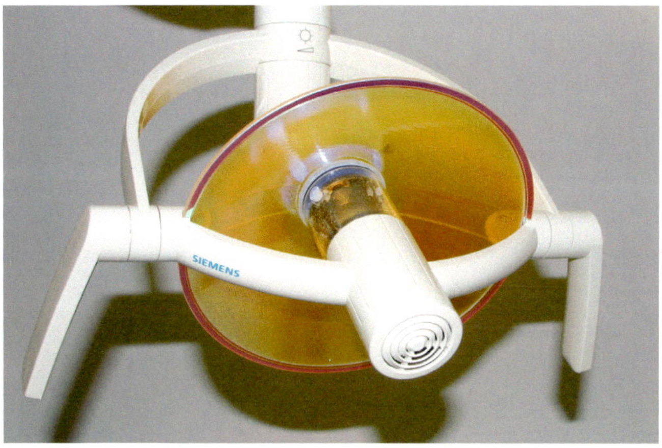

Fig 8-17 Operating light.

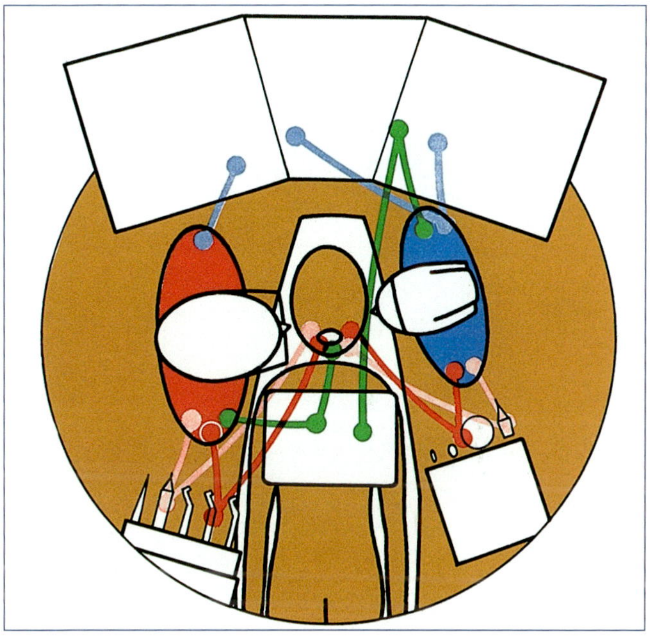

Fig 8-18a Everything is in easy reach with the split-unit concept.

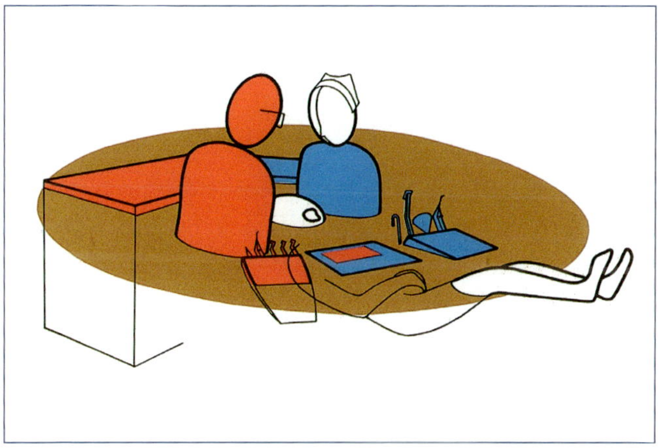

Fig 8-18b All instruments are on one level.

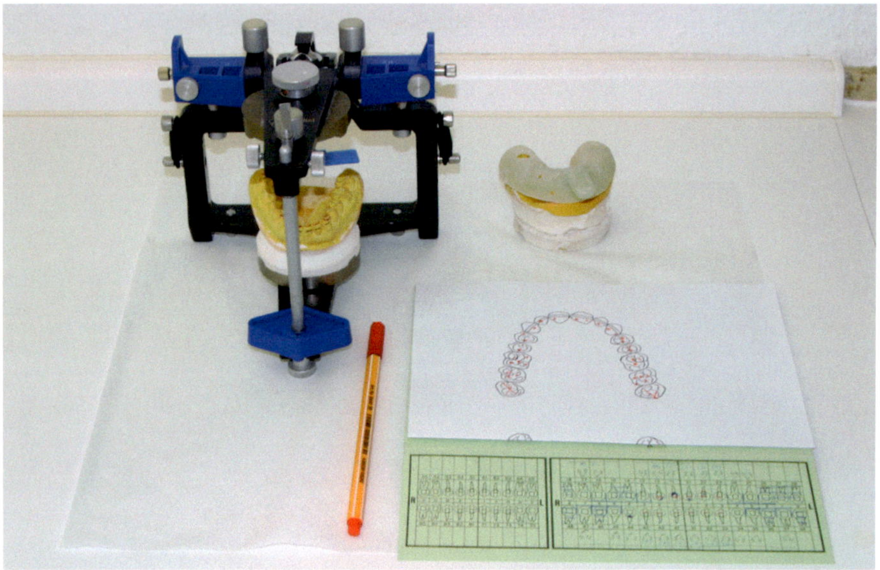

Fig 8-19a Working area D1.

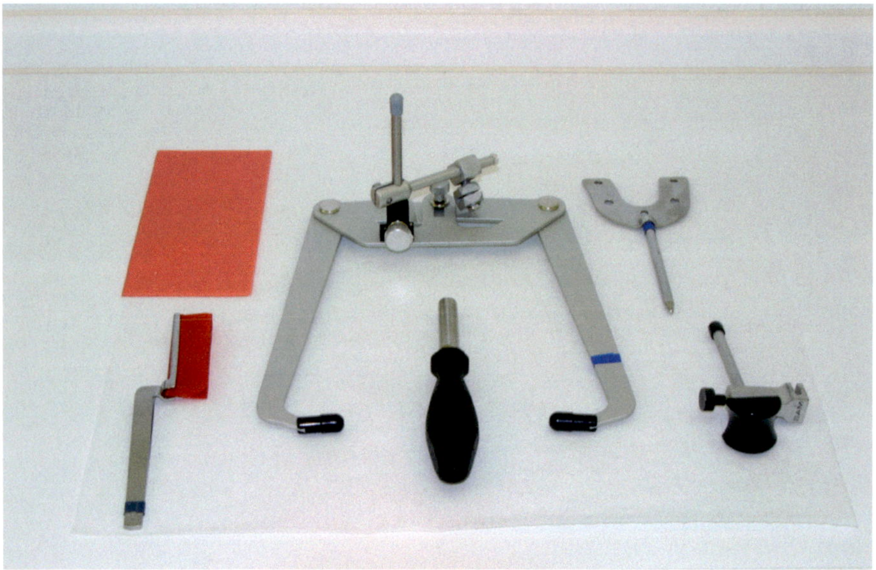

Fig 8-19b Working area D2.

Goal of workspace design

When the dentist's workspace is designed as discussed here, all of the equipment needed will be on one level and within reach, the patient will lie in a comfortable position, both the dentist and the assistant will sit upright comfortably, and the lighting will be good. Then, if a bit of pleasant background music is added and the atmosphere between the patient and the team is good, conditions will be right for successful and relaxed treatment. Dentists must realize that they are selling both personal attention and dental care.

A call to the dental industry

It would be outstanding if the dental industry would pay greater attention to the principles of ergonomics, physiology, and proper posture. The spines of many thousands of dentists and assistants would thank them for it. The author would be willing to contribute input, as would many colleagues who are active in the field of workspace design.

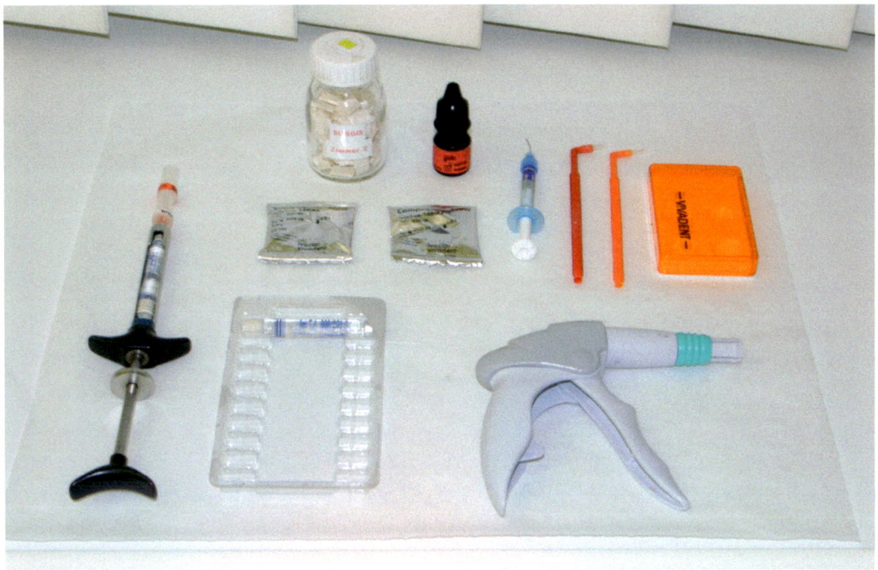

Fig 8-19c Working area A1.

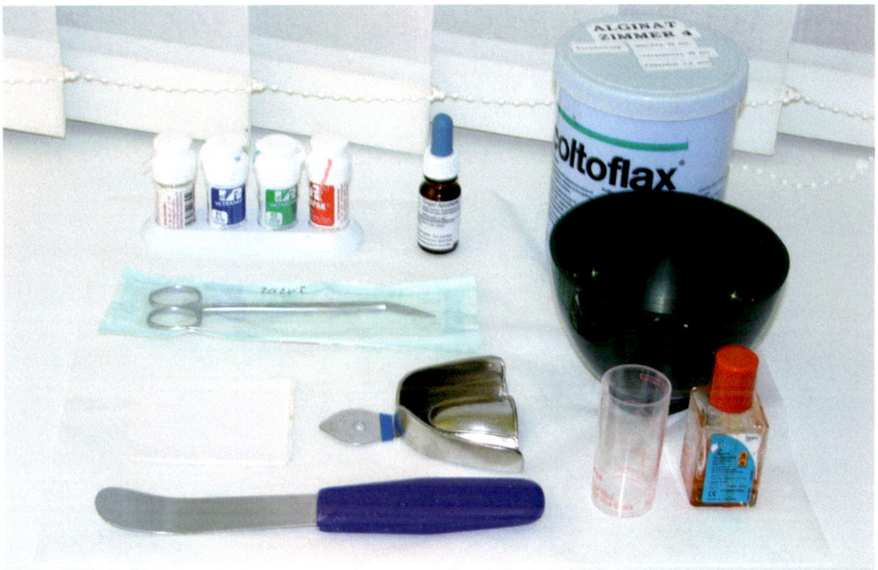

Fig 8-19d Working area A2.

Materials

Unfortunately, this book cannot cover all of the dental units and systems on the market. The author can only report on his own experiences in the world of dentistry, but it is always beneficial to be approachable and open minded about different kinds of information and technology. The following is a list of the units and instruments the author uses:

Siemens Sironette/Sirotesse (Sirona)
Siemens M1 dental unit (Sirona)
Sirona C2 (Sirona)
Neck and shoulder rest designed by Schön (Henry Schein)
Head rest (Böse Dental)
Cabinet suction and evacuation module (Dürr)
Drinking glasses for the patient (eg, Becht)
Hook for purses (available at tool stores; self-installed)
Shelf for glasses (available in automotive supply stores)

Dental Technique

Working position of the dental team

The dentist and the assistant arrange their work flow based on the principles of four-handed dentistry with a direct view of the patient in a reclining position. The concept used in the author's office is the split unit. The dentist's and assistant's working spaces are divided into halves following the concept designed by Kimmel et al.[2] Other concepts are certainly worthy of close consideration, but this is the one that the author has found to be most successful. Within arm's reach, the tray table is located in front of the patient; the dentist's unit is to the patient's right; the assistant's unit and evacuation unit are near the patient's head, and zones D1, D2, A1, and A2 are on the countertops (Figs 8-20a and 8-20b).

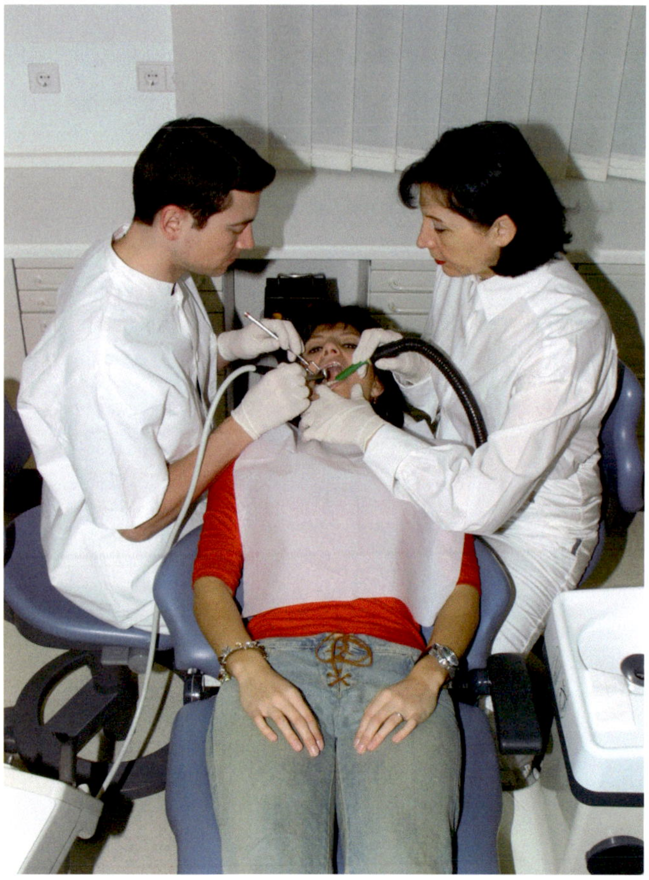

Fig 8-20a Dental team with the patient.

The members of the dental team all wear pants instead of skirts so that they are not impeded in their motion if they need to move in toward the patient's head (Fig 8-20c). The dentist's chair is positioned at a height that will allow the upper and lower leg to form an angle of 105 degrees whenever possible (Fig 8-20d). The assistant should sit somewhat higher, because he or she often has to look down into the patient's mouth from above at an angle. This allows the assistant a larger sitting angle. These factors, however, depend on the bodily proportions of the members of the team. The members of the team have to test their sitting positions so that they can set these positions and keep them. The foot pedal with touchpad should be pushed under the chair near the patient's head so that it can be accessed easily while the dentist sits in an upright position. The dentist's foot can rest comfortably on the lower ring of the chair (Fig 8-20e).

The working spaces of the dental team are divided into clock segments. The patient's head is at 12 o'clock, the dentist is at 9 o'clock, and the assistant is at 3 o'clock. This should be the starting position when treatment begins. In the course of individual treatments of different areas of the arch, the dentist may have to move between 9 and 12 o'clock, and the assistant may have to vary between 1 and 3 o'clock (Fig 8-20f).

Position of the patient

The patient begins by sitting down and is then brought into the appropriate position, depending on whether treatment involves the maxilla or mandible. If the dentist is working on the mandible, the patient's eyes and toes are at the same level (Fig 8-21a); if treatment involves the maxillary arch, the patient's head is stretched via a neck rest and leaned back as far as possible (Fig 8-21b). This flat and horizontal position is important for two reasons: it lets the dentist work with a direct view, and it prevents the patient's throat from closing and thus reduces the patient's risk of choking or aspirating foreign matter. Any position under 45 degrees poses the immediate threat of choking or aspirating.

The dentist should perform a water test once to experience this phenomenon. Water is carefully poured in the

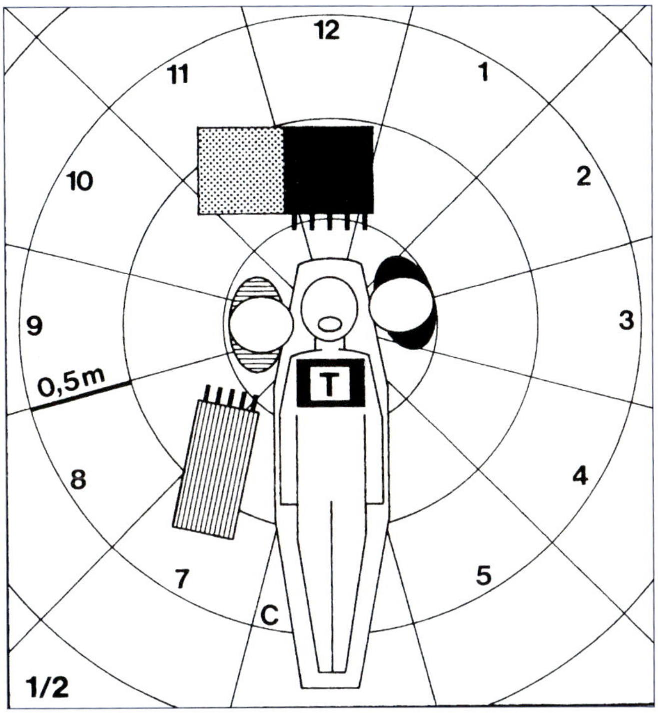

Fig 8-20b Treatment concept depicted as a clock. (From Hilger.[3] Reprinted with permission.)

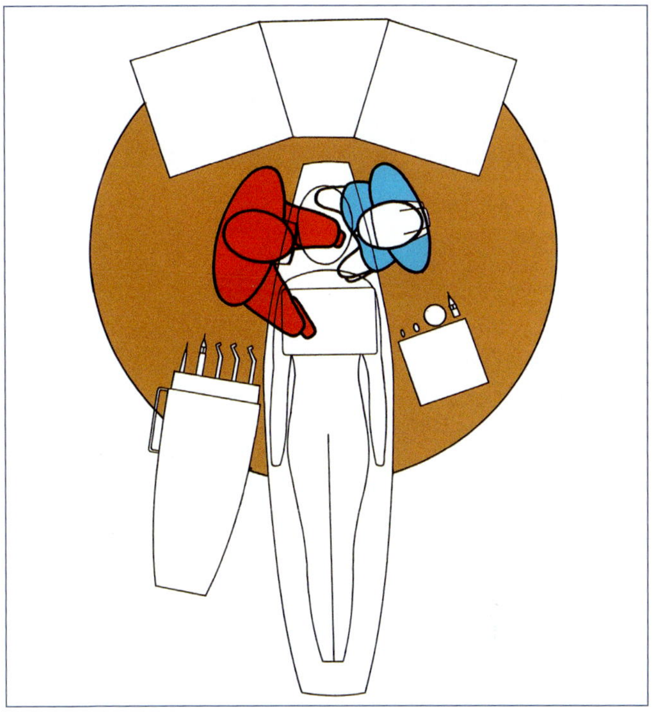

Fig 8-20c Sitting position of the dentist and assistant, both wearing pants. The dentist's knee is between the assistant's knees.

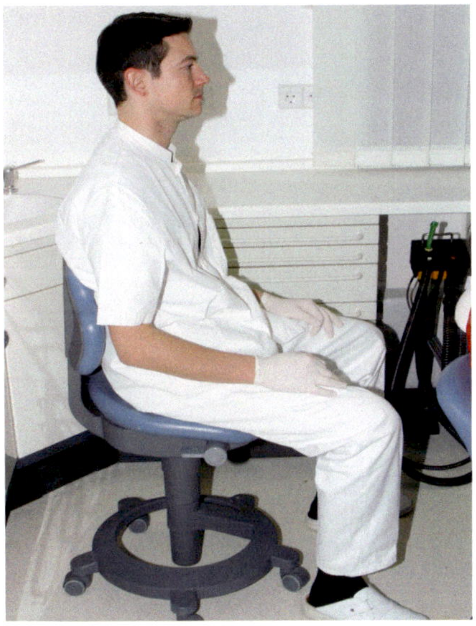

Fig 8-20d Dentist's sitting position: legs bent at an angle of 105 degrees.

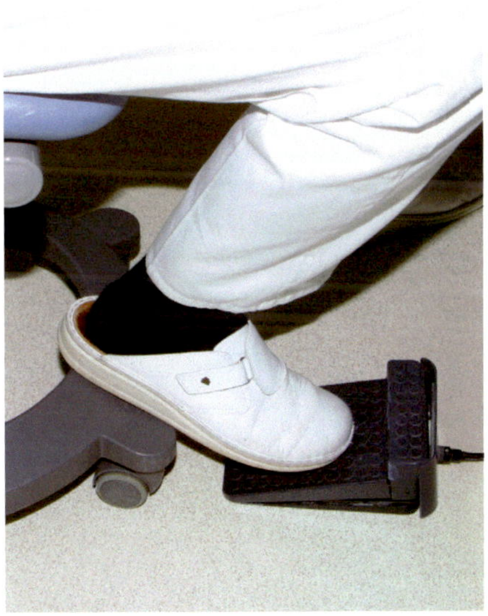

Fig 8-20e Position of the right leg on the pedal, with the foot resting on the ring of the chair base.

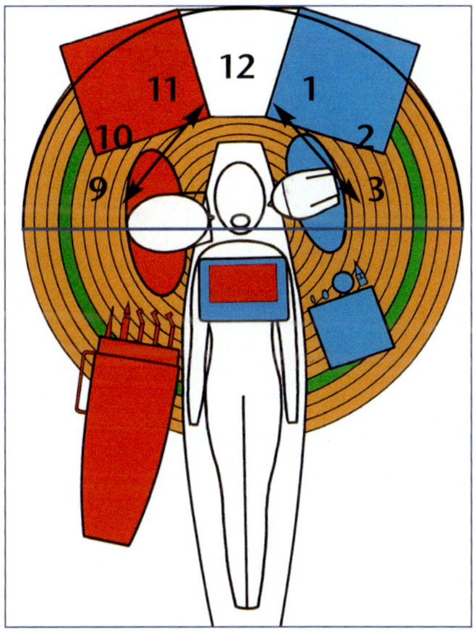

Fig 8-20f Range of the dentist's reach (9 to 12 o'clock) and assistant's reach (1 to 3 o'clock).

mouth of a person who is lying down. At this angle, the person will not swallow reflexively. Then the chair is tilted forward slowly but surely to continue the test. As soon as the person in the chair reaches an angle of 45 degrees, he or she will automatically swallow (Figs 8-21c to 8-21f). Keeping patients in a supine position is an important measure that protects them from swallowing and inhaling foreign matter accidentally.

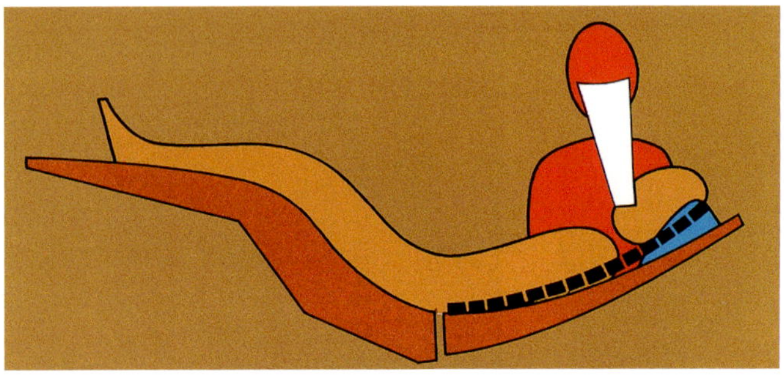

Fig 8-21a Patient's position during work on the mandible. (From Schön.[1] Reprinted with permission.)

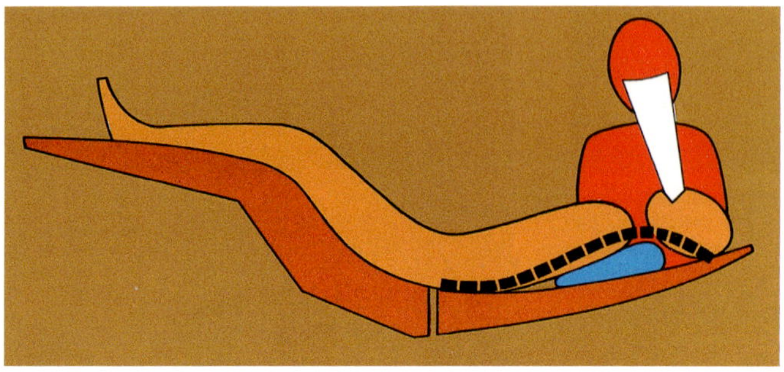

Fig 8-21b Patient's position during work on the maxilla. (From Schön.[1] Reprinted with permission.)

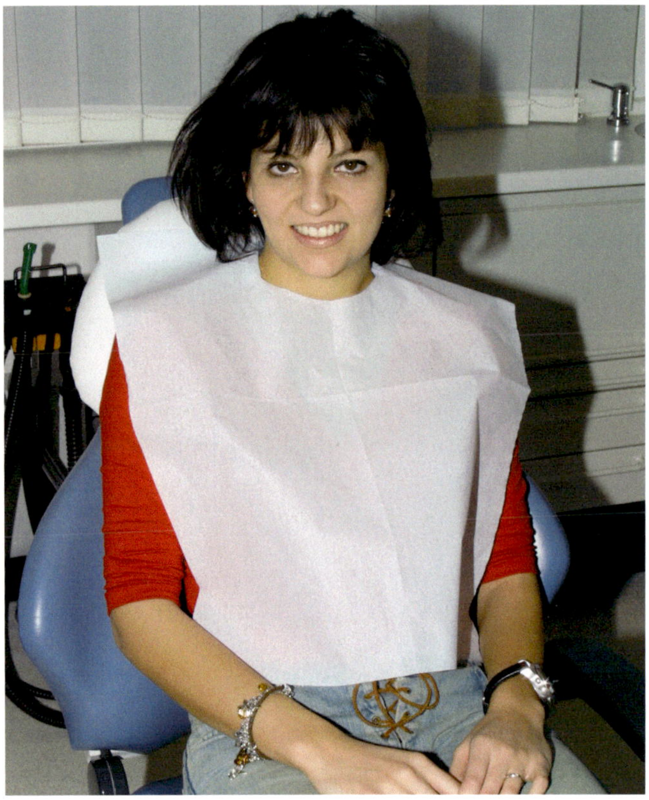

Fig 8-21c Patient in a seated position, wearing a lined, waterproof bib to protect her clothes.

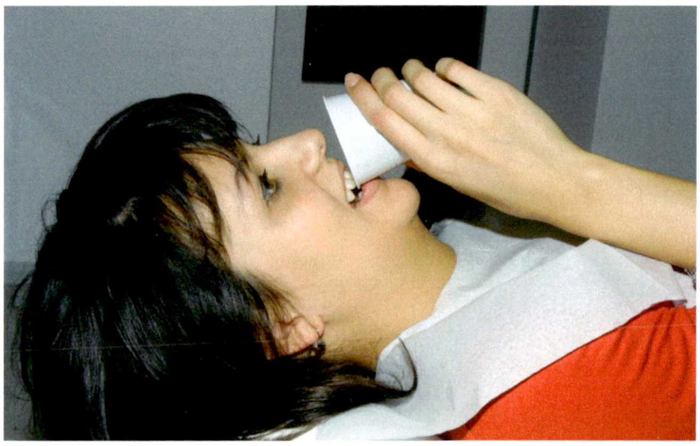

Fig 8-21d Water test.

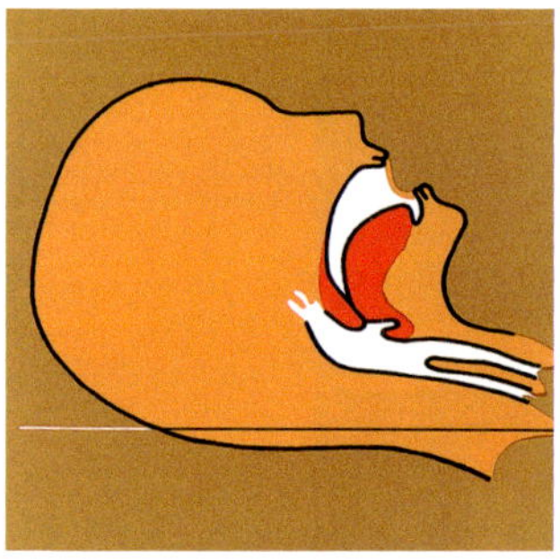

Fig 8-21e The tongue closes the throat when the patient lies down. (From Schön.[1] Reprinted with permission.)

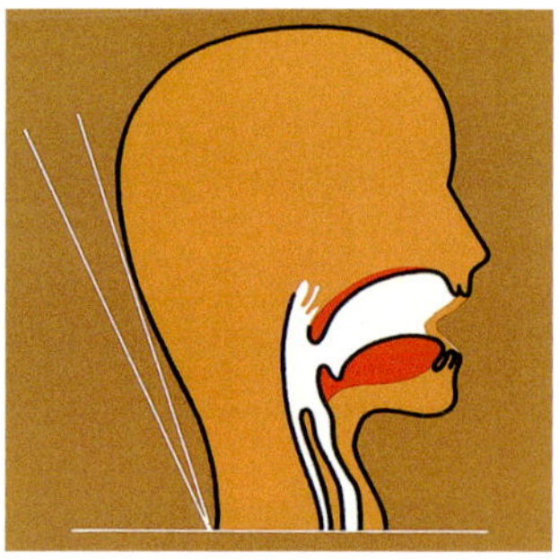

Fig 8-21f The throat is unobstructed when the patient sits. (From Schön.1 Reprinted with permission.)

Retraction technique

The fingers can be used to retract the cheeks and tongue and to expand the vestibule in the anterior region (Fig 8-22a), and a mirror can be used for the posterior region. A mirror with two stems is much more pleasant for the patient than a mirror with only one stem (Figs 8-22b and 8-22c). During long treatments, the corners of the patients mouth should be protected with petroleum jelly or salve.

Evacuation technique

Suction tips with a tongue guard have proven useful for keeping the tongue out of the way during evacuation. These tips are available in different colors (Figs 8-23a). A bright color should be selected to create a contrast to the tooth color; this is particularly important during treatment of anterior teeth.

These inflexible tips are too long if the assistant wants to rest and "cushion" the hand during suction and evac-

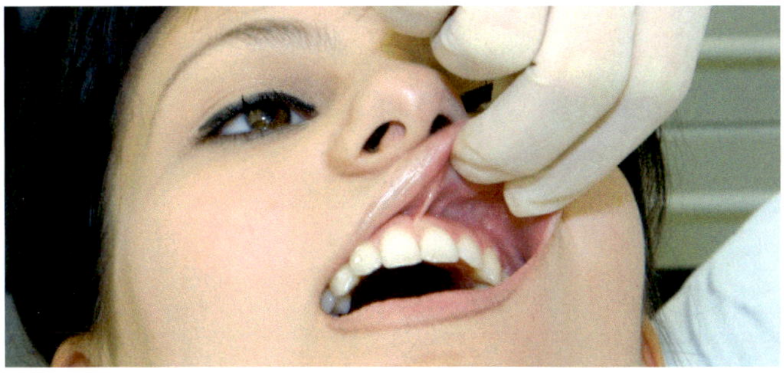

Fig 8-22a Retracting the upper lip with two fingers and a thumb.

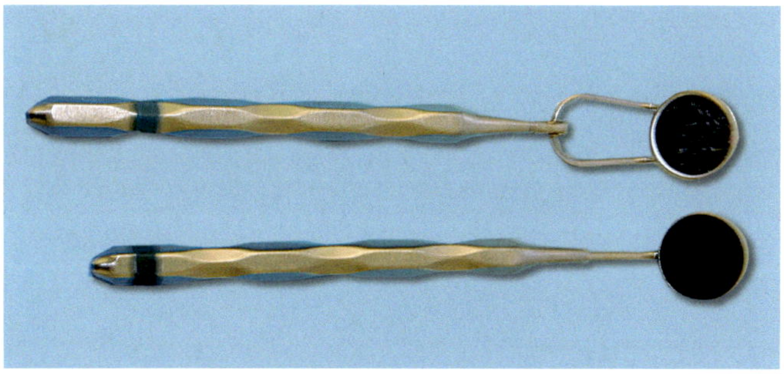

Fig 8-22b Single- and double-stemmed mirrors.

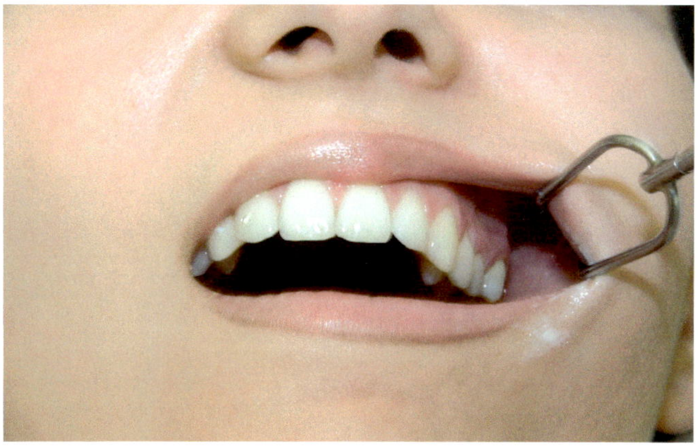

Fig 8-22c Example of retraction for access to the maxillary left posterior segment. Salve has been applied to the corners of the mouth.

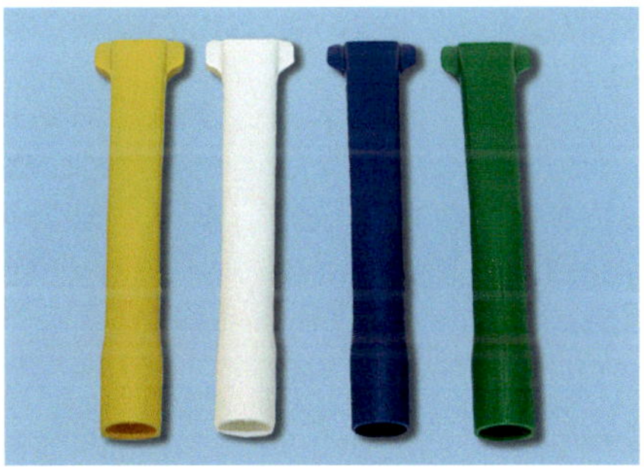

Fig 8-23a Suction tips of different colors.

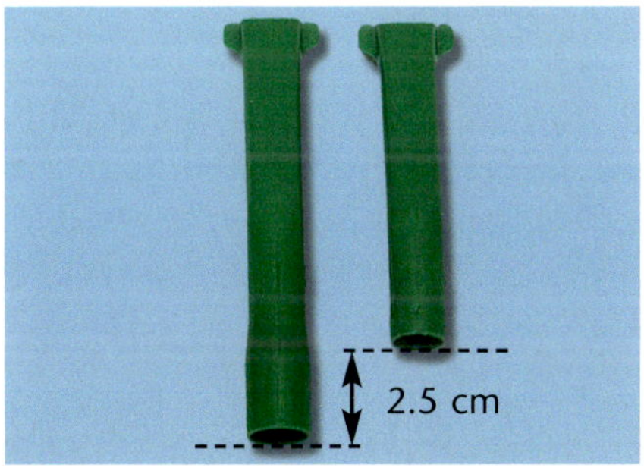

Fig 8-23b Full-length and shortened suction tips.

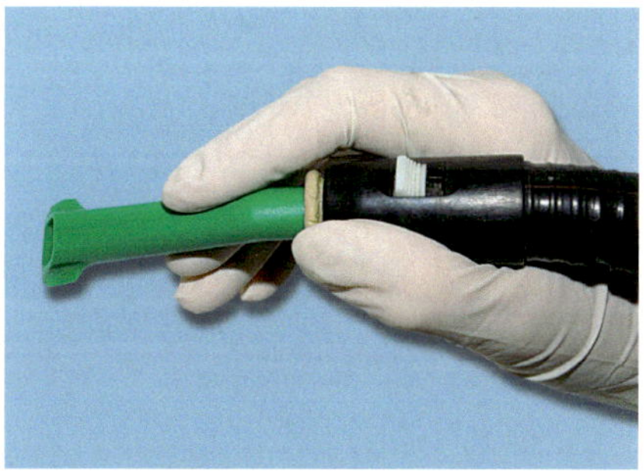

Fig 8-23c Cushioned hand position.

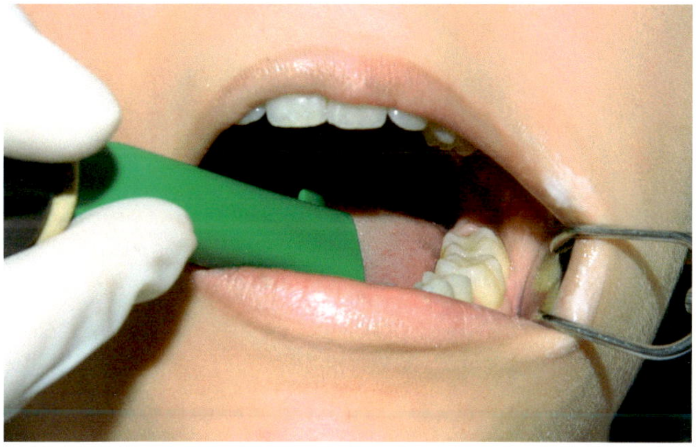

Fig 8-23d Cushioned hand position used on the patient (mandibular left quadrant).

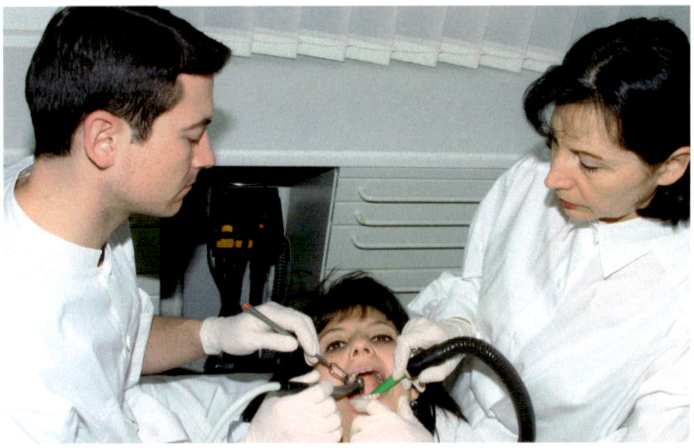

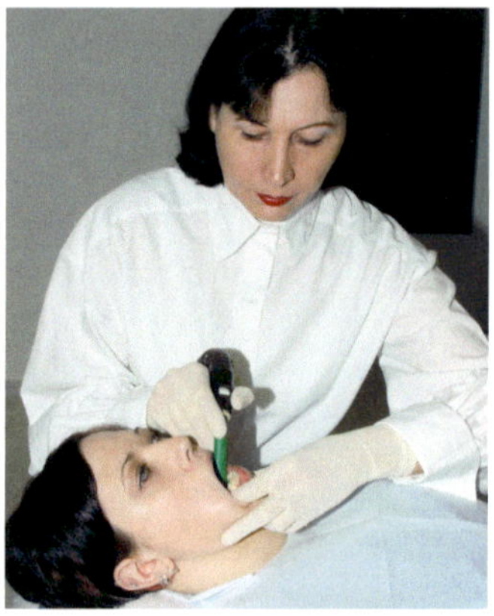

Fig 8-24a *(left)* Mandibular right posterior segment: overview showing the dental team.

Fig 8-24b *(right)* Mandibular right posterior segment: assistant's retraction and evacuation technique.

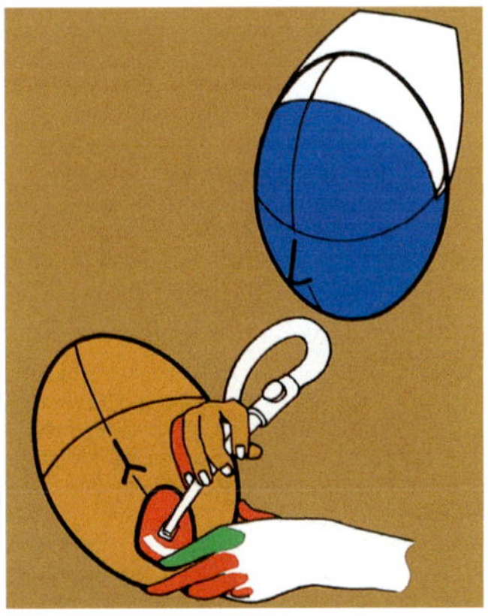

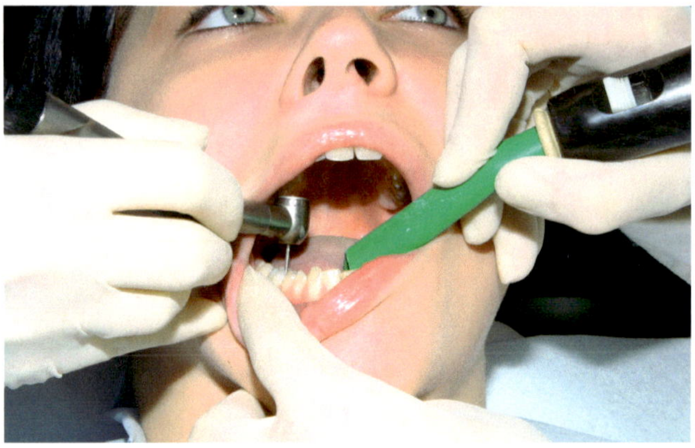

Fig 8-24c *(left)* Mandibular right posterior segment: drawing of the assistant's retraction and evacuation technique. *(red)* Support; *(green)* retraction. (From Schön.[1] Reprinted with permission.)

Fig 8-24d *(right)* Mandibular right posterior segment: dentist's preparation position.

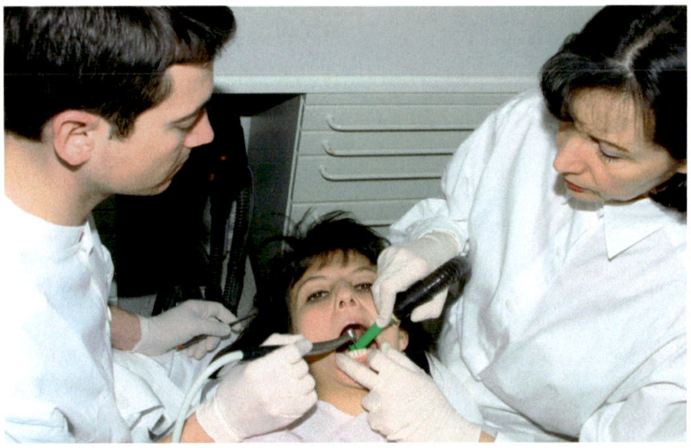

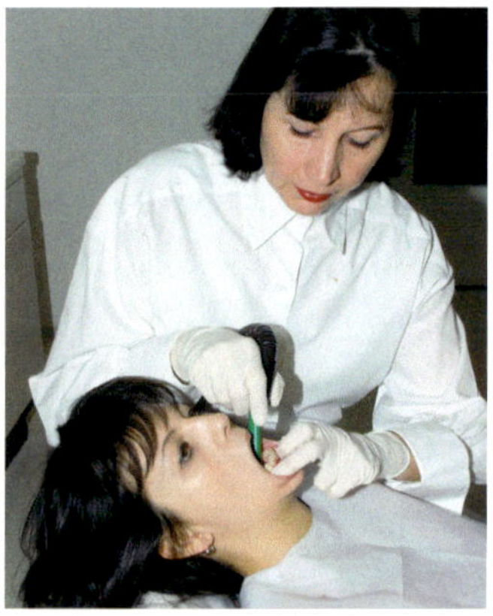

Fig 8-25a *(left)* Mandibular anterior teeth: overview showing the dental team.

Fig 8-25b *(right)* Mandibular anterior teeth: assistant's retraction and evacuation technique.

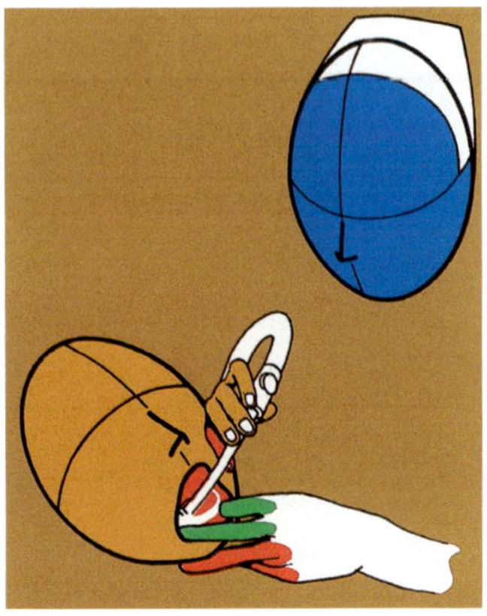

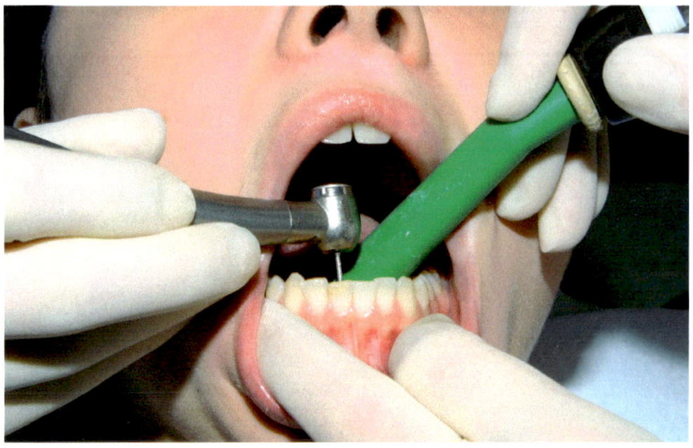

Fig 8-25c *(left)* Mandibular anterior teeth: drawing of the assistant's retraction and evacuation technique. *(red)* Support; *(green)* retraction. (From Schön.[1] Reprinted with permission.)

Fig 8-25d *(right)* Mandibular anterior teeth: dentist's preparation position.

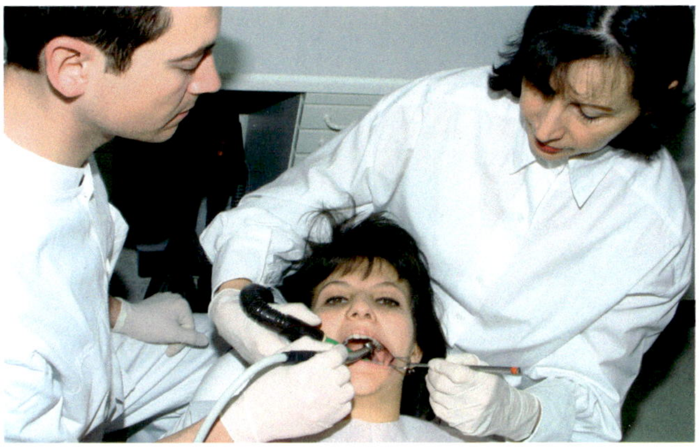

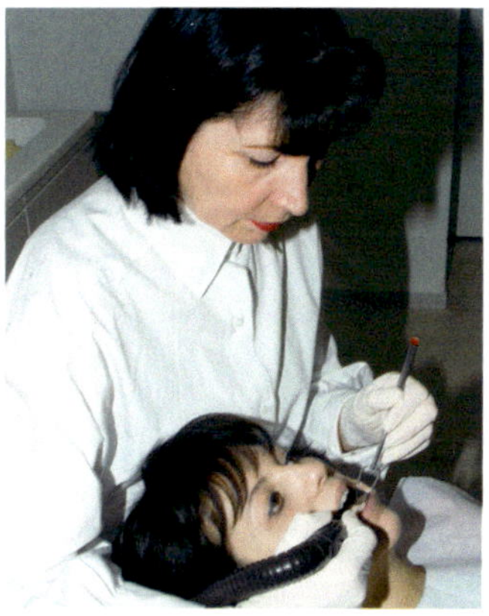

Fig 8-26a *(left)* Mandibular left posterior segment: overview showing the dental team.

Fig 8-26b *(right)* Mandibular left posterior segment: assistant's retraction and evacuation technique.

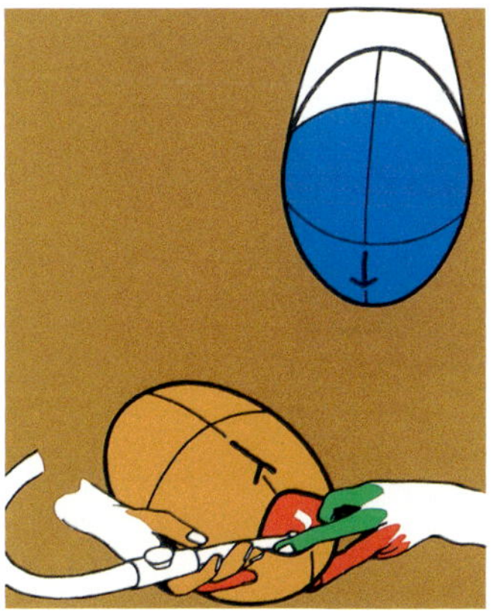

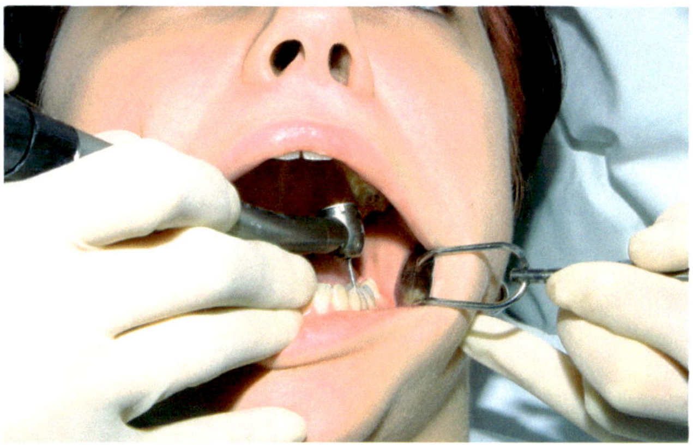

Fig 8-26c *(left)* Mandibular left posterior segment: drawing of the assistant's retraction and evacuation technique. *(red)* Support; *(green)* retraction. (From Schön.[1] Reprinted with permission.)

Fig 8-26d *(right)* Mandibular left posterior segment: dentist's preparation position.

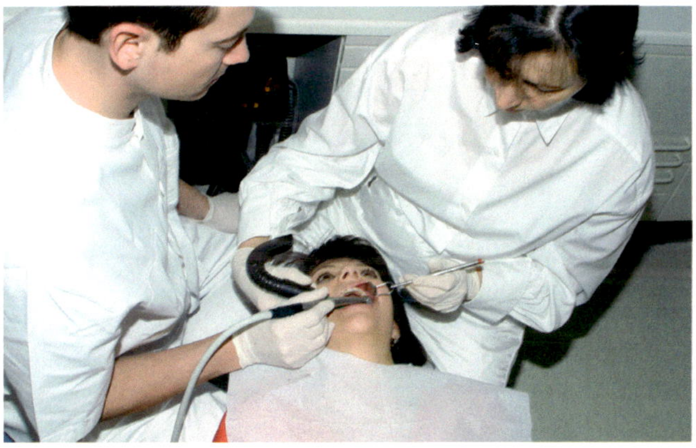

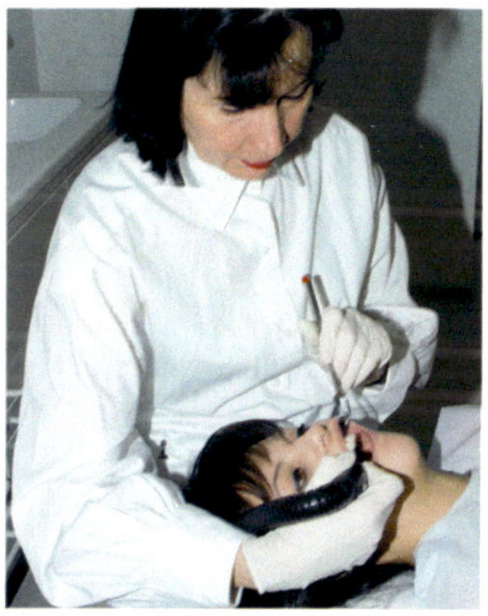

Fig 8-27a *(left)* Maxillary left posterior segment: overview showing the dental team.

Fig 8-27b *(right)* Maxillary left posterior segment: assistant's retraction and evacuation technique.

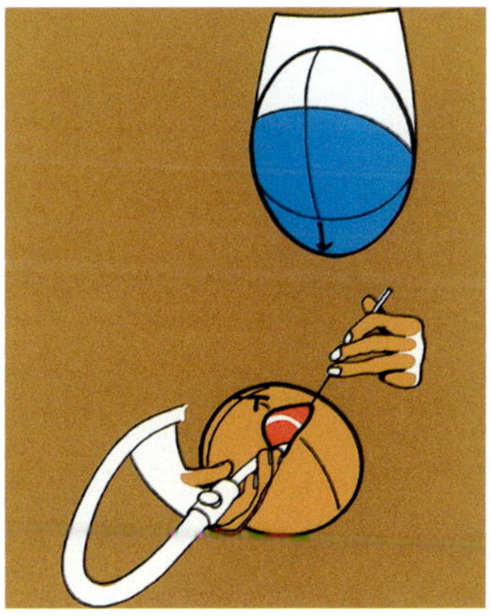

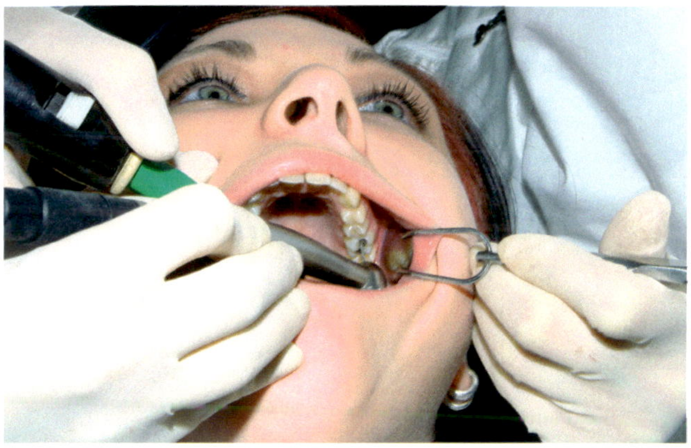

Fig 8-27c *(left)* Maxillary left posterior segment: drawing of the assistant's retraction and evacuation technique. (From Schön.[1] Reprinted with permission.)

Fig 8-27d *(right)* Maxillary left posterior segment: dentist's preparation position.

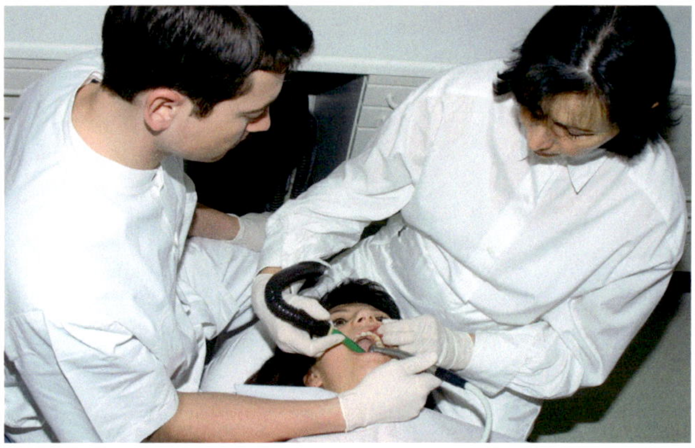

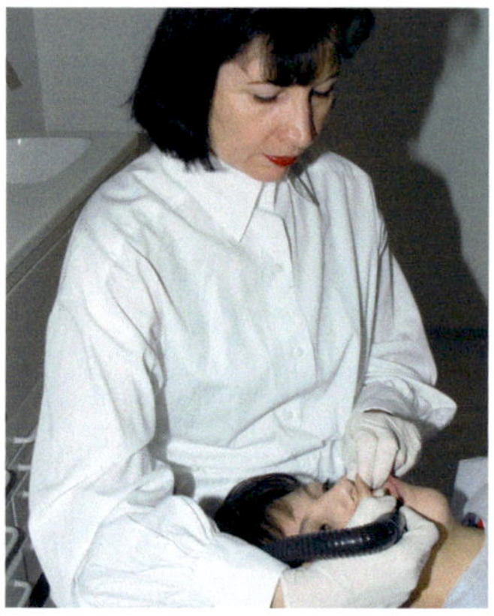

Fig 8-28a *(left)* Maxillary anterior teeth: overview showing the dental team.

Fig 8-28b *(right)* Maxillary anterior teeth: assistant's retraction and evacuation technique.

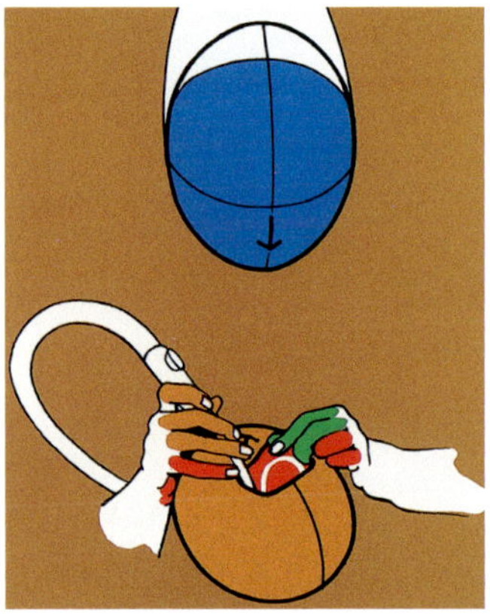

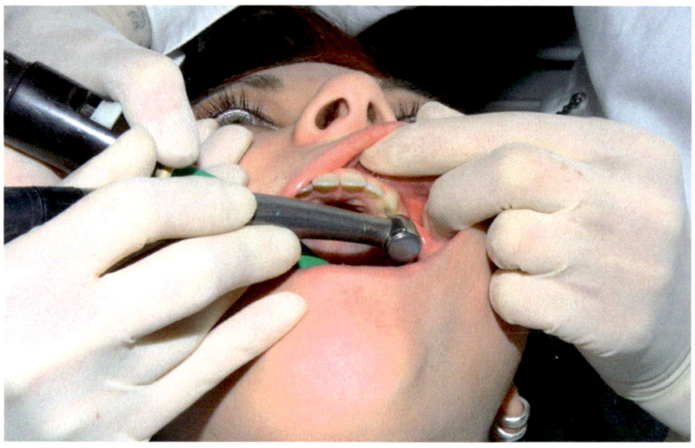

Fig 8-28c *(left)* Maxillary anterior teeth: drawing of the assistant's retraction and evacuation technique. *(red)* Support; *(green)* retraction. (From Schön.[1] Reprinted with permission.)

Fig 8-28d *(right)* Maxillary anterior teeth: dentist's preparation position.

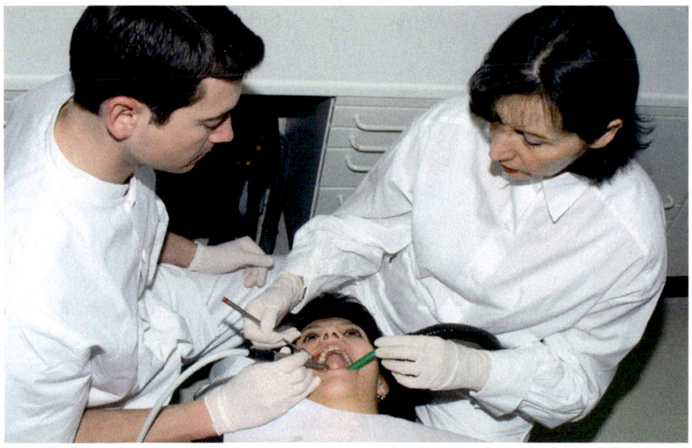

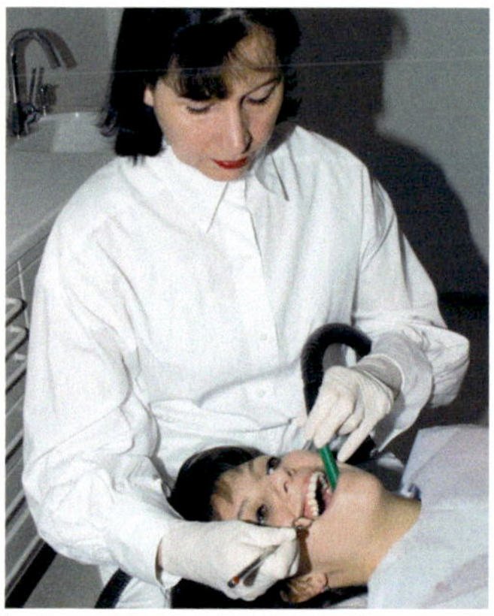

Fig 8-29a *(left)* Maxillary right posterior segment: overview showing the dental team.

Fig 8-29b *(right)* Maxillary right posterior segment: assistant's retraction and evacuation technique.

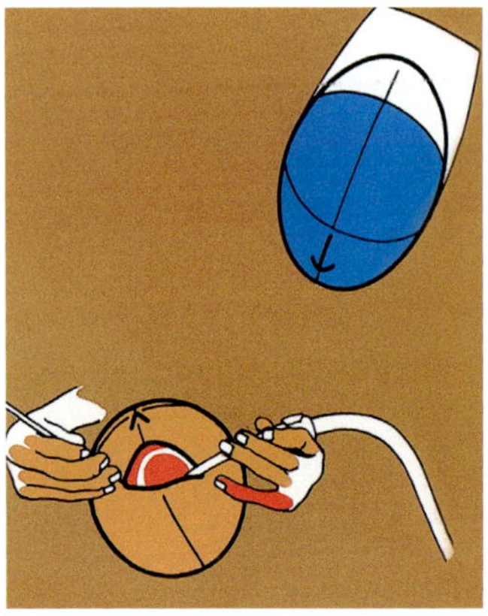

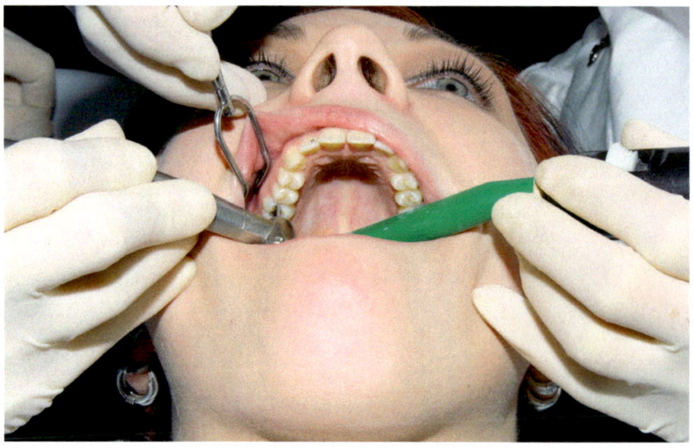

Fig 8-29c *(left)* Maxillary right posterior segment: drawing of the assistant's retraction and evacuation technique. *(red)* Support. (From Schön.[1] Reprinted with permission.)

Fig 8-29d *(right)* Maxillary right posterior segment: dentist's preparation position.

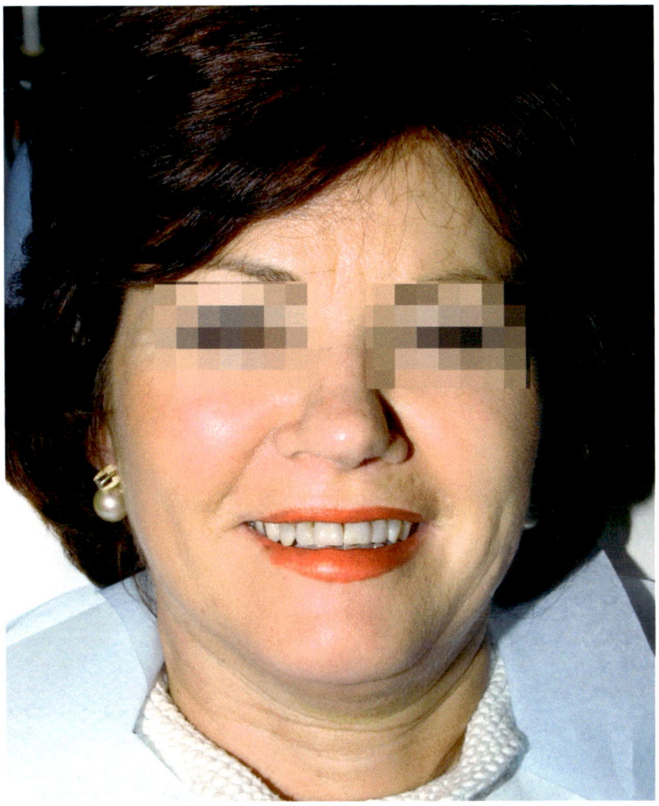

Fig 8-30a Patient wearing makeup.

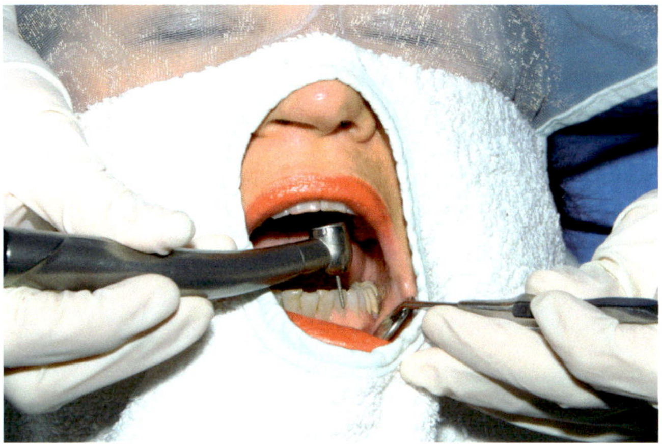

Fig 8-30b Mask to protect the patient's makeup.

uation, however, and have to be cut shorter (Figs 8-23b). The suction tip should be held at the wider end where it meets the tube, as if it were a pencil. By cushioning the shortened tip in the hand in this way, the assistant should be able to use his or her little finger to anchor the hand on the patient's face, which results in more control as well as a more relaxed position for evacuation (Figs 8-23c to 8-23d).

During evacuation, a bit of water should always be left in the patient's mouth so that he or she can still swallow but will not choke. This is for the safety of both the patient and the dentist.

To secure the patient's head, the assistant rests his or her hand in a cushioning position and guides the patient's head with the lower fingers. The assistant should imagine where the practitioner's field of vision is and then put the patient's head in the best position for that purpose. There should be no compromises here. It may be a bit unusual for the patient at first, but having the patient in the right position is extremely important so the team can perform its work directly and quickly while following a certain workflow and maintaining an ergonomically healthy position. The patient really only has two goals: for treatment to be as successful as possible and to go home as soon as possible.

Treatment positions for retraction and evacuation techniques

This section will present and illustrate the individual treatment positions. Each position is explained through an overview picture of the four-handed dental team, a picture of the assistant's holding and evacuation technique, a drawing showing the position of the fingers used to retract and support, and a picture of the dentist's preparation position.

Treatment positions for the mandible are divided into the mandibular right posterior segment (Figs 8-24a to 8-24d), mandibular anterior teeth (Figs 8-25a to 8-25d), and mandibular left posterior segment (Figs 8-26a to 8-26d). The same distinction is made for the maxilla: maxillary left posterior segment (Figs 8-27a to 8-27d), maxillary anterior teeth (Figs 8-28a to 8-28d), and maxillary right posterior segment (Figs 8-29a to 8-29d).

If treatment will be brief, it might be a good idea to offer a facial mask to patients who are wearing makeup, so that their makeup will not smear (Figs 8-30a and 8-30b). Patients should remove makeup before treatment, if the treatment session will be longer.

Materials

Siemens M1 Dental unit (Sirona)
Neck and shoulder rest designed by Schön (Henry Schein)
Evacuator tips; gloves (available at dental supply shops)
Lined patient drape (eg, Nordenta)
Double-stemmed mirror (eg, Lercher)
Petroleum jelly and panthenol salve (available at pharmacies)
Facial masks: Reusable Terry Face Drapes, washable (ProSafe Products)

9

Appendix

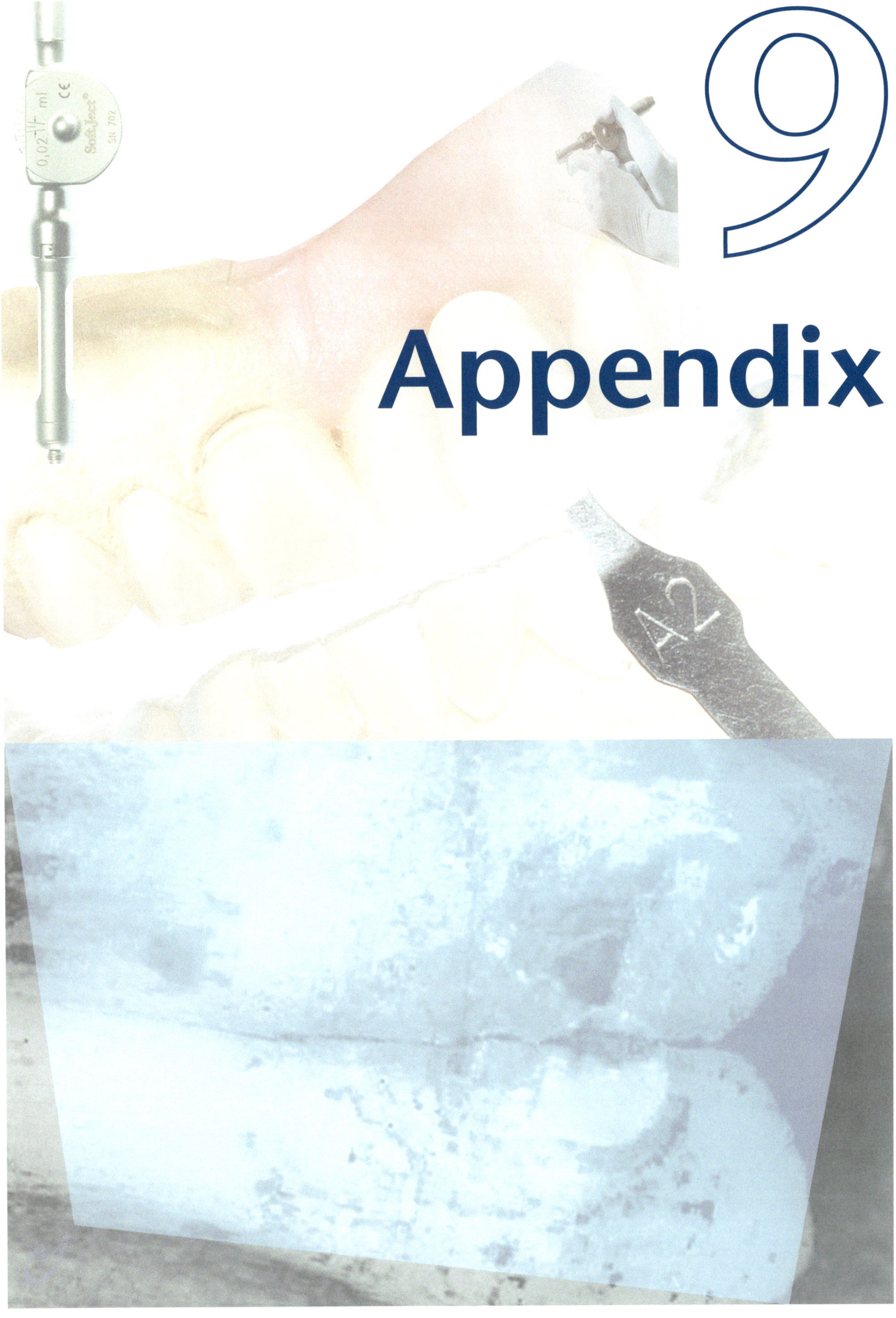

9

Index
References

Index

T

U

V

W

X

References

1 Prosthetic First Aid

Lost Abutment Teeth

Modular Transitional Implant System. Dentatus USA. A list of literature about the MTI system is available at http://www.dentatus.com/lit_mti2003.html, where some of the articles can also be downloaded.

2 Restorative Dentistry

Efficient Adhesive Bonding of Ceramic Inlays

I would like to thank my colleagues and friends of the (former) Berlin team: Prof Jean-François Roulet, Prof Michael Noack, and Dr Uwe Blunck. They made it possible for me to develop this method and have greatly enhanced its practical implementation with their scientific advice.
Readers should refer to the aforementioned researchers if they are interested in finding their way through the extensive amount of literature in the field of adhesive bonding. Even a bit of online surfing can yield an astonishing amount of scientific background information.

Diastema Closure with a Matrix System and Resin Composite

The quality of my digital photographs has often received numerous compliments from readers of my column and even the publishing house and the printers' shop. This I owe solely to the advice of my friend and colleague, Dr Wolfgang Bengel, from Bensheim, Germany. I heartily recommend his book, *Mastering Digital Dental Photography* (London: Quintessence Publishing, 2006).

3 Prosthodontics

Benefits of the Magnifying Loupe

1. Heinrich-Weltzien R, Kühnisch J, Senkel HI. Kann die Kariesrisiko-Einschätzung die Indikation zur Fissurenversiegelung beeinflussen? Quintessenz 1999;50:245–251.

Systematic Workflow in the Dental Laboratory and Office

Martignoni M, Schönenberger A. Precision Fixed Prosthodontics: Clinical and Laboratory Aspects. Chicago: Quintessence, 1990.
This book extensively covers the subject of precision between the dental laboratory and the dentist's office.

Adhesive Inlay/Onlay Supported Fixed Partial Dentures

2. Bücking W. Metallfreie Restaurationen mit glasfaserverstärkter Verbundtechnologie. Berlin: Quintessenz, 1999.

Causes of Bruxism

Dr Max Lüscher's extensive bibliography and a list of further reading as well as of the necessary materials (color test sheets, assessment forms, and assessment software) can be ordered from Lüscherdiagnostik, Mühlestiegstrasse 29, 4125 Riehen/BS, Switzerland or at http://www.luscher-color.com.

Fabrication of Centric Splints with Anterior Guidance

Suckert R. Okklusionskonzepte, ed 2. Munich: Neuer Merkur, 1999.

4 Periodontics

Interincisal Periodontal Splinting

1. Bücking W. Metallfreie Restaurationen mit glasfaserverstärkter Verbundtechnologie. Berlin: Quintessenz, 1999.

Predictable Papillary Regeneration

2. Gargiulo AW, Wentz FM, Orban B. Dimensions and relations of the dentogingival junction in humans. J Periodontol 1961;32:261–267.
3. Tarnow DP, Magner AW, Fletcher P. The effect of the distance from the contact point to the crest of bone on the presence or absence of the interproximal dental papilla. J Periodontol 1992;63:995–1004.
4. Kubein-Meesenburg D, Nägerl H, Bücking W. Die Biomechanik der Okklusion. In: Suckert R (ed). Okklusionskonzepte, ed 2. Munich: Neuer Merkur, 1999:231–278.
5. Kois JC. Altering gingival levels: The restorative connection. 1. Biologic variables. J Esthet Dent 1994;6:3-9.

6 Esthetic Dentistry

Functional Analysis of Lateral Cephalograms: Reestablishing the Vertical Dimension

1. Hasund A. Klinische Kephalometrie für die Bergen-Technik. Bergen, Norway: Bergen University, 1972.
2. Kubein-Meesenburg D, Nägerl H, Schwestka R, Jäger A. Wachstum des Gesichtsschädels und Biomechanik des stomatognathen Systems. Inf Orthod Kieferorthop 1990;22:7–23.
3. Schatz JP, Joho JP. Atlas der Anatomie im Fernröntgenbild. Berlin: Quintessenz, 1986.

Facial Profile Analysis

Determination and Reconstruction of Correct Anterior Tooth Length

4. Chiche GJ, Pinault A. Esthetics of Anterior Fixed Prosthodontics. Chicago: Quintessence, 1994.
5. Lee RL. Frontzahnführung. Hanser, Munich 1985.

6. Lehmann KM. Einführung in die Zahnersatzkunde. Munich: Urban und Schwarzenberg, 1988.
7. Rufenacht CR. Fundamentals of Esthetics. Chicago: Quintessence, 1990.
8. Mühlreiter E, de Jonge-Cohen TE. Mühlreiter's Anatomie des menschlichen Gebisses, ed 4. Leipzig: Arthur Felix, 1920.

Shade Matching

9. Henning G. Tipps zur fehlerfreien Farbbestimmung. Worksheet, available from Dr. G. Henning, Lörrach, Germany.
10. Ivoclar Vivadent: Chromascop – die Harmonie der Farben. Schaan, Liechtenstein.

Analysis and Transfer of the Midline

11. Goldstein RE. Change Your Smile, ed 3. Chicago: Quintessence, 1997.

Horizontal Facial Planes

12. Kois J. Research about the Dento-Facial Analyzer. Available from Gerd Loser, Leverkusen, Germany. E-mail: info@loser.de.

7 Orthodontics

Orthodontic Retainers

Bücking W. Metallfreie Restaurationen mit glasfaserverstärkter Verbundtechnologie. Berlin: Quintessenz, 1999.

8 Ergonomics

Dental Workspace

1. Schön F. Teamarbeit in der zahnärztlichen Praxis. Berlin: Quintessenz, 1972.
2. Kimmel K,Wagner B, Dombrowsky KJ. Die zahnärztliche Praxis. Cologne: Deutscher Ärzte-Verlag, 1978.
3. Hilger R. Arbeitssystem Zahnarztpraxis. Berlin: Quintessenz, 1988.